Modern Concepts
of
Gynecologic Oncology

Edited by
John R. van Nagell, Jr.
Hugh R. K. Barber

John Wright • PSG Inc
Boston   Bristol   London
1982

Library of Congress Cataloging in Publication Data
Main entry under title:

Modern concepts of gynecologic oncology.

    Bibliography: p.
    Includes index.
    1.   Generative organs, Female--Cancer.
I. Van Nagell, John R., 1939- . II. Barber,
Hugh R. K. 1918- . [DNLM: 1. Genital neoplasms,
Female. WP 145 M689]
RC280.G5M6   616.99′465   81-15983
ISBN 0-88416-268-0   AACR2

Published by:
John Wright • PSG Inc, 545 Great Road, Littleton,
Massachusetts 01460, U.S.A.
John Wright & Sons Ltd, 42–44 Triangle West,
Bristol BS8 1EX, England

Medicine is an ever-changing science. As new research and clinical experience broaden our knowledge, changes in treatment and drug therapy are required. The editors and the publisher of this work have made every effort to ensure that the treatment and drug dosage schedules herein are accurate and in accord with the standards accepted at the time of publication. Readers are advised, however, to check the product information sheet included in the package of each drug they plan to administer to be certain that changes have not been made in the recommended dose or in the indications and contraindications for administration. This recommendation is of particular importance in regard to new or infrequently used drugs.

Printed in Great Britain by John Wright & Sons (Printing) Ltd.
at The Stonebridge Press, Bristol.

International Standard Book Number: 0-88416-268-0

Library of Congress Catalog Card Number: 81-15983

ABOUT THE EDITORS

Dr. John R. van Nagell, Jr. is Professor of Obstetrics and Gynecology, and Director of Gynecologic Oncology at the University of Kentucky College of Medicine, Albert B. Chandler Medical Center in Lexington, Kentucky. Doctor van Nagell is a graduate of Harvard College and The University of Pennsylvania School of Medicine. He is a Fellow of the American College of Surgeons and the American College of Obstetricians and Gynecologists; and a Diplomate of the American Board of Obstetrics and Gynecology and is certified by the Division of Gynecologic Oncology. He is a member of 11 scientific societies including the Society of Gynecologic Oncologists, The American Society of Clinical Oncology, and The American Association of Cancer Research. Doctor van Nagell is the author of over 100 publications related to various aspects of gynecologic cancer, and is an American Cancer Society Professor of Clinical Oncology.

Dr. Hugh R. K. Barber is Professor and Chairman, Associate Dean for cancer programs at the New York Medical College, and Director of Obstetrics and Gynecology at Lenox Hill Hospital in New York City. Doctor Barber is a graduate of Columbia University and the College of Physicians and Surgeons of Columbia University. He is a Fellow of the American Association of Obstetricians and Gynecologists, American College of Surgeons, American College of Obstetricians and Gynecologists, Society of Gynecologic Oncologists; and a Diplomate of the American Board of Obstetrics and Gynecology. He has a subspecialty Board in Gynecologic Oncology. Doctor Barber is a member of 39 scientific societies, a founder member of the New York Gynecological Society and one of its past presidents, and past president of the American Cancer Society, New York City Division. Doctor Barber has lectured extensively throughout the United States and abroad. He is the author of more than 250 scientific articles, and the author of 12 books.

This book is dedicated to Betsy and Mary Louise with affection and appreciation for all their help.

John R. van Nagell, Jr., MD
Hugh R. K. Barber, MD

CONTRIBUTORS

Hugh R. K. Barber, MD
Professor and Chairman
Department of Obstetrics
 and Gynecology
New York Medical College
Director, Obstetrics and Gynecology
Lenox Hill Hospital
New York, New York

Elvis S. Donaldson, MD
Associate Professor
Department of Obstetrics
 and Gynecology
Associate Director Gynecologic
 Oncology
University of Kentucky
 College of Medicine
Albert B. Chandler Medical Center
Lexington, Kentucky

Stanley J. Dudrick, MD
Professor, Department of Surgery
The University of Texas Health
 Science Center at Houston
 Medical School
Houston, Texas

E. C. Gay
Research Associate
Division of Gynecologic Oncology
University of Kentucky
 College of Medicine
Albert B. Chandler Medical Center
Lexington, Kentucky

W. David Hager, MD
Clinical Associate Professor
Department of Obstetrics
 and Gynecology
University of Kentucky
 College of Medicine
Albert B. Chandler Medical Center
Lexington, Kentucky

Michael B. Hanson, MD
Assistant Professor
Division of Gynecologic Oncology
Department of Obstetrics
 and Gynecology
University of Kentucky
 College of Medicine
Albert B. Chandler Medical Center
Lexington, Kentucky

Yosh Maruyama, MD
Professor and Chairman
Department of Radiation Medicine
University of Kentucky
 College of Medicine
Albert B. Chandler Medical Center
Lexington, Kentucky

Edward J. Pavlik, PhD
Research Professor
Division of Gynecologic Oncology
Department of Obstetrics
 and Gynecology
University of Kentucky
 College of Medicine
Albert B. Chandler Medical Center
Lexington, Kentucky

Deborah F. Powell, MD
Professor, Department of Pathology
Director, Surgical Pathology
University of Kentucky
  College of Medicine
Albert B. Chandler Medical Center
Lexington, Kentucky

Charles T. Van Buren, MD
Associate Professor
Department of Surgery
The University of Texas Health
  Science Center at Houston
  Medical School
Houston, Texas

John R. van Nagell, Jr., MD
Professor and Director
Division of Gynecologic Oncology
Department of Obstetrics
  and Gynecology
American Cancer Society Professor
  of Clinical Oncology
University of Kentucky
  College of Medicine
Albert B. Chandler Medical Center
Lexington, Kentucky

CONTENTS

FOREWORD

Gynecologists have been vital to the great improvements in diagnosis and management of patients with malignant disease. They have led the way in the practical use of exfoliative cytology, advanced surgical techniques, the successful use of chemotherapy in such dread diseases as choriocarcinoma as well as the investigations into immunotherapy, while also caring for tremendous numbers of potential victims of cancer. These improvements are just beginning. Invasive cervical cancer, once such a frequent killer of women, can now be diagnosed in its earliest form of cellular aberration and obliterated by comparatively simple means. Indeed, it is entirely possible to eliminate invasive cervical cancer and to reduce significantly the incidence of other diseases, such as squamous cell cancer of the vagina and vulva, by the end of this century. That the future of gynecologic oncology is extremely promising is well recognized by physicians in training who, in ever-increasing numbers, seek fellowship leading to certification in this subspecialty. In addition, the recognition of gynecologic oncology as a subspecialty has given great impetus to interest in this area and indicated a need for a concise, authoritative, complete text on this subject.

This volume directed as it is to medical students, residents, Fellows and practicing oncologists, should play an important role in defining for them the natural history, demography, diagnosis, and managment of the diverse and unique diseases of this discipline. The various chapters in this text dealing with surgical procedures, radiation therapy, nutrition, chemotherapy, and immunology extend the range of interest to include not only gynecologic oncologists but all others interested in the correct management of patients with malignant neoplastic disease. While new specialty journals have been initiated and the older established ones have devoted increased space to gynecologic oncology, there has been a definite need for an organized presentation of the large volume of important new and established information as interpreted by experienced clinicians and teachers. Such has been the accomplished endeavor of this book. Its concise format and straightforward presentation give evidence of the authors' experience and the importance of this text and its subject to womankind.

Philip J. Krupp, MD
Medical Director
Oncology Center of
Greater New Orleans

PREFACE

Gynecologic oncology has evolved as a specialty over the past four decades. However, it was first identified as a subspecialty of obstetrics and gynecology on April 5, 1974. On that day the Division of Gynecologic Oncology of the American Board of Obstetrics and Gynecology examined candidates for special competence in gynecologic oncology. The Division of Gynecologic Oncology recognized the increasing importance of special knowledge areas, techniques, and skills within the discipline and specialty of obstetrics and gynecology.

Although the Division of Gynecologic Oncology has been firmly established as a discipline of obstetrics and gynecology, the greatest number of cases will be first seen, diagnosed, and treated by the nongynecologic oncologist. The purpose of this book is to establish guidelines to help the busy practitioner. The volume of material, the changing concepts, and the new advances in diagnosis and management make it difficult for the clinician engaged in a busy practice to keep abreast of the many changes sweeping over the specialty of oncology. The aim of this book is not originality but, rather, it is directed to bringing current concepts in gynecologic oncology together in a readable format. We have tried to make the presentation concise and practical without being superficial. The book is designed to serve both the needs of continuing education and the optimal delivery of health care.

The bibliographies have been chosen because they have historical value, represent an important point, or cover the most updated material that is available in gynecologic oncology. This provides a broad area of reference for those physicians desiring to explore a given phase of oncology in greater depth than is presented in the book.

A great number of physicians have been discouraged with the results of cancer therapy. However, significant advances have been made in the field of oncology. Among these advances have been: the wide application of the Pap smear, the conquest of gestational trophoblastic disease, the cure of eleven cancers with chemotherapy, the predictable control of eleven additional cancers and a great amount of palliation with chemotherapy, the treatment and rehabilitation of the patient with advanced gynecologic cancer, and the team approach and exciting research in the field of immune complexes and hybridomas.

Although the results, stage for stage, have improved only slightly, the overall mortality rate is decreasing because more patients are having their cancer diagnosed in an early stage of disease. This achievement is to the everlasting credit of the practicing physicians who have, by training and motivation, been successful in being able to advance both professional and public education. This is the keystone of early diagnosis and successful treatment.

The editors are grateful to their respective housestaff for the help, suggestions, and the stimulation they have provided. Colleagues have been most helpful by their interest and the advice that has been generated by our conversations with them. Each editor has some individual gratitude that must be expressed.

One editor (HRKB) wants to express his gratitude to Marcia Miller for her help and encouragement as well as her superb skill in the proofreading of this book. She has been ably helped by Ruzena Danek. Shirley Dansker and her library staff have been most helpful in supplying references, abstracts, and photocopies of important articles. My co-workers, Bridie McGuire and Ann McGuire, have lessened my burden by running my private practice office with their excellent handling of the problems that arise in any private office. To my wife, Mary Louise, I express my thanks and gratitude for her patience and help.

One editor (JRvN) would like to thank the members of the Department of Obstetrics and Gynecology, University of Kentucky Medical Center. To my wife, Betsy, I would like to express my gratitude for her help and encouragement throughout the preparation of this book.

The editors want to express their thanks to John Wright • PSG Inc for their help, support, and the opportunity to bring *Modern Concepts of Gynecologic Oncology* to our colleagues.

1 Incidence, Prevalence, and Median Survival Rates of Gynecologic Cancer

Hugh R. K. Barber

Gynecologic cancer is best divided into the lower and upper genital tracts. The lower genital tract includes the vulva, vagina, and cervix, while the upper genital tract includes the endometrium, tubes, and ovaries, as well as the breast.

Cancer continues to be the second overall cause of death in women in the United States, and is the primary cause in women from ages 35 to 54. The overall incidence of invasive cancer has decreased slightly in the past 25 years. The incidence decreased substantially for cancers of the stomach, uterus, rectum, and esophagus. In general, cancer between the ages of 20 and 40 is three times as common in women as men, but between the ages of 60 and 80, men account for more cancer cases. For women, a decrease in incidence has been noted for cancers of the uterus (both cervical and endometrial), bladder, and stomach. The incidence of breast and colon cancers remains unchanged, but lung cancer has steadily increased. For women, since 1950, the death rate has declined by 8% for blacks and 10% for whites. This is due mainly to a sharp reduction in deaths caused by cancer of the uterine cervix, which is attributed to increased use of Papanicolaou tests, regular checkup examinations, as well as improved antepartum and postpartum care. There was also a decline in stomach cancer.

However, the lung cancer rate has more than tripled from 4.0 per 100,000 in 1950 to 13.0 in 1975. The death rate increase of smokers of cigarettes over nonsmokers can be estimated by multiplying the number of cigarettes smoked per day by 0.5. Thus, 20 cigarettes smoked each day produces a tenfold increase in mortality from lung cancer. This smoking history is made more ominous by an early age of onset of smoking. The beginning of cigarette smoking at age 15 causes this mortality excess to be 2.5 times the risk of the smoker who has begun smoking at age 25, disregarding the slightly longer smoking history. It should be kept in mind that girls and young women are now among the heaviest smoking segments of our population. The proportion of smokers among girls in this age group increased by 5% from 1964 to 1975, a level of 27%. The number who smoke a pack or more of cigarettes a day quadrupled.

The American Cancer Society estimates that 76,400 new genital cancers will be reported in 1981, with invasive cancer of the cervix accounting for 16,000, endometrium 38,000, ovary 18,000 and other genital sites 4400. The deaths due to genital cancer in 1981 are estimated to total 22,700, with 7200 from cervical cancer, 3100 from endometrial, 11,400 from ovarian, and 1000 from other genital sites. It is estimated there will be 45,000 in situ cervical cancers reported in 1981.

In 1981 there will be 110,000 new breast cases reported, with 36,800 estimated deaths. Therefore, if the breast is considered part of the upper genital tract, there will be 186,400 new genital cancers and 59,500 deaths.

Exclusive of the breast, an estimated 11,000 plus patients will die in 1981 of genital cancer, who might have been saved by available methods of early detection followed by prompt, proper treatment. Seventy-two hundred patients died from cervical cancer, even though it is theoretically a preventable disease.

The prevalence rate includes the number of in situ and invasive cancers present in a given population at any specific period of time. The incidence rate indicates the numbers of cancers that are developing at any specified period of time. After the invasive cancers are removed, it is then possible to identify the number of individuals who are developing cancer.

The term "mean" (also called average) is the value which is derived by dividing the sum of the measurements by the total number of measurements, ie, 10, 20, 50, 80, 100 = 260 ÷ 5 = 52. The median is the value which lies in the middle of all values when they are placed in sequence, ie, 1, 3, 5, 8, 9, 10, 16, 30. Nine is in the middle and represents the median value. Mode is the value which occurs most frequently.

These measurements of a patient's survival include the observed survival rate, median survival time, and relative survival time. The observed survival time is a measure of the percentage of patients alive at the end of a specified interval of observation after the date of diagnosis. The actuarial or life table method of calculation is used because it utilizes all survival information accumulated to date. For example, the data available for a report included follow-up information into 1970 or 1971. By employing the life table method, it is possible to compute ten-year survival rates for patients diagnosed in the period of 1955 to 1964, even though the patients diagnosed in 1962, 1963, and 1964 were observed for less than a full ten years.

The median survival is reviewed above. It is the midway point in the survival experiences of a defined group of patients; half have died and half are still alive. For example, for women with cancer of the breast, the median survival is six years. This means that under present conditions a woman with breast cancer has a 50:50 chance of living at least six years after diagnosis.

The relative survival rate is the ratio of the observed survival rate to the survival rate expected in persons drawn from the population at a comparable time, with the same characteristics by race, sex, and age as the patient group.

CERVIX

On the basis of the incidence rates of cancer recorded in the Third National Cancer Survey, it has been calculated that 1.6% of newborn girls, about one out of 63, will develop invasive cancer of the cervix sometime during their lives.

The number of cancer cases diagnosed for a particular site in a given age group depends on the population at risk and the probability of developing that particular cancer at that age. The probability of developing invasive cancer of the cervix uteri increases with age until the menopause, then, after a slight dip, increases slightly and then levels off in older ages. However, the incidence then remains stable for the remainder of life.

The distribution of cases by age for cervical cancer shows the greatest number of cases is found in age groups 40–44 to 45–49 years. The mean age of cases of cervical cancer is 53.8 years, while the median age is 51.5 years.

The incidence rate for all ages in the Third National Cancer Survey compared to the 1947–1948 National Survey by the National Cancer Institute, shows a decrease in cervical cancer from 42.4 per 100,000 population to 17.8 per 100,000 population. The Third National Cancer Survey rates by race also declined. For white females, the rates were down to 15.3

per 100,000 population from 38.4, and, for black females, from 74.6 to 34.2 per 100,000 population. The incidence of cervical cancer is higher in low income groups. Puerto Rican immigrant women have about four times as much cervical cancer as mainland United States women.

Population-based data from the State of Connecticut show a reversal in the frequency of invasive versus in situ carcinomas of the cervix for the time periods 1955–1959 and 1965–1969. In the early period, two thirds of the cancers were invasive, whereas in the latest period two thirds of the cancers were diagnosed while still in situ. Among cancers diagnosed in 1969 and reported by the Third National Cancer Survey, the same relationship of two in situ cancers for each invasive cancer exists. The trend has continued up to the present time.

When the age distribution for patients with cervical cancer is considered, a distinct difference is noted between in situ and invasive diagnoses. Only 9% of women with invasive cancers are under the age of 35 at diagnosis, while 53% of the in situ carcinomas occur in women under age 35.

There has been little improvement in survival since 1950–1959 for patients with invasive cancer of the cervix. About half of these cancers continue to be diagnosed as localized disease and about one-third as regional disease. For black patients diagnosed from 1955 through 1964, the proportion diagnosed in the localized stage was only 40% compared to 52% for white patients, while the proportion of black patients diagnosed with regional involvement was 45% compared to 34% for white patients.

Unfortunately, there are no studies that directly count the mortality of cervical cancer patients with and without early detection. The evidence is less direct and depends on observations of the incidence and mortality of the disease in screened and unscreened populations. For example, if invasive cancer of the cervix is preceded by carcinoma in situ, and if early detection detects and treats carcinoma in situ, the incidence rate of invasive cancer of the cervix should drop. This has been observed in several studies. MacGregor examined women in Aberdeen, Scotland and found the incidence rate of invasive cancer of the cervix among screened women over age 30 to be 55 per 100,000, as opposed to 310 per 100,000 in unscreened women. Data from British Columbia show a similar pattern, with a difference of about 5 per 100,000 to 29 per 100,000 women over age 20. Many biases such as self-selection, immigration and emigration, and misregistration of patients confuse interpretation of these data, but they are very suggestive.

The observed median survival times by age for white patients are: All ages, 6.8 years; under 35, more than 10 years; 35–44, more than 10 years; 45–54, 8.6 years; 55–64, 5.5 years; 65 and over, 2.6 years. For black patients; All ages, 3.5 years; under 35, more than 10 years; 35–44, 7.2 years; 45–54, 2.9 years; 55–64, 2.8 years; 65 and over, 1.8 years.

VAGINA

Cancer of the vagina is the rarest of female genital cancers and is also among the rarest of all female cancers. It is less common than cancer of the vulva. In the Third National Cancer Survey, cancer of the vagina accounted for 0.2% of all female cancers, or a rate of 0.6% per 100,000 females.

Vaginal cancers (see Müllerian clear cell cancer below) are found predominantly in older women. Cancer of the vagina usually occurs after 70 years of age, and well over half of the women are over age 65 at the time of diagnosis.

There are about 300 deaths from cancer of the vagina annually, a rate of 0.2 per 100,000 females or about 0.2% of all female deaths. Since 1960, almost half of the vaginal cancers were diagnosed as localized. About one third of the patients had regional disease while one-sixth were diagnosed with distant metastases. The percentage of women who have localized disease decreases steadily as age increases, from 59% for patients under 45 years of age to 39% for patients 75 years of age and older.

The genital tract is divided into the lower and upper tracts. The lower tract includes the vulva, vagina, and cervix, while the upper tract includes the endometrium, Fallopian tubes, ovary, and the breast.

The observed median survival times by age for white patients are: All ages, 2.6 years; under 45, more than 5 years; 45–54, more than 5 years; 55–64, 2.2 years; 65–74, 2.3 years; 75 and over, 1.4 years. For black patients: All ages, 1.7 years; under 45, 55–64, 65–74, and 75 and over, not available.

VULVA

Cancer of the vulva is not a common cancer. Invasive squamous cell carcinoma accounts for 90% of all malignancy of the vulva. Only 1% to 4% of all female cancers are reported as occurring in the vulva. Melanomas are not included in these statistics. In the Third National Cancer Survey, cancer of the vulva accounted for 0.7% of all female cancers at the rate of 1.8 per 100,000 females. Cancer of the vulva occurs most frequently after the age of 65 years. Over three fourths of all patients with this disease are 55 years of age or older when the disease is diagnosed. Thirty percent of these cancers occur in women 75 years of age or older.

There are about 500 deaths annually in the United States, and the death rate is about 0.3 per 100,000 females or about 0.3% of all female cancer deaths.

The proportional distribution of patients by stage of the disease is that almost two-thirds are diagnosed as localized and about 30% are regional.

For all stages combined, women aged 45 to 54 at the time of diagnosis have the most favorable survival experience. This age group also has the highest proportion of patients, 77%, diagnosed with localized disease. When all patients with localized disease are considered, there is a clear trend of decreasing survival rates with increasing patient age.

The observed median survival times by age for white patients are: All ages, 5.8 years; under 45, more than 10 years; 45–54, more than 10 years; 55–64, more than 10 years; 65–74, 5.1 years; 75 and over, 1.7 years. For black patients: All ages, 6.8 years; under 45, 55–64, 65–74 and 75 and over, not available.

ENDOMETRIUM

Endometrial cancer is primarily a disease of mature women. Of approximately 49 million women 35 years of age or older, about 700,000 eventually will develop this type of cancer. Most cases are diagnosed in the 50–64 year age group. This year there will be about 38,000 new cases and 3100 deaths. Since these estimates are projections based on data from the Third National Cancer Survey, they do not reflect the increase which has occurred since then. Yet, three independent studies (Los Angeles Kaiser-Permanente Medical Center, University of Washington and California Department of Health, and Los Angeles County/Southern California Cancer Surveillance Program) have suggested that an upward trend in endometrial cancer may be developing in the United States. Two of the studies associated the increase with the use of estrogens; the third study reports an increased incidence of up to 10% in eight United States areas over a four-year period. A more recent study from Yale University disputes these reports.

On the basis of the incidence rates of cancer recorded in the Third National Cancer Survey, about 2.2% of newborn girls, or 1 in 45, will develop invasive cancer of the corpus uteri sometime during their lives. The current annual incidence rates show cancers of the uterine corpus occurring in about 20 per 100,000 women. Cancer of the endometrium accounts for about 7% of all cancers in women.

The greatest number of cases is found in age group 55–59 years. The mean age for cancer of the endometrium is 61.1 years, while the median age is 61.0 years, virtually the same. Cancer of the endometrium occurs more frequently in older women. Seventy percent of all patients are at least 55 years of age at the time of diagnosis.

Survival rates for all patients and for those with localized disease have been leveling off since the 1950s. Over three fourths of all patients are now diagnosed with localized disease. However, 10% of the patients have disease with regional spread, and for these women there is a trend of decreasing survival rates. There is a favorable median survival rate for patients under 65, but when the data is examined, one notes a steady decrease in both observed and relative survival rates as the age of the patient increases. An explanation may be that the percentage of patients with localized disease also decreases as age increases. However, even among women who have only localized disease, the age gradient seems to be a factor in patient survival.

Reagan has drawn attention to the increasing number of mixed adenosquamous cancers detected in the endometrium. These tumors constitute about 50% of the cancers of the endometrium reported from their service. This cancer has both malignant-appearing squamous and glandular components. Venous involvement is observed in one half of the cases, and blood vascular and transtubal routes may be involved in the dissemination of the neoplasm. In mixed adenosquamous cancer of the endometrium, the mean age at detection is 65.5 years. The duration of symptoms tends to be short, and abdominal or distant spread is observed more frequently than with endometrial adenocarcinoma or adenoacanthoma.

Adenosquamous tumors respond poorly to ionizing radiation. The five-year survival is 19.2%. This is significantly lower than the survival rates for the other types of endometrial cancer. The validity of this type of tumor has often been challenged. However, examination with the electron microscope has demonstrated keratohyalin-like granules and desmosomes with tonofilaments, structures regarded as characteristic of squamous cells.

The observed median survival times by age for white patients are: All ages, over 10 years; under 45, over 10 years; 45-54, over 10 years; 55-64, over 10 years; 65-74, 6.8 years; 75 and over, 2.4 years. For black patients: All ages, 1.7 years; under 45, over 10 years; 45-54, 5.2 years; 55-64, 1.8 years, 65-74, 1.2 years; 75 and over, 0.9 years.

BREAST

The breast is the most common site for cancer in women, constituting 28% of all cancer in women. One of every 13 females in this country develops the disease in her lifetime. About 110,000 new cases of breast cancer and 36,800 deaths from the disease is estimated in 1981. Breast cancer is the most common cause of death in women aged 39 to 44. Every 15 minutes a woman dies of breast cancer, with some 36,800 deaths per year.

The incidence of breast cancer increases with age. A woman at 70 has six times the chance of harboring a breast malignancy as has a woman at 40. The incidence of breast cancer has been increasing by 1% per year for at least the last ten years. A particularly steep rise has occurred in women under 40.

About one third of cases of breast cancer present to the physician in a stage too advanced to enable possible cure. It has been estimated that, in the United States today, not more than one fourth of women with breast cancer are alive and free of disease ten years after diagnosis.

The death rate from cancer of the breast has been stationary over the past 40 years in spite of advances in surgical, radiotherapeutic, and chemotherapeutic techniques.

About 47% of all breast cancers are now diagnosed as localized in the breast while another 40% of patients have disease which has spread to regional lymph nodes or tissues adjacent to the breast.

Almost half of all breast cancers occur in women of so-called middle age, 45 to 64 years. If the disease is localized, over 80% of these women live for at least five years (observed time). However, only 43% of the patients in this age group are diagnosed when the cancer is limited to the breast alone. Consequently, for all stages combined in this age group, only 60% are alive five years after diagnosis.

The observed median survival time by age is: All ages, 6 years; under 45, more than 10 years; 45–64, 9.5 years; 55–64, 6.5 years; 65–74, 5.2 years; 75 and over, 3.0 years.

FALLOPIAN TUBE

The rarest cancer of the female genital tract is primary carcinoma of the Fallopian tube. The reported incidence of primary tubal cancers has varied somewhat from as low as 0.1% to 1.1%. There are probably fewer than a thousand documented cases reported in the world literature. The difficulty in making an early diagnosis, the management, and the poor survival rate indicate that Fallopian tube carcinoma has many characteritics of ovarian cancer.

OVARY

Cancer of the ovary is the sixth leading cancer in women. On the basis of the Third National Cancer Survey data, about 1.4%, or one of every 70 newborn girls, will develop cancer of the ovary sometime during their lives. In 1981 there are 18,000 new cases of cancer of the ovary estimated.

The age specific incidence rates for ovarian cancer show a steady rise up to age 80 where they drop off slightly in the older ages. The greatest number of cases is found in age groups 50–54 through 55–59 years. The mean age was 62.3 while the median age was 59.0 years.

Among patients with common epithelial ovarian cancer, 70% to 80%

are in Stages III and IV at the time of diagnosis. Approximately 11,400 deaths from cancer of the ovary are estimated for 1981.

The observed median survival times by age for white patients are: All ages, 1.6 years; under 45, more than 5 years; 45-54, 1.9 years; 55-64, 1.5 years; 65-74, 0.9 years; 75 and over, 0.6 years. For black patients: All ages, 0.9 years; under 45, more than 5 years; 45-54, 2 years; 55-64, 0.7 years; 65-74, 0.5 years; 75 and over, 0.4 years.

BIBLIOGRAPHY

Barber HRK, Jones W: Lymphadenectomy in pelvic exenteration for recurrent cervix cancer. *JAMA* 215:1945, 1971.

Barber HRK, Kwon T: Management of gynecologic cancer, in Lawrence W Jr, Terz JJ (eds): *Cancer Management.* New York, Grune & Stratton, 1977, pp 397-448.

Cancer Facts and Figures 1980. *American Cancer Society,* New York City, 1979.

End Results in Cancer, report No. 4, *U.S. Department of Health, Education and Welfare, Public Health Service, National Institute of Health,* 1972.

Fidler HK, Boyes DA, Worth JA: Cervical cancer detection in British Columbia. *J Obstet Gynecol Br Commonw* 75:392, 1968.

Kirk ME: Gynecology: Progress in human pathology. *Human Path* 5:253, 1974.

Kistner RW: *Gynecology Principles and Practice* (ed 2). Chicago, Year Book Medical Publishers, Inc., 1975.

MacGregor JE: Evaluation of mass screening programs for cervical cancer in N.E. Scotland. *Tumori* 62:287, 1976.

Plentl AA, Friedman EA: *Lymphatic System of the Female Genitalia: The Morphologic Basis of Oncologic Diagnosis and Therapy.* Philadelphia, W.B. Saunders Co., 1971.

Reagan JW: The changing nature of endometrial cancer. *Gynecol Oncol* 2:144, 1974.

Silverberg E: *Gynecologic Cancer: Statistical and Epidemiological Information.* New York, American Cancer Society, 1975.

2 Staging and Classification

John R. van Nagell, Jr.

Although there have been recent advances in the treatment of gynecologic malignancies, many patients are either improperly evaluated prior to therapy or are not evaluated at all. Too often, physicians are unaware of the latest staging systems for gynecologic tumors, and therapy is decided upon without full knowledge of the extent or biologic behavior of the neoplasm. It is only by a thorough understanding of the stage and histology of a particular tumor that proper therapy can be individualized for the needs of each patient. In addition, uniform classification and staging of gynecologic cancers allows for more reliable statistical evaluation of treatment results from various institutions.

The classification and staging of tumors in the female pelvis has been considered by many organizations, including the Cancer Committee of the International Federation of Gynecology and Obstetrics (FIGO), the International Union Against Cancer (especially its TNM Committee), the Cancer Unit of the World Health Organization, the American Joint Committee, and the International Congress of Radiology. In the past, there were differences in the staging systems proposed by each of these organizations. In 1976, however, the American Joint Committee adopted the staging classification proposed by the Cancer Committee of FIGO. Likewise, the most recent revision of the recommendations of the TNM Committee has brought the TNM and FIGO definitions into full coformity with each other. At this time, therefore, all staging systems are substantially in full agreement both as to categories and details.

GENERAL RULES FOR CLINICAL CLASSIFICATION AND STAGING OF CARCINOMA OF THE CERVIX, CORPUS, VAGINA, AND VULVA (FIGO, 1976)

Every case of carcinoma of the uterus and vagina should be classified and staged prior to definitive therapy. Staging should be based on careful clinical examination and should be performed before any definitive therapy. It is desirable that the examination be performed by an experienced examiner and under anesthesia.

Clinical staging must under no circumstances be changed at a later date, and should never be postponed. It is never permitted to change the clinical staging on the basis of surgical and/or postmortem findings, even if there has been an obvious mistake in the staging. When it is doubtful to which stage a particular case should be allotted, the earlier stage should be chosen.

Opinions differ as to which findings should serve as a basis for clinical classification and staging of carcinoma of the uterus and carcinoma of the vagina. In order to obtain a correct and uniform classification and staging, the Cancer Committee of FIGO considers it important that only such examinations be used which can be carried out at any hospital by physicians and surgeons. The following examinations fulfill this requirement: palpation, inspection, colposcopy, endocervical curettage, hysterography, hysteroscopy, cytoscopy, proctoscopy, intravenous urography, and x-ray examinations of the lungs and skeleton.

Some clinicians prefer to supplement their examination with lymphography, arteriography, venography, laparoscopy, etc. The Cancer Committee does not recommend these latter examinations as a basis for staging. They may sometimes give information of importance, but it is evident that none of them is used routinely. Furthermore, opinions differ among roentgenologists about the interpretation of findings observed by, for instance, lymphography or venography.

The clinical staging of carcinoma of the cervix should be based on the examination methods noted above. A conization or amputation of the cervix should be regarded as a clinical examination, and an invasive carcinoma of the cervix diagnosed in this manner should be reported as invasive carcinoma. If, in a case of early invasive carcinoma, the gynecologist considers it appropriate only to perform an amputation or conization, this should be considered as therapy.

Cases of Stage Ia and Stage Ib "occ," which are revealed by histologic examination of the removed uterus, should be included in the therapeutic statistics concerning invasive carcinoma of the cervix.

Patients who have been operated upon under the wrong diagnosis, and where an advanced invasive carcinoma is found in the removed uterus, cannot be clinically staged. Such cases should not be included in therapeutic statistics, but it is desirable that they be reported separately.

DEFINITIONS OF THE DIFFERENT CLINICAL STAGES IN CARCINOMA OF THE CERVIX UTERI

Preinvasive carcinoma

Stage 0	Carcinoma in situ, intraepithelial carcinoma. Cases of Stage 0 should not be included in any therapeutic statistics for invasive carcinoma.
Stage I	Carcinoma strictly confined to the cervix (extension to the corpus should be disregarded).
Stage Ia	Microinvasive carcinoma (early stromal invasion).
Stage Ib	All other cases of Stage I. Occult cancer should be marked "occ."
Stage II	The carcinoma extends beyond the cervix, but has not extended onto the pelvic wall. The carcinoma involves the vagina, but not the lower third.
Stage IIa	No obvious parametrial involvement.
Stage IIb	Obvious parametrial involvement.
Stage III	The carcinoma has extended onto the pelvic wall. On rectal examination, there is no cancer-free space between the tumor and the pelvic wall. The tumor involves the lower third of the vagina. All cases with a hydronephrosis or nonfunctioning kidney.
Stage IIIa	No extension onto the pelvic wall.
Stage IIIb	Extension onto the pelvic wall and/or hydronephrosis or nonfunctioning kidney.
Stage IV	The carcinoma has extended beyond the true pelvis, or has clinically involved the mucosa of the bladder or rectum. A bullous edema, as such, does not permit a case to be allotted to Stage IV.
Stage IVa	Spread to adjacent organs.
Stage IVb	Spread to distant organs.

Notes About Staging Cervical Carcinoma

Stage Ia (microinvasive carcinoma) represents those cases of epithelial abnormalities in which histologic evidence of early stromal invasion is unambiguous. The diagnosis is based on microscopic examination of tissue removed by biopsy, conization, portio amputation, or of the removed uterus. Cases of early stromal invasion should thus be allotted to Stage Ia.

The remainder of Stage I cases should be allotted to Stage Ib. As a rule, these cases can be diagnosed by routine clinical examination.

Occult cancer is a histologically invasive cancer which cannot be diagnosed by routine clinical examination and is more than early stromal invasion. It is, as a rule, diagnosed on a cone, the amputated portio, or the removed uterus. Such cases should be included in Stage Ib and should be marked Stage Ib "occ."

As a rule, it is clinically difficult to estimate whether a cancer of the cervix has extended to the corpus or not. Extension to the corpus should therefore be disregarded.

A patient with a growth fixed to the pelvic wall by a short and indurated, but not nodular parametrium should be allotted to Stage IIb. It is impossible at clinical examination to decide whether a smooth and indurated parametrium is truly cancerous or only inflammatory. Therefore, a case should be placed in Stage IIIb only if the parametrium is nodular out on the pelvic wall, or the growth itself extends out on the pelvic wall.

The presence of hydronephrosis or a nonflunctioning kidney due to stenosis of the ureter by cancer permits a case to be allotted to Stage IIIb even if, according to the other findings, the case should be allotted to Stage I or Stage II.

The presence of a bullous edema as such should not permit a case to be allotted to Stage IV. Ridges and furrows in the bladder wall should be interpreted as signs of submucous involvement of the bladder if they remain fixed to the growth when palpated, ie, examination from the vagina or rectum during cystoscopy. A cytological finding of malignant cells in washings from the urinary bladder requires further examination and a biopsy from the wall of the bladder.

DEFINITIONS OF THE DIFFERENT CLINICAL STAGES IN CARCINOMA OF THE CORPUS UTERI

Stage 0 Carcinoma in situ. Histological findings suspicious of malignancy. Cases of Stage 0 should not be included in any therapeutic statistics.

Stage I	The carcinoma is confined to the corpus including the isthmus.
Stage Ia	The length of the uterine cavity is 8 cm or less.
Stage Ib	The length of the uterine cavity is more than 8 cm. Stage I cases should be subgrouped with regard to the histologic type of the adenocarcinoma as follows:
	G1 – highly differentiated adenomatous carcinoma.
	G2 – differentiated adenomatous carcinoma with partly solid areas.
	G3 – predominantly solid or entirely undifferentiated carcinoma.
Stage II	The carcinoma has involved the corpus and the cervix, but has not extended outside the uterus.
Stage III	The carcinoma has extended outside the uterus, but not outside the true pelvis.
Stage IV	The carcinoma has extended outside the true pelvis or obviously has involved the mucosa of the bladder or rectum. A bullous edema as such does not permit a case to be allotted to Stage IV.
Stage IVa	Spread of the growth to adjacent organs.
Stage IVb	Spread to distant organs.

Notes About Staging Endometrial Cancer

Studies on large series of endometrial carcinoma limited to the corpus have shown that the prognosis to some extent is related to the size of the uterus. However, enlargement of the uterus may be caused by fibroids, adenomyosis, etc. Therefore, the size of the uterus cannot serve as a basis for subgrouping Stage I cases. The length and the width of the uterine cavity may be related to the prognosis. The great majority of cases of corpus cancer belong to Stage I. A subdivision of these cases is desirable. Therefore, the Cancer Committee recommends a subdivision of the Stage I cases, especially with regard to the histopathologic examination of curettings.

The extension of the carcinoma to the endocervix is confirmed by fractional curettage, hysterography, or hysteroscopy. Scraping of the cervix should be the first step of the curettage, and the specimens from the cervix should be examined separately. Occasionally, it may be difficult to decide whether the endocervix is involved by the cancer or not. In such cases, the simultaneous presence of normal cervical glands and cancer in the same section will provide the final diagnosis. The presence of metastases in the vagina or ovary permits allotment of a case to Stage III.

DEFINITIONS OF THE DIFFERENT CLINICAL STAGES IN CARCINOMA OF THE VAGINA

Preinvasive carcinoma

Stage 0   Carcinoma in situ, intraepithelial carcinoma.

Invasive carcinoma

Stage I   The carcinoma is limited to the vaginal wall.
Stage II   The carcinoma has involved the subvaginal tissue, but has not extended onto the pelvic wall.
Stage III   The carcinoma has extended onto the pelvic wall.
Stage IV   The carcinoma has extended beyond the true pelvis, or has involved the mucosa of the bladder or rectum. Bullous edema as such does not permit a case to be allotted to Stage IV.
Stage IVa   Spread of the growth to adjacent organs.
Stage IVb   Spread to distant organs.

DEFINITIONS OF THE DIFFERENT CLINICAL STAGES IN CARCINOMA OF THE VULVA

The TNM classification shown below, and clinical staging of carcinoma of the vulva was adopted by the International Federation of Gynecology and Obstetrics in 1970.

T Primary Tumor

T1   Tumor confined to the vulva, 2 cm or less in larger diameter.
T2   Tumor confined to the vulva, more than 2 cm in diameter.
T3   Tumor of any size with adjacent spread to the urethra, and/or vagina, and/or perineum, and/or anus.
T4   Tumor of any size infiltrating the bladder mucosa and/or the rectal mucosa or both, including the upper part of the urethral mucosa, and/or fixed to the bone.

N Regional Lymph Nodes

N0   No nodes palpable.
N1   Nodes palpable in either groin, not enlarged, mobile (not clinically suspicious of neoplasm).
N2   Nodes palpable in either one or both groins, enlarged, firm, and mobile (clinically suspicious of neoplasm).
N3   Fixed or ulcerated nodes.

M Distant Metastases

M0   No clinical metastases.
M1a   Palpable deep pelvic lymph nodes.
M1b   Other distant metastases.

Clinical Stage Groups in Carcinoma of the Vulva

Stage 1	T 1	N 0	M 0
	T 1	N 1	M 0
Stage II	T 2	N 0	M 0
	T 2	N 1	M 0
Stage III	T 3	N 0	M 0
	T 3	N 1	M 0
	T 3	N 2	M 0
	T 1	N 2	M 0
	T 2	N 2	M 0
Stage IV	T 4	N 0	M 0
	T 4	N 1	M 0
	T 4	N 2	M 0
	T 1	N 3	M 0
	T 2	N 3	M 0

All other conditions containing M1a or M1b.

If cytology or histology of the lymph nodes reveals malignant cells, the symbol + (plus) should be added to N; if such examinations do not reveal malignant cells, the symbol − (minus) should be added to N.

CARCINOMA OF THE OVARY

Ovarian carcinoma is a common malignant tumor. It cannot be regarded as an entity. Therapeutic statistics on ovarian cancer are of limited value if attention is not paid to the histologic type of the growth. Experience has shown that there is no clear correlation between clinical and histologic malignancy in ovarian tumors. This holds true for various types of neoplasms, but especially for epithelial tumors, granulosa cell tumors, and virilizing tumors.

The Cancer Unit of the WHO has published a "histological typing of ovarian tumors," which helps to understand the pathology and behavior of ovarian neoplasms. The histopathologic classification of epithelial tumors adopted by the WHO corresponds in principle with that proposed by FIGO.

It should be noted that cases of germ-cell tumors, hormonal-producing neoplasms, and metastatic carcinomas should be excluded from therapeutic statistics on ovarian epithelial tumors.

Histologic Classification of the Common
Primary Epithelial Tumors of the Ovary

I   Serous cystomas
a) Serous benign cystadenomas.
b) Serous cystadenomas with proliferating activity of the epithelial cells and nuclear abnormalities, but with no infiltrative destructive growth (low potential malignancy).
c) Serous cystadenocarcinomas.

II   Mucinous cystomas
a) Mucinous benign cystadenomas.
b) Mucinous cystadenomas with proliferating activity of the epithelial cells and nuclear abnormalities, but with no infiltrative destructive growth (low potential malignancy).
c) Mucinous cystadenocarcinomas.

III Endometrioid tumors (similar to adenocarcinomas in the endometrium)
a) Endometrioid benign cysts.
b) Endometrioid tumors with proliferating activity of the epithelial cells and nuclear abnormalities, but with no infiltrative destructive growth (low potential malignancy).
c) Endometrioid adenocarcinomas.

IV Mesonephric tumors
a) Benign mesonephric tumors.
b) Mesonephric tumors with proliferating activity of the epithelial cells and nuclear abnormalities, but with no infiltrative destructive growth (low potential malignancy).
c) Mesonephric cystadenocarcinomas.

V   Concomitant carcinoma, undifferentiated carcinoma (tumors which cannot be allotted to one of the groups I, II, III, or IV).

VI No histology.

In some cases of inoperable widespread malignant tumor it may be impossible for the gynecologist and the pathologist to decide upon the origin of the growth. In order to evaluate the results obtained in the treatment of carcinoma of the ovary, it is, however, necessary that all patients be reported, including those who are thought to have a malignant ovarian tumor. If clinical examination cannot exclude the possibility that the lesion is a primary ovarian carcinoma, a case should be reported in the group "special category" (below), and it will then belong to either of the histologic groups V or VI.

Cases where explorative surgery has shown that an obvious ovarian malignant tumor is present, but where no biopsy has been taken, should be classified as ovarian carcinoma "No histology."

It is desirable to have a clinical stage-grouping of ovarian tumors similar to those already existing for other malignant tumors in the female pelvis. Sometimes it is impossible to make a final diagnosis by inspection or palpation, or by any of the other methods recommended for clinical staging of carcinoma of the uterus and vagina. Therefore, the Cancer Committee of FIGO has recommended that the clinical staging of primary carcinoma of the ovary should be based on clinical examination, ie, curettage and roentgenographic examination of the lungs and skeleton, as well as on findings by laparoscopy or laparotomy.

Stage-Grouping for Primary Carcinoma of the Ovary

This is based on findings at clinical examination and surgical exploration. The final history after surgery is to be considered in the staging, as is cytology as far as effusions are concerned.

Stage I	Growth limited to the ovaries.
Stage Ia	Growth limited to *one* ovary; no ascites.
	(i) No tumor on the external surface; capsule intact.
	(ii) Tumor present on the external surface and/or capsule ruptured.
Stage Ib	Growth limited to *both* ovaries; no ascites.
	(i) No tumor on the external surface; capsules intact.
	(ii) Tumor present on the external surface and/or capsules ruptured.
Stage Ic	Tumor either Stage Ia or Stage Ib, but with ascites* present or positive peritoneal washings.
Stage II	Growth involving one or both ovaries with pelvic extension.
Stage IIa	Extension and/or metastases to the uterus and/or tubes.
Stage IIb	Extension to other pelvic tissues, including the peritoneum and the uterus.
Stage IIc	Tumor either Stage IIa or Stage IIb, but with ascites* present, or positive peritoneal washings.
Stage III	Growth involving one or both ovaries with intraperitoneal metastases outside the pelvis, and/or positive retroperitoneal nodes. Tumor limited to the true pelvis with histologically proven malignant extension to small bowel or omentum.

---

*Ascites is defined as peritoneal effusion which, in the opinion of the surgeon, is pathologic and/or clearly exceeds normal amounts.

| Stage IV | Growth involving one or both ovaries with distant metastases. If pleural effusion is present, there must be positive cytology to allot a case to Stage IV. Parenchymal liver metastases equals Stage IV. |
| Special category | Cases which are thought to be ovarian carcinoma, but where it has been impossible to determine the origin of the tumor. |

BIBLIOGRAPHY

Acta Obstet Gynecol Scand 50:1-7, 1971.

Annual Report on Gynecological Cancer. FIGO, Stockholm, Sweden, vol 16, 1976.

Manual for Staging of Cancer, Chicago, American Joint Committee, 1977.

3 Cervical Intraepithelial Neoplasia

John R. van Nagell, Jr.
E. C. Gay
Deborah F. Powell

During the past decade, there have been significant advances in our knowledge concerning the pathogenesis and treatment of cervical intraepithelial neoplasia. The accessibility of the cervix to colposcopic visualization has permitted careful observation and histologic sampling of epithelial abnormalities as they occur. It is apparent that neoplastic change within the cervical epithelium can vary widely in anatomic extent and biologic behavior, and that therapy must be individualized accordingly. For organizational purposes, cervical dysplasia will be considered as a separate entity, distinct from carcinoma in situ. There is some disagreement as to the rate of progression of cervical dysplasia to carcinoma in situ. However, it is generally conceded that carcinoma in situ is an irreversible process which, if untreated, will often progress to invasive carcinoma.

ETIOLOGY AND EPIDEMIOLOGY

The reported prevalence (number of existing of cases in a population at a specific time) of cervical dysplasia has ranged from 5 to 37 per 1000

22

women screened (Briggs 1979). Prevalence of cervical neoplasia depends largely upon the socioeconomic status and age of the population, as well as on the existing level of cervical cytologic screening. The highest frequency of cervical dysplasia has been reported in previously unscreened teenage populations of low socioeconomic status (Feldman 1976). The prevalence of carcinoma in situ has varied from 3.6 to 8 per 1000, and has been directly related to the percentage of the at-risk population who are exposed to repeated cervical cytologic screenings. Christopherson (1969), for example (Figure 3-1), noted that, with successive cervical cytologic screenings, the prevalence of carcinoma in situ and invasive carcinoma decreased markedly, whereas the rate of dysplasia remained stable. Presumably, the cases of dysplasia appearing with each screening represented new cases in women who were cytologically normal on previous examinations. Therefore, these cases represent the *incidence* (number of new cases in the population over a given period of time) rather than *prevalence* of cervical dysplasia. The incidence of carcinoma in situ has

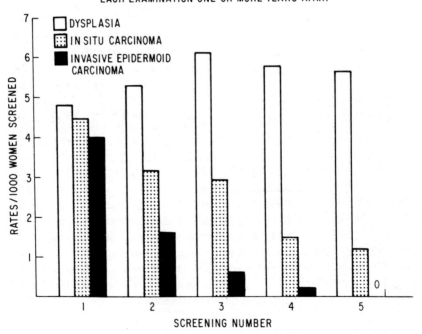

Figure 3-1   Declining rates of invasive cervical carcinoma and carcinoma in situ in a stable population with successive rescreenings. Note that the rate of cervical dysplasia is relatively constant. (Christopherson WM: *Obstet Gynecol Surv* 24:842–850, 1969.)

ranged from 1 to 5 per 100,000 women, and has not decreased in more recent studies. Therefore, it is safe to assume that etiologic agents responsible for cervical neoplasia have remained relatively constant in activity, and it is only by early detection methods that cervical epithelial abnormalities have been diagnosed at a potentially curable stage.

Existing data support the concept that abnormalities of the cervical squamous epithelium are related to a venereally-transmitted agent. Women with cervical cancer begin intercourse at an earlier age with a larger number of sexual partners then those without cervical cancer. Likewise, the incidence of cervical cancer is highest in women of low socioeconomic status who have had several marital partners. Women who develop cervical cancer are less likely to remain unmarried, tend to get married for the first time at a younger age, and are more likely to have had several marital partners than are patients without cervical cancer. Recently, Kessler (1976) has shown that the risk of developing cervical cancer is increased among the wives of men who, at some other times in their lives, were married to other women who developed cervical cancer.

The specific factor most consistently implicated in the etiology of cervical neoplasia is infection with genital herpesvirus (HSV-2). Evidence for the association between HSV-2 infection and subsequent cervical cancer is largely indirect, and is outlined in Table 3-1. Clinical evidence for venereal transmission of HSV-2 is derived largely from virus isolation or cytologic studies on the sexual contacts of males with confirmed HSV-2 penile infections. Nahmias et al (1969), for example, examined eight female sexual contacts of seven males with HSV-2 genital infections within one week of initial detection of herpetic lesions in their consorts. Seven of these eight contacts had clinically detectable HSV-2 infection of the vulva or cervix, and genital herpesvirus was isolated from each of them. Likewise, Rawls et al (1971) examined 30 female contacts of 30 male patients with clinically detectable, penile HSV-2 infections. Genital herpesvirus was isolated in 33% of these women as compared to 2% in a control population seen in the same clinic.

Seroepidemiologic studies have likewise suggested an association

Table 3-1
Indirect Evidence of Association Between
Herpesvirus Type 2 (HSV-2) Infection and Cervical Neoplasia

---

1. Venereal transmission of HSV-2
2. Seroepidemiologic studies
3. In vitro transformation of human cells by HSV-2
4. Herpesvirus-associated markers in cervical cancer cells
5. Induction of murine cervical cancer by HSV-2

---

between HSV-2 infection and cervical neoplasia. Numerous studies have shown that antibodies to herpes non-viron antigens are present in the sera of a significantly higher percentage of women with cervical cancer than in age-matched controls without cervical cancer. Hollinshead et al (1976), for example, reported that the sera of 88% of patients with invasive carcinoma of the cervix contained complement-fixing antibodies to herpesvirus tumor-associated antigens as compared to 11% in patients with nonsquamous carcinomas and 4% in normal patients. Likewise, Nahmias et al (1970) have shown that patients with carcinoma in situ and cervical dysplasia have higher titers of HSV-2 neutralizing antibodies than women without cervical neoplasia.

Another bit of indirect evidence implicating HSV-2 in the etiology of human cervical neoplasia has been the demonstration that this virus can transform cells in tissue culture and is oncogenic in experimental animals (Rapp and Reed 1976). HSV-2 viruses exposed to ultraviolet light have been shown to transform hamster embryo cells (Rapp and Duff 1974). These transformed cells, when transplanted in newborn hamsters, produced both fibrosarcomas and adenocarcinomas. Persistence of the viral genome in the transformed cells is supported by the presence of viral antigen in the cytoplasm and on the cell membrane. Recently, human embryonic lung cells have reportedly been transformed by temperature-sensitive mutants of HSV-2 (Darai and Munk 1973). Tumor induction in mice inoculated intravaginally with either inactivated or live HSV-2 has also been demonstrated. Wentz et al (1975), for example, noted that approximately 60% of mice developed intraepithelial lesions of the cervix or vagina after inoculation by inactivated HSV-2. In approximately one third of the animals studied, these lesions progressed to invasive cancer. Several recent studies have identified persistent HSV-2 virus or viral products in human cervical cancer. Infectious virus and viral antigens have been detected in spontaneously degenerating cell cultures derived from cervical carcinoma in situ. Likewise, Notter et al (1978) have been able to localize HSV tumor-associated antigens in biopsies of cervical cancer using a sensitive peroxidase-antiperoxidase system.

Finally, prospective studies provide further evidence of the association between genital herpetic infection and cervical neoplasia. Naib et al (1969) followed 44 patients with cytologic evidence of HSV-2 infection for four years. Twenty-five percent of these patients developed cervical dysplasia or carcinoma in situ as opposed to less than 2% in women of the same age and socioeconomic status without a detected herpes infection. Although these data suggest that HSV-2 infection may play an etiologic role in cervical oncogenesis, it is probable that other cocarcinogens are involved.

It is obvious that not all women with HSV-2 infections develop cervical neoplasia. The peak age of genital HSV-2 detection is approximately ten years earlier than that of carcinoma in situ, and over two thirds of women with genital HSV-2 infections will not develop epithelial abnormalities of the cervix.

Most investigators favor the concept that several etiologic factors are involved in cervical carcinogenesis. In certain patients, HSV-2 infection may initiate a multistep process which results in cervical intraepithelial neoplasia. However, the promotion of these lesions to invasive cancer probably depends upon additional factors which as yet have not been identified.

A second theory of the genesis of cervical neoplasia is that mutant spermatozoa themselves are the source of abnormal DNA. During the dynamic phase of metaplasia, this abnormal DNA is incorporated into the host epithelial-cell genome causing cellular neoplasia (Coppleson 1968). Reid (1965) labeled mouse spermatozoa with tritiated thymidine, and identified the labeled agent in regenerating stromal cells of the mouse uterus 17 hours after intrauterine injection. Autoradiography and electron microscopy demonstrated this agent in the nucleus of the host epithelial cell. Further studies by these investigators (Reid and Blackwell 1967) have demonstrated that an altered pattern of DNA in the host cell is produced by nuclear incorporation of spermatic DNA.

Chemical carcinogens have likewise been implicated in the production of cervical epithelial abnormalities in experimental animals. Christopherson and Broghamer (1962) were able to produce cervical dysplasia by applying methylcholanthrene to the cervices of mice. The number of mice developing cervical dysplasia or carcinoma in situ depended upon the frequency and duration of application of methylcholanthrene, the genetic strain of animals used, and the individual susceptibility or resistance of each host. Similarly, Patten et al (1963) noted the presence of cervical dysplasia in 22% of mice after intravaginal injection of *Trichomonas vaginalis*. Cellular evidence of dysplasia disappeared, however, following discontinuation of *Trichomonas* inoculation.

The protective role of circumcision in the prevention of cervical epithelial abnormalities is less certain. In support of the circumcision concept is the relatively low incidence of cervical cancer in Jewish and Moslem women (Wynder 1969). Likewise, smegma has been shown to be carcinogenic in experimental animals, despite the fact it does not contain the structure of any known chemical carcinogen (Pratt-Thomas et al 1956). Recent investigations, however, have not confirmed the protective effect of circumcision on the incidence of cervical epithelial abnormalities (Megafu 1979).

PATHOLOGY

The term "carcinoma in situ" was introduced by Broders (1932) to describe epithelial changes that were classified as preinvasive or noninvasive cancer. Likewise, Reagan et al (1953) defined the epithelial characteristics of atypical hyperplasia or dysplasia as similar to but less extensive than those characterizing carcinoma in situ. The specific definitions of both dysplasia and carcinoma in situ are clearly delineated in the World Health Organization monograph on the Histologic Typing of Female Genital Tract Tumors (1975).

Dysplasia and Carcinoma In Situ

Dysplasia and carcinoma in situ may at times be almost indistinguishable. Different degrees of dysplasia and carcinoma in situ are frequently present in the same cervix, and one may merge into the other. In determining the category to which the lesion belongs, the most severely affected areas have to be judged. Adequate sampling of the cervix is needed for accurate histologic diagnosis. Generally, these lesions have no characteristic naked-eye appearance.

Dysplasia   This is a lesion in which part of the thickness of the epithelium is replaced by cells showing varying degrees of atypia.

The epithelial abnormalities designated as dysplasia occur either in the squamous epithelium of the portio or in metaplastic epithelium of the endocervical mucosa. The changes may be observed in the cervical glands. The lesion may also accompany carcinoma in situ or invasive cervical carcinoma.

Dysplasia may be separated into three grades—mild, moderate, and severe, according to the degree of cellular atypia and epithelial architecture.

Mild dysplasia   (Figure 3-2A) Loss of polarity and of regular stratification are minimal. The nuclei are always enlarged, are often irregular, and are darkly stained. Mitoses are often found and are occasionally abnormal; they are confined to the lower third of the epithelium. The cytoplasm is generally well preserved and keratinization of single cells or of the epithelial surface is a common feature.

Moderate dysplasia   (Figure 3-2B) The degree of epithelial abnormality is intermediate between mild and severe dysplasia.

Severe dysplasia   (Figure 3-2C) Atypia is very pronounced. There is loss of polarity, and the crowded cells have large, darkly stained nuclei. Mitoses, occasionally including atypical forms, are seen. The abnormal cells tend to be present in the upper third, as well as the middle and lower thirds, of the epithelium. The superficial cells show a degree of maturation. A layer of flattened cells may form the surface.

Carcinoma In Situ   (Figure 3-2D) This is a lesion in which all or most of the epithelium shows the cellular features of carcinoma. There is no invasion of the underlying stroma.

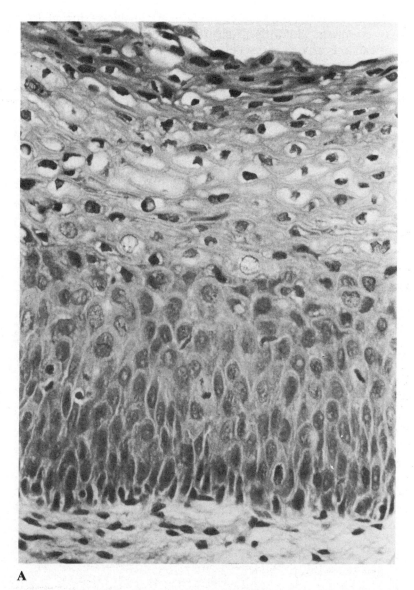

A

Figure 3-2 Cervical intraepithelial neoplasia. **(A)** Mild dysplasia — Abnormal cellular maturation with cellular and nuclear atypia extending from the basement membrane to involve the lower one third of the thickness of the epithelium. **(B)** Moderate dysplasia — Abnormal cellular morphology and altered maturation involving approximately two thirds of the thickness of the epithelium. **(C)** Marked dysplasia — Almost the entire thickness of the epithelium is replaced by abnormal cell growth, with evidence of epithelial maturation only in the most superficial layers. **(D)** Carcinoma in situ — The entire thickness of the squamous epithelium is replaced by proliferating abnormal cells. The basement membrane is intact.

28

In the classical form, small hyperchromatic nuclei are surrounded by scanty cytoplasm with little, if any, squamous differentiation. Orderly stratification is lacking and cellular polarity is often vertical or diagonal rather than horizontal. Mitoses, normal and abnormal, are found scattered throughout the epithelium. Flattened, parakeratotic cells may be present on the surface. The lesion often involves the cervical glands.

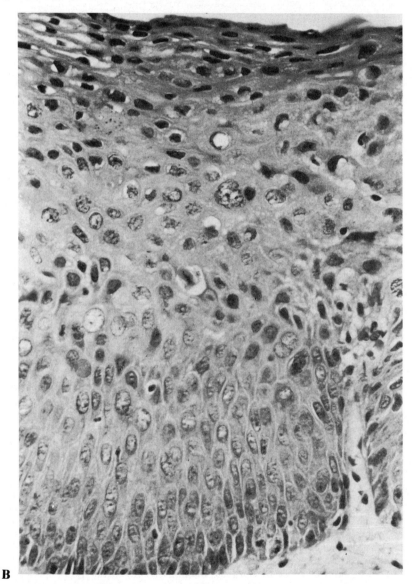

B

Figure 3-2 *(Continued)*

Variants of the classical form occur. These include a keratinizing type found characteristically in the portio, and a large cell nonkeratinizing form around the squamocolumnar junction or in the endocervix.

The histologic patterns of cervical dysplasia and carcinoma in situ have been associated with chromosomal abnormalities. For example, Kirkland (1969), utilizing the direct squash technique, noted that 30% of

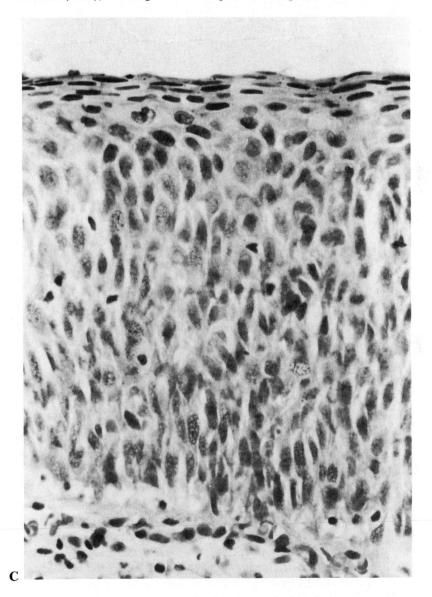

C

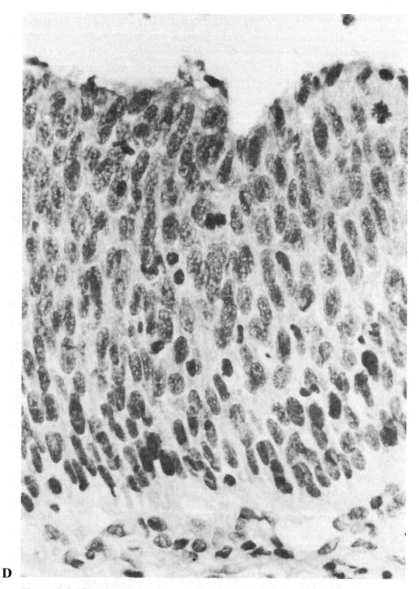

D

Figure 3-2 *(Continued)*

the cells with dysplasia had abnormal chromosomal patterns. Abnormal karyotypes were present in 40% of cells from carcinoma in situ and in 60% of the metaphase preparations from invasive carcinoma specimens. Microspectrophotometric techniques have also been used to study the DNA content of cells from cervical intraepithelial neoplasia (Wilbanks et al 1967). The nucleic acid content of cells derived from mild dysplasia is quite similar to that of normal cervical cells, whereas the DNA distribution of carcinoma in situ was essentially the same. The sequence of events involving the production of gross chromosomal changes is not clear. However, it is probable that these chromosomal abnormalities are of biological significance and that they are, in fact, an initial event in the neoplastic process.

A question of fundamental clinical importance is the rate of progression of dysplasia to carcinoma in situ, and from carcinoma in situ to invasive carcinoma. There is little doubt that the presence of cervical dysplasia places a patient at risk to develop carcinoma in situ. Stern and Neely (1963), for example, reported that the rate of new carcinomas in situ was 106 per 1000 in patients with dysplasia, as compared to a new population rate of 5.1 per 1000. Likewise, the rate of invasive carcinoma was 11 per 1000 in patients with dysplasia as compared with a rate of 1.5 per 1000 for a new population. There remains, however, considerable controversy as to the frequency of progression of cervical dysplasia to carcinoma in situ. Gray and Christopherson (1975) followed 111 patients with untreated, persistent cervical dysplasia for more than five years. During this time period, only 6% of these patients developed carcinoma in situ and 1% developed microinvasive carcinoma. Mild and moderate dysplasias commonly remained in the same phase or regressed when observed over many years. In contrast, Fox (1967) noted that 60% of mild or moderate dysplasias progressed to carcinoma in situ, 31% regressed, and 9% remained stable in a population of 278 patients followed from 15 to 90 months. The effect of cervical biopsies and the surrounding inflammatory and reparative processes in eradicating small areas of epithelial abnormality has been emphasized by Koss et al (1963). These investigators point out that the true natural history of cervical dysplasia can be ascertained only if dysplastic lesions are followed with cytologic sampling alone. In an effort to determine the transit times of mild, moderate, and severe dysplasia to carcinoma in situ, Barron and Richart (1968) followed 557 patients with cytologically diagnosed cervical dysplasia at three- to four-month intervals without biopsy or therapy. At each visit, samples were taken from the endocervix and exocervix, and the cervix was examined colpomicroscopically. If a patient had the cytologic diagnosis of carcinoma in situ, a conization was performed and she was discharged from the study. The results of this investigation are depicted in Figure 3-3. The mean transit time to carcinoma in situ was 86 months for a patient with very mild dysplasia, 58 months for mild dysplasia, 38 months for moderate dysplasia, and 44 months for all dysplasias taken together. Approximately 30% of dysplasias did not progress in severity during the time of this study. Unfortunately, there seems to be no reliable criteria on which to predict on an individual basis which dysplastic lesion will progress to carcinoma in situ. The risk for progression is greater with increas-

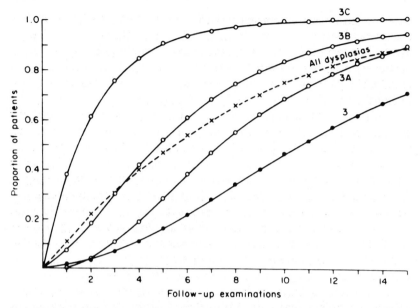

Figure 3-3 Rates of progression to carcinoma in situ in patients with cytologically diagnosed, very mild dysplasia (3), mild dysplasia (3A), moderate dysplasia (3B), and for all dysplasias. Follow-up intervals are one to four months. (Richart RM, Barron BA: *Am J Obstet* 105:386–393, 1969.)

ing histologic abnormality of the epithelium. However, there are few data to suggest that it is only those dysplasias with aneuploidy or an abnormal DNA distribution that will progress to carcinoma.

The biologic significance of carcinoma in situ is more clearly established. There is almost uniform agreement that carcinoma in situ of the cervix is a precursor of invasive carcinoma, and that spontaneous regression of carcinoma in situ is an extraordinarily rare event. Koss et al (1963), for example, followed 67 patients with carcinoma in situ from 6 to 84 months and noted that 50 (74%) persisted or progressed to invasive carcinoma. Spontaneous disappearance of carcinoma in situ occurred in only two patients. The remaining patients had regression or disappearance of carcinoma in situ following cervical biopsies or other forms of treatment. Similarly, Christopherson (1969) followed 29 patients with histologically confirmed carcinoma in situ from one to five years. Over one third of these lesions progressed to invasive cancer within a short period of time, and none reverted to normal.

DIAGNOSIS AND EVALUATION

The diagnosis of a cervical epithelial abnormality is most often made by cervical cytologic examination. Since Papanicolaou and Traut (1943) first reported the use of exfoliative cytology as an effective method in the diagnosis of cervical neoplasia, there has been little doubt that mass cytologic screening of "at risk" populations has been the single most important factor in decreasing the mortality from cervical cancer. Fidler et al (1968), reporting the effect of cervical cytologic screening in British Columbia, noted that the mortality from cervical cancer in the unscreened population was 29 per 100,000. Cervical cancer mortality in the same population after cytologic screening decreased to only 4 per 100,000. Similarly, Christopherson et al (1970) reported that the annual rate for invasive squamous cell carcinoma of the cervix in Louisville, Kentucky fell from 45 per 100,000 in 1955 to 30 per 100,000 in 1965 with progressive cytologic screening of the female population. In contrast, the number of cases of newly diagnosed carcinoma in situ during this 15-year time interval steadily increased. Thus, mass cytologic screening reversed the ratio of invasive squamous cell carcinoma to carcinoma in situ, and enabled women to be treated at an earlier stage in the biologic progression of cervical neoplasia.

The reliability of cervical cytology is dependent largely upon proper sampling techniques and accurate preparation and interpretation of the cytologic specimen. The relationship of the accuracy of cervical cytology to the site of sampling was thoroughly studied by Richart and Vaillant (1965). The results of their investigation are presented in Table 3-2). Vaginal pool sampling was totally inadequate for diagnosing any form of cervical neoplasia. Cytology was most accurate when external os aspiration was combined with cervical scraping. These findings have been confirmed by numerous investigators. Garite and Feldman (1978) stressed the need to add endocervical sampling to an ectocervical scrape in order to evaluate cells adequately at the squamocolumnar junction. These investigators noted that a significantly higher number of patients with cervical neoplasia had abnormal cervical cytology when these two sampling methods (endocervical swab and ectocervical scrape) were combined. Endocervical cells are normally present in the cytologic specimens of over

Table 3-2
False-Negative Rate Related to Method of Sampling
in Dysplasia, Carcinoma In Situ, and Invasive Cancer

Cell Sampling Method	Dysplasia (%)	Carcinoma in situ and Invasive Carcinoma (%)
External os aspiration	17	4
Cervical scraping	28	6
Vaginal pool aspiration	63	45
External os aspiration combined with cervical scraping	2	0

90% of women under the age of 45 (Gondos et al 1972), and their absence can be utilized to indicate the possibility of improper sampling. Self-collection methods such as vaginal irrigation have generally been unsatisfactory and are to be discouraged (Reagan and Lin 1967). Rubio (1977) has pointed out that instruments used in cell collection, such as cotton swab applicators and wooden spatulas, can actually trap abnormal cells, preventing their application to slides for fixation.

Another source of error is inaccurate interpretation of the cytologic specimen. Interpretation error is dependent upon the experience of each individual laboratory and has varied from 0.1% to 5%. Von Haam (1954), for example, reported that interpretation error was reduced from 9.5% to 2.7% with increasing experience of the same laboratory. Although some investigators report as great as a 10% error in the absolute correlation between cytologic and histologic findings, it is important to note the general reliability of cervical cytology in differentiating benign from malignant cervical disease. Van Nagell et al (1973) reported only four cases of carcinoma in situ and no case of invasive carcinoma in the hysterectomy specimens of 845 patients who had a negative cervical cytologic examination immediately prior to surgery. It is mandatory, therefore, that patients undergoing hysterectomy for benign disease have a cervical cytologic examination prior to surgery.

Since the majority of patients with cervical neoplasia are asymptomatic, a realistic plan for a regular cytologic screening of the population at risk is necessary. The frequency with which cervical cytologic examination should be performed is a subject of much recent discussion. Although some investigators have reported that cervical cytologic screening can be performed as infrequently as every three years following two negative smears (Walton 1976), there is considerable evidence to suggest that cervical cytology should be obtained annually. Fox (1968) reported that 195 of 547 patients with cervical dysplasia or carcinoma in situ had prior negative cytology. Furthermore, 140 of these patients developed varying degrees of cervical intraepithelial neoplasia within two years after a normal cervical cytologic examination. An additional 103 patients developed cervical dysplasia or carcinoma in situ within a one-year time interval, and one patient developed invasive carcinoma 14 months after a normal smear. Similarly, Pederson (1956) noted that invasive cancer developed in 26% of 127 untreated patients with carcinoma in situ within an average time period of only three to seven years. Annual cytologic screening in the United States can also be defended, using cost-benefit analysis (Coppleson and Brown, 1976).

Although the majority of cases of cervical intraepithelial neoplasia are first diagnosed by cytology, histologic confirmation is essential before treatment can be initiated. Any lesion that is apparent on visual inspection of the cervix should be biopsied. The application of Schiller's iodine solution to the cervix will often identify those areas at risk for cervical neoplasia. Normal glycogen-containing squamous epithelium stains brown after application of this solution, whereas areas of epithelial abnormality typically do not contain glycogen and are therefore nonstaining. Griffiths and Younge (1969) reported that nonstaining areas of the cervix were present in 83% of patients with carcinoma in situ. The importance of performing an endocervical curettage at the time of cervical biopsy cannot be overemphasized. Punch biopsies have been reported to be accurate in diagnosing carcinoma in situ in approximately 75% of cases when the area of epithelial abnormality was confined to the exocervix (van Nagell et al 1976). However, this accuracy fell to less than 60% when carcinoma in situ was located only in the endocervix. In a similar study, Selim et al (1973) reported that cervical biopsy combined with endocervical curettage accurately predicted the extent of histologic abnormality in over 90% of cases.

Colposcopy, first used in Germany by Hinselmann over 50 years ago, (Hinselmann 1925) has recently gained acceptance in the United States as a method to direct biopsies specifically to the site of cervical epithelial abnormalities. This technique provides stereoscopic observation of the cervix through an optical system which allows variable magnification of the field from 6- to 50-fold, depending upon the particular instrument used. Prior to colposcopic observation, the cervix is bathed in a dilute solution of 3% acetic acid and water. This not only removes the mucus from the epithelial surface, but transiently demarcates areas of abnormal epithelium. According to colposcopic theory, cervical neoplasia begins in the transformation zone, an area in which columnar epithelium is replaced by squamous epithelium through the process of metaplasia. During the active phase of metaplasia, the epithelial cell is particularly susceptible to the incorporation of foreign or abnormal genetic material, and it is in this zone that abnormal cellular change may occur. Epithelium in the atypical transformation zone is characterized by increased cellular and nuclear density, and appears more white and opaque than adjacent areas of normal epithelium (Coppleson et al 1971a). Neoplastic epithelium is also associated with changes in surface contour and vascular architecture. In general, native squamous epithelium is flat and smooth in contour, whereas atypical epithelium is often irregular. Specific vascular changes referred to as punctation or mosaicism are also present in areas of epithelial abnormality. In native cervical epithelium (Figure 3-4), alkaline phosphatase staining of stromal blood vessels indicates that terminal, looped capillaries project toward the epithelium in fingerlike stromal papillae. These vessels usually course tangential to the surface. In contrast, punctation (Figure 3-5) is characterized by twisted or coiled intraepithelial capillaries reaching obliquely to the surface, which provide increased blood flow to an area of increased cellular metabolism. Surface

36

vessels in an area of mosaic change (Figure 3-6) are often dilated, and are arranged in a honeycomb fashion separated by islands of epithelium. The third colposcopic change often present in the atypical transformation zone is an area of white epithelium (Figure 3-7). The epithelium appears white after application of acetic acid because there is often a thickened area of keratin above the epithelium, which obscures the underlying cervical vasculature. Changes in color, contour, topography, and vasculature are graded (Coppleson et al 1971c), and related to histologic changes

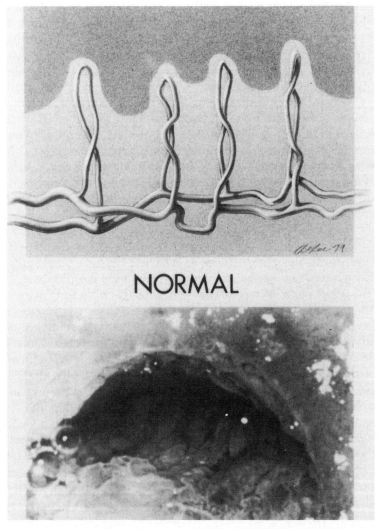

NORMAL

Figure 3-4 Colpophotograph of normal cervix. Capillary loops are regular and rise into the stromal papillae, but not to the surface.

in the cervical epithelium. It is impossible, however, to correlate one particular colposcopic pattern such as punctation with a specific degree of epithelial abnormality such as carcinoma in situ. Rather, colposcopy identifies the area at risk for epithelial neoplasia, and directs the clinician to biopsy that area.

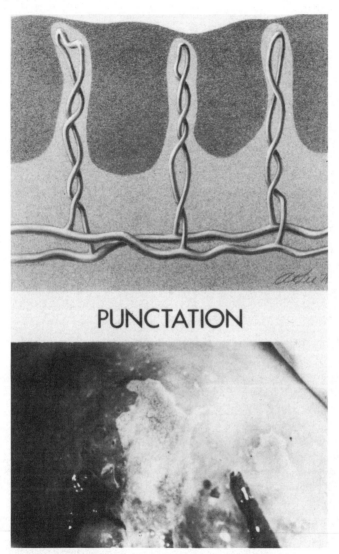

Figure 3-5 Colpophotograph of white epithelium with delicate punctation pattern on the anterior lip of cervix (courtesy of Dr Adolph Stafl, Milwaukee, Wisconsin). The intercapillary distance is very small, and the lesion is compatible with mild dysplasia. Note that the capillaries are twisted and extend nearly to the epithelial surface.

38

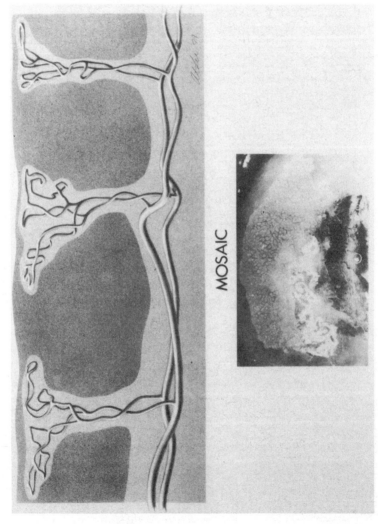

MOSAIC

Figure 3-6 Colpophotograph of small eversion of columnar epithelium to the portio. On the margins of this eversion, there is a large area of mosaic pattern with slightly increased intercapillary distance (courtesy of Dr Adolph Stafl, Milwaukee, Wisconsin). The biopsy of this lesion revealed moderate dysplasia in the epithelium with mosaic changes. Stromal capillaries are often branched and extend nearly to the surface.

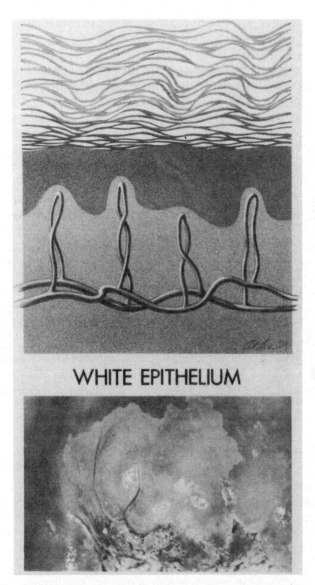

Figure 3-7 Colpophotograph of white epithelium after application of acetic acid to the cervix (courtesy of Dr Adolph Stafl, Milwaukee, Wisconsin). The borders are irregular, and the lesion is compatible with mild dysplasia. A directed biopsy revealed mild dysplasia.

The accuracy of colposcopy depends upon complete visualization of the transformation zone. The anatomic location of this zone changes with age, sexual activity, and parity of the patient (Figure 3-8). Coppleson (1971b) has documented that the squamocolumnar junction is most often located on the exocervix and even on the portio vaginalis in newborn females. At puberty, the vaginal pH decreases, and the exposed columnar epithelium undergoes metaplasia to squamous epithelium. With increasing age and parity, the squamocolumnar junction moves further cephalad, so that in postmenopausal women it may lie within the endocervical canal. Therefore, most investigators routinely perform an endocervical curettage at the time of colposcopically-directed biopsy. The performance of an endocervical curettage is an essential adjunct to exocervical biopsy, particularly when a lesion extends into the endocervical canal. This is exemplified by the study of Treadway et al (1972) in which there was absolute correlation between colposcopically-directed biopsy and conization findings in over 95% of cases when endocervical curettage was negative. When the endocervical curettage was positive, however, the histologic findings of directed biopsy and conization were in agreement in only 62% of the cases. Likewise, Ronk et al (1977) reported that colposcopically-directed biopsies failed to diagnose microinvasive or invasive cancer in only 2% of patients when endocervical curettage was negative.

The use of colposcopy has been particularly effective in the evaluation of pregnant patients with cervical epithelial abnormalities. The physiologic eversion of the cervix during pregnancy allows for excellent colposcopic visualization of the transformation zone (Ostergard and Nieberg 1979). Also, conization during pregnancy is associated with a significant risk of hemorrhage, premature delivery, and cervical incompetence (Daskal and Pitkin 1968; Averette et al 1970). Stafl and Mattingly (1973) reported the successful use of colposcopy in 89 pregnant patients with abnormal cervical cytology. The transformation zone was completely visualized in all patients, and directed biopsies were obtained in those patients with abnormal colposcopic findings. There were no complications of directed biopsy, and conization was avoided in all patients.

Perhaps the most controversial aspect of colposcopy has been the proper definition of indications for its use. For many years, cytology and colposcopy were considered competitive techniques. It is apparent, however, that cytology is the most practical method for screening patients with cervical neoplasia. Colposcopy actually complements cytology, and is recommended as the next step in the evaluation of a patient with an abnormal Papanicolaou smear. It also allows for continuous observation and understanding of the cervix as a dynamic organ progressing through normal and abnormal change. It is important to emphasize that the technique of colposcopy is only as good as the person who is performing

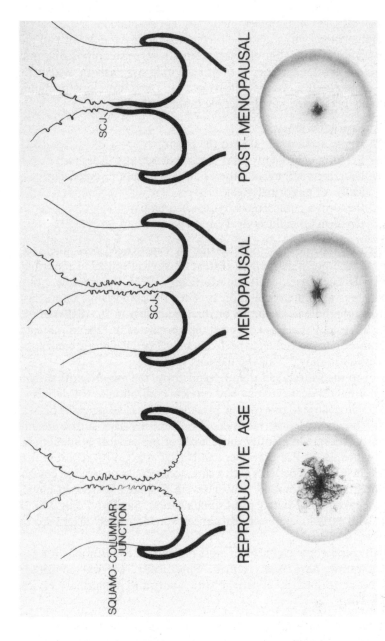

Figure 3-8 Anatomic variation of the squamocolumnar junction related to patient age. Note that, with increasing patient age, the squamocolumnar junction migrates up the endocervical canal. Complete visualization of the transformation zone is therefore most difficult in the postmenopausal patient.

it. Specific training is required to learn the technique, and constant practice is necessary to maintain a high level of accuracy. Colposcopy is, therefore, best suited to an institution or group practice in which a large number of patients with cervical neoplasia are evaluated.

Ideally, colposcopy should be performed on all patients with abnormal cervical cytology, although some centers perform colposcopy only when there is cytologic evidence of at least mild dysplasia persistent for three or more months, or moderate dysplasia. The following steps should be routinely performed in colposcopic examination:

1. Repeat cytology
2. Apply acetic acid (3%) to the cervix
3. Perform colposcopy (and colpophotography if desired)
4. Describe anatomically the extent and location, colposcopically, of abnormal areas
5. Perform a colposcopically-directed biopsy
6. Perform an endocervical curettage

When utilized in the proper setting by experienced personnel, colposcopy is accurate in defining the extent of cervical epithelial abnormality in over 80% of cases. Stafl and Mattingly (1977), for example, noted that there was absolute correlation between the colposcopic impression and the histopathologic diagnosis on directed biopsy in 560 (85%) of 659 patients. Histology was less advanced than predicted in 12% of patients, and was more advanced than expected in only 3%. Diagnostic conization was necessary in only 5% of the patients studied.

Prior to the widespread use of colposcopy, the majority of patients with abnormal cervical cytology had cervical conization as the definitive diagnostic procedure to rule out the presence of invasive cancer. This was necessary because cervical biopsies of Schiller-negative sites were not sufficiently accurate to identify those areas of the cervical epithelium involved by neoplasia. For example, van Nagell et al (1976) reported that only 253 (76%) of 334 patients with a carcinoma in situ on cervical conization had either carcinoma in situ or severe dysplasia present in biopsy specimens taken immediately prior to conization. Similarly, only 7 of 24 patients with early invasive cervical cancer were accurately diagnosed by nondirected biopsies.

With colposcopy available to most patients, the indications for cervical conization have been refined. Specifically, cervical conization should be performed in a patient with confirmed abnormal cervical cytology when:

1. no cervical epithelial abnormality is seen colposcopically,
2. the full anatomic extent of the area of epithelial abnormality cannot be seen,

3. the transformation zone is not completely visualized,
4. there is a persistent discrepancy between the findings of cervical cytology and those of colposcopically directed biopsy, and
5. microinvasive carcinoma is diagnosed on cervical biopsy.

It is recommended that colposcopy be performed prior to cervical conization on all patients. In this way, the extent of the transformation zone and the area of epithelial abnormality can be defined. Also, those cases in which a lesion involves the vaginal epithelium will be identified. If colposcopy is not available, the cervix should be stained with Schiller's solution so that all nonstaining areas can be included in the conization specimen. Conization for a lesion which is entirely endocervical (Figure 3-9) should remove far less tissue than a lesion with both exocervical and endocervical involvement.

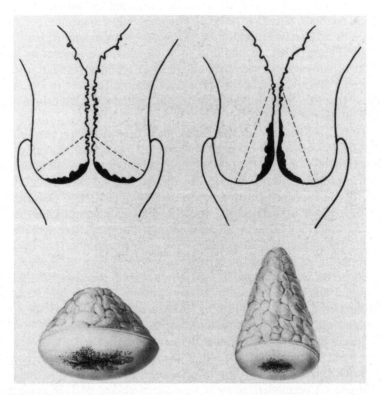

Figure 3-9 Conization size related to anatomic location of the cervical lesion. A cervical epithelial abnormality involving the exocervix requires a different type of conization than a similar lesion confined to the endocervix. Colposcopy should be performed prior to cervical conization in order to define the full extent of each cervical lesion.

The following guidelines should be adhered to when performing cervical conization:

1. Extensive preoperative preparation of the vagina and cervix should be avoided, since this procedure could damage cervical epithelium.
2. Perform colposcopy or Schiller's staining of the cervix and vagina prior to conization.
3. Perform conization using a cold-knife.
4. The surgical specimen should include all areas of colposcopically-defined, abnormal epithelium on the endocervix and within the endocervical canal.
5. The cervix should then be dilated, and an endocervical curettage performed.

The conization specimen should be processed by radical or sagittal cutting methods (Burghardt 1973).The conization specimen is usually divided into 12 sections, and three to four levels are examined from each section (Figure 3-10). In addition, any block with a suspicious lesion should be subjected to step-sectioning. Most recent investigations have reported a diagnostic error for cervical conization from 1% to 3%, and it is likely that this error could be further reduced by strict adherence to the above guidelines.

During the past decade, the technique of frozen-section examination of conization specimens has been utilized with increasing frequency. This method involves cutting the conization specimen into 3- to 4-mm sections which are frozen on a microtome disc. Frozen sections are then cut, using a microtome cryostat at temperatures of $-10°C$ to $-40°C$ (Kaufman et al 1962). Slides are examined, and the findings communicated to the surgeon while the patient is still anesthetized. The usual time necessary to prepare and examine all slides varies from 20 to 40 minutes. If no evidence of neoplastic invasion of the cervical stroma is present, a hysterectomy can be performed immediately, thereby avoiding the risks of a second anesthesia and the postoperative complications of cervical conization. Kaufman et al (1962) reviewed the findings of 210 conization specimens evaluated with the frozen section technique. Fourteen patients (7%) had differences between frozen-section diagnosis and the final diagnosis made from paraffin blocks of the same specimen. However, one patient, diagnosed as having severe dysplasia on frozen section, had microinvasive carcinoma on permanent section. In a larger review of 1136 conization specimens examined by the cryostat technique, Powell et al (1968) reported that there was a discrepancy between frozen and permanent section diagnosis in only 12% of the cases. Frozen-section examination of conization specimens, therefore, can be accurate when used by patholo-

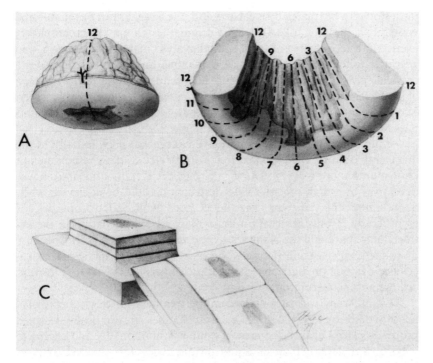

Figure 3-10 Processing the cone biopsy specimen. **(A)** The cone biopsy, tagged with a suture at 12 o'clock, is opened at this position and pinned flat to a board, mucosal side up, for fixation. **(B)** The opened and fixed cone is sectioned with a sharp blade into approximately 12 equal slices, and each slice is embedded in paraffin. **(C)** Sections of the paraffin blocks are cut 6 μ thick at three different levels of the block to insure adequate evaluation of the embedded material.

gists familiar with the method. However, further therapy should be deferred until completion of permanent section diagnosis in any patient in whom the extent of cervical epithelial abnormality is questionable on frozen section.

THERAPY

The method of treatment of cervical intraepithelial neoplasia depends upon the anatomic extent of the lesion and the degree of histologic abnormality. Too often, a particular therapeutic method is utilized because of its familiarity, rather than because it is indicated specifically in the treatment of a certain lesion. If there is a focal area of epithelial abnormality which is present only on the exocervix, local excision with a knife or biopsy forceps may be curative. It should be emphasized, however, that the extent of the lesion must be defined by colposcopy, and the transformation zone should be fully visualized. Also, if the lesion is to be treated by local excision, the patient must be reliable and willing to return for follow-up. The original lesion may be incompletely excised or a second area of focal epithelial abnormality may develop, and adequate follow-up examinations are essential. Following treatment for a cervical epithelial abnormality, it is recommended that the patient be seen at least every three months for two years, and every six months thereafter. Should an area of epithelial neoplasia recur, more frequent examinations may be indicated.

Although cryotherapy for invasive cancer was used initially in the nineteenth century, the thermal effects of extreme cold on tissue were not known until more recently. During the past decade, instrumentation was developed by which precise tissue destruction could be achieved, while maintaining the inherent anesthetic and hemostatic properties of cryotherapy. Tissue destruction takes place by ice formation in the extracellular space and the resultant hypertonic state which occurs because of solute concentration (Underwood et al 1976). The increased, extracellular osmotic pressure causes a loss of intracellular water and leads to cell membrane disruption.

Cryotherapy was first utilized in the treatment of cervical epithelial abnormalities by Crisp (1967). One of a number of specifically designed probes is placed against the area of epithelial abnormality and cooled to $-60°C$ with liquid freon or liquid nitrous oxide for a period of three minutes. This is followed by a three-minute thaw, and refreezing again to $-60°C$ for three minutes. Most investigators have attempted to include a 2-mm margin of normal epithelium in the treated area, due to the rapid dissipation of effective temperature. Within minutes following cryotherapy, an area of erythema and tissue necrosis develops as defined by the probe depth and temperature. The area of tissue necrosis usually sloughs within two weeks and re-epithelialization is completed by ten weeks.

This method of therapy has been particularly effective in the treatment of mild and moderate cervical dysplasias limited to the exocervix. The major advantage of this method of therapy is that it can be performed without analgesia in an outpatient facility, thereby avoiding the expense of hospital admission and the risks of a general anesthetic. In general, the failure rate of cryotherapy increases with increasing severity of the histologic abnormality. Treadway et al (1972) reported a cryotherapy failure rate of 13% in patients with mild dysplasia. This failure rate increased to 31% in patients with severe dysplasia or carcinoma in situ. The overall failure rate for cryotherapy is presented in Table 3-3. Unfortunately, very few studies present data concerning the recurrence rates of cervical epithelial abnormalities many years after cryotherapy. Perhaps cryotherapy is only postponing the progression of cervical neoplasia. The importance of the specific duration and method of cryotherapy has been emphasized by Creasman et al (1973). These authors reported a cryotherapy failure rate of 48% in patients with severe dysplasia or carcinoma in situ, who were treated by a single freeze technique ($-60°C$ for three minutes). In contrast, this failure rate decreased to only 10% with the freeze-thaw-refreeze technique previously described.

Table 3-3
Failure Rate of Cryotherapy in Treatment of Patients with Cervical Dysplasia and/or Carcinoma In Situ

Reference	Year	No. of Patients	Failure Rate (%)
Creasman and Parker	1975	431	22
Crisp	1972	123	13
DiSaia et al	1974	166	10
Gray and Christopherson	1975	66	25
Kaufman et al	1973	190	10
Ostergard	1972	147	7.6
Townsend and Ostergard	1971	35	8.4
Treadway et al	1972	118	19
Underwood et al	1976	64	6

The hazards of the indiscriminate use of cryotherapy have been emphasized recently by Sevin et al (1979). These investigators reported eight cases of invasive cervical cancer discovered after one or more courses of cryotherapy for presumably noninvasive cervical lesions. Carcinoma had spread to the pelvic lymph nodes in four patients, and three died from their disease 7 to 24 months following definitive therapy. Five patients had abnormal cytology prior to cryotherapy, and four were incompletely evaluated prior to cryotherapy. One of the major criticisms of this method is that colposcopic evaluation of cervical epithelium is particularly difficult following cyrotherapy since the squamocolumnar junction is high in the endocervical canal. It is therefore recommended that cryotherapy be restricted for the present to those centers where there is existing expertise in cytology, pathology, and colposcopy, and where adequate long-term follow-up of patients can be achieved. Fortunately, cryosurgery has been associated with minimal morbidity or posttherapy complications. Since the procedure depresses fibroblastic activity, scarring is minimal and the incidence of subsequent infertility is low. Crisp (1972), for example, reported no cervical stenosis or increased incidence of infertility in 123 patients with cervical dysplasia treated by cryotherapy. The only adverse symptom noted was the slight discomfort associated with cervical dilatation.

A second outpatient method used in the treatment of cervical intraepithelial neoplasia is electrocautery. Utilization of this method was based on the historical observation that the incidence of cervical cancer was markedly reduced in patients who had undergone cervical cauterization for chronic cervicitis. The cervical lesion, as well as the entire transformation zone, is destroyed by electrocoagulation diathermy. Coagulation usually extends into the lower endocervical canal, including the glandular crypts. In certain cases this procedure may require regional anesthesia. Richart and Sciarra (1968) reported successful eradication of the area of cervical neoplasia with the first course of electrocautery in 89% of patients with cervical dysplasia. Likewise, Hollyock and Chanen (1976) noted an apparent primary cure rate of 94% for this method of treatment in 450 patients with cervical dysplasia or carcinoma in situ. These authors restricted treatment by electrocautery to those patients with a cervical lesion fully visible by colposcopy. Unfortunately, electrocautery produces pain or discomfort in a significant percentage of patients (Creasman and Parker 1975). In addition, cervical stenosis has been reported following cautery in at least 5% of patients. For these reasons, most investigators have favored the use of cryosurgery rather than electrocautery.

Recently, there has been much interest in the application of the carbon dioxide laser to the treatment of cervical intraepithelial neoplasia. The term "laser" is an abbreviation for "light amplification by stimulated emission of radiation." The carbon dioxide laser has a wavelength of 10.6 μ, which can be focused in a constant beam by a series of mirrors to produce high-power density (Adducci 1978). Sophisticated instrumentation has allowed the laser to be combined with a colposcope or operating microscope. The beam is directed by colposcopic visualization to a 2-mm area of the cervical epithelium which is being treated. When the beam strikes the cervical epithelium, the cells absorb the energy, are heated to 100°C, and are vaporized. Below the vaporized epithelium, an area of stromal necrosis is produced by absorption of infrared energy and thermal burn. The depth of the stromal burn can be controlled by exposure time to the beam, but is generally much less than that produced by electrocautery. When laser surgery is used in the treatment of cervical intraepithelial neoplasia, the following guidelines should be adhered to:

1. The entire lesion should be confined to the visible portion of the cervix, with no evidence of endocervical extension.
2. The squamocolumnar junction should be fully visualized.
3. There should be no colposcopic or cytologic evidence of invasive cervical cancer.

Using the above criteria, Stafl et al (1977) treated 46 patients with cervical or vaginal neoplasia. Treatment failures occurred in five patients (10%), and were due to inadequate depth of destruction. Postoperative complications were minimal, and the treated area was healed within one month after therapy. The major advantage of laser therapy over cryosurgery or electrocautery is that it produces more localized destruction of a particular lesion, and is associated with minimal scarring and stenosis. Also, laser therapy does not cause transportation of the squamocolumnar junction of the endocervical canal. Consequently, patients can be adequately followed by colposcopy after laser surgery. The most significant disadvantage of laser therapy is the cost of the instrument. Also, the use of the laser in the treatment of cervical neoplasia requires a skilled clinician who is both an excellent colposcopist and well trained in laser therapy. Consequently, laser surgery is available in those relatively few centers where such personnel exist, and where there is a sufficiently large group of patients with cervical epithelial abnormalities to evaluate the efficacy of this form of treatment.

Cervical conization has been the therapeutic method most commonly utilized in patients with cervical intraepithelial neoplasia desiring to preserve childbearing function. This procedure is specifically indicated in the treatment of those patients with endocervical dysplasia or carcinoma in situ. Colposcopy is particularly useful in determining the anatomic extent and location of the lesion which must be removed by conization. In general, the size of the conization specimen is not related to the incidence of postconization complications (Rubio et al 1975), so the amount of tissue excised should be as large as may be necessary to include the area of abnormality as well as a margin of normal epithelium. The importance of removing an area of surrounding normal tissue has been emphasized by several investigators. Ahlgren et al (1975), for example, reported a cure rate of 98% when histologic evaluation indicated that conization margins were free of disease. In contrast, the cure rate decreased to 70% in those cases in which the surgical margins of the conization specimen were involved by the neoplastic process. Similarly, Bjerre et al (1976) reported a significantly higher cure rate if the resection margins of the conization specimen were free of pathologic epithelium. The overall recurrence rate of cervical neoplasia following conization for carcinoma in situ is illustrated in Table 3-4. This is somewhat surprising, since the reported incidence of residual neoplasia in the cervix following conization varies from 22% to 29% (Creasman and Rutledge 1972, van Nagell et al 1976). It is therefore quite possible that the inflammatory reaction at the conization site actually destroys areas of residual neoplasia apparent on examination of the hysterectomy specimen. Conization should be used as the definitive method of treatment only in women who are willing to return for regular follow-up examinations. A complete pelvic examination, including cervical cytology, should be obtained every three months for five years and every six months thereafter.

Cervical conization is a major surgical procedure requiring general anesthesia and hospitalization. It has also been associated with a signifi-

Table 3-4
Recurrence Rate of Cervical Neoplasia
Related to Treatment Method for Carcinoma In Situ

Author	Conization		Hysterectomy	
	No. of Patients	No. Recurring (%)	No. of Patients	No. Recurring (%)
Ahlgren et al (1975)	343	24 (7.0)	NA	NA
Bjerre (1976)	1500	200 (13)	NA	NA
Boyes (1970)	808	31 (3.8)	2849	24 (0.9)
Creasman and Rutledge (1972)	65	5 (7.7)	642	17 (2.4)
Kolstad (1976)	795	26 (3.2)	238	8 (3.3)
van Nagell et al (1976)	109	7 (6.4)	374	5 (1.1)
Total	3620	293 (8.1)	4103	54 (1.3)

NA = not available.

cant incidence of postoperative complications. The most common complication of cervical conization is hemorrhage, which has been reported to occur in 10% to 15% of cases. The majority of patients with postconization hemorrhage respond adequately to resuturing, but 1% to 2% require hysterectomy (Bjerre et al 1975). An additional 10% of patients have cervical stenosis following conization, and a smaller number (1.3%) experience pelvic cellulitis or abscess (Hester and Read 1960). In the pregnant patient, hemorrhagic complications of cervical conization are even more severe. Averette et al (1970) reported that nearly 10% of pregnant women undergoing cervical conization required blood transfusion. In addition, there is an increased risk of abortion or fetal loss after conization. Daskal and Pitkin (1968), for example, reported that there was a 6.6% incidence of fetal loss associated with cervical conization itself. The most significant late complication of conization is cervical stenosis. Byrne (1966) reported that 29% of patients experienced cervical stenosis following conization, and that infertility occurred in approximately one-half that number.

Hysterectomy remains the definitive surgical procedure in the management of carcinoma in situ, particularly in patients who have completed childbearing function. Recurrent vaginal epithelial abnormalities occur in approximately 1% of patients following hysterectomy (Table 3-4). This recurrence rate is higher in patients with residual carcinoma in situ in the uterine specimen (van Nagell 1976). There is little evidence that the routine surgical removal of a 3-cm segment of vaginal cuff with the hysterectomy specimen decreases the incidence of recurrent vaginal neoplasia. Creasman and Rutledge (1972), in a study of 642 patients with intraepithelial cervical carcinoma, could find no relationship between the size of the vaginal cuff removed at hysterectomy and subsequent recurrence of vaginal neoplasia. Rather, colposcopic evaluation of the vagina should be performed on all patients undergoing hysterectomy for carcinoma in situ. In that way, those cases with coexistent vaginal epithelial abnormalities can be identified, and the appropriate colposcopically localized area removed surgically. Complications of vaginal or abdominal hysterectomy performed as therapy for cervical carcinoma in situ are generally the same as those associated with hysterectomy in general.

In a series of 246 patients undergoing vaginal hysterectomy following conization for carcinoma in situ, van Nagell et al (1972) reported that pelvic cellutitis occurred in 12% of patients. The incidence of pelvic infection was significantly higher when the conization-hysterectomy interval was two days than when it was six weeks. Examination of the uterine specimens in the two-day group revealed that a marked degree of inflammatory response with extension of lymphocytic infiltration through the full thickness of the specimen was present in over 80% of the cases. This same degree of inflammatory cell infiltration was present in only 5% of the surgical specimens when the conization-hysterectomy interval was six weeks. It is therefore recommended that hysterectomy be performed either immediately after cyrostat examination of the conization specimen or six weeks later. Following hysterectomy for cervical carcinoma in situ, pelvic examination, including a vaginal cytologic specimen, should be performed every three months for two years, and every six months thereafter.

A systematic approach to the diagnosis and therapy of cervical intraepithelial neoplasia is presented in Figure 3-11. Colposcopy with endocervical curettage is performed on essentially all patients with abnormal cervical cytology. If colposcopy is inadequate because of incomplete visualization of the lesion or the transformation zone, or if there is a persistent discrepancy between cytologic and colposcopic findings, cervical conization is performed. If colposcopy indicates a focal exocervical lesion, and the endocervical curettage is negative, then the lesion is treated by surgical excision, cryosurgery, or laser therapy. When there is an endocervical component of cervical neoplasia, conization is recommended as the therapeutic method of choice. In a patient who desires childbearing, but has carcinoma in situ present in the conization specimen, cervical cytology is obtained at three-month intervals. Recurrence of abnormal cytology is followed by repeat colposcopy, conization, or hysterectomy.

A similar management protocol for pregnant patients with cervical epithelial abnormalities is illustrated in Figure 3-12. As has been previously stated, the physiologic eversion of the cervix during pregnancy allows for adequate colposcopic visualization of the endocervix, and directed biopsy eliminates the necessity for routine endocervical curettage

52

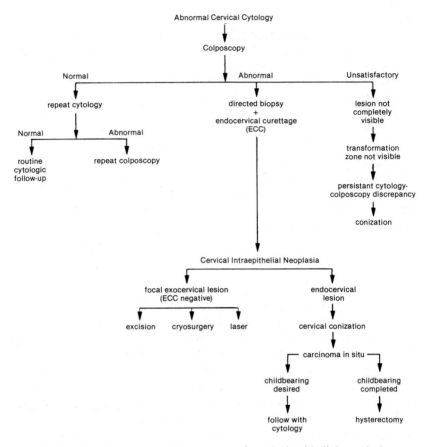

Figure 3-11 Evaluation and treatment of cervical epithelial neoplasia.

(Ostergard and Nieburg 1979). If directed biopsy shows dysplasia or carcinoma in situ, the patient is allowed to deliver vaginally, and further evaluation and therapy is postponed until six weeks following delivery. When colposcopically-directed biopsy indicates microinvasive carcinoma in the first two trimesters, excision of the lesion or conization is recommended. Cesarean section, however, is indicated in a patient with biopsy-diagnosed microinvasive carcinoma in the third trimester, and cervical conization is performed six weeks postpartum. Should a pregnant patient be found to have histologically confirmed invasive cervical cancer, appropriate therapy is undertaken immediately. Pregnant patients with abnormal cervical cytology, but no histologic or colposcopic evidence of an epithelial abnormality, are followed at monthly intervals with colposcopy, and allowed to deliver vaginally.

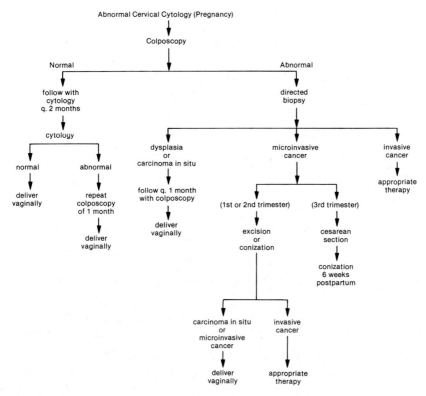

Figure 3-12 Evaluation and treatment of cervical epithelial neoplasia in pregnancy.

BIBLIOGRAPHY

Adducci JE: Gynecologic surgery using the CO_2 laser. *Int Surg* 63:72–74, 1978.

Ahlgren M, Ingemarsson I, Lindberg LG, et al: Conization as treatment of carcinoma in situ of the uterine cervix. *Obstet Gynecol* 46:135–140, 1975.

Averette HE, Nasser N, Yonkow SL, et al: Cervical conization in pregnancy: Analysis of 180 operations. *Am J Obstet Gynecol* 106:543–549, 1970.

Barron BA, Richart RA: A statistical model of the natural history of cervical carcinoma based on a prospective study of 557 cases. *J Nat Cancer Inst* 41:1343–1353, 1968.

Bjerre B, Eliasson G, Linell F, et al: Conization as only treatment of carcinoma in situ of the uterine cervix. *Am J Obstet Gynecol* 125:143–152, 1976.

Briggs RM: Dysplasia and early neoplasia of the uterine cervix. *Obstet Gynecol Surv* 34:70–99, 1979.

Broders AC: Carcinoma in situ contrasted with benign penetrating epithelium. *JAMA* 99:1670–1674, 1932.

Burghardt E: *Early Histological Diagnosis of Cervical Cancer.* Trans EA Friedman, Stuttgart, Thieme, 1973.

Byrne GD: Cone biopsy—A survey of 100 cases. *Aust NZ J Obstet Gynaecol* 6:266–270, 1966.

Christopherson WM: Concepts of genesis and development in early cervical neoplasia. *Obstet Gynecol Surv* 24:842–850, 1969.

Christopherson WM, Broghamer WL: A study of the reversibility of dysplasia of the uterine cervix. *Proceedings of the First International Congress of Exfoliated Cytology.* Philadelphia, JB Lippincott Co, 1962, pp 269–273.

Christopherson WM, Mendes WM, Ahirja EM, et al: Cervix cancer control in Louisville, Kentucky. *Cancer* 26:29–38, 1970.

Coppleson LW, Brown B: The prevention of carcinoma of the cervix. *Am J Obstet Gynecol* 125:153–159, 1976.

Coppleson M: The etiology of squamous carcinoma of the cervix. *Obstet Gynecol* 32:432–436, 1968.

Coppleson M, Pixley E, Reid B: *Colposcopy: A Scientific and Practical Approach to the Cervix in Health and Disease.* Springfield, Ill, Charles C Thomas, 1971a, p 36; 1971b, p 77; 1971c, p 265.

Creasman WT, Rutledge F: Carcinoma in situ of the cervix: An analysis of 861 patients. *Obstet Gynecol* 39:373–380, 1972.

Creasman WT, Weid JC, Curry SL, et al: Efficacy of cryosurgical treatment of severe cervical intraepithelial neoplasia. *Obstet Gynecol* 41:501–506, 1973.

Creasman WT, Parker RT: Management of early cervical neoplasia. *Clin Obstet Gynecol* 18:233–245, 1975.

Crisp WE, Asadourian L, Romberger W: Application of cryosurgery to gynecologic malignancy. *Obstet Gynecol* 30:668–673, 1967.

Crisp WE: Cryosurgical treatment of neoplasia of the uterine cervix. *Obstet Gynecol* 39:495–499, 1972.

Darai G, Munk K: Human embryonic lung cells abortively infected with herpes hominis Type 2 show properties of cell transformation. *Nature New Biol* 241:268–269, 1973.

Daskal JL, Pitkin RM: Cone biopsy of the cervix during pregnancy. *Obstet Gynecol* 32:1–4, 1968.

Feldman MJ, Linzey EM, Srebnik A: Abnormal cervical cytology in the teenager: A continuing problem. *Am J Obstet Gynecol* 126:418–421, 1976.

Fidler HK, Boyes DA, Worth AJ: Cervical cancer detection in British Columbia. *J Obstet Gynecol Br Commonw* 75:392–404, 1968.

Fox CH: Biologic behavior of dysplasia and carcinoma in situ. *Am J Obstet Gynecol* 99:960–972, 1967.

Fox CH: Time necessary for conversion of normal to dysplastic cervical epithelium. *Obstet Gynecol* 31:749–754, 1968.

Garite TJ, Feldman MJ: An evaluation of cytologic sampling techniques: A comparative study. *Acta Cytol* 22:83–85, 1978.

Gondos B, Marshall D, Ostergard D: Endocervical cells in cervical smears. *Am J Obstet Gynecol* 114:833–834, 1972.

Gray LA, Christopherson WM: The treatment of cervical dysplasia. *Gynecol Oncol* 3:149–153, 1975.

Griffiths CT, Younge PA: The clinical diagnosis of early cervical cancer. *Obstet Gynecol Surv* 24:967–975, 1969.

Hester LL, Read RA: An evaluation of cervical conization. *Am J Obstet Gynecol* 80:715–721, 1960.

Hinselmann H: Verbesserung der inspektionsmoglichkoit von vulva, vagina, und portio. *München Med Wchnschr* 77:1733, 1925.

Hollinshead AC, Chretien PB, O'Bong L, et al: In vivo and in vitro measurements of the relationship of human squamous carcinoma to herpes simplex virus tumor-associated antigen. *Cancer Res* 36:821–828, 1976.

Hollyock VE, Chanen W: Electrocoagulation diathermy for the treatment of cervical dysplasia and carcinoma in situ. *Obstet Gynecol* 47:196–199, 1976.

Kaufman RH, Abbott JP, Scheihing WC: Use of the refrigerated microtome for rapid diagnosis of cervical conization specimens. *Am J Obstet Gynecol* 84:107–112, 1962.

Kessler I: Human cervical cancer as a venereal disease. *Cancer Res* 36:783–791, 1976.

Kirkland JA: The study of chromosomes in cervical neoplasia. *Obstet Gynecol Surv* 24:784–794, 1969.

Koss LG, Stewart FW, Foote FW, et al: Some histological aspects of behavior of epidermoid carcinoma in situ and related lesions of the uterine cervix: A long-term prospective study. *Cancer* 16:1160–1211, 1963.

Megafu U: Cancer of the genital tract among the Ibo women in Nigeria. *Cancer* 44:1875–1978, 1979.

Nahmias AJ, Dowdle WR, Naib ZM, et al: Genital infection with Type 2 herpes virus hominis: A commonly occurring venereal disease. *Br J Vener Dis* 45:294–298, 1969.

Nahmias AJ, Josey WE, Naib ZM, et al: Antibodies to herpes virus hominis Types 1 and 2 in humans: II. Women with cervical cancer. *Am J Epidemiol* 91:547–552, 1970.

Naib Z, Nahmias A, Josey W, et al: Genital herpetic infection. *Cancer* 23:940–945, 1969.

Notter MFD, Docherty JJ, Mortel R, et al: Detection of herpes simplex virus tumor-associated antigen in uterine cervical tissue: Five case studies. *Gynec Oncol* 6:574–581, 1978.

Ostergard DC, Nieburg R: Evaluation of abnormal cervical cytology during pregnancy with colposcopy. *Am J Obstet Gynecol* 134:756–758, 1979.

Papanicolaou GN, Traut HF: *Diagnosis of Uterine Cancer by the Vaginal Smear.* New York, The Commonwealth Fund, 1943, p 47.

Patten SF, Hughes CP, Reagan JW: An experimental study of the relationship between *Trichomonas vaginalis* and dysplasia in the uterine cervix. *Acta Cytol* 7:187–195, 1963.

Pederson O: Spontaneous course of cervical precancerous conditions. *Am J Obstet Gynecol* 72:1063–1071, 1956.

Powell J, Jones FS, Daugherty RE, et al: Cervical carcinoma correlation of microtome, cryostat, cytologic, and histologic diagnosis. *Obstet Gynecol* 33:476–481, 1968.

Pratt-Thomas HR, Heins HC, Latham E, et al: The carcinogenic effect on human smegma: An experimental study. *Cancer* 9:671–680, 1956.

Rapp F, Duff R: Oncogenic conversion of normal cells by inactivated herpes simplex virus. *Cancer* 34:1353–1362, 1974.

Rapp F, Reed C: Experimental evidence for the oncogenic potential of herpes simplex virus. *Cancer Res* 36:800–806, 1976.

Rawls WE, Gardner HL, Flanders RW, et al: Genital herpes in two social groups. *Am J Obstet Gynecol* 110:682–689, 1971.

Reagan JW, Seidemand S: The cellular morphology of carcinoma in situ and dysplasia or atypical hyperplasia of the uterine cervix. *Cancer* 6:224–235, 1953.

Reagan JW, Lin F: An evaluation of the vaginal irrigation technique in the detection of uterine cancer. *Acta Cytol* 11:374–382, 1967.

Reid BL: Interaction between homologous sperm and somatic cells of the uterus and peritoneum in the mouse. *Exp Cell Res* 40:679–683, 1965.

Reid BL, Blackwell PM: Evidence for the possibility of nuclear uptake of polymerised deoxyribonucleic acid of sperm phagocytosed by macrophages. *Aust J Exp Biol Med Sci* 45:323–326, 1967.

Richart RM, Vaillant HW: Influence of cell collection techniques upon cytological diagnosis. *Cancer* 18:1474–1478, 1965.

Richart RM, Sciarra JJ: Treatment of cervical dysplasia by out-patient electrocauterization. *Am J Obstet Gynecol* 101:200–205, 1968.

Ronk DA, Jimesson GK, Merrill JA: Evaluation of abnormal cervical cytology. *Obstet Gynecol* 49:581–586, 1977.

Rubio CA, Thomassen P, Kock Y: Influence of the size of cone specimens on postoperative hemorrhage. *Am J Obstet Gynecol* 122:939–944, 1975.

Rubio CA: A trap for atypical cells. *Am J Obstet Gynecol* 128:687–688, 1977.

Selim MA, So-Bosita JL, Blair OM, et al: Cervical biopsy versus conization. *Obstet Gynecol* 41:177–182, 1973.

Sevin BU, Ford JH, Girtanner RD, et al: Invasive cancer of the cervix after cryosurgery: Pitfalls of conservative management. *Obstet Gynecol* 53:465–471, 1979.

Stafl A, Mattingly RF: Colposcopic diagnosis of cervical neoplasia. *Obstet Gynecol* 41:168–176, 1973.

Stafl A, Wilkinson EJ, Mattingly RF: Laser treatment of cervical and vaginal neoplasia. *Am J Obstet Gynecol* 2:128–136, 1977.

Stern E, Neely PM: Carcinoma and dysplasia of the cervix: A comparison of rates in new and returning populations. *Acta Cytol* 7:357–361, 1963.

Treadway DR, Townsend DE, Hovland DN, et al: Colposcopy and cryosurgery in cervical intraepithelial neoplasia. *Am J Obstet Gynecol* 114:1020–1024, 1972.

Underwood PB, Lutz MH, Van Fletcher R: Cryosurgery: Its use for the abnormal pap-smear. *Cancer* 38:546–552, 1976.

van Nagell JR, Roddick JW, Copper RM, et al: Vaginal hysterectomy following conization in the treatment of carcinoma in situ of the cervix. *Am J Obstet Gynecol* 113:948–951, 1972.

van Nagell JR, Hager WD, Roddick JW: Reliability of the cervical cytologic smear as a screening procedure in patients undergoing gynecologic surgery for benign disease. *Am J Obstet Gynecol* 116:111–114, 1973.

van Nagell JR, Parker JC, Hicks LP, et al: Diagnostic and therapeutic efficacy of cervical conization. *Am J Obstet Gynecol* 124:134–139, 1976.

van Nagell JR, Donaldson ES, Gay EC: Evaluation and treatment of patients with invasive cervical cancer. *Surg Clin North Am* 58:67–85, 1978.

von Haam E: Some observations in the field of exfoliative cytology. *Am J Clin Path* 24:652–662, 1954.

Walton RJ: The task force on cervical cancer screening programs. *Can Med Assoc J* 114:1033, 1976.

Wentz WB, Reagan JW, Heggie AD: Cervical carcinogenesis with herpes simplex virus, Type 2. *Obstet Gynecol* 46:117–122, 1975.

Wilbanks GD, Richart RM, Terner JY: DNA content of cervical intraepithelial neoplasia studies by two-wavelength Fuelgen cytophotometry. *Am J Obstet Gynecol* 98:792–799, 1967.

World Health Organization: *Monograph on the Histologic Typing of Female Genital Tract Tumors.* Geneva, WHO, 1975.

Wynder EL: Early cervical neoplasia. *Obstet Gynecol Surv* 34:1697–1711, 1969.

4 Invasive Cervical Cancer

John R. van Nagell, Jr.
E. C. Gay
Deborah F. Powell
Yosh Maruyama

Although the incidence of cervical cancer has been steadily declining over the past 30 years, it is estimated that over 15,000 new cases of invasive carcinoma will be diagnosed annually in the United States, and that over 7000 patients will die each year of this disease. This is particularly disturbing, since regular, cervical cytologic screening has been reported to reduce mortality from cervical cancer effectively. In fact, several investigators (Cramer 1974, Chistopherson et al 1976) have shown that the death rate from cervical cancer is inversely proportional to the level of cytologic screening in a population. Recently, it has become apparent that there are many histologic and anatomic variations of cervical cancer and that these variants often have quite different biologic and prognostic implications. More than ever, it is necessary to identify the specific histologic and anatomic configurations of cervical cancer, and to select the appropriate method of therapy for each patient based on a thorough knowledge of these factors.

ETIOLOGY AND EPIDEMIOLOGY

The etiology of cervical intraepithelial neoplasia has been discussed in detail in Chapter 3, and there is little evidence to suggest that those agents responsible for the genesis of cervical carcinoma in situ are different from those causing invasive cervical cancer. Consequently, this material will be presented only in summary form. Available data support the concept that cervical carcinoma is related to a venereally transmitted agent. Women with cervical cancer begin sexual intercourse at an earlier age and have a greater number of sexual partners than women without cervical cancer (Kessler 1976). Likewise, women with cervical cancer tend to marry at an earlier age and are more likely to have several marital partners than women who do not develop cervical cancer. Squamous cell carcinoma of the cervix is also exceedingly rare in virginal women.

The infectious agent most closely associated with cervical cancer is genital herpesvirus (HSV-2). Evidence for this association includes: 1) retrospective seroepidemiologic studies showing a significantly higher incidence of complement-fixing antibodies to HSV-2-associated antigens in the sera of patients with cervical cancer than in age-matched controls, 2) the known sexual transmission of HSV-2, and 3) the ability of HSV-2 to cause malignant transformation of embryonic cells in tissue culture.

There is little doubt that the major reduction in cervical cancer mortality is due to effective cervical cytologic screening. In the United States, the annual death rate from cervical cancer has fallen from over 20 per 100,000 in 1930 to less than 7 per 100,000 at the present time (Silverberg 1980). Although the precise relationship between carcinoma in situ and invasive cervical carcinoma is unknown, it is quite likely that the majority of cases of invasive cervical cancer are preceded by carcinoma in situ. Cytologic screening has allowed for detection of cervical neoplasia at an intraepithelial stage when it is curable by surgery alone. The annual rate of cytologic screening of the at-risk population in the United States varies from 5% to 25%, depending upon the geographic location and socioeconomic status of the population. There is a direct relationship between the annual percentage of the population screened annually and the percent decrease in cervical cancer incidence (Cramer 1974). It is important to note that about 10% of women in the United States have never had a Pap smear. This figure rises to as high as 25% in black women who live in rural areas (Rochat 1976). The prevalence of cervical cancer screening is also directly related to the educational status and mean income of the population. Twenty-four percent of women with a grade school education have never been screened cytologically whereas only 4% of college graduates have never had a Pap smear. The woman at highest risk for the development of cervical cancer is typically of low socioeconomic status and education, who has had sexual intercourse at an early age with a number of different partners. It is obvious, therefore, that many of the women who need cytologic screening most have never had a Pap smear.

The mean age at diagnosis of patients with invasive cervical cancer has varied from 48 to 55 years, depending upon the population studied. Although the mean age of patients with carcinoma in situ is at least ten years less than that of patients with invasive carcinoma, (Figure 4-1), it should not be concluded that it takes ten years for carcinoma in situ to progress to invasive cervical cancer in an individual patient. The cellular biology of a particular tumor, as well as the immune status of the host, plays an important role in determining the rate of progression of a given intraepithelial lesion. Prompt therapy of carcinoma in situ has undoubtedly been a major factor contributing to the observed decrease in mortality from cervical cancer.

EVALUATION

Perhaps the most serious deficiency in the management of patients with invasive cervical cancer is the lack of a detailed evaluation system which is uniformly applied to all patients. It is no longer sufficient to classify a lesion according to stage alone. There are wide variations of lesion size and anatomic location within each stage, and accurate definition of these variables is of prognostic significance to the patient. In addition, histomorphologic criteria, such as cell type and lymph-vascular space invasion by tumor cells, are directly related to patient survival, and should be evaluated in all cases prior to therapy.

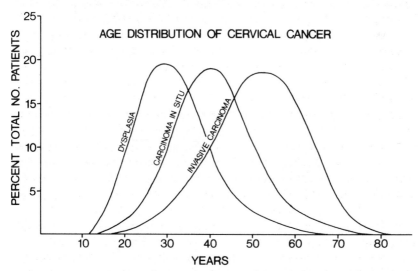

Figure 4-1 Age distribution of patients with cervical dysplasia, carcinoma in situ, and invasive cancer.

Although cervical cytology is the most common method of diagnosing cervical epithelial abnormalities, therapy should not be instituted without histologic confirmation of invasive cancer. A cervical biopsy should include sufficient tissue to establish accurately the cell type of the lesion as well as the presence of lymph-vascular space invasion by tumor cells.

Essential to proper evaluation of cervical cancer is a complete understanding of the anatomic pathways of spread of the disease. Cervical cancer spreads both by direct invasion into adjacent tissues and by embolization into lymphatic channels, resulting often in lymph nodal disease. There are three major pathways of direct invasion by cervical cancer (Figure 4-2):

1. Superiorly, cervical cancer cells spread in the stromal lymphatics to invade the lower uterine segment and myometrium. This type of spread is not recognized in the International Federation of Gynecology and Obstetrics (FIGO) Staging System. As a result, the prognostic significance of this finding has not been thoroughly investigated. The incidence of uterine involvement by cervical cancer has varied in the literature from 4% to 17% (Wentz and Jaffe 1966, Perez et al 1975), and is directly related to the size of the lesion.

2. Inferiorly, cervical cancer spreads to the vaginal stroma and epithelium. This is not surprising, since there is a rich anastomatic network between the lymphatics of the cervix and those of the upper vagina. Biopsy-proven extension of cervical cancer to the upper two thirds of the vagina places the lesion into FIGO Stage IIa. Further extension of tumor in the lymphatic channels within the endopelvic fascia of the lower one third of the vagina results in the lesion being classified as Stage IIIa.

3. Laterally, cervical cancer spreads via the paracervical and parametrial lymphatics to involve the ureter and lateral pelvic wall structures. This is the most common pathway of spread of cervical cancer (Plentyl and Friedman 1971).

The four primary regional lymph node groups to which cervical cancer most often metastasizes are the: 1) internal iliac, 2) obturator, 3) external iliac, and 4) common iliac lymph nodes. Plentyl and Friedman (1971) summarized the distribution of lymph node metastases in over 700 patients with cervical cancer. Lymph nodal metastases varied directly with extent of the disease, and were present in 15% of patients with Stage I disease, 29% of patients with Stage II disease, and 47% of patients with Stage III disease. In patients with lymph nodal metastases, the external iliac group was involved in 23% of cases, the obturator nodes in 19%, the internal iliac nodes in 17%, and the common iliac group in 12%. An additional 21% of patients had either parametrial or paracervical lymph nodes involved by metastatic cervical cancer.

Once histologic confirmation of invasive cervical cancer has been established, the lesion should be staged. Staging can be defined as a clinical estimation of the extent of disease, and should be performed on all patients prior to therapy. Staging is important in that it: 1) provides a clinical approximation of the anatomic configuration of a tumor which must be considered in treatment planning, 2) allows comparison of different treatment modalities in the therapy of clinically similar lesions, and 3) is directly related to patient prognosis.

Various staging systems for cervical cancer have been utilized over the past 50 years. However, the most useful has been the International Federation of Gynecology and Obstetrics Staging System (Table 4-1). It is important to note that a patient's stage of disease cannot be changed even if more extensive tumor is found at the time of operation. Intravenous pyelography, chest x-ray, cystoscopy, and sigmoidoscopy can be used in addition to clinical examination in determining the stage of cervical cancer. The anatomic proximity of the ureters to the cervix makes examination of the lower urinary tract mandatory in patients with cervical cancer.

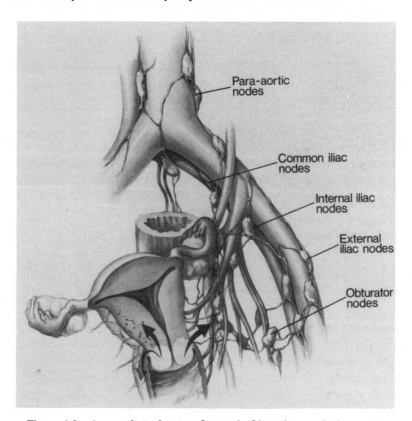

Figure 4-2 Anatomic pathways of spread of invasive cervical cancer.

Table 4-1
International Federation of Gynecology and Obstetrics
Staging System for Invasive Cervical Cancer

Stage I	Carcinoma strictly confined to the cervix (extension to the corpus should be disregarded).
Stage Ia	Microinvasive carcinoma (early stromal invasion).
Stage Ib	All other cases of Stage I. Occult cancer shoud be marked "occ."
Stage II	Extension of the carcinoma beyond the cervix, but not the lower third.
Stage IIa	No obvious parametrial involvement.
Stage IIb	Obvious parametrial involvement.
Stage III	Extension of the carcinoma onto the pelvic wall. On rectal examination, there is no cancer-free space between the tumor and the pelvic wall.
Stage IIIa	No extension onto the pelvic wall.
Stage IIIb	Extension onto the pelvic wall and/or hydronephrosis or nonfunctioning kidney.
Stage IV	Extension of the carcinoma beyond the true pelvis, or clinical involvement of the mucosa of the bladder or rectum. A bullous edema as such does not permit a case to be allotted to Stage IV.
Stage IVa	Spread of the growth to adjacent organs.
Stage IVb	Spread to distant organs.

The prognostic significance of ureteral obstruction prior to surgery is illustrated in Table 4-2. The average five-year survival of patients with ureteral obstruction was 18%, as compared to over 50% in patients without this finding. Therefore, intravenous pyelography should be performed

Table 4-2
Five-Year Survival Rates of Patients
With and Without Ureteral Obstruction by Cervical Cancer

Investigator	No. of Patients	Patients Without Ureteral Obstruction (%)	Patients With Ureteral Obstruction (%)
Aldridge and Mason (1950)	333	59	16
Burns et al (1960)	365	62	24
Barber et al (1963)	503	22	7
Kotteimer (1964)	1402	56	8.8
Bosch et al (1973)	990	51	33
	3593 (total)	50 (average)	18 (average)

prior to therapy in all patients with cervical cancer, and those cases with ureteral obstruction should be placed into Stage IIIb. The relationship of ureteral obstruction to initial stage in cervical cancer was reported by van Nagell et al (1975), and is presented in Table 4-3. It is interesting to note that 4 out of 181 patients (2.8%) with palpable evidence of Stage Ib disease actually had ureteral obstruction by tumor.

Table 4-3
Ureteral Obstruction Related to Stage in Cervical Cancer

Stage Prior to Intravenous Pyelography	No. of Patients	Patients with Obstruction on Intravenous Pyelography	
		Unilateral (%)	*Bilateral (%)*
I	181	4 (2.2)	0
IIa	40	0	0
IIb	159	12 (7.5)	0
IIIa	9	1 (11.1)	1 (11.1)
IIIb	115	32 (27.8)	6 (5.2)
IV	79	24 (30.4)	6 (7.6)

The role of cystoscopy in the evaluation of patients with invasive cervical cancer is less clear. Some investigators advocate the routine use of cystoscopy in evaluating all patients with cervical cancer, whereas others favor its use only in the presence of palpable visible extension of the tumor toward the bladder. Cystoscopic findings in 583 previous patients with cervical cancer who had cystoscopy were reported by van Nagell et al (1975), and are illustrated in Table 4-4. Bladder biopsies were performed

Table 4-4
Cystoscopic Findings in Patients with Cervical Cancer

Stage prior to Cystoscopy	No. of Patients	Patients with Abnormalities				
		Invasive Cancer	*Mass Elevating Bladder*	*Bullous Edema*	*Bladder Inflammation*	*Vesicovaginal Fistula*
I	177	0	0	1	4	0
IIa	40	0	2	0	0	0
IIb	147	0	6	5	3	0
IIIa	7	0	1	0	0	0
IIIb	133	27	41	6	0	0
IV	79	18	5	1	0	2
Totals	583	45	55	13	7	2

in 120 patients, and histologic confirmation of invasion of the bladder mucosa by cervical cancer was obtained in 45. No patient with Stage I or Stage II disease had extension of invasive cervical cancer to the bladder mucosa. The incidence of biopsy-proven bladder invasion was 20% in patients with Stage IIIb cervical cancer. Fifty-five patients were found to have a mass elevating the bladder, but no evidence of mucosal invasion. The significance of this finding has not been evaluated, and is not considered in the present FIGO Staging System. It is therefore recommended that cystoscopy be performed on all patients with Stage IIb disease or greater, or in any lesion with palpable or visible extension toward the bladder. Histologic evidence of bladder mucosal invasion is prerequisite to inclusion in Stage IVa.

In addition to staging each cancer, every effort should be made to record the dimensions of the cervical lesion. Patient survival is directly related to lesion size, and complete knowledge concerning the size and anatomic location of each tumor is helpful in determining optimal therapy, particularly in patients with Stage Ib disease. Piver and Chung (1975) reported that the five-year survival of patients with Stage Ib lesions less than 3 cm in diameter was 88%, as opposed to 65% in patients with cervical lesions larger than 3 cm in diameter. These authors suggested that primary surgical therapy was most effective in patients with Stage Ib disease whose tumors were less than 3 cm in diameter. Likewise, van Nagell et al (1977) noted a recurrence rate of only 9% in patients with cervical lesions less than 2 cm in diameter. In contrast, women with Stage Ib lesions greater than 2 cm experienced a 44% recurrence rate when treated by surgery alone. It is not sufficient simply to stage each lesion before deciding upon the appropriate therapy. Numerous other variables including cell type, lesion size, and the extent and location of extrapelvic metastases, are prerequisite to a complete understanding of the biologic behavior of each tumor. It is only by a thorough understanding of all of these variables that an appropriate treatment plan can be devised which will meet the needs of each patient and therefore maximize survival.

The correlation between clinical staging and intraoperative findings is 70% at best (van Nagell et al 1971), and a significant number of patients have more advanced disease than can be appreciated on pelvic examination. In addition, the incidence of extrapelvic lymph node metastases in patients with Stages III and IV disease has been reported to be as high as 30% (Averette et al 1972, Lepanto et al 1975, Buchsbaum 1979). As a result, several investigators have recommended the use of certain adjunctive procedures in addition to staging in order to evaluate the extent of disease prior to therapy more completely.

The first of these is lymphangiography. The accuracy of this procedure in determining the presence of disease of the lymph nodes has varied widely in the literature. Piver and Barlow (1973) found that 23 of

24 patients with positive lymphangiographic findings actually had histologic evidence of tumor metastases in the paraaortic nodes. Likewise, Fuchs and Rosenberg (1975) noted an 85% accuracy rate of lymphangiography in patients with cervical cancer. Nevertheless, up to 15% of nodes thought to be negative on lymphangiography were actually found to contain small foci of metastatic disease (Piver and Barlow 1973, Brown et al 1979). Therefore, it is suggested that pretherapy lymphangiography is utilized specifically in those patients with a potentially high incidence of lymph node metastases. This would include patients with bulky Stage IIb lesions and all cases with Stage III and IV disease. Patients having a lymphangiogram compatible with paraaortic lymph node metastases should undergo further diagnostic procedures such as percutaneous needle biopsy or lymph node biopsy.

To confirm the presence of nodal disease, two approaches to pretherapy selective lymph node biopsy have been utilized. The intraperitoneal approach has provided more complete exposure of the pelvic lymph nodes, but has been associated with a significant incidence of complications when followed by radiation therapy. According to this method (Buchsbaum 1972), a paramedian incision is extended approximately 5 cm cephalad and 5 cm caudad from the umbilicus. This allows for exposure of the anterior and lateral lymph node chains along the entire length of the abdominal aorta. More recently, a retroperitoneal approach to the paraaortic lymph nodes has been advocated (Schellhas 1975, LaGasse et al 1979). This method involves a right, midrectus abdominal incision with reflection of the posterior peritoneum anteriorly and medially to expose the paraaortic nodes. This method does not allow for extensive exploration of the lower pelvic nodes, but has been associated with extremely few postradiation complications. Percutaneous transperitoneal lymph node biopsy, utilizing a small gauge needle, has been reported in a small number of patients with cervical cancer (Zornoza et al 1977, Wallace et al 1977). Needle biopsy is guided by fluoroscopy or ultrasound, and has been effective in confirming the presence of metastatic carcinoma in the external iliac, common iliac, and paraaortic lymph node groups. This procedure has not been associated with major complications (Holm et al 1975), and has the advantage of not requiring a general anesthetic. Furthermore, radiation following needle aspiration of lymph nodes has not been associated with the high incidence of enteric complications reported in patients undergoing extended field irradiation after intraabdominal surgery (Wharton et al 1977).

Other noninvasive techniques are presently being used to determine the extent and location of cervical cancer prior to therapy. These methods include computer-assisted tomography (CAT scan), ultrasonography, and radioimmunodetection methods utilizing radiolabeled antibodies to antigens produced by the cervical tumor itself. At present, these methods are experimental, but there is substantial evidence to indicate that they provide a more precise estimation of the extent of the primary tumor and its metastases than is available by clinical examination alone.

The role of biochemical markers as a means of monitoring the response rate of cervical cancer to therapy is presently being investigated. Recent studies have indicated that rising plasma CEA levels often precede the clinical diagnosis of recurrence by up to six months (Khoo and Mackey 1973, van Nagell et al 1978). Immunohistochemical detection of antigens in tumor tissue sections obtained from biopsy specimens prior to treatment identifies the antigen profile for each tumor (Primus et al 1975). Those antigens present in highest concentrations in tumor tissue can then be measured serially in the plasma, following treatment, as a method to predict occult recurrence. Plasma antigen determinations should be performed before therapy and at monthly intervals thereafter. The subject of tumor markers in gynecologic cancer will be discussed more completely in Chapter 21.

PATHOLOGY

Before discussing the histologic classification of invasive cervical cancer, it is pertinent to review the definition of microinvasive cancer. In the past, there have been many definitions of microinvasive cancer, and the reported incidence of lymph node metastases in patients with this diagnosis has varied from 0% to 4.8% (Ruch 1970, Boronow 1977). In order to have therapeutic relevance, a definition of microinvasive cancer should preclude the possibility that metastatic cancer is present in the regional lymph nodes. In 1974, the Society of Gynecologic Oncologists adopted a definition of microinvasive cancer which included only those cases in which invasion was limited to a depth of less than 3 mm of the stroma without evidence of lymph-vascular space invasion by tumor cells (Figure 4-3). Using this definition, Boronow (1977) reported that there was no evidence of lymph node metastases in 35 patients with microinvasive cancer who had a radical hysterectomy with pelvic lymphadenectomy. The incidence of positive lymph nodes was 21% in patients with more extensive invasion of the cervical stroma. It should be emphasized that the diagnosis of microinvasive cervical cancer can be made only from a conization specimen in which an adequate number of sections have been taken to rule out the presence of coexisting invasive cancer. Careful examination of these tissue sections for the presence of lymph-vascular space invasion should also be made. Provided that these criteria are strictly fulfilled, the above mentioned definition of microinvasive cervical cancer is complete and should provide accurate histologic data on which to base therapeutic decisions.

The diagnosis of invasive cervical cancer should be made only after unequivocal histologic evidence of stromal invasion by tumor cells to a depth greater than 3 mm. Tumors should be classified as follows, according to the criteria of Reagan et al (1957):

1. Large cell nonkeratinizing cancer (Figure 4-4). This tumor is characterized by large cells with a high nuclear-cytoplasmic ratio,

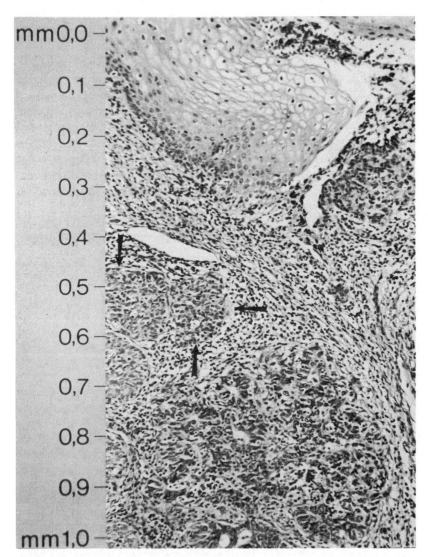

Figure 4-3 Microinvasive cervical cancer. Nests of tumor cells with irregular borders (arrows) extend to a depth of no more than 3 mm below the epithelial basement membrane, as measured by ocular micrometer.

coarse, granular nuclear chromatin, basophilic cytoplasm, and limited pleomorphism.

2. Keratinizing squamous cell carcinoma (Figure 4-5). This tumor contains large cells with a high degree of pleomorphism. The production of structured keratin material (eg, keratin pearls) is essential for inclusion into this category.

3. Small cell carcinoma (Figure 4-6). This tumor is identified by the presence of small primitive cells with dark, coarsely granular nuclei. These cells are remarkably uniform in size and have the highest nuclear-cytoplasmic ratio of all cervical squamous carcinomas.

4. Adenocarcinoma (Figure 4-7). These tumors are characterized by glandular elements often containing mucicarmine-positive material. Special tumor types included in this category are those containing squamous elements such as adenocanthoma, in which the malignant glandular component is associated with benign squamous metaplasia, and adenosquamous carcinoma, in which both the glandular and squamous components are malignant. Other rare adenocarcinomas of the cervix are the clear-cell carcinoma and the adenocystic carcinoma, which is thought to arise from malignant transformation of the basal cell layer of the cervix (Hoskins et al 1979).

In addition to cell type, histologic specimens of invasive cervical cancer should be examined for the presence of lymph-vascular space inva-

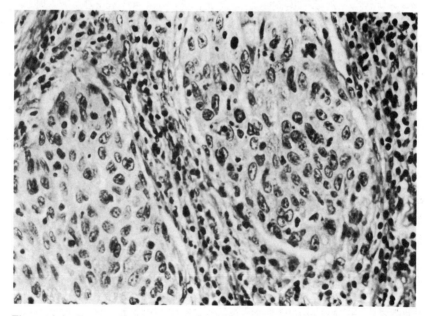

Figure 4-4 Large-cell nonkeratinizing cancer of the cervix. Tumor contains sheets of cells with abundant cytoplasm and no keratin formation.

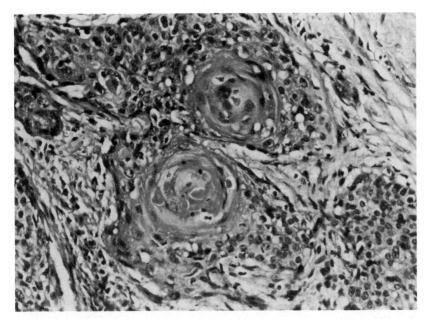

Figure 4-5 Keratinizing squamous cell carcinoma of the cervix. Tumor contains large cells forming numerous keratin pearls.

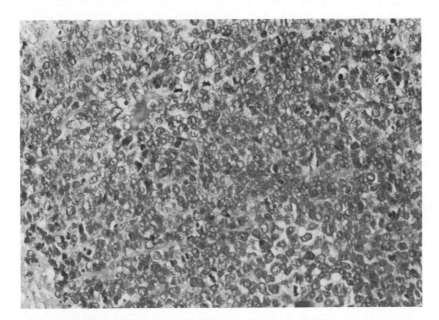

Figure 4-6 Small-cell carcinoma of the cervix. Tumor contains sheets of small cells with markedly altered, nuclear cytoplasmic ratio and scant cytoplasm. Cells are only slightly larger than lymphocytes.

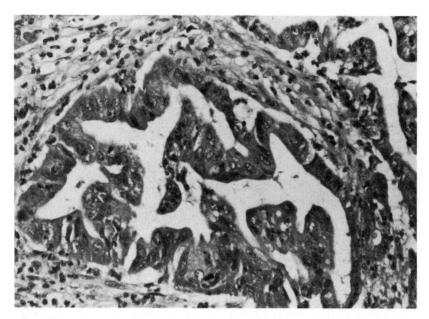

Figure 4-7 Adenocarcinoma of the cervix. Tumor consists of malignant glands, often with demonstrable cytoplasmic mucin infiltrating the cervical stroma.

sion by tumor cells (Figure 4-8). This finding has been shown to be of prognostic significance (Barber et al 1978), and is important in treatment planning. The degree of lymphocytic infiltration around tumor cells is of experimental interest, since it has been correlated with host cellular immunity (Bloom and Field 1971). However, the relationship of this finding to recurrence rate and patient survival has not been established.

THERAPY

Microinvasive Cancer

The appropriate treatment of microinvasive carcinoma has been somewhat controversial since different definitions of this entity have been utilized. As previously stated, we recommend the definition of microinvasion first proposed by the Society of Gynecologic Oncology, namely, cervical carcinoma in which invasion is limited to a depth of less than 3 mm without lymph-vascular space invasion. This diagnosis can be made only from a conization specimen which has been sectioned adequately and examined with a micrometer to establish the depth of stromal invasion. If these criteria are adhered to, the optimal therapy for microinvasive carcinoma of the cervix is total abdominal hysterectomy. Abdominal hysterectomy is preferable to vaginal hysterectomy in that any enlarged lymph node suspicious of malignancy can be readily biopsied and sent for frozen-section examination. Colposcopy should be performed prior to surgery so that any area of vaginal extension can be identified and excised at the time of hysterectomy. Should there be any doubt as to whether the depth of stromal invasion extends beyond 3 mm, or whether lymph-vascular space invasion by tumor cells exists, a radical hysterectomy with pelvic lymphadenectomy should be performed.

Invasive Cancer

The basic requirement of any therapeutic method used in the treatment of invasive cervical cancer is that it treat both the primary tumor and the regional pelvic lymph nodes to which the primary tumor might metastasize. Historically, different investigators have advocated either radical surgery or irradiation as the therapeutic method of choice for patients with cervical cancer. However, very few prospective randomized studies using both these methods in patients with the same stage of disease have been reported. In a randomized study of 100 patients with all stages of cervical cancer treated alternatively with surgery or radiation therapy, Roddick and Greenlaw (1971) reported that survival was generally higher in the radiation therapy group. Survival was equal, however, in patients with Stage I disease treated

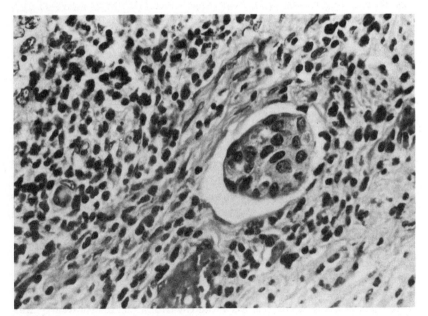

Figure 4-8 Lymph-vascular space invasion by cervical cancer. Note tumor cells in space lined by flattened endothelial cells.

either by radical hysterectomy and pelvic lymphadenectomy, or radiation therapy. Likewise, Masubuchi et al (1969) reported no significant differences in the survival of 448 patients with Stage I cervical cancer treated either by radical surgery or radiation therapy.

More recently, certain investigators have proposed analytical methods to determine those patients whose tumors are best treated by radical surgery. These methods are based on results which show that the effectiveness of radical surgery as a treatment method markedly decreases when cervical cancer has spread beyond the cervix to involve regional pelvic lymph nodes. Webb and Symmonds (1979), for example, noted that only 57% of patients treated by radical hysterectomy and pelvic lymphadenectomy survived five years when pelvic lymph nodes were involved by metastatic cervical cancer. Piver and Chung (1975) reported a direct correlation between the size of the cervical lesion and lymph nodal metastases. Thirty-five percent of patients with Stage Ib lesions greater than 3 cm in diameter had metastatic disease in the pelvic lymph nodes. In contrast, lymph node metastases were present in only 21% of patients whose lesions were less than 3 cm in diameter. Five-year survival following radical surgery was 90% in patients with Stage Ib lesions less than 3 cm in diameter, but fell to 66% in patients with larger lesions. These authors concluded that radical surgery was most effective in Stage Ib lesions less than 3 cm in diameter, and should not be employed in patients with Stage IIa disease. In a similar study, van Nagell et al (1979) reported that only 6% of patients with Stage Ib cervical cancers less than 2 cm in diameter had positive pelvic lymph nodes as opposed to 18% in larger lesions. Patient survival was slightly higher when these small cervical tumors were treated with radical surgery than with radiation therapy.

Cell type has also been useful in determining the optimal method of therapy for each patient, as previously noted. Small-cell carcinomas of the cervix have been shown to metastasize early to regional pelvic lymph nodes. Van Nagell et al (1978) reported that lymph node metastases were present in over 50% of patients with Stage Ib small-cell cancers. Recurrent carcinoma developed in 54% of patients with small-cell carcinoma treated with radical surgery, as opposed to 31% in patients treated with radiation therapy. This difference occurred despite the fact that the larger cervical lesions generally were treated with radiation therapy. These investigators suggested that small-cell carcinomas should be preferentially treated with radiation therapy, and that the field size of external radiation should be extended as indicated on the basis of selected lymph node biopsy findings.

Finally, the presence of lymph-vascular space invasion by tumor cells should be considered when determining optimal therapy for an individual lesion. Barber et al (1978) reported that the tumor cell invasion of lymph-vascular spaces in the cervical stroma decreased the five-year survival in patients with Stage Ib cervical cancer from 90% to 60%. Similarly, van Nagell et al (1979) noted that lymph-vascular space invasion was associated with a 30% increase in recurrence rate in patients with Stage Ib disease. Over one half of these recurrences were confined to the pelvis. The finding of lymph-vascular space invasion alone should not mandate primary treatment with radiation therapy. However, it is indicative of an increased risk for regional and even systemic spread of the primary tumor.

It would seem, therefore, that primary radical hysterectomy and pelvic lymphadenectomy is the treatment of choice in young, healthy patients with Stage Ib large cell squamous cancers less than 3 cm in diameter. The advantage of radical surgery over radiation therapy in these patients is that ovarian and vaginal function can be preserved, while the bowel and bladder complications of radiation therapy can be avoided. Although there are few objective data concerning the efficacy of radiation therapy in the treatment of lymph node metastases found at the time of radical surgery, the authors favor its use. A certain number of patients have only microscopic disease in the intervening lymphatics after surgical removal of positive lymph nodes. Theoretically, these microscopic tumor metastases are susceptible to irradiation at a dose which can be tolerated by normal, lateral, pelvic wall structures. It is therefore recommended that all patients with lymph node metastases receive postoperative external radiation to the pelvis. A dose of 5000 to 6000 rad of external therapy is given to a field size including the area from which positive lymph nodes were removed. Dose fractionation is often increased due to lowered tissue tolerance following surgery, so that radiation therapy is given at a rate of 160 to 200 rad per day. Buchsbaum (1979) reported that over one third of patients with paraaortic lymph node metastases actually had a spread to the scalene lymph nodes. Patients with positive paraaortic lymph nodes should have a scalene lymph node biopsy. If metastatic cervical cancer is present in the scalene or mediastinal lymph nodes, chemotherapy should be combined with pelvic radiation as the primary therapeutic method.

Although pregnant patients with early stage cervical cancer traditionally have been treated with radical surgery (Ulfelder et al 1970, Dudan 1973), there is little evidence to indicate that the biology of this tumor is actually changed during pregnancy (Bosch 1966, Mikuta 1967). Therefore, the same histologic and clinical variables should be considered in the pregnant and nonpregnant patient with cervical cancer when trying to determine proper therapy. In the first two trimesters of pregnancy, therapy should be instituted immediately without consideration of fetal outcome. In patients with Stage Ib large-cell lesions less than 3 cm in diameter, radical hysterectomy and pelvic lymphadenectomy is the treatment of choice. Usually, surgical exposure is sufficient, and this operation can be performed without prior hysterotomy. Patients with more advanced stage disease should be treated primarily with radiation therapy. External therapy is given prior to intracavitary radiation, and spontaneous abortion usually occurs three to six weeks after initiation of treatment (Bosch 1966). After 32 weeks gestation, fetal maturation studies should be obtained every two weeks, and cesarean section performed when these studies, including amniotic fluid lecithin and sphingomyelin concentrations, indicate fetal maturity. In patients with Stage Ib disease, radical hysterectomy and pelvic lymphadenectomy can be performed at the time of cesarean section. Radiation therapy is the preferred treatment in patients with more advanced stage disease.

As has been previously stated, surgery is the primary treatment of choice in selected patients with Stage Ib cervical cancer. The specific operation utilized is radical abdominal hysterectomy and pelvic lymphadenectomy.

Radical hysterectomy and pelvic lymphadenectomy has undergone numerous modifications since its original description by Clark in 1895. The purpose of this operation is the removal en bloc of the cervical tumor, uterus, parametria, and upper vagina, together with the obturator, internal iliac, external iliac, and common iliac lymph nodes. The ureters are dissected free of parametrial lymphatic tissue from the pelvic brim to their entrance into the bladder. Complete excision of the internal iliac artery and vein was once performed as part of this operation. However, it was associated with increased blood loss and fistula formation, and has consequently been abandoned by most surgeons. Kolbenstvedt and Kolstad (1974), utilizing preoperative and postoperative lymphangiography, reported that pelvic lymphadenectomy was often incomplete. Specificially, the lateral sacral nodes of the internal iliac group were the nodes most often missed. These authors stress the necessity of having complete knowledge of pelvic anatomy, and meticulous lymph node removal on the part of the surgeon performing this operation.

Recent advances have been made in the medical management of patients undergoing radical hysterectomy and pelvic lymphadenectomy. Prophylactic antibiotics have been beneficial in reducing the incidence of postoperative pelvic infection, and are utilized by most surgeons. Likewise, techniques for the rapid infusion of blood intraoperatively have protected the patient from the complications of hypovolemia. A rare, but severe, complication of rapid blood replacement is a hemolytic transfusion reaction, being reported in one of every 2500 to 6000 units transfused (Bluemle 1965, Pineda et al 1978). Symptoms of a transfusion reaction include a sudden increase in body temperature ($> 2°F$), hypotension, oliguria and, in severe cases, disseminated intravascular coagulopathy with excessive bleeding. Unfortunately, the patient experiencing this complication is often anesthetized, making diagnosis particularly difficult. Laboratory values diagnostic of a hemolytic transfusion reaction include: 1) free hemoglobin in the plasma or urine, 2) elevated unconjugated serum bilirubin, and 3) decreased serum haptoglobin. Coagulation studies indicative of disseminated intravascular coagulopathy are prolonged bleeding and prothrombin times, decreased serum fibrinogen and platelet count, and blood clot lysis. Treatment of this complication is directed toward reversal of the intravascular coagulopathy and prevention of renal cortical damage (Table 4-5).

Table 4-5
Treatment of Acute Hemolytic Transfusion Reaction

1. Terminate transfusion
2. Retype patient + Units administered
3. Vigorous fluid therapy
4. Diuretics to increase renal blood flow
5. Heparin to reverse intravascular coagulopathy

The use of prophylactic anticoagulants following radical hysterectomy is somewhat more controversial. Although thromboembolic disease remains one of the most common complications after radical hysterectomy (Webb and Symmonds 1979), the extensive dissection implicit in the operation often results in a denuded area in the retroperitoneal space, which could potentially bleed with the administration of anticoagulants. Consequently, a prospective investigation needs to be undertaken to determine if the benefits of anticoagulation outweigh its complications in radical surgery.

There have also been several technical advances in the operation of radical hysterectomy and pelvic lymphadenectomy. These include: 1) vaginal vault closure with peritonealization of the bladder base, rectum, and ureters, 2) retroperitoneal suction drainage, and 3) suprapubic bladder drainage. Symmonds and Pratt (1961) reported that the combination of vaginal cuff closure and retroperitoneal suction drainage caused a significant decrease in the incidence of vesicovaginal fistulas, ureterovaginal fistulas, and lymphocysts following radical hysterectomy and pelvic lymphadenectomy. Drains are placed in the iliac fossae after removal of the surgical specimen and closure of the vaginal vault (Figure 4-9). The drains are then brought out through stab wounds in the lower abdominal quadrants, and pelvic reperitonealization is completed. Roddick et al (1973) measured the protein and electrolyte concentrations of retroperitoneal suction drainage. Sodium, potassium, and chloride concentrations were slightly higher in the drainage fluid than in the serum, whereas protein concentrations were slightly lower. The mean drainage volume was approximately 300 ml during the first postoperative day, and decreased to less than 50 ml on the sixth day following surgery. Accurate quantitation of protein and electrolyte concentrations in suction drainage allows these losses to be replaced, thereby avoiding postoperative fluid and electrolyte abnormalities.

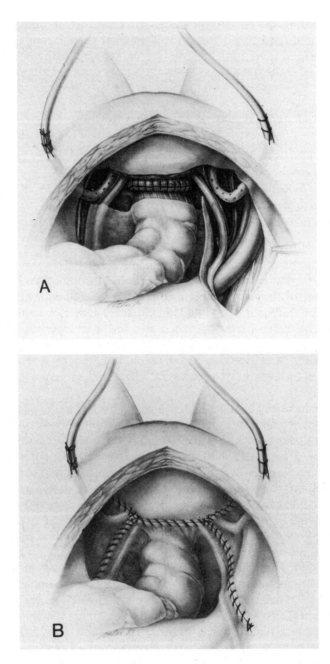

Figure 4-9 Technique of insertion of pelvic drains following radical hysterectomy and pelvic lymphadenectomy. **(A)** Drains inserted into retroperitoneal space after removal of surgical specimen. **(B)** Reperitonealization of pelvis with drains in place.

With extensive dissection of the bladder base and paravesical spaces at the time of radical hysterectomy, there is often damage to the autonomic fibers, resulting in increased myogenic tone and bladder hypertonicity. This phase usually occurs during the immediate postoperative period and is characterized by: 1) diminution of vesical capacity, 2) elevation of resting bladder pressure, and 3) increased residual volume (Seski et al 1977). Bladder hypertonicity is often followed by a hypotonic phase due to the partial interruption of sympathetic fibers which provide bladder sensation. During this phase, overdistention of the bladder can occur, thereby increasing the risk of fistula formation. For this reason, prolonged postoperative bladder drainage is indicated. Green et al (1962), in a study of over 600 patients, reported a 50% reduction in major ureteral complications when constant bladder drainage was increased from two to six weeks following radical hysterectomy. The use of suprapubic bladder drainage following radical hysterectomy and pelvic lymphadenectomy was reported by van Nagell et al (1972). A small incision is made in the bladder at the time of surgery and a No. 18 Foley catheter inserted (Figure 4-10). The catheter is brought out through a stab wound lateral to the midline abdominal incision and connected to straight drainage. The patient is instructed to begin intermittent clamping of the

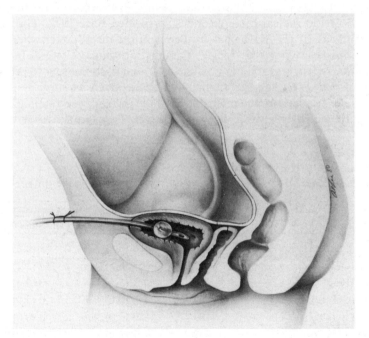

Figure 4-10 Suprapubic bladder drainage following radical hysterectomy with pelvic lymphadenectomy.

catheter during the third postoperative week, and the catheter is removed when the postvoiding bladder drainage has been associated with a decrease in the incidence of postoperative urinary tract infection and fistulae, and is more comfortable for the patient than a urethral catheter.

The most common complications of radical hysterectomy and node dissection continue to be those related to the urinary tract. Urinary tract infection has been reported to occur in approximately 15% of patients following radical hysterectomy (Webb and Symmonds 1979). The aforementioned bladder hypotonicity which often follows this operation is associated with an increase in urinary residual volume and infection. Patients should be maintained on a urinary antibacterial agent as long as a catheter remains in the bladder. The incidence of urinary tract fistulae following radical hysterectomy is summarized in Table 4-6. The incidence of ureterovaginal and vesicovaginal fistulae has decreased progressively over the past two decades, and these complications presently occur in less than 3% of patients following radical hysterectomy. For example, Green et al (1962) reported an overall ureteral fistula rate of 8.5% in patients undergoing radical hysterectomy and pelvic lymphadenectomy from 1939 to 1961. In 1966, however, these same investigators noted a reduction in the incidence of ureteral fistulae to 1.5% by the use of ureteral suspension to the anterior division of the internal iliac artery, and prolonged postoperative bladder drainage. Sall et al (1979) reported no ureteral fistulae in 130 radical hysterectomies performed since 1972. The most common site of ureterovaginal fistulae is in the distal ureter where the ureter has been dissected from its parametrial tunnel. Ureteral fistulae should be repaired as soon as possible after diagnosis in order to prevent upper urinary tract damage. In many instances, extensive surgical dissection of the distal ureter and interruption of the ureteral blood supply make fistula repair extremely difficult, and ureteral resection with ureteroneo-

Table 4-6
Incidence of Ureterovaginal and Vesicovaginal Fistulae
Following Radical Hysterectomy with Pelvic Lymphadenectomy

Investigator	No. of Patients	Ureterovaginal Fistula (%)	Vesicovaginal Fistula (%)
Liu and Meigs (1955)	473	28 (5.9)	3 (0.6)
Green et al (1962)	623	53 (8.5)	14 (2.2)
Green (1966)	65	1 (1.5)	0 (0.0)
Averette (1969)	44	0 (0.0)	0 (0.0)
Park et al (1973)	189	0 (0.0)	0 (0.0)
Sall et al (1979)	349	7 (2.0)	3 (0.9)
Webb et al (1979)	564	15 (2.6)	13 (2.3)

cystotomy is the procedure of choice. In the rare instance in which a ureteral fistula occurs above the pelvic brim, a transuretero-ureterostomy may be necessary.

A second potentially severe complication is ureteral stricture. This complication is rare, being reported in less than 1% of patients following radical hysterectomy. Ureteral stricture is frequently asymptomatic and is diagnosed by postoperative intravenous pyelography. Ureteral dilatation is often successful in correcting the area of stenosis, but occasionally surgical resection of the stricture area with ureteroneocystotomy is required.

Vesicovaginal fistulae have been much less common than ureteral fistulae due to intraoperative recognition and repair of bladder lacerations. It is recommended that the bladder be inflated with approximately 300 ml saline following removal of the surgical specimen. The procedure allows the surgeon to recognize small defects in the bladder so that they can be repaired immediately before a fistula develops. Vesicovaginal fistulae often cannot be repaired immediately because of necrosis and infection at the fistula sites. The patient should be placed on antibiotics and the fistula site cleaned prior to attempting surgical repair. Cystoscopy should be performed to define the location of the fistula accurately, as well as its anatomic relationship to the ureteral orifices. In the absence of previous radiation therapy, repair of vesicovaginal fistulae, from either a vaginal or intravesical approach, is almost always successful, and urinary diversion or nephrectomy can be avoided.

Although some investigators (Rampone et al 1973) have advocated the use of radical hysterectomy and pelvic lymphadenectomy following radiation therapy, the combination of two radical therapeutic methods is generally associated with an increased incidence of major postoperative complications without improving survival. The extensive retroperitoneal dissection associated with pelvic lymphadenectomy often causes devascularization of the distal ureter and bladder base. When the effects of radiation on the microcirculation are added to these surgically induced changes, the risk of major injury to normal pelvic organs is increased. In an earlier study, Gray et al (1958) treated 61 patients with a combination of preoperative radiation and radical hysterectomy and pelvic lymphadenectomy. Major urinary tract or enteric complications occurred in 12% of the patients, and it was concluded that the morbidity and mortality associated with radical surgery after radiation did not justify this combined approach.

Several investigators (Nelson et al 1975, Rutledge et al 1976) have reported the efficacy of extrafascial hysterectomy following radiation therapy for Stage Ib and IIb barrel-shaped lesions. These lesions characteristically contain a large volume of hypoxic malignant cells (Burghardt 1978), and their anatomic configuration is such that the endocervical component of the tumor is often outside the isodose curve of curative radiation therapy (Figure 4-11). Consequently, if radiation therapy alone is used, there is a high incidence of central recurrence (Jampolis et al 1975). In a series of 137 patients with Stage I and II cervical cancer who had radical surgery after radiation therapy, Crawford et al (1965) reported that residual cancer was present in the uterus of 27 patients (20%). Fletcher and Rutledge (1962) first proposed the addition of extrafascial hysterectomy to radiation therapy in the treatment of bulky Stages I and II tumors. External therapy was reduced to 4000 rad, and was followed by one radium implant of 4000 to 5000 mg-hours and extrafascial hysterectomy. Nelson et al (1975) reported the results of this treatment method on 212 patients with large central lesions. The five-year survival of these patients was comparable to that of patients with nonbulky Stage I and II tumors, and the incidence of isolated central recurrence was reduced to 2%. Severe urinary tract or bowel complications occurred in only 7% of cases, as compared to 17% in patients treated at the same institution with radiation followed by radical hysterectomy and pelvic lymphadenectomy.

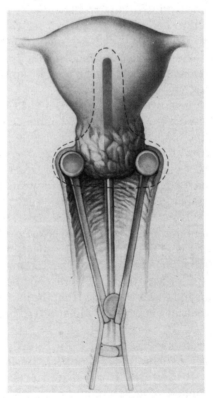

Figure 4-11 Barrel-shaped cervical cancer with intracavitary implant in place. Note that a portion of the tumor is outside the curative isodose curve.

In a more recent study, van Nagell et al (1979) reported that the addition of extrafascial hysterectomy to radiation therapy significantly reduced the recurrence rate in all Stage Ib tumors greater than 5 cm in diameter. Careful clinical observation of the response of all Stage I and II cervical cancers to radiation therapy may also indicate the need of additional surgery in selected patients. Marcial et al (1970) noted that the degree of radiation-induced tumor regression was directly related to the incidence of local recurrence in cervical cancer patients. Patients whose tumors regressed completely by the end of external therapy had an excellent three-year survival. In contrast, tumors with incomplete regression after completion of radiation often recurred. It would appear, therefore, that the addition of extrafascial hysterectomy to radiation therapy is indicated in bulky Stage Ib and IIb tumors, as well as in selected, smaller early-stage lesions which do not respond clinically to irradiation.

Radiation therapy is presently the therapeutic method of choice in most patients with Stage Ib lesions greater than 3 cm in diameter, and in patients with more advanced-stage disease. This is based generally on the assumption that radiation therapy is more effective than radical surgery in treating disease which has spread beyond the cervix to involve the pelvic lymph nodes. In patients with lymph node disease, there is a high probability that microscopic metastases are present in the intervening lymphatics which are not visible. It is therefore extremely difficult, if not impossible, to eradicate this microscopic disease surgically. The reported low survival of patients with advanced-stage disease who were treated primarily with radical surgery has confirmed these assumptions (Brunschwig and Daniel 1962, Roddick and Greenlaw 1971).

A complete discussion of the theory of radiation therapy and its application to the treatment of cervical cancer is presented in Chapter 5. Basically, radiation therapy is given as a combination of external therapy and one or two intracavitary implants. External therapy, in a dose of 4000 to 5000 rad, is given from a linear accelerator or a cobalt-60 source. The field size is usually confined to the pelvis, but may be extended to include specific tumor configurations or areas of lymph node metastases. The standard pelvic field is 15 × 15 cm and has an upper level at the L-5 vertebral body. When the paraaortic lymph nodes contain metastatic cervical cancer, the field size is usually extended upward to a level of the L-1 interspace. This extended field is given a total of 4500 to 5000 rad. External radiation is provided at a dosage rate of 160 to 200 rad per day, depending upon the vascular status of the patient (van Nagell et al 1974, van Nagell et al 1977). Most therapists prefer to give external irradiation prior to intracavitary therapy, since it reduces tumor bulk and enhances the ability of intracavitary sources to eradicate the remaining pelvic disease. Dosimetry is computerized, and the dose, both to the tumor and to normal tissues throughout the pelvis, can be accurately determined.

Through a combination of external and intracavitary therapy, the tumor is given 10,000 to 15,000 rad, the paracervical area (point A) 8000 rad, and the lateral pelvic wall structures 5500 to 6000 rad. The major limiting factor to the amount of radiation given is the tolerance of normal tissues adjacent to the cervix. In general, the bladder and ureters should receive no more than 7000 rad, the rectum and sigmoid colon no more than 6000 rad, and the small bowel no more than 4500 rad.

Complications from radiation therapy are generally related to vascular damage caused by ionizing radiation. Radiation causes capillary endothelial proliferation and progressive lumenal narrowing. Consequently, there is decreased tissue perfusion, localized hypoxia, and, eventually, cell death. This effect is particularly pronounced in patients with preexisting vascular disease such as hypertension or diabetes mellitus. In addition, radiation therapy has been reported to depress endothelial regeneration and retard collagen synthesis (Edwards and Dunphy 1958). Radiation complications are dose-related and increase markedly when normal tissue tolerance is exceeded. Sophisticated computerized dosimetry techniques are utilized in most centers to provide maximal doses to the tumor, while minimizing radiation to adjacent normal structures. Consequently, severe radiation complications, including enteric or urinary tract fistulae, are relatively rare, being reported in less than 5% of patients treated (Fletcher 1971, van Nagell et al 1974). A more complete discussion of the incidence and treatment of radiation related complications is presented in Chapter 5.

There are few data concerning the use of chemotherapy as an adjunct to the primary treatment of cervical cancer. Most reports present the response rate of recurrent cervical cancer to a specific chemotherapeutic agent or combination of agents. A complete response is defined as the total disappearance of tumor, whereas a partial response is defined as a reduction in measurable tumor dimensions of at least 50% for a period of one month or more.

The response of cervical cancer to single-agent chemotherapy, is shown in Table 4-7. Only 2% of patients obtained complete tumor remission, whereas about 20% experienced partial remission of their disease. Although the number of reported patients is small, cisplatin appears to be a relatively effective drug, in that over 40% of treated cases have achieved some form of remission.

Recently, several investigators have reported the efficacy of multiple-drug regimens in the therapy of metastatic cervical cancer (Table 4-8). Combinations of bleomycin and mitomycin C (Miyamoto et al 1978, Baker et al 1978) have been particularly useful, resulting in a significant incidence of total remission. It is important to emphasize that the reported response rates for chemotherapy have been achieved in patients with widely metastatic or recurrent disease often present in extrapelvic

Table 4-7
Responses of Cervical Cancer to Single-Agent Chemotherapy

Investigator	Drug	Complete Response (%)		Partial Response (%)	
Malkasian et al (1964)	fluorouracil	0/22	(0)	5/22	(23)
Moore et al (1968)	mercaptopurine	0/18	(0)	1/18	(5)
Smith (1969)	cyclophosphamide	0/91	(0)	18/91	(20)
Moore et al (1968)	chlorambucil	1/26	(4)	6/26	(23)
Thigpen et al (1979)	cisplatin	3/25	(12)	8/25	(32)
Stolinsky et al (1973)	hexamethylmelamine	0/21	(0)	8/21	(38)
Slavik (1975)	doxorubicin	0/20	(0)	3/20	(15)
Mathé (1970)	bleomycin	1/18	(5)	5/18	(28)
Totals		5/241	(2)	54/241	(22)

organs. There is a definite need for the design of prospective trials in which single or multiple agents are used in association either with surgery or radiation therapy in the primary therapy of certain types of cervical cancer. Two such high-risk groups are patients with small-cell carcinoma and those with advanced-stage disease who have histologically confirmed

Table 4-8
Response of Cervical Cancer to Multiple-Agent Chemotherapy

Investigator	Drug Combination	Complete Response (%)		Partial Response (%)	
Papavasilou (1969)	methotrexate and cyclophosphamide	3/23	(13)	7/23	(30)
Piel et al (1973)	methotrexate and bleomycin	3/8	(37)	2/8	(25)
Conroy et al (1976)	methotrexate and bleomycin	0/20	(0)	12/20	(60)
Barlow et al (1973)	doxorubicin and bleomycin	0/15	(0)	2/15	(13)
Day et al (1978)	doxorubicin-methyl CCNU	9/31	(29)	5/31	(16)
Miyamoto et al (1978)	bleomycin and mitomycin	12/15	(80)	2/15	(13)
Baker et al (1978)	bleomycin, mitomycin, and vincristine	8/50	(16)	22/50	(44)
Totals		35/162	(22)	52/162	(32)

metastases to the paraaortic lymph nodes. Several studies utilizing a combination of chemotherapy and immunotherapy in patients with cervical cancer are in progress, but to date the results of these investigations have not been reported.

SURVIVAL AND FOLLOW-UP

The overall five-year survival rate of patients with cervical cancer treated at various centers throughout the world has been presented in the annual reports on the results of treatment in carcimona of the uterus, vagina, and ovary. The survival statistics of the most recent Annual Report (1973) are illustrated in Table 4-9. Five-year survivals ranged from over 80% in patients with Stage I disease to less than 10% in patients with Stage IV cancer. It should be pointed out that significantly higher patient survival rates have been reported by individual institutions. In general, the best cure rates have been attained at centers with both excellent radical surgery and radiation therapy capabilities. Therapy is jointly decided upon after complete review of each case by gynecologic oncologists, radiation therapists, and pathologists.

Table 4-9
Five-Year Survival Rates Related to Stage,
in Treated Patients with Invasive Cervical Cancer

Stage	No. of Patients	5-Year Survival (%)
I	18,440	14,829 (80.4)
II	22,482	13,231 (58.9)
III	17,290	5668 (32.8)
IV	2934	208 (7.1)
Totals	61,146	33,936 (55.5)

Approximately one half of patients who develop recurrent cervical cancer do so within one year following therapy (van Nagell et al 1979). An additional 25% of recurrences are noted during the second year after treatment, and only 5% of patients develop recurrent disease more than five years after therapy. Therefore, patients should be seen at monthly intervals during the first year after therapy, every two months for the next year, and every six months thereafter. Careful pelvic examination and cervical cytologic sampling should be performed at the time of each visit. In addition, intravenous pyelography and chest x-ray should be performed once yearly for the first five years after treatment.

BIBLIOGRAPHY

Annual Report on the Results of Treatment in Carcinoma of the Uterus, Vagina, and Ovary. Stockholm, 1973, vol 16.

Aldridge CW, Mason JT: Ureteral obstruction in carcinoma of the cervix. *Am J Obstet Gynecol* 60:1272–1280, 1950.

Averette HE, LaPlatney DR, Little WA: Current role of radical hysterectomy as primary therapy for invasive carcinoma of the cervix. *Am J Obstet Gynecol* 105:79–89, 1969.

Averette HE, Dudan RC, Ford JH: Exploratory celiotomy for surgical staging of cervical cancer. *Am J Obstet Gynecol* 113:1090–1093, 1972.

Baker LH, Opipari MI, Wilson H, et al: Mitomycin C, vincristine, and bleomycin therapy for advanced cervical cancer. *Obstet Gynecol* 52:146–158, 1978.

Barber HRK, Roberts S, Brunschwig A: Prognostic significance of preoperative non-visualizing kidney in patients receiving pelvic exenteration. *Cancer* 16:1614–1615, 1963.

Barber HRK, Sommers SC, Rotterdam H, et al: Vascular invasion as a prognostic factor in Stage Ib cancer of the cervix. *Obstet Gynecol* 52:343–348, 1978.

Barlow J, Piver M, Chuang J, et al: Adriamycin and bleomycin alone and in combination in gynecologic cancers. *Cancer* 32:735–743, 1973.

Bloom HJ, Field SR: Impact of tumor grade and host resistance on survival of women with breast cancer. *Cancer* 28:1580–1589, 1971.

Bluemle LW: Hemolytic transfusion reactions causing acute renal failure: Serologic and clinical considerations. *Postgrad Med* 38:484–489, 1965.

Boronow RC, Rutledge F: Vesicovaginal fistula, radiation, and gynecologic cancer. *Am J Obstet Gynecol* 111:85–90, 1971.

Boronow RC: Stage I cervix cancer and pelvic node metastases. *Am J Obstet Gynecol* 127:135–137, 1977.

Bosch A, Marcial VA: Carcinoma of the uterine cervix associated with pregnancy. *Am J Roentgol Radium Ther Nucl Med* 96:92–99, 1966.

Bosch A, Frias Z, deValda G: Prognostic significance of ureteral obstruction in carcinoma of the cervix uteri. *Acta Radiol* 12:47–56, 1973.

Bricker EM: Bladder substitution after pelvic evisceration. *Surg Clin North Am* 31:1511–1521, 1950.

Broders AC: Carcinoma-grading and practical application. *Arch Path Lab Med* 2:376–381, 1926.

Brown RC, Buchsbaum HJ, Twefik HH, et al: The accuracy of lymphangiography in the diagnosis of para-aortic lymph node metastases from carcinoma of the cervix. *Obstet Gynecol* 54:571–575, 1979.

Brunschwig A, Pierce V: Necropsy findings in patients with carcinoma of the cervix: Implications for treatment. *Am J Obstet Gynecol* 56:1134–1137, 1948.

Brunschwig A, Daniel WW: The surgery of pelvic lymph node metastases from carcinoma of the cervix. *Am J Obstet Gynecol* 83:389–392, 1962.

Brunschwig A: Surgical treatment of carcinoma of the cervix, recurrent after irradiation or combination of irradiation and surgery. *Am J Roentgol Radium Ther Nucl Med* 99:365–370, 1967.

Buchler DA, Kline JC, Peckham BM, et al: Radiation reactions in cervical cancer therapy. *Am J Obstet Gynecol* 111:745–750, 1971.

Buchsbaum HJ: Para-aortic lymph node involvement in cervical carcinoma. *Am J Obstet Gynecol* 113:942–947, 1972.

Buchsbaum HJ: Extrapelvic lymph node metastases in cervical carcinoma. *Am J Obstet Gynecol* 133:814–821, 1979.

Burghardt E, Pickell H: Local spread and lymph node involvement in cervical cancer. *Obstet Gynecol* 52:138–145, 1978.

Burns BC, Everett HS, Brack CB: Value of urologic study in the management of carcinoma of the cervix. *Am J Obstet Gynecol* 80:997–1003, 1960.

Castro JR, Issa P, Fletcher GH: Carcinoma of the cervix treated by external irradiation alone. *Radiology* 95:163–166, 1970.

Chau PM, Fletcher GH, Rutledge RN, et al: Complications in high dose whole pelvis irradiation in female cancer. *Am J Roentgol Radium Ther Nucl Med* 87:22–40, 1962.

Christopherson WM, Lundin FE, Mendez WM, et al: Cervical cancer control: A study of morbidity and mortality trends over a twenty-one year period. *Cancer* 38:1357–1366, 1976.

Clark JG: A more radical method of performing hysterectomy for cancer of the uterus. *Johns Hopkins Bull* 53:120–128, 1895.

Conroy J, Lewis G, Brady L, et al: Low dose bleomycin and methotrexate in cervical cancer. *Cancer* 37:660–670, 1976.

Cramer DW: The role of cervical cytology in the declining morbidity and mortality of cervical cancer. *Cancer* 34:2018–2027, 1974.

Crawford EJ, Robinson LS, Vaught J: Carcinoma of the cervix: Results of treatment by radiation alone and by combined radiation and surgical therapy in 335 patients. *Am J Obstet Gynecol* 91:480–487, 1965.

Day T, Wharton J, Taylor J, et al: Chemotherapy for squamous carcinoma of the cervix: Doxorubicin-methyl CCNU. *Am J Obstet Gynecol* 132:545–548, 1978.

Dudan RC, Yon J, Ford J, et al: Carcinoma of the cervix and pregnancy. *Gynecol Oncol* 1:283–289, 1973.

Durrance FY, Fletcher GH, Rutledge FN: Analysis of central recurrent disease in Stages I and II squamous cell carcinomas of the cervix on intact uterus. *Am J Roentgol Radium Ther Nucl Med* 126:831–838, 1969.

Easley JD, Fletcher HG: Analysis of the treatment of Stage I and Stage II carcinomas of the uterine cervix. *Am J Roentgol Radium Ther Nucl Med* 111:243–238, 1971.

Edwards LC, Dunphy JE: Wound healing: Injury and repair. *N Engl J Med* 259:275–285, 1958.

Fletcher GH, Rutledge FN, Chau PM: Policies of treatment in cancer of cervix uteri. *Am J Roentgol Rad Ther Nucl Med* 87:6–21, 1962.

Fletcher GH: Cancer of the uterine cervix. Janeway lecture, 1970. *Am J Roentgol Ther Radium Nucl Med* 111:225–242, 1971.

Fuchs WA, Rosenberg GS: Lymphography in carcinoma of the uterine cervix. *Acta Radiol* 16:353–361, 1975.

Gellman D: Cervical cancer screening programs. I. Epidemiology and natural history of carcinoma of the cervix. *Can Med Assoc J* 114:1003–1012, 1976.

Gray MJ, Gusberg SB, Guttmann R: Pelvic lymph node dissection following radiotherapy. *Am J Obstet Gynecol* 76:629–633, 1958.

Green TH, Meigs JV, Ulfelder H, et al: Urologic complications of radical Wertheim hysterectomy: Incidence, etiology, management and prevention. *Obstet Gynecol* 20:293–312, 1962.

Green TH: Ureteral suspension for prevention of ureteral complications following radical Wertheim hysterectomy. *Obstet Gynecol* 28:1–11, 1966.

Halpin TF, Frick HC, Munnell EG: Critical points of failure in the therapy of cancer of the cervix: A reappraisal. *Am J Obstet Gynecol* 114:755–764, 1972.

Henriksen E: The lymphatic spread of carcinoma of the cervix and of the body of the uterus: A study of 420 necropsies. *Am J Obstet Gynecol* 58:924–942, 1949.

Holm HH, Pedersen JF, Kristersen JK, et al: Ultrasonically guided percutaneous puncture. *Rad Clin North Am* 13:493–503, 1975.

Hoskins WJ, Averette HE, Ng ABP, et al: Adenoid cystic carcinoma of the cervix uteri: Report of six cases and review of the literature. *Gynecol Oncol* 7:371–384, 1979.

Hrenshchyshyn MM, Sheehan FR: Lymphangiography in advanced gynecologic cancer. *Obstet Gynecol* 24:525–529, 1964.

Jampolis S, Andras EJ, Fletcher GH: Analysis of sites and causes of failures of irradiaiton in invasive squamous cell carcinoma of the intact uterine cervix. *Radiology* 115:681–685, 1975.

Kessler I: Human cervical cancer as a venereal disease. *Cancer Res* 36:783–791, 1976.

Khoo SK, Mackey EV: Carcinoembryonic antigen in cancer of the female reproductive system: Sequential levels and effects of treatment. *Aust NZ J Obstet Gynecol* 13:1–7, 1973.

Kolbenstvedt A, Kolstad P: Pelvic lymph node dissection under preoperative lymphographic control. *Gynecol Oncol* 2:39–59, 1974.

Kottmeier HL: Ten year end results, radiological treatment of carcinoma of the cervix. *Acta Obstet Gynecol* 111:195–203, 1962.

Kottmeier HL: Complications following radiation therapy in carcinoma of the cervix and their treatment *Am J Obstet Gynecol* 88:854–866, 1964.

Kottmeier HL: Surgical and radiation treatment of carcinoma of the uterine cervix. *Acta Obstet Gynecol Scand* (suppl) 43, 1964.

LaGasse LD, Ballon SC, Berman ML, et al: Pretreatment lymphangiography and operative evaluation in carcinoma of the cervix. *Am J Obstet Gynecol* 134:219–224, 1979.

Lepanto P, Littman P, Mikuta J: Treatment of para-aortic nodes in carcinoma of the cervix. *Cancer* 35:1510–1513, 1975.

Liu W, Meigs JW: Radical hysterectomy and pelvic lymphadenectomy: A review of 473 cases including 244 for primary invasive carcinoma of the cervix. *Am J Obstet Gynecol* 69:1–32, 1955.

Malkasian GD, Decker D, Mussey E, et al: Preliminary observations of carcinoma of the cervix treated with 5-fluorouracil. *Am J Obstet Gynecol* 88:82–85, 1964.

Marcial VA, Bosch A: Radiation-induced tumor regression in carcinoma of the uterine cervix: Prognostic significance. *Cancer* 108:113–123, 1970.

Martzloff KH: Carcinoma of the cervix uteri: A pathologic and clinical study with particular reference to the relative malignancy of the neoplastic process as indicated by the predominant cell type of cancer cell. *Johns Hopkins Bull* 34:141–155, 1923.

Masubuchi K, Tenjin Y, Kubo H: Five year cure rate for carcinoma of the cervix uteri. *Am J Obstet Gynecol* 103:567–574, 1969.

Mathe G: Study of the clinical efficacy of bleomycin in human cancer. *Br Med J* 2:643, 1970.

Mikuta J: Invasive carcinoma of the cervix in pregnancy. *South Med J* 60:843–847, 1967.

Miyamoto T, Takabe Y, Watanabe M, et al: Effectiveness of a sequential combination of bleomycin and mitomycin C on the advanced cervical cancer. *Cancer* 41:403–414, 1978.

Moore G, Bross I, Ausman R: Effects of 6-mercaptopurine (NSC-755) in 290 patients with cancer. *Cancer Chemother Rep* 52:655–660, 1968.

Moore G, Bross I, Ausman R: Effects of chlorambucil (NSC-3088) in 374 patients with advanced cancer. *Cancer Chemother Rep* 52:661–666, 1968.

Nelson AJ, Fletcher GH, Wharton JT: Indications for adjunctive conservative extrafascial hysterectomy in selected cases of carcinoma of the uterine cervix. *Am J Roent* 123:91–99, 1975.

Ng ABP, Reagan JW: Microinvasive carcinoma of the uterine cervix. *Am J Clin Path* 52:511–529, 1969.

Papavasilou C, Angelaskis P, Gouvalis P, et al: Treatment of cervical carcinoma by methotrexate (NSC-740) combined with cylophosphamide. *Cancer Chemother Rep* 52:225–261, 1969.

Parente JT, Silberblatt W, Stone M: Infrequency of metastasis to ovaries in Stage I carcinoma of the cervix. *Am J Obstet Gynecol* 90:1362, 1964.

Park RC, Patow WE, Rogers RE, et al: Treatment of Stage I carcinoma of the cervix. *Obstet Gynecol* 41:117–122, 1973.

Parker RT, Wilbanks GD, Yowell RK, et al: Radical hysterectomy and pelvic lymphadenectomy with and without preoperative radiotherapy for cervical cancer. *Am J Obstet Gynecol* 99:933–943, 1967.

Paunier JP, Delclos L, Fletcher GH: Causes, time of death, sites of failure in squamous-cell carcinoma of the uterine cervix on intact uterus. *Radiology* 88:555–562, 1967.

Perez CA, Zivnuska F, Askin J: Prognostic significance of endometrial extension from primary carcinoma of the uterine cervix. *Cancer* 35:1493–1504, 1975.

Perez CA, Breaux S, Askins F, et al: Irradiation alone or in combination with surgery in Stage Ib and IIa carcinoma of the uterine cervix: A nonrandomized comparison. *Cancer* 43:1062–1072, 1979.

Piel I, Slayton R, Perlia CP, et al: Combination chemotherapy with bleomycin and methotrexate in recurrent and disseminated cervical carcinoma: A preliminary study. *Gynecol Oncol* 1:184–190, 1973.

Pineda A, Brzica S, Tasvell H: Hemolytic transfusion reactions. *Mayo Clin Proc* 53:738–790, 1978.

Piver MS, Barlow JJ: Para-aortic lymphadenectomy, aortic node biopsy, and aortic lymphangiography in staging patients with advanced cervical cancer. *Cancer* 32:367–370, 1973.

Piver MS, Chung WS: Prognostic significance of cervical lesion size and pelvic node metastases in cervical carcinoma. *Obstet Gynecol* 46:507–512, 1975.

Plentyl AA, Friedman E: *Lymphatic System of the Female Genitalia. The Morphologic Basis of Oncologic Diagnosis and Therapy. Vol. 2.* Philadelphia, W.B. Saunders Co, 1971.

Primus FJ, Wang RH, Sharkey RM, et al: Detection of carcinoembryonic antigen in tissue sections by immunoperoxidase. *J Immunol Methods* 8:267–276, 1975.

Rampone JF, Klem V, Kolstad P: Combined treatment of Stage Ib carcinoma of the cervix. *Obstet Gynecol* 41:163–167, 1973.

Reagan JW, Hamonic MJ, Wentz WB: Analytical study of cells in cervical squamous cell cancer. *Lab Invest* 6:241–250, 1957.

Rochat R: The prevalence of cervical cancer screening in the United States in 1970. *Am J Obstet Gynecol* 125:478–483, 1976.

Roddick JW, Greenlaw RH: Treatment of cervical cancer. *Am J Obstet Gynecol* 109:754–764, 1971.

Roddick JW, van Nagell JR, Bell RM: Protein and electrolyte content of retroperitoneal junction. Drainage after radical hysterectomy with pelvic lymphadenectomy. *Gynecol Oncol* 1:149–153, 1973.

Rutledge FN, Fletcher GH, MacDonald EF: Pelvic lymphadenectomy as an adjunct to radiation therapy in treatment for cancer of the cervix. *Am J Roentgol Radium Ther Nucl Med* 95:607–614, 1965.

Rutledge FN, Wharton JT, Fletcher GH: Clinical studies with adjunctive surgery and irradiation therapy in treatment of carcinoma of the cervix. *Cancer* 38:596–602, 1976.

Sall S, Pineda AA, Calanog A, et al: Surgical treatment of Stages Ib and IIa invasive carcinoma of the cervix by radical abdominal hysterectomy. *Am J Obstet Gynecol* 135:442–446, 1979.

Schellhas H: Extraperitoneal para-aortic node dissection through an upper abdominal incision. *Obstet Gynecol* 46:444–447, 1975.

Seski JC, Diokno AC, Anderson DG: Bladder dysfunction after radical hysterectomy. *Am J Obstet Gynecol* 128:643–651, 1977.

Silverberg E: Cancer statistics, 1979. *Cancer* 30:23–38, 1980.

Slavik M: Adriamycin (NSC-123127) activity in genitourinary and gynecologic malignancies. *Cancer Chemother Rep* 6:297–303, 1975.

Smith JP, Rutledge F, Burns B, et al: Systemic chemotherapy for carcinoma of the cervix. *Am J Obstet Gynecol* 97:800–807, 1967.

Stolinsky D, Bateman J: Further experience with hexamethylmelamine (NSC-13875) in the treatment of carcinoma of the cervix. *Cancer Chemother Rep* 57:497–499, 1973.

Strockbine MJ, Hancock JE, Fletcher GH: Complications in 831 patients with squamous cell carcinoma of the intact uterine cervix treated with 3,000 rads or more whole pelvis irradiation. *Am J Roentgol Radium Ther Nucl Med* 108:293–304, 1970.

Swan DS, Roddick JW: A clinical-pathological correlation of cell type classification of cervical cancer. *Am J Obstet Gynecol* 116:666–670, 1973.

Symmonds RE, Pratt JH: Prevention of fistulas and lymphocysts in radical hysterectomy. *Obstet Gynecol* 17:57–63, 1961.

Thigpen T, Shingleton H, Homesley H, et al: cis-Dichlorodiammineplatinum (II) in the treatment of gynecologic malignancies: Phase II trials by the gynecologic oncology group. *Cancer Treat Rep* 63:1549–1555, 1979.

Ulfelder H, Smith CJ, Costello JB: Invasive carcinoma of the cervix during pregnancy. *Am J Obstet Gynecol* 98:424–428, 1967.

van Nagell JR, Roddick JW, Lowin DM: The staging of cervical cancer: Inevitable discrepancies between clinical staging and pathologic findings. *Am J Obstet Gynecol* 110:973–978, 1971.

van Nagell JR, Parker JC, Maruyama Y: Bladder or rectal injury following radiation therapy for cervical cancer. *Am J Obstet Gynecol* 119:727–732, 1974.

van Nagell JR, Sprague AD, Roddick JR: The effect of intravenous pyelography and cystoscopy on the staging of cervical cancer. *Gynecol Oncol* 3:87–93, 1975.

van Nagell JR, Donaldson ES, Parker JC, et al: The prognostic significance of cell type and lesion size in patients with cervical cancer treated by radical surgery. *Gynecol Oncol* 5:142–151, 1977.

van Nagell JR, Donaldson ES, Gay EC: Evaluation and treatment of patients with invasive cervical cancer. *Surg Clin North Am* 58:67–85, 1978.

van Nagell JR, Donaldson ES, Gay EC, et al: Carcinoembryonic antigen in carcinoma of the uterine cervix: I. The prognostic value of serial plasma determinations. *Cancer* 42:2428–2434, 1978.

van Nagell JR, Donaldson ES, Wood EG, et al: The significance of vascular invasion and lymphocytic infiltration in invasive cervical cancer. *Cancer* 41:228–234, 1978.

van Nagell JR, Donaldson ES, Gay EC, et al: Carcinoembryonic antigen in carcinoma of the uterine cervix. II. Tissue localization and correlation with plasma antigen concentration. *Cancer* 44:944–948, 1979.

van Nagell JR, Rayburn W, Donaldson ES, et al: Therapeutic implications of patterns of recurrence in cancer of the uterine cervix. *Cancer* 44:2354–2361, 1979.

Wallace S, Jing BS, Zornoza J: Lymphangiography in the determination of the extent of metastatic carcinoma: The potential value of percutaneous lymph node biopsy. *Cancer* 39:706–718, 1977.

Webb MJ, Symmonds, RE: Wertheim hysterectomy: A reappraisal. *Obstet Gynecol* 54:140–145, 1979.

Wentz WB, Lewis GC: Correlation of histologic morphology and survival in cervical cancer following radiation therapy. *Obstet Gynecol* 26:228–232, 1965.

Wentz WB, Jaffe RM: Squamous cell carcinoma of the cervix with higher uterine involvement. *Obstet Gynecol* 28:271–272, 1966.

Wharton JT, Jones HW, Day TG, et al: Pre-irradiation celiotomy and extended field irradiation for invasive carcinoma of the cervix. *Obstet Gynecol* 49:333–338, 1977.

Wheeless CR: Small bowel bypass for complications related to pelvic malignancy. *Obstet Gynecol* 92:661–666, 1973.

Yagi H: Extended abdominal hysterectomy with pelvic lymphadenectomy for carcinoma of the cervix. *Am J Obstet Gynecol* 69:33–47, 1955.

Zornoza J, Wallace S, Goldstein JM, et al: Transperitoneal percutaneous retroperitoneal lymph node aspiration biopsy. *Radiology* 122:111–115, 1977.

Zornoza J, Lukeman JM, Jing BS, et al: Percutaneous retroperitoneal lymph node biopsy in carcinoma of the cervix. *Gynecol Oncol* 5:43–51, 1977.

5 Radiation Therapy in the Treatment of Cervical Cancer

Yosh Maruyama
John R. van Nagell, Jr.

The majority of patients with cervical cancer are treated by radiation therapy, either alone or in combination with surgery. During the past two decades, advances in radiation sources and methods have allowed maximal doses to be delivered to the cervical tumor and its regional pelvic lymph nodes while minimizing doses to adjacent normal structures. As a result, significant improvements have been achieved in the cure rate of cervical cancer, and the incidence of radiation-related complications has been reduced. In analyzing treatment results, it is evident that the diagnosis of cervical cancer in an early stage is extremely important. Radiation therapy, like other methods, is most effective in the treatment of early stage lesions, whereas the frequency of both local and extrapelvic recurrence is highest in bulky, advanced stage lesions. In many patients, optimal therapy involves a combination of radiation therapy and surgery. Therefore, the highest cure rates for patients with cervical cancer are generally achieved in centers in which there is a coordinated effort by gynecologic oncologists and radiation oncologists to individualize therapy to the needs of each patient. Such a coordinated program includes uniform evaluation and staging, mutual decisions as to appropriate therapy, and coordinated follow-up.

This chapter will present 1) a brief history of radiation therapy in the treatment of cervical cancer, 2) specific parameters essential in evaluation of patients undergoing radiation therapy, 3) principles of radiation treatment planning in cervical cancer, 4) treatment of early and advanced stage cervical cancer, 5) complications of treatment, and 6) survival of cervical cancer patients treated with radiation.

HISTORY OF RADIATION THERAPY
IN THE TREATMENT OF CERVICAL CANCER

Roentgen rays were discovered in 1895 and radium was isolated three years later by Marie and Pierre Curie. Becquerel described the biological effects of radiation in man, and in 1903, radium was used in the treatment of cervical cancer (Cleaves). In 1913, Abbe reported the cure of cervical cancer by radium application. Domenici developed a system of filtering therapeutic radiation through a series of platinum layers that effectively removed all beta particles. Cervical tumors could then be treated by pure gamma irradiation. Regaud (1927) was the first to develop time-dose relationships for radium which were used to calculate tumoricidal doses to the cervix without producing necrosis of normal pelvic tissues. Therapists at the Curie Foundation in Paris advocated the delivery of low intensity irradiation to the cervix over one week. This work was extended by Patterson and colleagues at Manchester (1948), who studied the effects of combined external therapy and intracavitary radium in the treatment of cervical cancer. These investigators advocated the delivery of low intensity radium to the cervix over a prolonged time period, and utilized point A (2 cm lateral and 2 cm superior to the external cervical os) as a reference point to measure paracervical radiation. In contrast, therapists at Stockholm (Radiumhemmet) utilized short application of more heavily loaded radium applicators delivering high intensity irradiation to the pelvis two or three times in three weeks. The M.D. Anderson Hospital System developed by Fletcher (1969, 1973) was based on advanced treatment planning methods integrating external megavoltage therapy with intracavitary radium implants. Various therapeutic combinations were utilized, and specific treatment plans were developed according to the individual needs of each patient. Conclusions of clinical studies performed at these institutions have served as the basis of subsequent therapeutic systems in many radiation oncology centers throughout the world. These include:

1) In patients with Stage I cervical cancer, radium therapy alone is as effective as radium and x-ray therapy (76.1% *vs* 73.9% five-year survival)-Paterson and Russell, 1963.

2) In patients with Stage II cervical cancer, the combination of radium and x-ray therapy produces a higher cure rate than radium therapy alone (58.7% *vs* 53.3% five-year survival)-Paterson and Russell, 1963.

3) In patients with Stage III cervical cancer, radium therapy given after x-ray treatment produces a higher survival than radium therapy given before x-ray treatment (48.1% *vs* 33.3% five-year survival)-Schwarz, 1969.

4) In patients with Stages I and II disease, supplemental sidewall radiation with a radiation beam having a broad and flat parametrial isodose produces a higher five-year survival than when supplemental sidewall radiation is given from narrow radiation beam (Stage I 79.6% *vs* 76.1%, Stage II 61.5% *vs* 53.3%)-Cole, 1973.

5) In patients with Stages I and II cervical cancer, flattening the pelvic x-ray isodose curves to 8 cm lateral to the midline produces a similar survival rate regardless of the x-ray modality or the beam energy used (Cole 1973).

6) In patients with advanced stage cervical cancer, high dose (5000 to 6000 rad) external therapy to the pelvis using megavoltage beams significantly improves five-year survival (Castro 1970, and Fletcher 1971).

7) In all stages of cervical cancer, implant therapy following external beam radiation produces a higher five-year survival than external beam therapy alone (Schwarz 1969).

The discovery of induced radioactivity by Frederic and Irene Joliot-Curie in 1934 served as the basis for the later development of high activity cobalt-60, which opened prospects for fractionated teletherapy of deep-seated tumors. Based on these principles, other sources such as cesium-137 and californium-252 were successfully adopted for use in intracavitary therapy.

The development of high energy accelerators, and their application to cervical cancer therapy was also a major therapeutic advance. The first betatron was constructed by Kerst in 1943 and since that time many of these machines have been constructed. Linear accelerators were first used in England in the radiation therapy of pelvic tumors (Miller 1962). These high intensity sources made it possible to deliver tumoricidal doses of radiation to virtually any site in the pelvis.

Finally, the development of afterloading systems (Suit et al 1963, Joelsson and Backstrom 1970) have minimized radiation exposure of personnel involved in implant therapy. Afterloading is the insertion of radioactive sources into applicators that are prepositioned in the tumor-bearing region. This technique has allowed precise positioning of sources within the patient, and has improved dosimetry while protecting the therapist from excessive radiation exposure (Wilson and Maruyama 1974).

EVALUATION OF PATIENTS WITH CERVICAL CANCER UNDERGOING RADIATION THERAPY

A detailed evaluation system for patients with cervical cancer has been presented in Chapter 4. However, certain aspects of evaluation in patients undergoing radiation therapy deserve emphasizing. Every lesion should be staged according to the International Federation of Gynecology and Obstetrics (FIGO) Staging System (Table 5-1). The uniform acceptance of this system is not only important in determining the most appropriate therapy for each patient, but is also necessary for proper evaluation of cases treated at different institutions. In addition to stage, the size and anatomic configuration of each tumor should be evaluated. Cervical cancers can generally be described as exophytic, infiltrative, or ulcerative, and each of these anatomic patterns has specific therapeutic requirements.

Table 5-1
International Federation of Gynecology and Obstetrics Staging System for Invasive Cervical Cancer

Stage I	Carcinoma strictly confined to the cervix (extension to the corpus should be disregarded).
Stage Ia	Microinvasive carcinoma (early stromal invasion).
Stage Ib	All other cases of Stage I. Occult cancer should be marked "occ."
Stage II	The carcinoma extends beyond the cervix, but not the lower third.
Stage IIa	No obvious parametrial involvement.
Stage IIb	Obvious parametrial involvement.
Stage III	The carcinoma has extended on to the pelvic wall. On rectal examination there is no cancer-free space between the tumor and the pelvic wall.
Stage IIIa	No extension onto the pelvic wall.
Stage IIIb	Extension onto the pelvic wall and/or hydronephrosis or nonfunctioning kidney.
Stage IV	The carcinoma has extended beyond the true pelvis or has clinically involved the mucosa of the bladder or rectum. A bullous edema as such does not permit a case to be allotted to Stage IV.
Stage IVa	Spread of the growth to adjacent organs.
Stage IVb	Spread to distant organs.

The cell type of each cervical tumor should be recorded prior to therapy. Although there have been numerous systems for the histologic classification of cervical cancer, the one proposed by Reagan and colleagues (1957) is the most prognostically significant. According to this system, cervical cancers are divided into large cell nonkeratinizing carcinoma, keratinizing squamous cell carcinoma, small cell carcinoma, and adenocarcinoma. There is increasing evidence to suggest that keratinizing squamous cell carcinoma is more resistant to radiation therapy than large cell nonkeratinizing carcinoma (Wentz 1961, van Nagell et al 1979). Similarly, small cell carcinomas are associated with a higher incidence of metastases and a poorer survival than the other cell types of squamous cell carcinoma (Wentz and Lewis 1965, van Nagell 1977).

An accurate description of lesion size is also extremely important. In patients with Stage Ib cervical cancer and a lesion diameter of more than 3 cm there is recent evidence to suggest that radiation therapy may be the therapeutic method of choice (Piver and Chung 1975, van Nagell et al 1979). Likewise, Stage Ib lesions in excess of 5 cm diameter often contain a relatively radioresistant core requiring surgical removal following radiation therapy. Finally, the response of each lesion during radiation therapy is directly related to recurrence rate (Marcial and Bosch 1970), and tumor regression is best estimated by serial measurements of the cervical lesion throughout treatment.

The importance of a thorough evaluation of the pelvic and para-aortic lymph nodes in patients undergoing radiation therapy for cervical cancer cannot be overemphasized. The incidence of extrapelvic lymph nodal metastases may be as high as 30% in patients with bulky, advanced stage disease, and these metastases would not be included in the traditional fields of radiation therapy. Patients with bulky Stage Ib and IIb tumors as well as all patients with more advanced stage disease should have lymphangiography and CT scans to identify lymph nodal metastases. Patients with suspicious or positive findings on these noninvasive methods should have further evaluation, including fine needle biopsy (Zornoza et al 1977) or retroperitoneal lymph node sampling (Lagasse 1979) to histologically confirm these findings.

In addition to those studies required in the evaluation of tumor biology, there are a number of variables related directly to radiation complications which must be studied. All patients should be questioned concerning a history of pelvic inflammatory disease. Pelvic inflammatory disease has been shown to produce reactive vasculitis and fibrin thrombosis in the small vessels of the bowel and bladder (van Nagell et al 1977). Radiation-induced vascular endothelial proliferation often causes localized hypoperfusion and hypoxia in these organs, and the combination of radiation therapy and pelvic inflammation has been associated with a high incidence of enteric complications. Likewise, prior abdominal surgery is often associated with intraperitoneal adhesions and fixation of the bowel within the pelvis. Consequently, radiation therapy following surgery is associated with an increased incidence of bowel or urinary tract injury, and a history of prior pelvic surgical procedures should be noted.

The nutritional status of the patient is also related to the subsequent incidence of radiation-induced complications. Cervical cancer patients who are underweight according to standard height and weight charts have been reported to have a higher incidence of enteric injury following radiation therapy (van Nagell et al 1974). Similarly, Copeland (1977) has shown that patients suffering from malnutrition often have delayed wound healing and increased morbidity following cancer therapy. For this reason, any evidence of recent weight loss or malnutrition should be carefully documented in patients undergoing radiation therapy. Finally, radiation-related enteric complications have been shown to occur with increased frequency in patients with underlying vascular disease, such as diabetes mellitus or hypertension (van Nagell et al 1974, Maruyama et al 1974). Patients with a history of vascular disease should be thoroughly evaluated in an effort to quantitate the severity of small vessel disease. Van Nagell and co-workers (1979) reported a direct correlation between the status of the retinal and pelvic arterioles. Consequently, fundoscopic examination with retinal photography is indicated in patients with severe hypertension or diabetes mellitus as a means to objectively define the extent of vascular disease.

RADIATION BIOLOGY RELATED
TO CERVICAL CANCER THERAPY

A complete discussion of the principles of radiation biology is presented in Chapter 19. However, those definitions and concepts which are relevant to the therapy of cervical cancer will be emphasized herein. Before discussing these concepts, it is pertinent to review the definitions of a number of terms which are commonly used in radiation biology.

Definition of Terms

Brachytherapy	— Refers to all techniques using radioactive sources at less than a 5 cm distance from the tumor.
Endocurie therapy	— Refers to all techniques using radioactive sources embedded in the tumor.
Teletherapy	— Refers to all techniques using radioactive sources at a distance of more than 5 cm from

the tumor irrespective of the energy of characteristics of the radiation.

Atomic Number	— The number of protons in the nucleus as well as the number of electrons outside the nucleus.
Atomic Weight	— The sum of the neutrons and protons in the nucleus.
Ionization	— Removal of an electron from an atom.
Ionizing Radiation	— Radiation which produces ionization.
Gamma Rays	— Electromagnetic radiation emitted from an excited nucleus. Gamma rays and x-rays are both photons. However, x-rays originate outside the nucleus.
Linear Energy Transfer (LET)	— The energy lost by a particle per micron of path length expressed in keV/μ.
Half Life	— The time necessary for one half of the atoms from a radioactive source to disintegrate.
Electron Volt (eV)	— The amount of energy released when an electron falls through a potential difference of one volt.
keV	— 1000 eV
meV	— 1,000,000 eV
Dose	— The amount of energy absorbed per gram of tissue.
Dosimetry	— Measurement and calculation of the dose received by the patient.
Isodose Curves	— Lines of equal absorbed dose within a patient.
Source-Skin Distance (SSD)	— The distance along the central ray between the source of radiation and the patient's skin.
Field Size	— The size of the field of irradiation measured at the stated source—skin distance.
Inverse Square Law	— The intensity of radiation from a point source is inversely related to the square of the distance from that source.

Half Value Layer (HVL)	— Thickness of a specified material required to attenuate a radiation beam to one half its original intensity.
Oxygen Enhancement Ratio (OER)	— The ratio of maximum sensitivity in oxygen to sensitivity in the absence of oxygen.
Rad	— A unit of absorption. 1 rad = 100 ergs/cm.
RBE	— Relative biological effectiveness compared to orthovoltage.
Roentgen	— A unit of exposure. 1 roentgen = 2.58 × 10^{-4} coul/kg air.

Elemental particles used in the therapy of cervical carcinomas are illustrated in Table 5-2. The majority of patients with cervical cancer are treated with gamma irradiation, although neutrons are being used with increasing frequency in advanced stage disease (Hussey et al 1977). Radionuclides commonly utilized in radiation therapy are presented in Table 5-3. At present, cesium-137, cobalt-60, and californium-252 are the most

Table 5-2
Nuclear Elemental Particles and Radiation Used in Radiotherapy of Cervical Cancer

Particle	Mass	Charge	Properties
Electron (e)	0.000548	−1	Every atom contains electrons outside the nucleus. The electron is also called a beta particle.
Neutron (n)	1.008986	0	The neutron is an uncharged particle that has nearly the same mass as a proton.
Proton (p)	1.007597	+1	The proton is the nucleus of the hydrogen atom. It is positively charged.
Pi Mesons (π)	$273m_0$	−1	Pi mesons may have a positive or negative charge, but those used in pelvic radiation therapy are negatively charged. They are produced by the bombardment of matter with high energy protons or photons.
Gamma Ray (γ)	0	0	The gamma ray is a photon emitted from an excited nucleus. It travels at the speed of light.

frequently used sources in intracavitary implants. Radium-226 has largely been replaced by sources with shorter half-lives. Californium-252 is a source of both gamma irradiation and fast neutrons (Krishnaswamy 1971, Anderson 1973). Iridium-192 and tantalum-182 wires are most often used as interstitial sources which are implanted directly into the tumor. Radiation therapy produced from machines, which is used in the treatment of cervical cancer, can be divided into orthovoltage radiation (150 to 500 keV) and megavoltage radiation ($\geqslant$ 1 mcV). Orthovoltage x-rays are produced in an x-ray tube that consists of 1) a hooded copper anode into which a tungsten target has been placed, and 2) a cathode assembly consisting of a filament inside a glass envelope (Figure 5-1).

A high voltage transformer accelerates electrons from the cathode to the anode, and these high velocity electrons are directed into the target. X-rays are produced by the deceleration of these electrons passing into the surface layers of the target, and are directed through a port. The maximal radiation dose from orthovoltage therapy is concentrated in the skin surface. Therefore, orthovoltage radiation given through a vaginal cone can

Table 5-3
Radionuclides Used in Radiation Therapy of Cervix Carcinomas

Isotope	Beta Energy	Important Gamma Energy	Half-Life
Sealed			
Radium-226	Filtered	Many 0.05–2.43 meV (0.8 meV av)	1620 years
Radon-222	Filtered	0.3–0.85 (0.8 meV av)	3.83 days
Cesium-137	Filtered	0.66 meV	30 years
Cobalt-60	Filtered	1.17, 1.33 meV	5.3 years
Californium-252	Filtered	Many γ-rays 0.5–1 meV; fast neutron emitter	2.65 years
Unsealed			
Gold-198 (liquid or seed)	0.28–1.37 meV	0.41, 0.67 meV	2.69 days
Iridium-192 (wire)	0.06	0.32–0.48 meV	74 days
Phosphorus-32 (liquid)	1.71 meV		14.3 days
Tantalum-182 (wire)	0.36 – 0.51 meV	0.05–1.24 meV (1.18 meV av)	115 days
Iodine-125 (seed)		0.035 meV	60 days

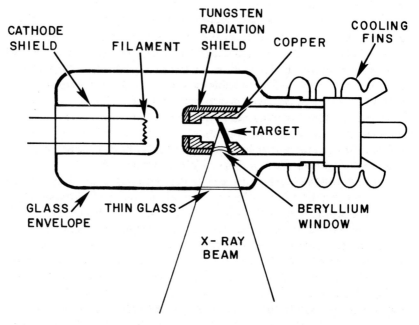

A

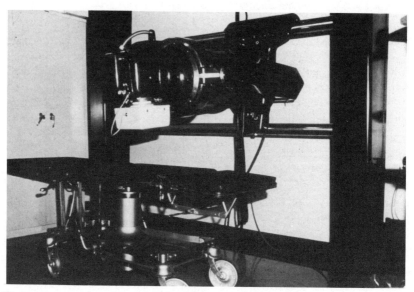

B

Figure 5-1 **(A)** Schematic representation of x-ray tube producing orthovoltage x-rays. **(B)** Photograph of orthovoltage machine (use now limited in cervical cancer therapy).

be used in the treatment of superficial cervical cancers as a method to stop surface hemorrhage. In addition, orthovoltage therapy can be used in the intraoperative treatment of lymph nodal metastases from cervical cancer.

Teletherapy machines using cobalt-60 as the source of gamma rays have been the mainstay of cervical cancer therapy for the past two decades. These machines consist of a lead-filled steel container at the center of which is placed a cobalt-60 source, as well as a wheel-type device for bringing this source into a position opposite an opening in the head so that an effective beam of radiation may emerge (Figure 5-2). The beam is controlled by a multiplane collimator which is made of a series of moving lead diaphragms. These lead bars define the field size and sharpen the beam. The cobalt-60 source is usually replaced every five years to maintain adequate gamma ray intensity. Most of the units constructed recently are designed for rotation about a central axis, and the source and collimator are balanced by a radiation shield and counterweight.

The betatron is a device for accelerating electrons that are bent into a circular path by an alternating current magnetic field. Electrons achieve extremely high velocities and are then directed into a target to produce x-rays. The efficiency of x-ray production is high and a water-cooling mechanism is required. High energy x-ray irradiation can be generated using this device with the optimum energy for therapy being 20 to 50 meV. Betatrons are particularly useful in the treatment of advanced stage cervical cancers.

Linear accelerators (Linacs) are machines that use radio frequency waves as a means to accelerate particles into a target. A power supply produces these waves which increase in velocity as they pass down the tube (Figure 5-3). Electrons are injected at the top of the tube and are carried forward with increasing speed on the crest of each wave. The electrons are then directed into a target with the subsequent production of x-rays. Both the electrons and x-rays produced in the linear accelerator can be used for therapeutic purposes. The majority of Linacs provide x-ray beam energies of 4 to 25 meV. The fact that more than 70% of the maximum dose can be delivered at a depth of 8 cm allows these machines to be used for many of the treatment techniques presently employed in cobalt-60 teletherapy units. Linacs also have large field size capabilities, a low penumbra, and facilities for precise beam positioning (Dobson et al 1977). Recently, high-energy (700 meV) linear accelerators have been used to accelerate protons into a carbon target producing negatively charged pi mesons (Feola and Maruyama 1971). These pions interact extensively with carbon, nitrogen, and oxygen molecules in the cell, and are presently being studied in the therapy of cervical cancer.

The central axis depth-dose distribution of cobalt-60, gamma rays, and megavoltage x-rays within the patient are illustrated in Figure 5-4. Treatment to greater depths and with a greater depth of maximum dose

Co-60 SOURCE CARRIED IN HEAVY METAL SLIDER

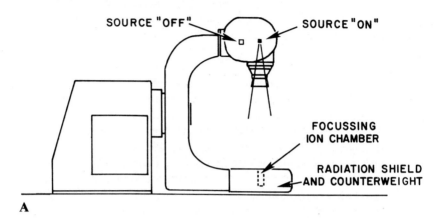

A

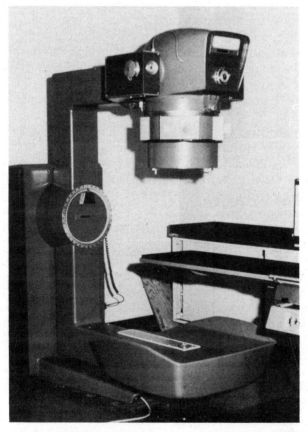

B

Figure 5-2 **(A)** Schematic representation of cobalt-60 machine. **(B)** Photograph of cobalt-60 machine currently used in treatment of cervical cancer.

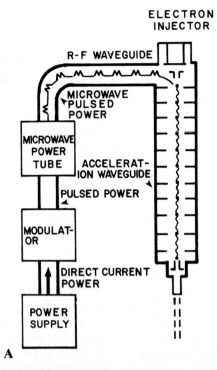

ELECTRON
INJECTOR

R-F WAVEGUIDE

MICROWAVE
PULSED
POWER

MICROWAVE
POWER
TUBE

ACCELERAT-
ION WAVEGUIDE

PULSED POWER

MODULAT-
OR

DIRECT CURRENT
POWER

POWER
SUPPLY

A

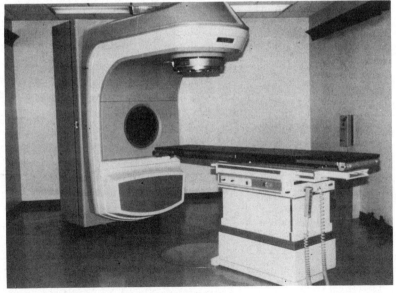

B

Figure 5-3 **(A)** Schematic representation of electron acceleration by linear accelerator. **(B)** Photograph of linear accelerator currently used in cervical cancer
therapy.

buildup is possible with the use of higher beam energies. The sophisticated megavoltage therapy units now available allow precise positioning of the beam and patient, enable beam size to be limited to tumor site, and facilitate accurate measurement of the dose delivered.

The radiation exposure of personnel operating megavoltage machines or performing intracavitary implants is a subject of continuing concern. For this reason, the National Council on Radiation Protection has established standards for the maximum permissible dose equivalent allowed for occupational exposure. The concept of dose equivalent (DE) was adopted, since a dose of one type of radiation may produce a much larger biological effect than the same dose of a different type of radiation. The unit of dose equivalent is the *rem*. Dose equivalent can be calculated using the following formula:

$$DE \text{ (rem)} = D \text{ (rad)} \times QF \times (DF_1) \times (DF_2)$$

where QF is a quality factor and DF_1 and DF_2 represent various distribution factors. One parameter used in determining the quality of a beam is the linear energy transfer (LET). In general, heavy particle irradiation (high LET) has a greater biological effect than low LET irradiation. For example, if neutrons produce ten times the biological effect as electrons for the same dose then a quality factor (QF) of ten would be used in calculating the dose equivalent. Likewise, differential distribution of a radioactive source is not uniform and may produce an unusually large biologic effect. A summary of the dose-limiting recommendations for occupational exposure and for the public in general in presented in Table 5-4.

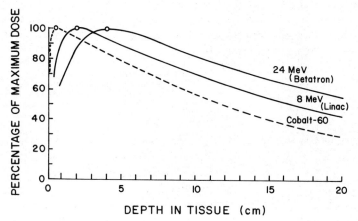

Figure 5-4 Central axis depth dose distribution of cobalt-60 gamma rays, and x-rays from an 8 meV linear accelerator and a 24 meV betatron. Note greater depth dose penetration with higher energy photons.

Table 5-4
Dose Limits of Radiation Exposure

Category	Dose Limit
Combined whole body occupational exposure	5 rem/year
Long-term accumulation to age N-years	$(N -18) \times 5$ rem
Specific Organs	
gonads	5 rem/year
lens of eye	5 rem/year
bone marrow	5 rem/year
skin	15 rem/year
hands	75 rem/year
Dose limits for family of patients	
individual < age 45	0.5 rem/year
individual ≥ age 45	5 rem/year

The combined whole body exposure of personnel involved in providing radiation therapy to patients should not exceed 5 rem/year (NRC Report, 1971). Dose limits for individuals receiving radiation under the age of 45 is 0.5 rem in any one year, whereas those over the age of 45 are allowed 5 rem annually. Personnel monitoring is usually performed using film badges that yield an adequate measurement of radiation received to the body surface near the monitor. In order to reduce the dosage rate from radiation scatter or leakage, barriers of lead or concrete are placed in the walls of rooms containing radiation machines. In addition, radioactive sources are maintained in sealed lead containers, and afterloading procedures minimize personnel exposure. Qualified safety officers carry out thorough radiation surveys of each new installation and make periodic follow-up reports to insure the full maintenance of safety standards (Wilson and Maruyama 1974).

Cellular Effects of Ionizing Radiation

Gamma rays and x-rays eject fast electrons from atoms within the cell. These electrons lose energy by interactions with other molecules within the cell causing further ionization and damage. According to the target theory, the ionizing event directly involves a target molecule for cellular inactivation. The ionization of water in a cervical cancer cell, for example, produces hydrogen and hydroxyl free radicals. These free radicals are highly unstable and react chemically with cellular constituents causing irreversible damage to nuclear DNA, cytosol enzyme systems, and the cell membrane. Cell death after irradiation occurs most commonly by mitotic inhibition. Characteristically, lethally irradiated cells may appear normal but degenerate because they are unable to undergo continued cellular division. Other cells may undergo several normal divisions and then, due to subtle damage in their genetic material, enter abnormal mitosis and make no further attempt to divide. These cells may continue synthetic and metabolic functions, but appear to swell, and eventually degenerate. Cytologic evidence of radiation injury to cervical cancer cells include: cytoplasmic vacuolization and amphophilia, nuclear and cytoplasmic enlargement, prominent nucleoli, and localized disruption of the cell membrane. This process may take numerous cell cycles and explain why radiation effects on cervical tumor tissue may not be apparent for several weeks.

Histologic findings indicative of radiation injury include: capillary endothelial and intimal proliferation, neovascularization with vascular ectasia, and nuclear atypia in epithelial cells and fibroblasts. In addition, there is a nonspecific inflammatory cell infiltrate that is similar to that seen in other types of tissue injury. This inflammatory response is particularly intense during the first three weeks after therapy. The skin may become erythematous and, if the vascular changes are severe, ulceration and fibrosis with delayed healing may occur. For this reason, it is generally recommended that surgical procedures be performed no sooner than four weeks after completion of radiation therapy.

Radiosensitivity of Cervical Cancer

In order to obtain maximal results in the treatment of cervical cancer, it is important to know the intrinsic sensitivity of cervical cancer cells to radiation as well as the sensitivity of those normal structures adjacent to the cervix. For a particular tumor, the radiation dose required for tumor control and the tissue tolerance of normal adjacent structures can be defined. Tumors such as ovarian dysgerminomas or testicular seminomas are eradicated by relatively low doses of radiation, and the therapeutic ratio for these tumors is high. Carcinomas of the cervix require much higher radiation doses for control than seminomas. However, the radioresistance of the normal cervix and vagina is also quite high so that tissue tolerance is acceptable. Cervical tumors are also readily accessible to clinical examination such that the radiation source can be placed directly adjacent to the tumor. In cervical cancer, radiation sensitivity is related to tumor size, cell type, anatomic configuration, and the percent of hypoxic or noncycling cells within the tumor.

Although some investigators have concluded that adenocarcinomas are more resistant to radiation than squamous cell carcinoma, there is little objective data to support this conclusion. Rather, cervical adenocar-cinomas have a different growth pattern than squamous cell carcinomas, which results in an anatomic configuration that is unfavorable for therapy. Adenocarcinomas arise in the endocervix and tend to spread up into the lower uterine segment and myometrium. Consequently, these tumors often reach a large volume without appearing to be that extensive (Lu et al 1976). A significant percent of these cells are hypoxic and therefore relatively radioresistant. Also, tumor cells in the myometrium are at a greater distance from the intracavitary source than are cells con-fined to the cervix and consequently receive a smaller radiation dose. It is probable that the observed difference in survival between adenocar-cinoma and squamous cell carcinoma of the cervix is more related to tumor volume than to an inherent resistance of adenocarcinoma to radiation. There is more evidence to suggest that specific cell types of squamous cell carcinoma may have differential sensitivity to radiation. Several in-vestigators (Wentz and Reagan 1959, Swan and Roddick 1973) have re-ported that patients with large cell nonkeratinizing carcinomas have a significantly higher five-year survival than those with keratinizing squamous cell carcinomas when treated with radiation. The difference in survival of patients with keratinizing and nonkeratinizing tumors has not been observed when they are treated with radical surgery, suggesting that the relative radiation resistance of keratinizing tumors may explain the reported variation of prognosis with this cell type (van Nagell 1977). In contrast, small cell carcinomas of the cervix have been shown to have a higher rate of both local and distant recurrences independent of the treat-ment method employed.

As has been previously mentioned, the anatomic configuration of the tumor is also related to radiation sensitivity. Small exophytic tumors con-taining a high percent of well-oxygenated, cycling tumor cells are relatively sensitive to radiation therapy. Large endophytic tumors in which the ma-jority of cells are hypoxic and in resting phases of the cell cycle are quite radioresistant.

The role of the hypoxic tumor cell as a reason for radioresistance and the problem of trying to overcome this resistance is one of the most im-portant problems in current cancer research. In 1953, Gray proposed that oxygen effect was the major reason for the radioresistance of certain human tumors. Thomlinson and Gray (1956) showed that the appearance of cells in cords of tumor from human lung cancers changed according to their proximity to capillaries. Viable tumor cells surrounded blood vessels and were aligned adjacent to them for approximately 100 μ. Beyond this point (150 μ toward the center of the tumor) necrosis and dying cells were evident. This histologic observation was ascribed to the fact that each cell removes a fraction of the available oxygen and nutrients as they diffuse away from the vessel (Figure 5-5). At a critical distance toward the center of the tumor no more oxygen remains and cell death occurs. This oxygen effect is particularly prominent in advanced stage cervical cancers and has been shown by a variety of methods (Bush et al 1978, Evans et al 1965, Kolstad 1971, Maruyama et al 1980).

The radiosensitivity of cervical tumors is in part determined by the proportion of oxic and hypoxic cells. Oxygenated cells are approximately three times more radiosensitive than hypoxic tumor cells. Hypoxic cells may constitute only a fraction of the tumor cells present. However, the radiosensitivity of the hypoxic cell population determines the radiation dose necessary for tumor control. For example, if 6000 rad is necessary to control a fully oxic tumor of the cervix, 18,000 rad would be necessary to control a totally hypoxic identical tumor. The spatial distribution of these cells within the tumor is illustrated in Figure 5-6. In this example, a critical tumor cell-capillary distance of 100 to 150 μ is essential to maintain the p0^2 gradient necessary for tumor viability. Each cell measures about 10 to 15 μ in diameter and abuts on its edges with neighboring cells. Since diffusion is the only means by which oxygen and nutrients are made available to the cell, the central and innermost cells become increasingly hypoxic and ultimately nonviable. The principal force creating this gradient is the uncontrolled cell division of the fully oxic cells adjacent to the blood supply.

A hypoxic tumor cell can return from an oxygen deficient state to a fully oxic state. This transition is designated "reoxygenation" and was originally described by Kallman (1972). In a solid tumor, radiation or chemotherapy may destroy well-oxygenated cells, allowing hypoxic cells to move closer to vessels and to a source of oxygen supply. Subsequently,

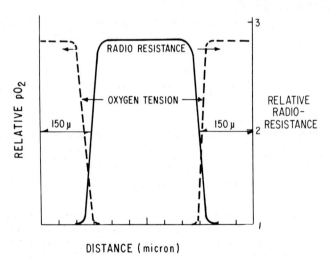

DISTANCE (micron)

Figure 5-5 Radioresistance and tumor hypoxia is present deep in the tumor cord where the tumor cell-capillary distance is in excess of 100 μ. It is these oxygen-deprived cells which are radioresistant.

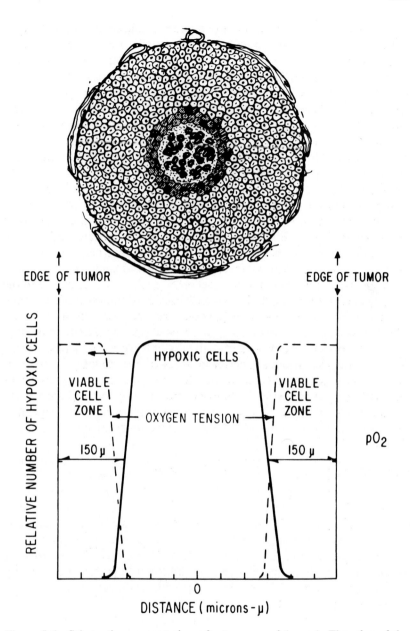

Figure 5-6 Schematic representation of a tumor cord (upper). The edge of the cord is close to capillaries and oxygenation is normal (lower figure). The center of the tumor becomes progressively more hypoxic (dark line) and it is at the center of the cord at distances greater than 150 μ from the vasculature that necrotic regions appear. Hypoxic (black and shaded) cells represent about 10% to 15% of the usual tumor and are distributed deep in the core of the tumor (solid line—lower figure and black cells).

110

these cells exhibit varying sensitivities indicating a transition from a hypoxic state to a heterogenous oxygenation state to an oxic state, that is, a "reoxygenation shift" (Figure 5-7). A number of clinical observations support this concept: 1) the decreased responsiveness of cervical tumors to radiation therapy in patients whose hemoglobin and oxygen-carrying capacity are reduced (Evans et al 1965), 2) the increased response of cervical tumors to radiation therapy in patients whose anemia has been corrected by blood transfusion (Bush et al 1978), 3) the progressive increase in pO^2 in most tumors during radiation therapy (Koller 1963, Bergsjo et al 1968), 4) the improved response rate of cervical tumors when treated in high pressure oxygen (Watson et al 1978), and 5) the difference in radiosensitivity exhibited by the early or delayed application of fast neutron-emitting californium-252 therapy in a fractionated radiotherapy course (Maruyama 1979). This indicates that improved oxygen-carrying capacity of the blood, high pressure oxygen (HPO) therapy, and effective antihypoxic tumor therapy all lead to the improved response of cervical cancer to radiation therapy.

A final cause of radiation resistance in cervical tumors is the presence of noncycling tumor cells. A noncycling tumor cell ceases to traverse the cell cycle and enters into a resting or nonproliferating (G_0) state (Figure 5-8). These noncycling cells are spatially distributed in a similar fashion to hypoxic cells, ie, in poorly perfused areas of the tumor remote from sources of oxygen and nutrients. Since these cells are in a nonmetabolizing state, they are quite resistant to any type of therapy directed against cycling cells (Schabel 1975). Although it is easy to assume that the hypoxic and noncycling cell are one and the same, it would be erroneous to do so. Although a cell is in a nonproliferating (NP) state, it may be potentially able to return to an actively cycling phase causing tumor recurrence. Therefore, therapeutic efforts are properly directed toward reducing the number of noncycling cells in the tumor. In general, the number of noncycling cells is directly related to the size of the tumor. Therefore, combination therapy designed to achieve tumor debulking generally decreases the number of noncycling cells (Maruyama and Feola 1976). In addition, certain phase-specific drugs, such as hydroxyurea (HU) when used in combination with radiation therapy, induces tumor cell recycling by destroying those cells in the relatively radioresistant S phase (Hreshchyshyn et al 1979).

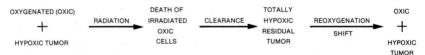

Figure 5-7 Illustration of progressive reoxygenation shift that occurs during radiation therapy.

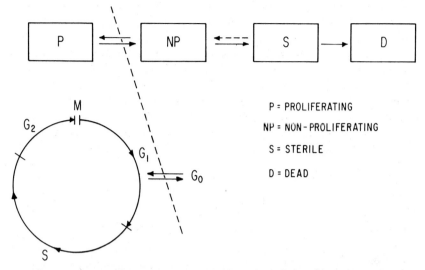

Figure 5-8 Cell cycle parameters in a tumor. A proliferating cell (P) is actively cycling (see left lower figure). Nonproliferating (NP) cells can be resting or quiescent, sterile (S) or dead (D). These noncycling states are often referred to as G_0 but can take place in the G_1 or G_2 phase of the cell cycle.

Biologic Effect of Dose, Fractionation, and Time on Tissue Response

In general, the limits of radiation dose to the tumor are set by the radiation tolerance of adjacent normal tissues. Strandquist (1944) first established the concept that an absolute cancerocidal dose for each tumor did not exist. He constructed curves relating total dose to percent tumor control and found that they were sigmoid in shape (Figure 5-9). Similar sigmoid curves related radiation dose to normal tissue damage. The goal of therapy is to obtain maximal tumor control while minimizing damage to normal structures. Therefore, it is often impossible to give the tumor a dose that would achieve 100% control because the complication rate would be too high.

Fractionation refers to the number of fractions or individual treatments over which the total dose is given. Dose refers to the quantity of radiation given in each fraction. The biologic effect of radiation depends on total dose, fractionation, dose rate, and treatment time. For example, the biologic effect of 1000 rad given in one treatment is significantly greater than if it is given in five fractions. In general, external irradiation for cervical cancer is given at a dose rate of 200 rad/day for five treatments each week. However, this dose rate may be reduced to 160 rad/day in patients with underlying vascular disease. When the same radiation dose is given over a greater time period, there is more time for

112

both normal and tumor tissue recovery, and hence less radiation complications. Similarly, a specific dose given to a small radiation field is better tolerated than the same dose given to a large field. It is by the manipulation of these variables that the radiation therapist seeks to obtain maximum tumor effect while limiting complications.

In an effort to standardize the biologic effect achieved by various combinations of external and intracavitary therapy, Ellis devleoped the concept of Nominal Standard Dose (NSD). Nominal Standard Dose, expressed in *ret*, takes into consideration total dose, treatment time, and fractionation, and is described in the following formula:

$$NSD \text{ (ret)} = \frac{D}{T^{0.11} \times F^{0.24}}$$

where D = total dose (rad), T = time (days), and F = number of fractions. This system equates the biologic effect of a nominal single dose expressed in ret to that of a complete fractionated radiation therapy course. The biologic effect of both intracavitary and external therapy can be added in this system, allowing comparison of a number of different radiation systems thoughout the world. The ret dose required for tumor control varies with the size of the tumor (Shukovsky 1970). The normal tissue tolerance of connective tissue has been demonstrated to be 1800 to 1900 ret (Ellis 1971, Fletcher 1973) so that each treatment plan can be designed to approach normal tissue tolerance.

Orton and co-workers (1973) have proposed the concept of partial tolerance (*PT*) based on *NSD* and the number of fractions given.

$$PT = n/N \text{ (NSD)}$$

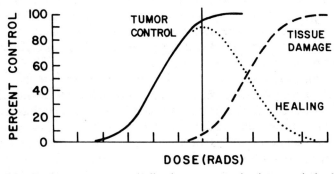

Figure 5-9 Dose-response curve indicating a progressive increase in both tumor control and normal tissue damage with increasing dose. Vertical line indicates optimal dose at which tumor control is maximal and tissue damage is minimal (after Strandquist, 1944).

where N = number of fractions to reach tolerance dose, and n = actual number of fractions given, Tolerance (Tol) would then be reached by the total of PT courses given.

$$Tol = (PT)_1 + (PT)_2 + \ldots (PT)_n$$

The advantage of using a combination of time (T), total dose (D), and number of fractions (F) for schedules of interrupted therapy is that TDF tables have been prepared for a large variety of treatment schedules that can easily be related to tissue tolerance. Thus, one fraction per week or five fractions per week for a dose per fraction of 20 to 1000 rad are all easily used.

Similarly, TDF tables have been prepared for low dose rate therapy from a variety of radionuclides used in intracavitary implants.

THERAPY

The concept central to effective radiotherapy is that the radiation dose given should obtain the maximum frequency of tumor control with the minimum of normal tissue complications. Most treatment plans are designed to give doses that will produce no more than a 5% normal tissue complication rate.

Treatment planning is based upon dose surveillance of a number of standard reference points as well as a thorough knowledge of the normal tissue tolerance of various pelvic and abdominal organs. Points A and B in the Manchester System, though arbitrary, represent meaningful reference points for the estimation of the biological effect of treatment. Additional points used in dose surveillance are summarized in Table 5-5 and illustrated in Figure 5-10. Briefly, these include the anterior rectal wall, posterior bladder wall, and sigmoid colon, which can be localized using appropriate contrast media and orthogonal radiographs. Point T is 1 cm above the cervix marker and 1 cm lateral to the tandem. This point more often represents the tumor itself than does point A. Point V represents the vaginal surface and is particularly important in cases where cervical carcinoma has extended to involve the vagina. Finally, point C represents the external iliac nodes at the lateral pelvic wall. Sophisticated computerized methods can reliably calculate the dose given to these and other points throughout the pelvis (Maruyama et al 1976).

Tissue tolerance for relevant pelvic and abdominal structures is illustrated in Table 5-6. It is difficult, however, to accurately define a true tolerance dose when a combination of external and intracavitary therapy is used. For example, the generally recognized volume tolerance for the bladder is 7000 rad. However, the tolerance of a single point on the

114

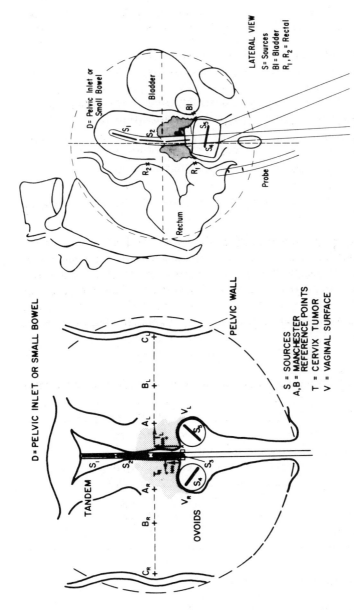

Figure 5-10 A-P reference points used for optimized intracavitary implant therapy. Lateral view of reference point array. (Reproduced with permission from: Maruyama Y, van Nagell JR, Wrede DE, et al: Approaches to optimization of dose in radiation therapy of cervix carcinoma. *Radiology* 120:389–398, 1976.)

Table 5-5
Reference Points for Dose Surveillance in Implant Radiotherapy

Point A	—	2 cm above and lateral to external os, fornix, or cervicovaginal junction (whichever is highest)
Point B	—	3 cm lateral to point A
Point C	—	Lateral pelvic wall
Point T	—	Tumor dose at cervix,1 cm above and lateral to fornix or cervicovaginal junction
Lateral Vagina Mucosa	—	Lateral walls at ovoid level (V_R, V_L)
Vagina Mucosa	—	Anterior and posterior walls at ovoid level (V_A, V_P)
Rectum	—	Anterior wall of rectum
Bladder	—	Posterior wall of trigone
Point D	—	Pelvic inlet dose, 1 cm above tip of tandem

posterior bladder wall may be higher. Similarly, the dose rate of implant therapy directly affects tissue tolerance and consequently the incidence of radiation-induced complications. All systems use a combination of external beam and intracavitary therapy. Optimal combinations vary, but preimplant radiotherapy by external megavoltage beams greatly reduces tumor bulk and facilitates effective intracavitary therapy (Swartz 1969), Maruyama et al 1976).

Table 5-6
Radiation Tissue Tolerance of Normal Pelvic and Abdominal Structures

Tissue	Tolerance Dose (Rad)
Kidney	2000
Liver	3000
Small Bowel	4500
Large Bowel	6000
Rectum	6000
Bladder	7000
Ureter	7500

External Beam Pelvic Radiotherapy

The primary purpose of whole pelvis irradiation is to decrease tumor volume and to reduce the gross anatomical distortion produced by invasion of normal pelvic structures. In patients with Stages IB and IIA

116

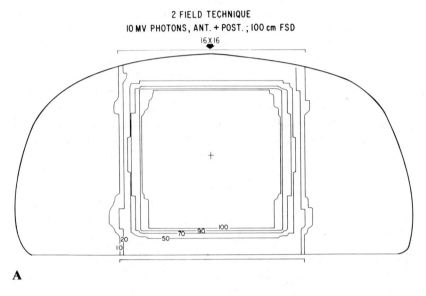

2 FIELD TECHNIQUE
10 MV PHOTONS, ANT. + POST. ; 100 cm FSD

A

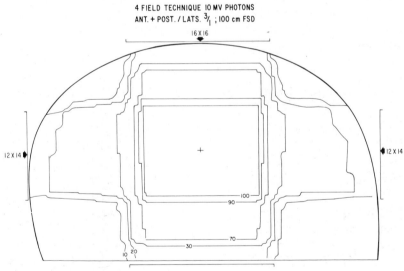

4 FIELD TECHNIQUE 10 MV PHOTONS
ANT. + POST. / LATS. $^3/_1$; 100 cm FSD

B

Figure 5-11 **(A)** Isodose curves for two-field treatment technique (upper figure) with 10 meV x-rays from linear accelerator treated at a focus-skin distance of 100 cm. **(B)** Isodose curves of four-field treatment technique (lower figure) using 10 meV x-rays from a linear accelerator. This method is useful for patients with A-P diameter ⩾24 cm.

disease, 4000 rad external therapy is given at a dose rate of 180 to 200 rad/day. Patients with more advanced stage disease are treated with a total of 4000 to 5000 rad whole pelvis therapy given over five to seven weeks. Any patient with prior abdominal surgery, pelvic inflammatory disease, or severe vascular disease is treated at a reduced dose rate of 160 rad/day. Field size is individualized but is generally 256 cm² (16 cm × 16 cm). Patients with a small anterior-posterior (A-P) diameter (< 20 cm) are treated with two opposing A-P ports. However, large patients are usually treated with an arrangement of two A-P/P-A and two lateral ports producing optimal pelvic dose distribution (Figure 5-11). At least two fields are treated per day to reduce the given dose per field per day. Midline shielding is used, with the width of the shielded area varying from 3 to 6 cm, depending upon the implant isodose pattern. At doses in excess of 4000 rad, the midline shield is extended cephalad to the top of the field in order to reduce the dose to the small bowel (Figure 5-12). A pelvic sidewall boost of 500 to 1000 rad is often given depending upon the stage and configuration of the tumor. When external therapy is given at a dose rate of 800 to 900 rad per week, most patients are asymptomatic. A dose rate of 1000 rad external therapy per week may produce mild symptoms, such as dysuria or proctitis, in approximately 15% of patients. However, few patients will require breaks in their treatment schedule as a result of these symptoms.

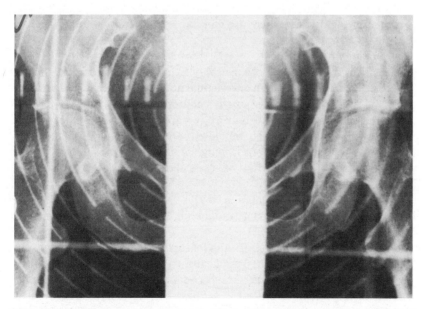

Figure 5-12 Simulator port of lateral pelvic boost field. Entire midline is shielded to avoid high enteric radiation dose.

Implant Irradiation Methodology

In radiation implantation therapy, five factors are important in achieving tumor control within the limits of normal tissue tolerance. These are: 1) dose, 2) time interval between implants, 3) number of implants, 4) dose rate, and 5) external beam dose and number of fractions or treatments. These factors must be considered as they relate to the methods and technique of implantation therapy.

External dose When external beam and internal therapy are applied, the use of unblocked external fields to pelvic viscera delivers dose to radiosensitive structures and decreases the residual tissue tolerance to implant therapy. The change is roughly inverse to the magnitude of the external whole pelvic dose. Partially blocked fields as previously described are useful for the reduction of bowel and bladder dose.

Contrast media and localization of adjacent structures It is difficult to consider dosage in closely adjacent structures without the use of radiography and contrast media to accurately localize the bladder and rectum (Maruyama et al 1976). Dose in these sites is easily calculated by current computerized methods.

Probe monitors of radionuclide dosage This is a simple and rapid means of checking the correctness of the radium loading and of representative dose in adjacent organs (Maruyama et al 1974). It permits greater confidence in computer calculated doses (Gustafsson et al 1962, Hoskins et al 1975). Probe monitors are used less frequently in most clinics at the present time. However, their use can allow a clinic to standardize and calibrate a treatment system.

Packing and placement Tight, properly placed vaginal packs can displace sensitive sites and organs away from radiant sources in the applicators. The uterine tandem and vaginal applicators should be in proper position and conform to the patient's anatomy.

Afterloading This not only allows greater personnel safety in the use of radioactive materials, but also permits the therapist access to the sources for removal, repositioning, or change in the intensity of the various sources. This important advance allows tremendous flexibility in individualized treatment.

Computer assisted planning This permits a large variety of loadings to be considered (Maruyama et al 1976) as well as optimization (Tai et al 1978).

Accessibility of sources in applicators Analysis or radiographs showing the relationship of the applicator to the position of bowel, bladder, and other adjacent structures permits consideration of alternative loading arrangements (Figure 5-13); these can be individualized based upon the configuration and location of the disease as well as that of normal tissue (Maruyama et al 1976).

External manipulability of applicator position   Although this can be done by reapplication, repacking, or removal of an unsatisfactory application, it is also clear that external change of the applicator position is often easily accomplished, provided it is accessible to the therapist for manipulation (Maruyama et al 1976).

Afterloading capability, accessibility of a variety of applicators for external manipulation, and computer treatment planning allow individualized treatment to be given to each patient. It is also possible to load sources of different activity in different positions within the applicators to obtain optimal doses at tumor reference points (Maruyama et al 1976).

In studies from this institution based upon computer-optimized treatment of cervix carcinoma (Hoskins et al 1975) it was possible to use many different loading arrangements and to obtain isodose curves identical to those obtained by standard loading methods. Computer-optimized treatment planning requires: 1) the use of reference points stated above, 2) specifications of tolerance dosage for radiosensitive organs, 3) the use of at least five radioactive sources in the applicators with a constraint that no source be of zero strength, 4) approximately half of the activity placed in a linear arrangement in the uterine tandem and the remainder in the vagina, and 5) a rad/mg hour ratio = 1.0 (at point A). Computer-optimized loadings cannot correct a technically, badly placed applicator system. If necessary, repositioning, proper placement of packs, anteflexion of the tandem, or anteversion of a retroflexed uterus needs to be performed first (Maruyama et al 1976). These procedures are best performed in a designated Implant Suite situated in the Radiotherapy Department. Under these circumstances, alternative methods of applicator placement using analgesia rather than anesthesia can be performed with great reduction in lost patient time and morbidity (Maruyama et al 1979).

Several changes in applicator position or loading involved in dose optimization are shown in the following figures. Figure 5-14 demonstrates that identical doses can be delivered to point A and the tumor point T, while reducing sigmoid colon dose by leaving the tip of the tandem unloaded. In a second illustration (Figure 5-15) anteflexion of the tandem itself produced optimal dose distribution to the tumor. In another example, the dose to the bladder and rectum was reduced by simply unloading the ovoids (Figure 5-16).

Dosage to the pelvic organs and tumor depends upon distance from the radioactive source. In Figure 5-17, the sources S_1 to S_5 have been shown schematically. S_1 treats the fundus of the uterus and contributes to dose at point A. S_2 is usually closest to point A and loadings at this position readily control the dose at point A. S_3 is positioned in the cervical canal and dominates the dose contributed by the implant to point T. S_4

and S₅ are sources in the ovoids and treat the lateral vaginal mucosal surfaces. S_3, S_4, and S_5 contribute the largest dose to the rectum and bladder, and also to the tumor. If the ovoids are widely spaced, the doses at V_3 and V_4 are low and "hanging" source can be placed in between the ovoids to keep dose at therapeutic levels. Systems that sit high in the pelvis, sometimes from overly generous vaginal packing, can irradiate small bowel excessively. An overly anteflexed system will usually deliver high dosage to the bladder, whereas a retroverted system often delivers an excessive dose to the rectum. In a system that uses multiple implants, a poor dose distribution evident at the first implant may be corrected by a subsequent application.

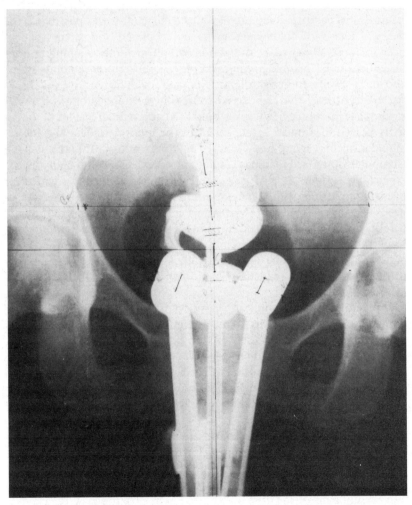

A

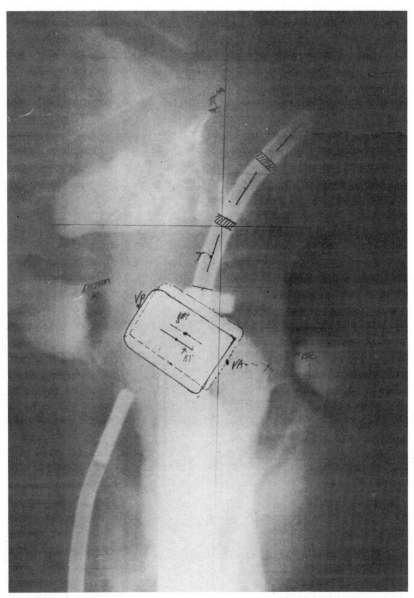

B

Figure 5-13 (A) A-P radiograph of pelvis showing method used to localize pelvic structures. Thin barium sulfate is used in rectum and lower sigmoid colon. Diazotrozoatic is placed in Foley balloon, air in bladder, and a thin barium-soaked pack in vagina. (Reproduced with permission from Maruyama Y, van Nagell JR, Wrede DE, et al: Approaches to optimization of dose in radiation therapy of cervix carcinoma. *Radiology* 120:389–398, 1976.) **(B)** Lateral radiograph.

122

The use of the optimization concept in this clinic has virtually eliminated radiogenic high dose complications in radiosensitive pelvic organs. It has also permitted the use of novel radionuclides, such as the neutron-emitting isotope californium-252, in advanced cervical cancer without causing undue complications. A 5% major complication rate has been reduced to less than 1% by individualized cervical cancer therapy. The control rate achieved by this system is comparable to those published by other major cancer treatment centers. Thus, attention to the type of details inherent in the individualized therapy concept appears to lead to a beneficial outcome for cervical cancer patients.

NON LOADING OF TIP

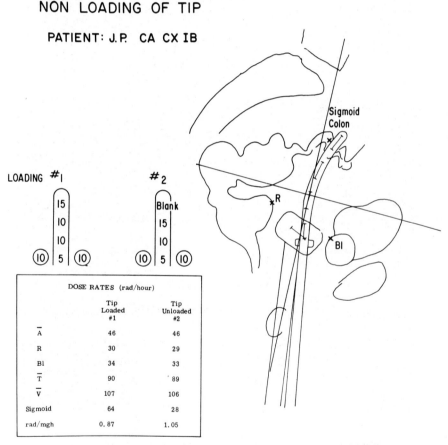

DOSE RATES (rad/hour)	Tip Loaded #1	Tip Unloaded #2
$\overline{A}$	46	46
R	30	29
Bl	34	33
$\overline{T}$	90	89
$\overline{V}$	107	106
Sigmoid	64	28
rad/mgh	0.87	1.05

Figure 5-14 Optimization of tumor dose for Stage Ib tumor by nonloading to tip of elongated system in patient with 8 cm uterine canal. Still higher actual tumor volume (point T) doses can be obtained by placing a source of higher activity at the S₃ position. (Reproduced with permission from: Maruyama Y, van Nagell JR, Wrede DE, et al: Approaches to optimization of dose in radiation therapy of cervix carcinoma. *Radiology* 120:389–398, 1976.)

Management Program for Cervical Cancer

A specific management program for cervical cancer related to stage is presented in Table 5-7. Microinvasive cervical cancer (Stage Ia) is usually treated by surgery, but may also be effectively treated using two radionuclide implants providing a dose of 8000 rad to point A. As has been previously discussed (Chapter 4), Stage Ib lesions less than 3 cm in diameter can be treated either with radical hysterectomy and pelvic lymphadenectomy or radiation therapy. Radical surgery may also be indicated in patients with 1) pelvic inflammatory disease, 2) uterine myomata that preclude satisfactory intracavitary therapy, or 3) severe vaginal stenosis preventing optimal implant application.

Z-AXIS ANTEFLEXION OF TANDEM

PATIENT: M.H.   CA CX II A

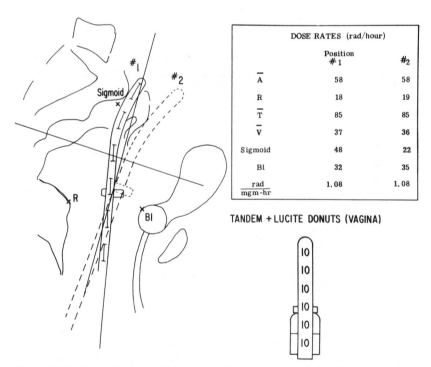

	DOSE RATES (rad/hour)	
	Position #1	#2
$\bar{A}$	58	58
R	18	19
$\bar{T}$	85	85
$\bar{V}$	37	36
Sigmoid	48	22
Bl	32	35
$\frac{rad}{mgm\text{-}hr}$	1.08	1.08

TANDEM + LUCITE DONUTS (VAGINA)

Figure 5-15 Optimization of dose by anteflexion of tandem. Higher tumor doses can be delivered by higher activity in the S_{3-4} (third and fourth tandem source from tip) position. (Reproduced with permission from: Maruyama Y, van Nagell JR, Wrede DE, et al: Approaches to optimization of dose in radiation therapy of cervix carcinoma. *Radiology* 120:389–398, 1976.)

124

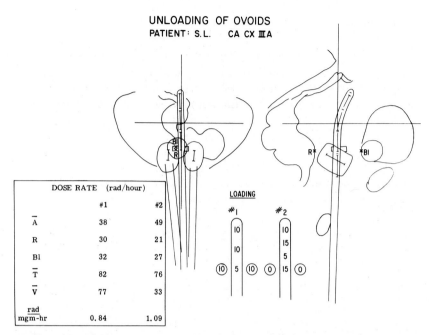

UNLOADING OF OVOIDS
PATIENT: S.L.   CA CX ⅢA

LOADING

DOSE RATE	(rad/hour)	
	#1	#2
A̅	38	49
R	30	21
Bl	32	27
T̅	82	76
V̅	77	33
rad/mgm-hr	0.84	1.09

Figure 5-16 Optimization of reducing dose in radiosensitive structures by fractionated unloading of system, eg, unloading of ovoids. (Reproduced with permission from: Maruyama Y, van Nagell JR, Wrede DE, et al: Approaches to optimization of dose in radiation therapy of cervix carcinoma. *Radiology* 120:389–398, 1976.)

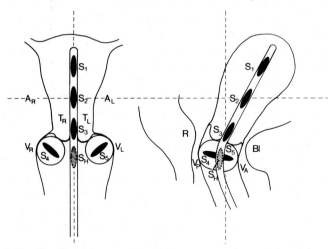

Figure 5-17 Configuration of sources in applicators. In afterloaded system all sources can potentially be moved in the tandem, removed, changed in position, and strength of activity to best achieve tumor control while limiting dose to normal tissues. Hanging source can be used for widely spread ovoid system to treat V_a and V_p, which receive low dose under those conditions.

Table 5-7
Radiation Therapy of Cervical Cancer
According to Stage (University of Kentucky System)

Stage	Intracavitary Therapy (Point A dose)	Whole Pelvis External Therapy (Rad)	Pelvic Sidewall Boost (Midline Shielding)	Total Dose (Rad) Pt. T	Pt. A
Ia	2 implants (8000 rad)	---	---	12,000	8000
Ib	2 implants (4000 rad)	4000	1000	12,000-15,000	8000
IIa IIb (<5 cm diameter)	2 implants (4000 rad)	4000	2000	12,000-15,000	8000
IIb (Bulky) IIIa IIIb	2-3 implants* (3500-4500 rad)	4000-5000	500-1000 (variable by tumor pattern)	12,000-15,000	8000-9000
IVa IVb	2-3 implants* (3500-4500 rad)	4000-5000	500-1000 (variable by tumor pattern)	12,000-15,000	8000-9000

*See section on californium-252

Radiation therapy for Stage Ib cervical cancer includes a combination of 4000 rad whole pelvis external therapy followed by two radionuclide implants ($\sim$ 50 rad/hr dose rate) two weeks apart providing a total dose of 8000 rad to point A and 12000 to 15000 rad to point T. An additional 1000 rad parametrial boost is given to a split field using midline shielding. In patients with bulky, or barrel-shaped Stage Ib lesions >5 cm in diameter, combined preoperative radiation therapy followed by extrafascial hysterectomy is indicated. In these cases, external therapy in doses of 4000 to 5000 rad to the whole pelvis is followed by one implant providing a total dose of 6500 rad to point A, 9000 to 11000 rad to point T, and 8000 to 9000 rad to the surface of the vagina (V_L and V_R). An extrafascial hysterectomy with bilateral salpingo-oophorectomy is then performed four to six weeks later (Rutledge et al 1976, van Nagell et al 1979). A lateral pelvic sidewall boost of 1000 rad may be given postoperatively depending upon the findings at surgery. However, complications have been shown to rise sharply when doses in excess of 8000 rad are given to point A (Peckham et al 1969). At doses over 4000 rad, the upper border of the pelvic port is reduced 3 cm to decrease small bowel doses.

Additional surgery may also be indicated in patients with Stage Ib cervical cancer whose lesions fail to respond during radiation therapy. Of all the parameters used to monitor tumor response to radiotherapy, the most important is tumor regression or decrease in tumor size. Marcial and co-workers (1970) carefully studied the regression patterns of cervical cancers during radiation therapy. Those patients with tumors demonstrating significant regression by the end of the external beam therapy (4500 rad) had a 96% three-year survival as opposed to a 2% survival rate for patients whose tumors never regressed during therapy (Table 5-8). In a more recent study, Hardt and colleagues (1981) confirmed these findings. Patients having no palpable or visible evidence of disease one month following completion of therapy had a 95% five-year survival. Conversely, patients with residual gross tumor at this time had a recurrence rate of 80%. Response to therapy was related directly to stage but the recurrence rate in Stage Ib lesions not regressing during therapy was 60%. For this reason, patients with Stage Ib cervical cancers not responding to radiation therapy should be considered for adjunctive extrafascial hysterectomy.

Table 5-8
Tumor Regression by Fractionated External Beam Radiotherapy
Followed by Radium Implant and Three-Year Survival

Regression	Ib	IIa	IIb	IIIa	IIIb	IVa	IVb	Total
Early or by end of external therapy	44/45	23/24	4/4	1/2	1/1	—	—	73/76 (96%)
At radium insertion	11/13	15/22	9/13	4/5	0/1	—	0/1	39/55 (71%)
Within 3 mo postradium	23/25	40/51	41/63	22/38	14/26	4/9	1/1	145/213 (68%)
Very delayed (>3 mo postradium)	—	10/11	16/20	14/21	6/9	1/6	0/1	47/68 (69%)
No regression	0/1	0/5	0/10	0/7	0/13	0/7	0/3	1/46 (2%)

Adapted from Marcial and Bosch 1970.

The management of Stage IIa and small (<5 cm diameter) Stage IIb lesions is similar to that for bulky Stage Ib tumors. Whole pelvis therapy (4000 rad) is followed by two implants two weeks apart, providing 8000 rad to point A. An additional parametrial and pelvic sidewall boost of 2000 rad is given through a reduced port (3 cm off upper border) with midline shielding. In selected Stage IIb lesions that demonstrate regression of parametrial disease during external therapy, the addition of extrafascial hysterectomy may be beneficial (Rutledge et al 1976). The treatment of advanced stage disease (bulky Stage IIb to Stage IVb) is complicated by the fact that these tumors contain a high percent of hypoxic cells that are relatively radioresistant. In these tumors, whole pelvis external and sidewall therapy is given over five to seven weeks. In addition, a pelvic boost of 500 to 1000 rad may be given to either one or both sidewalls depending upon the anatomic configuration of the tumor. Following completion of external therapy, two or three implants are given at two-week intervals. The total dose to point A is kept as near 8000 rad as possible, but may be higher in individual cases. The tumor (point T) receives 12000 to 15000 rad using this methodology. Recently, californium-252 has been substituted for cesium-137 in clinical trials as an intracavitary source in the treatment of bulky or advanced stage cervical tumors at this institution. A brief discussion of californium-252 and the results of preliminary clinical trials will be presented in a subsequent section. Randomized prospective clinical trials are important to improve the outcome of new treatments for advanced stage disease (Palmer Saunders 1978, Comroe 1978).

Extended Field Radiation

The para-aortic lymph nodes are a common site of extrapelvic metastases in advanced cervical cancer, and the optimal treatment of these nodes represents an area of current interest in radiation therapy. The incidence of para-aortic metastases varies with stage and tumor volume, and may be as high as 40% in advanced stage disease (Buchsbaum 1972, Nelson et al 1974, Piver et al 1977). The diagnosis of extrapelvic lymph nodal metastases is usually made by lymphangiography or CT scanning, but must be confirmed histologically by fine needle aspiration or retroperitoneal lymph node sampling prior to therapy. When disease is found to involve the para-aortic lymph nodes, the radiation field is reduced in width and extended upwards from the pelvic field (L_4-L_5 interspace) to the level of the T_{12} vertebral body. A total dose of 5000 to 5500 rad is delivered, usually in continuity with the pelvic radiation field (Fletcher et al 1972, Lepanto et al 1975, Piver et al 1977). The dose per fraction has varied from 150 to 200 rad/day. Major enteric complications have been reported in 20% to 40% of patients receiving extended field irradiation after exploratory laparotomy (Piver et al 1977, Wharton et al 1976). Long-term survival statistics on significant numbers of patients with positive para-aortic nodes treated with radiation therapy are unavailable. However, preliminary results suggest that the five-year survival of these patients may be as high as 20% (Hughes et al 1980).

Carcinoma of the Cervical Stump

Squamous cell carcinomas of the cervical stump are still common because of the practice of supracervical hysterectomy, which was advocated frequently in the past. Treatment is complicated by the fact that the cervical canal will usually accommodate only one source. Whole pelvis radiotherapy in a dose of 4000 rad is followed by standard applicator positioning with the placement of a 25 mg radium equivalent radionuclide source in the cervical canal (Fletcher 1973). A 1:1 cervical canal-to-vaginal ovoid radionuclide loading will usually give a satisfactory dose to point A, the vaginal surfaces (V_R and V_L), and the tumor (T). Treatment planning should vary with stage of disease in the usual manner as shown in Table 5-7.

Carcinoma of the Cervix in Pregnancy

Radiation therapy is generally the treatment of choice for pregnant patients with Stage IIa or greater disease. As expected, treatment varies with tumor stage and the duration of pregnancy (Bosch et al 1966, Creasman 1970, Gustafsson et al 1962). In general, the uterus, cervix, and pelvic structures are highly vascular, and the condition of the pregnancy must be taken into consideration. In the first or second trimester, whole pelvis radiotherapy in a dose of 4000 rad is given, usually producing spontaneous abortion of the fetus. Two radionuclide implants are then performed as previously described, providing a total of 8000 rad to point A. In the third trimester, treatment may be delayed two to four weeks until fetal lung maturation has occurred. A cesarean section is then performed leaving the uterus in place for later intracavitary therapy. A full course of external beam therapy precedes two radionuclide implants delivering essentially the same tumor dose as that given in a nonpregnant state.

Radiation Following Surgery for Cervical Cancer

Postoperative radiation therapy is most commonly performed for two indications. The first of these is in patients following hysterectomy in which occult invasive cervical carcinoma has been found in the surgical specimen. The prognosis for these patients is excellent when therapy is started in the immediate postoperative period. If there is evidence of only microscopic disease in the cervix, the patient can be treated with local intracavitary therapy providing approximately 10000 to 12000 rad surface dose to the vaginal vault. More advanced lesions are treated with whole pelvis radiation to a dose of 4000 to 5000 rad. This dose is fractionated over five to seven weeks and followed by two vaginal vault implants providing a total vaginal surface dose of 10000 to 12000 rad (Durrance 1968). Postoperative radiation is also given following radical hysterectomy and pelvic lymphadenectomy when metastatic disease is present in the pelvic or para-aortic lymph nodes. Whole pelvis radiotherapy in a dose of 6000 rad is given in an effort to achieve local tumor control. However, the dose per fraction is reduced to 150 to 160 rad in order to lessen the radiation effect on normal tissues whose blood supply has been compromised by prior surgery. Para-aortic or extended field radiation may also be indicated according to the specific site of lymph nodal metastases. The treatment plan utilized for para-aortic irradiation has been discussed previously.

Reirradiation in Recurrent Cervical Cancer

After a full course of radiotherapy, additional pelvic radiation has little except a palliative role in the management of recurrent cervical carcinoma (Jones et al 1970). In the previously inadequately treated patient, a moderately radical course can be contemplated but must be highly individualized in planning and implementation. Small localized recurrences may be treated with coned ports over the region or with interstitial implants. In general, iodine-125 has been a very satisfactory radionuclide to use for interstitial therapy. Unfortunately, retreatment is often associated with severe complications and tumor persistence is common (Einhorn 1975).

Adjuvant Chemotherapy and Radiation

Clinical trials using combinations of adjuvant chemotherapy and radiation therapy in the treatment of cervical cancer are in progress. At the present time, the most effective agent used in combination with radiation is hydroxyurea (HU). In a controlled clinical trial in which hydroxyurea was given at three-day intervals during a fractionated course of external whole pelvis therapy (5000 to 6000 rad), complete tumor regression was increased from 48% to 68% ($p < .05$) (Hreschchyshyn et al 1979). Both survival and duration of progression-free interval were significantly increased in patients receiving hydroxyurea. In this study, bone marrow depression was also more common and severe in the HU group. These results show that a combination of radiation therapy and a chemotherapeutic agent such as hydroxyurea, which is specifically cytotoxic to cells in the S-phase of the cycle, can lead to improved tumor control. It is thought that these agents produce a perturbation in resting cell kinetics such that tumor cells are recruited from a resting to a proliferating phase of the

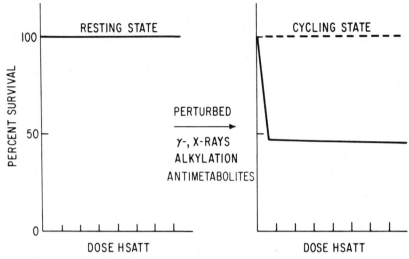

Figure 5-18 Effect of pertubation of a cell population. A resting cell population (left side of figure) is insensitive to the effects of high specific activity tritiated thymidine (HSATT) and no decrease in survival occurs. Once perturbed, cells begin to enter a cycling phase. At that time, flash exposures of the population to HSATT results in uptake by cycling cells and therefore detects the fraction in DNA-S phase by killing them. Hydroxyurea has an action identical to HSATT.

cycle (Figure 5-18). This change increases the radiation sensitivity of the tumor and facilitates radiation-induced tumor regression.

EXPERIMENTAL RADIOTHERAPY IN CERVICAL CANCER

Experimental studies in the radiation therapy of cervical cancer have been directed largely at the problem of tumor cell hypoxia. As has been previously stated, advanced stage cervical cancers contain a high percent of hypoxic cells many of which are noncycling and quite resistant to radiation therapy. In order to counteract this "oxygen effect" in bulky cervical tumors, several experimental approaches have been attempted. The first of these is the use of high pressure oxygen (HPO) during therapy. High pressure oxygen administered to patients in special lucite chambers at 3 atm of pressure (hyperbaric) has been studied as a means to increase the oxygen tension of cervical tumors during fractionated external therapy (Figure 5-19). Different fraction sizes and total doses combined with intracavitary therapy were studied in a randomized clinical trial by the British Medical Research Council on hyperbaric oxygen therapy (Watson et al 1978). Advanced stage cervical tumors were treated by conventional schedules at the participating centers, either in air or in HPO tanks.

Tumors were significantly better controlled when treated in hyperbaric oxygen (Table 5-9). However, normal tissue complications also occurred more frequently in HPO (Table 5-10) suggesting that perhaps some hypoxic cells present in normal tissue were radiosensitized. The effect of hyperbaric oxygen in decreasing tumor recurrence was most pronounced when external therapy was given over six to ten fractions (Table 5-11). The use of hyperbaric oxygen significantly reduced the incidence of pelvic recurrence from 39% to 17%.

The second experimental approach in the therapy of cervical cancer has been the use of high LET particles, such as fast neutrons or negative pions. The most promising of these clinical trials has involved the use of

Table 5-9
Local Recurrence Free Rates for Advanced Carcinoma of the Cervix British Medical Research Council Trial Five-Year Tumor Free Probability of Significant Difference

	Patients	Percent Control	Significance
HPO	161	67	
AIR	159	47	p < .001

Adapted from Watson, Halnow, and Dische et al 1978.

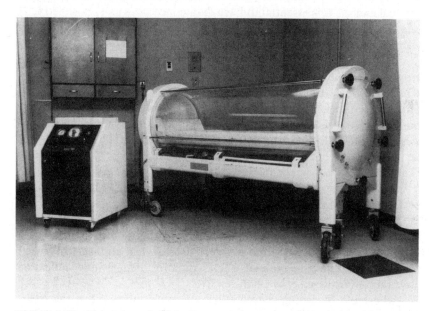

Figure 5-19 Examples of High Pressure Oxygen (HPO) tank used in HPO Therapy. Patients are placed in the tank, the tank pressurized to 3 atm of 100% oxygen, the patients allowed time for tissue saturation to occur, and then radiotherapy is given. (Courtesy of Dr. Henry Plank, LDS Hospital, Salt Lake City, Utah.)

Table 5-10
Treatment Morbidity of Patients Treated Under HPO

	Patients	Complications
HPO	161	42 (26%)
AIR	159	30 (19%)

Adapted from Watson, Halnow, and Dische et al 1978.

californium-252 brachytherapy. Californium-252 is a radionuclide that emits 1) a fission spectrum of neutrons with an average energy of 2.1 to 2.3 meV, and 2) gamma photons with an energy of 0.5 to 1.0 meV. At the present time, californium-252 is being considered for use as an alternative to cesium for intracavitary radiotherapy for advanced stage cervical cancer. The rationale for its use is based in part upon its oxygen enhancement ratio (OER), which is significantly lower than that of radium-226 or Cesium-137 (Hall et al 1975, Kal et al 1976). Californium-252 is therefore advantageous for treating tumors in which the success of present therapy is limited by the presence of hypoxic cells. Neutrons also have a higher relative biological effect (RBE) than gamma radiation and therefore are more effective for hypoxic cell killing (Maruyama et al 1978). In order to design meaningful treatment plans for californium-252 in the therapy of cervical cancer, it is essential to have data concerning its 1) dosimetry, 2) relative biological effectiveness (RBE), 3) oxygen enhancement ratio (OER), and 4) dose rate effect.

Accurate dosimetry of the mixed flux of neutrons and gamma rays from californium-252 is difficult to measure. Basically, paired detectors sensitive either to neutrons, or to gamma rays are used. From the differential response of these detectors, the neutron and gamma ray components of the radiation can be determined. From available data, it is clear that the biological effect of californium-252 is almost entirely due to neutrons, and that low dose gamma rays contribute only minimally (Table 5-12).

The relative biologic effectiveness (RBE) of the californium-252 neutron components has been determined with dose rates of 10 to 279 rad/hr to be in the range of 3.9 to 11.2 (mean $\sim$ 6.0). This increase in the RBE of californium-252 compared to photon radiation, particularly at a reduced dose rate, is very important clinically when applied to cervical cancer therapy since its biologic effect on tumor tissue is independent of dose rate (Maruyama et al 1980).

The most favorable characteristic of californium-252 in the treatment of bulky cervical tumors is its low oxygen enhancement ratio (OER). Currently available fast neutron or particle beams exhibit OERs which are 1.7 or greater. In low dose rate californium-252 neutron therapy, OER values of 1.4 have been reported for mammalian cells. Thus, a therapeutic

Table 5-11
Actuarial Recurrence-Free Survival Rate for Stage III Carcinoma of Cervix

Center	Treatment Service	Ext. Rad Dose	No. Fractions	Time (days)	Radium	Five-Year Survival	Recurrence-Free Five-Year Survival	Significant Probability
Portsmouth	HPO AIR	3500-3600 rad (max)	6-7	18-22	−	42 8	58 18	p=.07
Oxford	HPO AIR	4250 rad (max)	10	31	+	35 0	46 13	p=.15
Glasgow	HPO AIR	4250-4500 rad (mod)	20	28	+	31 28	80 57	p=.011
Mt. Vernon	HPO AIR	5500 rad (min)	27	38	+	30 38	69 40	p=.037
All Patients: 119 124	HPO AIR							

Adapted from Watson, Halnow, and Dische et al 1978.

134

Table 5-12
Calculated Neutron and Gamma-Ray Dose Rates* and n/γ Ratios for Carcinoma of the Cervix (Two Implants)

Reference Point	Neutrons (rad/hr)	Rays (rad/hr)	n/γ	rem/hr**
A	18.1	9.7	1.87	118.3
B	3.5	2.8	1.25	23.8
C	3.8	3.0	1.27	25.8
D	11.5	4.8	2.40	73.8
R	14.4	7.6	1.90	94.0
BL	13.9	7.7	1.81	91.1
T	44.2	21.5	2.06	286.7
V_{rl}	17.6	9.3	1.89	114.9
V_{ap}	16.6	9.0	1.84	108.6

*The RBE for neutrons was assumed to be ∿6.
**The University of Kentucky Pelvic Reference System.
Source: Tai and Maruyama (1979).

gain factor of 1.56 or 56% may result from the use of californium-252 neutron brachytherapy.

Based on the theoretical advantages of californium-252, a clinical trial was initiated at the University of Kentucky in 1976 to determine efficacy of this source of treatment of patients with advanced cervical cancer (Maruyama et al 1980). Results of these trials have indicated that this form of local neutron therapy is well tolerated and is readily combined with external therapy from either cobalt-60 or other forms of external beam radiotherapy (Castro et al 1973, Maruyama 1981) (Figure 5-20). It also can be combined with surgery, or other conventional radionuclides used in intracavitary therapy (cesium-137 or radium-226) without a significant incidence of pelvic complications (Maruyama et al 1981). Advanced stage carcinomas of the cervix were noted to regress more rapidly and clearance of these tumors was more complete when neutron brachytherapy was combined with fractionated whole pelvis radiotherapy (Maruyama 1979).

An important new consideration is the sequence in which the californium-252 is applied in relation to external therapy. In a clinical trial, it was found that intracavitary therapy with californium-252 when given prior to external beam radiotherapy was significantly more effective in producing tumor control than when given after fractionated radiotherapy (Maruyama 1981). Moreover, with a subsequent whole pelvis radiation dose of 4500 to 5000 rad, the two modalities interacted optimally and because of tumor reoxygenation, the fractionated radiotherapy resulted in a more favorable outcome, ie, 90% frequency of local tumor clearance (Table 5-13). Standard external beam radiotherapy is usually administered preceding intracavitary implants since it reduces tumor bulk and enhances the effectiveness of implant therapy by concentrating dose near the residual pelvic disease. Thus, the preexternal beam application of californium-252 represents a major deviation from this schedule. The efficacy of californium-252 appears to be highest during the time in tumor therapy when tumor bulk and number of hypoxic tumor cells is maximal (Maruyama et al 1980).

Table 5-13
Californium-252 Therapy in Advanced Carcinoma of Cervix — Local Control By Early or Delayed Implant

Relationship of Implant To External Therapy	Local Tumor Control	Tumor Persistence	Total
Pre- or Early	19	2	21
Post- or Delayed	10	11	21
	29	13	

Chi Square $X^2 = 6.69$
$P < .01$

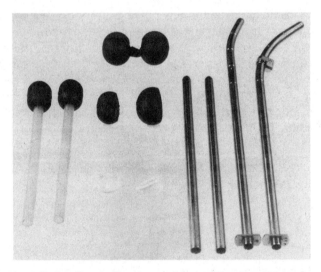

Figure 5-20 Afterloading applicators used for californium-252 implant therapy. The isodose curves around each californium-252 source is less truncated on the ends because the end of the source does not attenuate neutrons as much as it does the gamma rays. Tandems only can be used for advanced uterocervicovaginal disease but for more localized advanced tumors of the cervix or uterus, a tandem and ovoid arrangement can be used. For the destroyed vault, a single tube was satisfactory. Stainless steel uterine tandems, Manchester ovoids, either intact or split into hemiovoids (mixed sizes were often used), stainless steel vaginal tandems (used for destroyed fornix), plastic tubes, finger cots or condom (to hold ovoid or tandems), Lucite rings (not shown) were also used.

In a subsequent study in which patients with bulky Stage Ib or IIb cervical tumors were treated with intracavitary californium-252 and external therapy prior to extrafascial hysterectomy, there was no evidence of residual tumor in the surgical specimen in 15 of 24 cases (63%). There were no major complications of treatment and the four-year survival of these patients was 80% (Maruyama et al 1981).

Presently available data from clinical trials using californium-252 brachytherapy in the treatment of cervical cancer allows the following conclusions to be made.

1) Californium-252 intracavitary therapy has been used safely in combination with external photon beam therapy. The oxygen enhancement ratio (OER) of californium-252 is approximately 1.4 and its relative biologic effectiveness (RBE) is $\sim$ 6.0.

2) Californium-252 is most effective when used in combination with fractionated external therapy.

3) Preliminary data suggests that optimal tumor regression occurs when californium-252 intracavitary therapy precedes rather than follows external therapy.

4) A combination of preoperative californium-252 brachytherapy and fractionated external therapy followed by extrafascial hysterectomy produced rapid clearance of bulky Stage Ib and IIb cervical tumors. The four-year survival rate of patients with these lesions was 80%.

Recent clinical investigation shows promise in the treatment of hypoxic tumors by the identification of compounds that selectively sen-

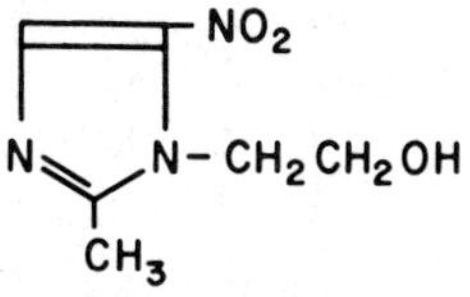

METRONIDAZOLE (FLAGYL)

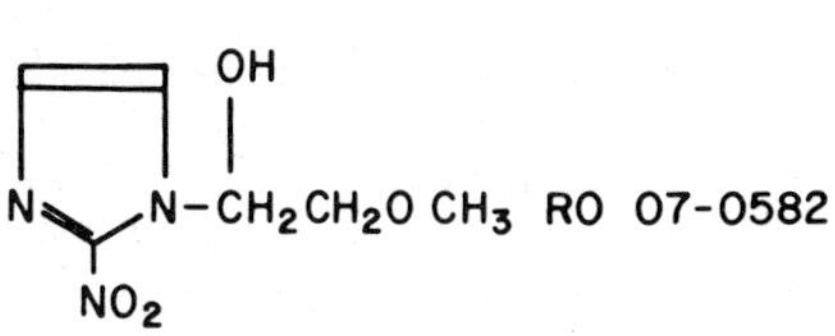

MISONIDAZOLE

Figure 5-21 Chemical structure of nitroimidazole compounds used as hypoxic radiosensitizers. These compounds mimic the effect of oxygen as a radiosensitizer in tumors and hypoxic regions.

sitize hypoxic cells to the effects of radiation. This approach has emphasized isolation of oxygen substitutes that can diffuse into poorly vascularized, and hypoxic tumor areas without being metabolized like oxygen. To date, the most effective radiosensitizing agents have been the nitroimidazole compounds (Figure 5-21) of which metronidazole is one example. Clinical trials using these compounds as radiosensitizing agents with radiation therapy were begun as early as 1974 in Canada, and preliminary data suggest that improved tumor control has been obtained in glioblastomas (Urtasun et al 1976). However, controlled clinical trials of these agents in cervical cancer have yet to be reported.

RADIATION COMPLICATIONS

General Principles

Radiation-induced complications in patients undergoing therapy for cervical cancer are generally dose related. Wall and colleagues (1966) for example, reported an increase in major bladder or rectal complications from 5% to 10% when external therapy was raised from 4000 rad to 6000 rad. Likewise, Kottmeier and Gray (1961) in a study of 500 cervical cancer patients treated at the Radiumhemmet, reported that there was a direct correlation between measured bladder and rectal doses and complications. There were no radiation-related injuries to these organs when the measured dose was less than 4000 rad. Generally, the complication rate is higher when a large volume of tissue is irradiated than when an equal dose of radiation is given to a small field. All complications are more common when chemotherapy is added to radiotherapy (Phillips 1978).

Patients at high risk to develop radiation complications are those with 1) poor nutritional status and a history of recent weight loss, 2) previous pelvic or abdominal surgery, 3) severe vascular disease, or 4) pelvic inflammatory disease. In patients with poor nutritional status, tissue response to all forms of injury is generally decreased (Copeland et al 1977). Patients with prior pelvic surgery often have dense intraperitoneal adhesions with fixation of bowel in the pelvis. Consequently, abnormally high doses are given to these enteric structures with an ensuing high complication rate. Patients with diabetes mellitus or hypertension often have a significant systemic microangiopathy with medial thickening and lumenal narrowing in the small vessels of the bowel or bladder (Figure 5-22). The superimposed capillary endothelial and intimal thickening caused by radiation (Figure 5-23) accentuates lumenal narrowing, causing hypoperfusion and local necrosis (van Nagell et al 1974). Similarly, pelvic inflammatory disease causes a reactive vasculitis of small vessels in the bowel and bladder, which are then particularly susceptible to radiation damage (van Nagell et al 1977).

138

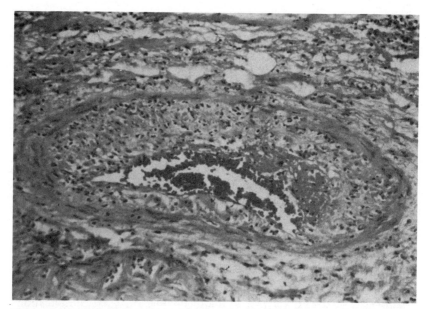

Figure 5-22 Diabetic vascular changes, like other preexisting vascular abnormalities, can accentuate the effects of radiation injury. This small dermal artery from a diabetic patient shows medial hypertrophy. H & E stain, magnification 400 X.

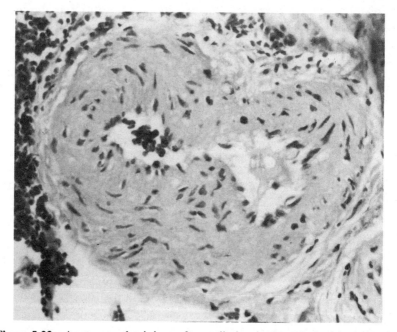

Figure 5-23 Acute vascular injury after radiation is characterized by necrosis, early fibrin thrombus formation and acute inflammation of the vessel wall. H & E stain, magnification 400 X.

Finally, Buchler (1974) has shown that patients experiencing severe radiation reactions during therapy are at high risk for the subsequent development of severe enteric or urinary tract injuries. Therefore, dose rate reduction or brief skips in treatment should be considered in patients with severe cystitis or sigmoiditis during radiation therapy.

The specific complications reported in recent large series of patients undergoing radiation for cervical cancer are summarized in Table 5-14. For organizational purposes, these will be discussed according to organ site.

Skin and Subcutaneous Tissue

With the use of megavoltage therapy, the incidence of severe skin reactions has markedly decreased. Since the peak dose from these sources (D max) is distributed well below the skin surface, there is a significant "skin-sparing" effect. Radiation dose to the skin should be limited to 5000 rad since subcutaneous fibrosis and panniculitis occur with doses of 6000 to 7000 rad. In patients with A-P diameters in excess of 22 cm, rotational or multiple field therapy may be required in order to obtain proper dosimetry while limiting the skin dose. Intertriginous skin reactions are best managed by careful hygiene, daily Sitz baths, and application of cornstarch to the involved areas.

Cervix

Radiation reactions of the cervix are quite common and usually involve sloughing of the tumor site. In extensive lesions, cervical and upper vaginal vault necrosis can occur. This complication is best treated conservatively with peroxide douches three times per day and steroid suppositories. Several months may be required for reepithelialization to occur.

Vagina

Vaginal stenosis with varying degrees of shortening occurs in over 70% of patients undergoing radiation therapy for cervical cancer (Abitbol and Davenport 1974). This complication is best avoided by 1) encouraging vaginal use after treatment or 2) utilization of vaginal dilators following completion of radiation therapy.

Bladder

Following high-dose external beam therapy and intracavitary implants, both acute and delayed bladder reactions can occur. Acute hemor-

Table 5-14
Complications of Radiation Therapy in Patients Treated for Cervical Cancer

	Patients	Sigmoiditis	Rectal Stricture	Rectovaginal Fistula	Small Bowel Obstruction	Ureteral Stricture	Hemmorrhagic cystitis	Vesicovaginal Fistula
Chau et al 1962	741	42(5.7%)		8(1.0%)	6(0.8%)	11(1.5%)	18(2.4%)	4(0.5%)
Peckham et al 1969	346	18(5.2%)		4(1.2%)	16(1.7%)	6(1.7%)	16(4.6%)	1(0.2%)
Shingleton et al 1969	1107					10(0.9%)		
Moller et al 1970	923	60(6.5%)	17(1.8%)	25(2.7%)				
Nieminen et al 1970	461			25(5.4%)				16(3.5%)
Strockbine et al 1970	831	76(9.1%)	5(0.6%)	18(2.2%)	36(4.3%)		6(0.7%)	16(1.9%)
Joelsson et al 1971	3075				15(0.5%)			
Slater et al 1971	1416		1(<0.1%)	3(0.2%)	18(1.3%)			4(0.3%)
Mikal et al 1972	305	26(8.5%)	9(2.9%)	12(3.9%)	9(2.9%)	4(1.3%)	33(11%)	6(2.0%)
Villasanta et al 1972	641	61(9.5%)		18(2.8%)	10(1.6%)	13(2.0%)	36(5.6%)	6(0.9%)
Friburg et al 1973	83	1(1.2%)	9(11%)		2(2.4%)		12(14.1%)	
Lang et al 1973	860			3(0.3%)			6(0.7%)	37(4.3%)
Buchler et al 1974	31							
van Nagell et al 1974	271			4(1.5%)	8(3.0%)			2(0.7%)
Punnonen et al 1976	279	18(6.5%)	3(1.0%)	2(0.7%)	1(0.4%)	2(0.7%)	1(0.4%)	
Bosch 1977	1139	86(7.5%)	9(0.8%)	9(0.8%)	5(0.4%)	1(<0.1%)	25(2.2%)	3(0.3%)
Underwood et al 1977	100					4(4.0%)		
van Nagell et al 1977	348				15(4.3%)			
Combined Series		(7.3%)	(1.1%)	(1.6%)	(1.5%)	(1.1%)	(3.0%)	(1.4%)

rhagic cystitis is reported in approximately 3% of patients (Figure 5-24), and is best treated by a combination of fluids, phenazopyridine hydrochloride 100 mg tid, and appropriate antibiotics. In more severe cases, bladder ulceration and necrosis with fistula formation occurs. These patients are usually quite ill and require nutritional support, antibiotics, and analgesics. Hydrogen peroxide douches are used to keep the fistula site clean but urinary diversion is required to facilitate healing. Surgical repair of a small vesicovaginal fistula may be successful provided that the fistula is clean and that a new source of blood supply, such as the omentum, is transplanted to the operative site. However, the success rate of surgical repair of large radiation-induced vesicovaginal fistulas is low.

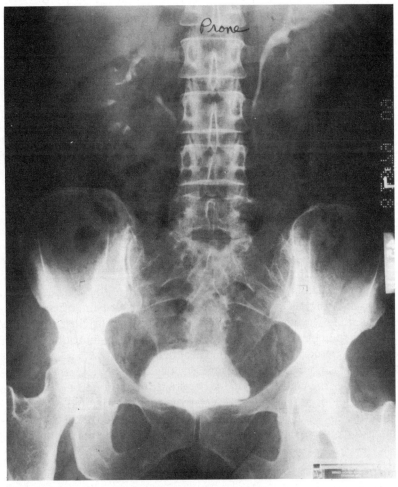

Figure 5-24 Acute radiation cystitis in patient treated for residual carcinoma of cervix after partial hysterectomy. Sources lay close to the bladder and cystitis developed with edematous bladder mucosa, as shown by IVP study.

Rectum

The rectum is more susceptible to radiation injury than any other organ because of its close proximity to the vagina and cervix. Consequently, the normal tissue tolerance of this organ to radiation is often approached. The symptoms of radiation proctitis include frequent bowel movements, tenesmus, pain, and rectal bleeding. Radiation proctitis should be treated by a low-residue diet and medication with Kaopectate or Lomotil. In severe cases, reduction of radiation dose or temporary suspension of treatment may be required. Ulceration of the rectum occurs almost exclusively on the anterior wall at the level corresponding to the maximum dose from the vaginal implant (Strockbine et al 1970). Rectal ulceration will often heal with conservative treatment including steroid enemas. However, persistent ulcers should be biopsied to rule out the presence of recurrent disease. Rectovaginal fistula occurs in approximately 1% of patients undergoing radiation therapy for cervical cancer, and is caused by necrosis of the anterior rectal wall. Proctoscopy and a barium enema should be performed in order to rule out recurrent disease or other associated fistulas. A diverting colostomy should be performed to facilitate healing at the necrotic fistula site. Prior to attempts at surgical correction, the margins of the fistula should be clean with evidence of a reasonable blood supply. As in the repair of vesicovaginal fistula, the surgical correction of a rectovaginal fistula requires transposition of a new source of blood supply to the operative site.

Sigmoid Colon

Sigmoiditis is a relatively common complication of pelvic radiation therapy and is associated with high doses of external therapy (5000 to 6000 rad), particularly when a relatively fixed loop of sigmoid lies close to the implant system. Symptoms of sigmoiditis include pain, often with intermittent diarrhea and constipation. In its severe form, the patient may experience almost constant pain, weakness, and malnutrition. Milder forms of sigmoiditis respond to medical management with a low-residue diet, antispasmodics, and cortisone enemas. However, severe cases require a diverting colostomy and general nutritional support. A rare late complication of radiation is severe narrowing of the sigmoid colon causing partial or complete bowel obstruction (Figure 5-25). This complication also requires performance of a proximal diverting colostomy.

Small Bowel

The mucosa of the small bowel is quite sensitive to radiation, and the patient receiving high doses ($\sim$ 5000 rad) of whole pelvis or extended field radiation may experience ileitis with pain and watery diarrhea. Mild cases respond to Lomotil and antispasmodics, but more severe injury requires temporary interruption of therapy. The terminal ileum is the most common site of small bowel injury because it is fixed at the ileocecal junction and has a relatively poor blood supply. The incidence of small bowel injury is highest in small habitus patients who have had 1) previous surgery with resultant pelvic adhesions, 2) pelvic inflammatory disease,

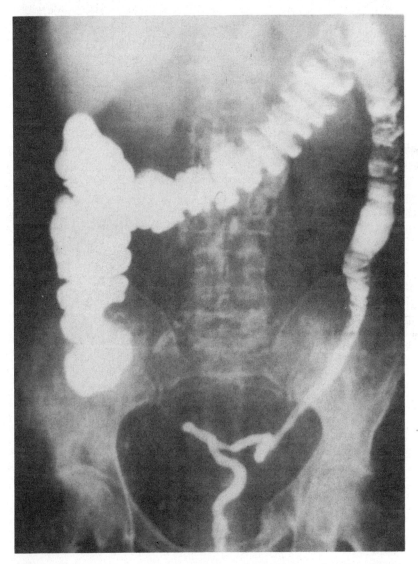

Figure 5-25 Marked stenosis of rectum and sigmoid in patient heavily overtreated for low stage cervical cancer. Patient had chronic diarrhea and "pencil" stools.

144

or 3) severe vascular disease such as hypertension, diabetes or arteriosclerosis (van Nagell et al 1974). Delayed or late small bowel injuries manifest themselves as progressive intermittent bowel obstruction and fistula formation, with or without perforation (Figure 5-26). The patient often presents with postprandial nausea and crampy pain which is relieved by vomiting. Eventually, the patient experiences severe weight

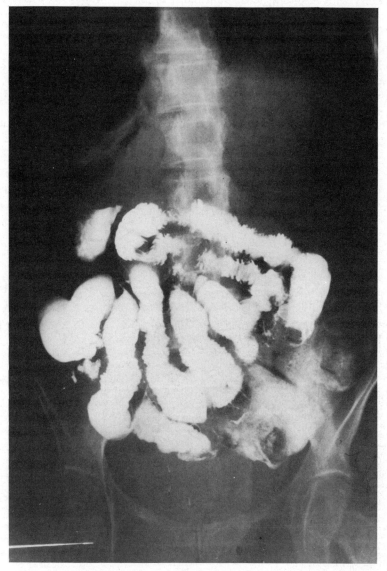

Figure 5-26 Radiation enteritis after high dose pelvic irradiation for cervical carcinoma. Patient had malabsorption syndrome and intermittent small bowel obstruction.

loss and multiple nutritional deficiencies. The diagnosis of small bowel obstruction is confirmed by flat and upright abdominal radiograms. Patients with mild degrees of intermittent obstruction should be treated with conservative measures and nutritional support if possible. When complete small bowel obstruction is diagnosed, however, surgical intervention is required as soon as possible to prevent perforation. A left shift in the white blood count is often indicative of bowel wall necrosis and impending perforation. The area of small bowel obstruction and necrosis may be quite localized (Figure 5-27), indicating a vascular basis for its genesis.

At present there is controversy in the literature concerning the surgical procedure of choice in treating radiation-induced small bowel obstruction. Wheeless (1973) has advocated bypassing the involved segment with the creation of mucous fistulas (Figure 5-28). In contrast, Schmitt and Symmonds (1981) favor excision of the necrotic small bowel with primary anastomosis to the cecum or ascending colon (Figure 5-28). In cases where there is massive pelvic necrosis and fistulization, excision may be impractical. However, in cases of isolated segmental obstruction, primary resection with anastomosis of the ileum to the ascending colon is indicated.

Ureter

Ureteral complications are extremely rare unless very high dose whole pelvis radiation has been given (Slater et al 1971, Villasanta 1972).

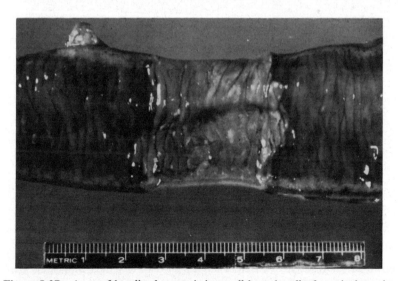

Figure 5-27 Area of localized necrosis in small bowel wall of surgical specimen from patient with radiation-induced small bowel obstruction.

146

Any ureteral abnormality or obstruction that develops following radiation therapy should be considered as evidence of recurrent disease (Bosch
1973, Van Dyke et al 1975). In rare instances, a radiation-related ureteral
stricture can be relieved by incision of dense adhesions around the ureteral
sheath.

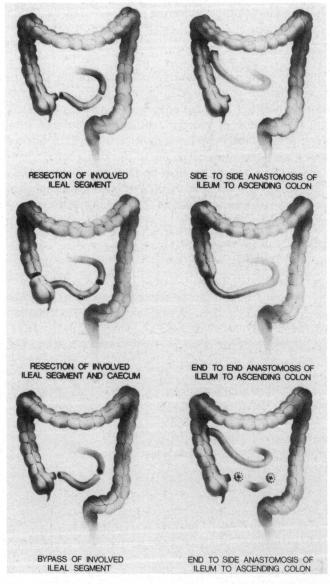

Figure 5-28   Illustration of different surgical procedures in the treatment of small
bowel obstruction with perforation. The procedure of choice must be individualized
to the needs of each patient.

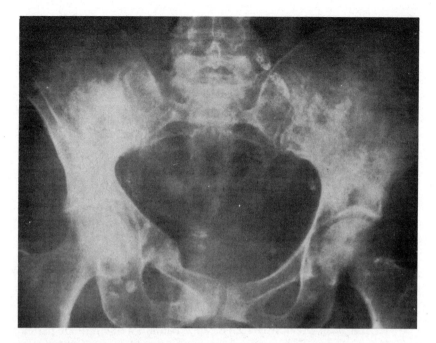

Figure 5-29   Severe osteoradionecrosis of pelvis from orthovoltage radiotherapy of cervical carcinoma. Patient had multiple bone fractures of pelvis.

Skeleton

Femoral neck fractures and pelvic osteoradionecrosis (Figure 5-29) are most commonly seen following orthovoltage therapy. Since megavoltage radiation spares the bone, this complication is rare in present treatment regimens. The treatment of these rare complications must be individualized after orthopedic consultation. Leukemia is rare after radiotherapy (Zippin et al 1971).

SURVIVAL AND FOLLOW-UP

The five-year survival of patients recently treated for invasive cervical cancer in selected cancer centers is presented in Table 5-15. In these centers, the survival is slightly higher, stage for stage, than that compiled and reported from the entire recent literature by the Annual Report on the Results of Treatment in Carcinoma of the Uterine Cervix (see Chapter 4). Although not specifically shown in these statistics, it is pertinent to note that the addition of extrafascial hysterectomy to radiation therapy has produced an increase in the survival of selected patients with bulky, barrel-shaped Stage Ib lesions (van Nagell et al 1979).

Table 5-15
Five-Year Results in Carcinoma of Cervix Uteri

Institution	Cases	Percent Survival by Stage			
		I	II	III	IV
Cancer Institute Hospital (Japan)*	2627	92**	76	49	18
Radiumhemmet (Sweden)*	3767	88	59	21	7
M. D. Anderson T.I. (USA)*	2281	84	61	29	14
The Christie Hospital (England)*	4046	82	55	28	7
Massachusetts General Hospital, Pondville State Hospital (USA)*	803	82	56	19	10
Gustave Roussy (France)*	1299	78	64	29	8
Institute du Radium, Paris (France)*	1087	69	59	27	0
University of Kentucky (USA)†	526	86	70	48	29

* Sixteenth Annual Report on the Results of Treatment in Carcinoma of the Uterus and Vagina (1976) for the period 1959 to 1968.
** Both surgery and radiation are used for Stage I and early Stage II.
† van Nagell and Maruyama, 1979.

As has been previously stated, approximately one half of patients who develop recurrent cervical cancer do so within one year following therapy, and an additional 25% within the second year after treatment. Cure is achieved with 95% certainty in five to seven years (Easson 1973). For this reason, it is recommended that patients be seen at monthly intervals during the first year following therapy, every two months for the next year, and every six months thereafter. Pelvic examination and cervical cytologic sampling should be performed at the time of each visit.

BIBLIOGRAPHY

Abbe R: The use of radium in malignant disease. *Lancet* 2:524, 1913.

Abitbol M, Davenport JH: The irradiated vagina. *Obstet Gynecol* 44:249-256, 1974.

Adams GE: Chemical radiosensitizers of hypoxic cells. *Br Med Bull* 29:48-53, 1973.

Alfert HJ, Gillenwater JY: The consequences of ureteral irradiation with special reference to subsequent ureteral injury. *J Urol* 107:369-371, 1972.

Anderson LL: Status of dosimetry for 252-Cf medical neutron sources. *Phys Med Biol* 18:779-799, 1973.

Andrews JR: The oxygen effect, in *The Radiobiology of Human Cancer Radiotherapy*. Philadelphia, W.B. Saunders Co., 1968, pp 105-147.

Averette HE, Dudan RC, Ford JH, et al: Staging of cervical cancer. *Clin Obstet Gynecol* 18:215-232, 1975.

Baker HRK, Sommers SC, Rotterdam H, et al: Vascular invasion as a prognostic factor in Stage Ib cancer of the cervix. *Obstet Gynecol* 52:353-358, 1978.

Baud J: Carcinoma of the cervix (Stage I) treated intracavitarily with radium alone. *JAMA* 138:1138-1142, 1948.

Bergsjo P, Evans JC: Oxygen tension of cervical carcinoma during the early phases of external radiation. I. Measurements with a Clark Microelectrode. *Scand Clin Lab Invest* 22:159–166, 1968.

Bergman JL, Lagasse LD, Watring W, et al: The operative evaluation of patients with cervical carcinomas by an extraperitoneal approach. *Obstet Gynecol* 50:658–664, 1977.

Bewley DK, Fowler JF, Morgan RL, et al: Experiments on the skin of pigs with fast neutrons or 8 meV x-rays including some effects of dose fractionation. *Br J Radiol* 36.107–115, 1963.

Bewley DK: Pretherapeutic experiments with the fast neutron beam from the medical research council cyclotron. II. Physical aspects of the fast neutron beam. *Br J Radiol* 36:81–88, 1963.

Boag JW: Maximum likelihood estimates of the proportion of patients cured by cancer therapy. *J R Statis Soc* 11:15, 1949.

Boronow RC: Management of radiation-induced vaginal fistulas. *Am J Obstet Gynecol* 110:1–8, 1971.

Boronow RC, Rutledge FN: Vesicovaginal fistula, radiation and gynecologic cancer. *Am J Obstet Gynecol* 111:85–90, 1971.

Bosch A, Marcial VA: Carcinoma of the uterine cervix associated with pregnancy. *Am J Roent* 96:92–99, 1966.

Bosch A, Frias Z: Complications after radiation therapy for cervical carcinoma. *Acta Radiol Ther Phys Biol* 16:53–62, 1977.

Bosch A, Frias Z, deValda G: Prognostic significance of ureteral obstruction in carcinoma of the cervix uteri. *Acta Radiol* 47–56, 1973.

Breitenecker G, Tatra G: Histoautoradiographische untersuchungen wahrend der strahlentherapi des zervixkarzinoms. *Strahlentherapie* 146:664–670, 1973.

Buchler DA, Kline JC, Carr WF: Intracavitary dosimetry for carcinoma of the cervix and subsequent complications. *Am J Obstet Gynecol* 120:83–90, 1974.

Buchler DA, Kline JC, Peckham BM, et al: The relationship of NSD to reactions and complications following treatment for malignant uterine cervical neoplasms. *Rad Biol* 110:687–690, 1974.

Buchsbaum JJ: Para-aortic lymph node involvement in cervical carcinoma. *Am J Obstet Gynecol* 113:942–947, 1972.

Burch WD, Arnold ED, Chetham-Stone A: Production of transuranium elements. *Nuc Sci Eng* 17:438–442, 1963.

Bush RS, Jenkin DT, Allt WEC, et al: Definitive evidence for hypoxic cells influencing cure in cancer therapy. *Br J Cancer* 37 (suppl 3):302–306, 1978.

Caderao JB, Hussey DH, Fletcher GH, et al: Fast neutron radiotherapy for locally advanced pelvic cancer. *Cancer* 37:2620–2629, 1976.

Carlson L, Delcos L, Fletcher GH: Distant metastases in squamous cell carcinoma of the uterine cervix. *Radiol* 88:961–966, 1967.

Castro JR, Issa P, Fletcher GH: Carcinoma of the cervix treated by external irradiation alone. *Radiology* 95:163–166, 1970.

Castro JR, Oliver GD, Withers HR, et al: Experience with californium-252 in clinical radiotherapy. *Am J Roent* 117:182–194, 1973.

Catterall M: The results of randomized and other clinical trials of fast neutrons from the medical research council cyclotron, London. *Int J Rad Onc Biol Phys* 3:247–253, 1977.

Catterall M, Suthercard I, Bewley DK: First results of a randomized clinical trial of fast neutron compared with x- or gamma rays in treatment of advanced tumors of the head and neck. *Br Med J* 21:653–666, 1975.

Caldwell WL, Durand RE: *Clinical Prospects for Hypoxic Cell Sensitizers and Hyperthermia.* Madison, WI, University of Wisconsin, October 1978.

150

Chau PM, Fletcher GH, Rutledge FN, et al: Complications in high dose whole pelvis irradiation in female pelvic cancer. *Am J Roent* 97:22-40, 1962.

Christopherson WM, Lundin FE, Mendez WN, et al: Cervical cancer control: A study of morbidity and mortality trends over a 21-year period. *Cancer* 38:1357-1366, 1976.

Christopherson WM, Parker JE: Relation of cervical cancer to early marriage and childbearing. *N Engl J Med* 273:235-239, 1965.

Cleaves MA: Radium with a preliminary note on radium rays in the treatment of cancer. *J Adv Ther* 21:667-682, 1903.

Cole MP: Radiotherapy for cervical cancer – x-rays, in Easson EC (ed): *Cancer of the Uterine Cervix.* London, WB Saunders, 1973, pp 53-75.

Colvett RD, Rossi HH, Krishnaswamy V: Dose distributions around a californium-252 needle. *Phys Med Biol* 17:356-364, 1972.

Committee for Radiation Oncology Studies: Proposal for a program in particle-beam radiation therapy in the United States. *Cancer Clin Trials* 1:160-165, 1978.

Comroe JH: Experimental studies designed to evaluate the management of patients with incurable cancer. *Proc Natl Acad Sci USA* 75:4543, 1978.

Conroy J, Lewis GC, Brady LW, et al: Low dose bleomycin and methotrexate in cervical cancer. *Cancer* 37:660-664, 1976.

Copeland EM, Daly JM, Dudrick SJ: Nutrition as an adjunct to cancer treatment in the adult. *Cancer Res* 37:2451-2456, 1977.

Creasman WT, Rutledge FN, Fletcher GH: Carcinoma of the cervix associated with pregnancy. *Obstet Gynecol* 36:495-501, 1970.

Creasman WT, Rutledge FN: Preoperative evaluation of patients with recurrent carcinoma of the cervix. *Gynecol Oncol* 1:111-118, 1972.

Daly JW: Vesicovaginal fistula after radiation therapy. *J Fla Med Assoc* 58:25-26, 1971.

Day T, Wharton J, Taylor J, et al: Chemotherapy for squamous carcinoma of the cervix: Doxorubicin methyl CCNU. *Am J Obstet Gynecol* 132: 545-548, 1978.

DeCosse JJ, Rodes RS, Wentz WB, et al: The natural history and management of radiation-induced injury of the gastrointestinal tract. *Ann Surg* 170:369-383, 1969.

Del Regato JA: Transvaginal roentgen therapy in carcinoma of the cervix. *Radiol* 49:413-414, 1947.

Dische S: The hyperbaric oxygen chamber in the radiotherapy of carcinoma of the uterine cervix. *Br J Radiol* 47:99-107, 1974.

Dobson J, Kalberer JT, George FW: Megavoltage radiation-therapy equipment: Performance characteristics and operational costs. *Appl Radiol* 6:105-108, 1977.

Durrance FY, Fletcher GH, Rutledge FN: Analysis of central recurrent diseases in Stages I and II squamous cell carcinoma of the cervix on intact uterus. *Am J Roent* 106:831-838, 1969.

Durrance FY: Radiotherapy following simple hysterectomy in patients with Stage I and II carcinoma of the cervix. *Am J Roent* 102:165-169, 1968.

Easson EC, Russell MH: *Uterine Cervix in the Curability of Cancer in Various Sites.* Baltimore, MD, Williams and Wilkins, 69-75, 1968.

Easson EC: *Cancer of the Uterine Cervix.* London, W.B. Saunders, 1973.

Einhorn N: Frequency of seven complications after radiation therapy for cervical carcinoma. *Acta Radiol Ther Phys Biol* 14:42-48, 1975.

Ellis F: Nominal standard dose and the ret. *Br J Radiol* 44:101-108, 1971.

Evans JC, Bergsjo P: Influence of anaemia on the results of radiotherapy in cancer of the cervix. *Radiology* 84:709-716, 1965.

Fairchild RG, Drew RN, Atkins HL: Dose rate effects for various dose rates of 252-Cf radiation on hela cells in culture. *Radiology* 96:171–174, 1970.

Feola J, Maruyama Y: Radiobiological considerations for pions in radiotherapy. *Oncology* 25:536–557, 1971.

Fletcher GH: Background of present dose-time fractionation practice, in *Time and Dose in Radiotherapy*. Brookhaven Symposium, 1969, pp 260–267.

Fletcher GH: Current views on radiotherapy of cancer of the uterine cervix, in *Cancer of the Uterus and Ovary*. MDAH Symposium. Chicago, Yearbook Medical Publishers Inc, 183–194, 1969.

Fletcher GH: Cancer of the uterine cervix. *Am J Roent* 111:225–242, 1971.

Fletcher GH, Rutledge FN: Extended Field Technique in the Management of the Cancers of Uterine Cervix. *Am J Roent* 114:116–122, 1972.

Fletcher GH: Clinical dose response of human malignant epithelial tumors. *Br J Radiol* 46:1–12, 1973.

Fowler JR, Morgan RL, Wood CAP: Pretherapeutic experiments with the fast neutron beam from the medical research council cyclotron. I. The biological and physical advantages and problems of neutron therapy. *Br J Radiol* 36:77–80, 1963.

Friberg LG, Johnsson JE: Bladder and intestinal injuries following intracavitary irradiation of carcinoma of the uterine cervix. *Acta Radiol Ther* (Stockholm) 13:288–296, 1974.

Fu KK, Philips TL, Rowe JR: The RBE of neutrons in vivo. *Cancer* 34:48–53, 1974.

Gothlin JH: Postlymphographic percutaneous fine needle biopsy of lymph nodes guided by fluoroscopy. *Radiology* 120:205–207, 1976.

Gray LH, Conger AD, Ebert M, et al: The concentration of oxygen dissolved in tissue at the time of irradiation as a factor in radiotherapy. *Br J Radiol* 26:638–648, 1953.

Grossman J, Kurohara SS, Webster JH, et al: The prognostic significance of tumor response during radiotherapy in cervical carcinoma. *Radiology* 107:411–415, 1973.

Gustafsson DC, Kottmeier HL: Carcinoma of the cervix associated with pregnancy. Study of Radiumhemmets' series of cases during the period 1953-1956. *Acta Obstet Gynecol Scand* 41:1–21, 1962.

Gusberg SB, Fish SA, Wang YY: The growth pattern of cervical cancer. *Obstet Gynecol* 2:557–561, 1953.

Gusberg SB: The diagnosis and treatment of cancer, in Clark RL, Cumley RW, et al (eds): *Oncology Vol IV*. Chicago, Yearbook Medical Publishers Inc, 1970, pp 250–256.

Guthrie RT, Buchsbaum HJ, White AJ, et al: Para-aortic lymph node irradiation in carcinoma of the uterine cervix. *Cancer* 34:166–168, 1974.

Hall EJ, Rossi HH: The potential of californium-252 in radiotherapy. Preclinical measurements in physics and radiobiology. *Br J Radiol* 48:477–490, 1975.

Hansen LH, Collins CG: Multicentric squamous cell carcinomas of the lower female genital tract. *Am J Obstet Gynecol* 98:982–986, 1967.

Hardt N, van Nagell JR, Hanson M, et al: Radiation-induced tumor regression as a prognostic factor in patients with invasive cervical cancer. *Cancer* (In press).

Hartman P, Diddle AW: Vaginal stenosis following irradiation therapy for carcinoma of the cervix uteri. *Cancer* 30:426–429, 1972.

Henriksen E: The lymphatic spread of carcinoma of the cervix and of the body of the uterus. *Am J Obstet Gynecol* 58:924–942, 1949.

Henriksen E: Distribution of metastases in Stage I carcinoma of the cervix. *Am J Obstet Gynecol* 80:919–932, 1960.

Herbst AL, Scully RE, Robboy SJ, et al: Stilbestrol-induced abnormalities of the genital tract in young women. *Prog Gynecol* 6:647–668, 1975.

Hoskins B, Wrede DE, Maruyama Y, et al: Computer dosimetry based upon pelvic simulation. *Acta Radiol* 14:362–368, 1975.

Hreshchyshyn MM: Experiences with chemotherapy in gynecologic cancer. *NY State J Med* 64:2431–2434, 1964.

Hreshchyshyn MM, Aaron BS, Boronow RC, et al: Hydroxyurea or placebo combined with radiation to treat Stages IIIb and IV cervical cancer confined to the pelvis. *Int J Rad Onc Biol Phys* 5:317–322, 1979.

Hughes R, Brewington K, Hanjani P, et al: Extended field irradiation for cervical cancer based on surgical staging. *Oncology* 9:153–161, 1980.

Hussey DH, Parker RG, Eager CC: Evolution of dosage schedules at the fast neutron therapy facilities in the United States. *Int J Rad Onc Biol Phys* 3:255–267, 1977.

Jampolis S, Andres J, Fletcher GH: Analysis of sites and causes of failure of irradiation in invasive squamous cell carcinoma of the intact uterine cervix. *Radiology* 115:681–685, 1975.

Joelsson I, Backstrom A: Applicators for remote afterloading technique for optimum pelvic dose distribution in carcinoma of the uterine cervix. *Acta Radiol Ther Phys Biol* 9:233–238, 1970.

Joelsson I, Raf L, Soderberg G: Stenosis of the small bowel as a complication in radiation therapy of carcinoma of the uterine cervix. *Acta Radiol Ther Phys Biol* 10:593–604, 1971.

Joelsson I, Ruden BI, Corta A, et al: Determination of dose distribution in the pelvis by measurement and by computer in gynecologic radiation therapy. *Acta Radiol Ther Phys Biol* 11:289–304, 1972.

Johnson JE, Noldberg UB: Dosimetry of combined intracavitary and external irradiation of carcinoma of the uterine cervix. *Acta Radiol* 14:251–256, 1975.

Johnson JE: Squamous cell carcinoma of the uterine cervix. *Acta Radiol* 16:33–51, 1977.

Jones TK, Levitt SH, King ER: Retreatment of persistent and recurrent carcinoma of the cervix with irradiation. *Radiology* 95:167–174, 1970.

Kademian MT, Busch A: Staging laparotomy and survival in carcinoma of the uterine cervix. *Acta Radiol Ther Phys Biol* 16:314–327, 1977.

Kal HB, Barendsen GW: The OER at low dose rates. Letters to the Editor. *Brit J Radiol* 49:1049–1051, 1976.

Kallman RF: The phenomenon of reoxygenation and its implications for fractionated radiotherapy. *Radiology* 105:134–142, 1972.

Kerst DW: The betatron. *Radiology* 40:115–120, 1943.

Kline JC, Schultz AE, Vermund H, et al: High dose radiotherapy for carcinoma of the cervix. *Am J Obstet Gynecol* 104:479–484, 1969.

Kline JC, Buchler DA, Boone ML, et al: The relationships of reactions to complication in radiation therapy of cancer of the cervix. *Radiology* 105:413–416, 1977.

Koller O: *A Colpophotographic Study of the Vascular Pattern of the Uterine Cervix with Special Reference to Precancerous Lesions and Cancer.* Oslo, Sweden, Oslo Universitetsforlaget, 1963.

Kolstad P: *Vascularization, Oxygen Tension and Radiocurability in Cancer of the Cervix.* Norwegian Monograph on Medical Science, Scandanavian University Books, Oslo, Sweden, Oslo Universitetsforlaget, 1964.

Kottmeier HL, Gray MJ: Rectal and bladder injuries in relation to radiation-dosage in carcinoma of the cervix. *Am J Obstet Gynecol* 82:74–82, 1961.

Kottmeier HL: Complications following radiation therapy in carcinoma of the cervix. *Am J Obstet Gynecol* 88:854–866, 1964.

Kottmeier HL: Surgical and radiation treatment of carcinoma of the uterine cervix. *Acta Obstet Gynecol Scand* 43:1–48, 1964.

Kottmeier HL: Surgical and radiation treatment of carcinoma of the uterine cervix. *Gynecol Clin Radiumhemmet* 43:1–48, 1964.

Kottmeier HL: Evaluation of treatment of recurrence after surgery and radiotherapy for carcinoma of the cervix, in *Cancer of the Uterus and Ovary.* MDAH Symposium. Chicago, Yearbook Medical Publishers Inc, pp 283–295, 1969.

Kottmeier HL: *Annual Report on the Results of Treatment in Carcinoma of the Uterus, Vagina, and Ovary,* vol 16. International Federation of Gynecology and Obstetrics, Stockholm, Sweden, 1976.

Krishnaswamy V: Calculation of the dose distribution about californium-252 needles in tissue. *Radiology* 98:155–160, 1971.

Kurohara SS, Vongtama VY, Webster JH, et al: Post-irradiation recurrent epidermoid carcinoma of the uterine cervix. *Am J Roent* 111:249–259, 1971.

Lacassagne A: La radiotherapie des epitheliomas du col uterin a l'Inst du Radium, Paris. *Arch de l'Inst du Radium* 2:95–132, 1930.

Lagasse LD, Ballon SC, Berman ML, et al: Pretreatment lymphangiography and operative evaluation in carcinoma of the cervix. *Am J Obstet Gynecol* 134:219–224, 1979.

Lang EK, Wood M, Brown R, et al: Complications in the urinary tract related to treatment of carcinoma of the cervix. *South Med J* 66:228–236, 1973.

Lepanto P, Littman P, Mikuta J, et al: Treatment of para-aortic nodes in carcinoma of the cervix. *Cancer* 35:1510–1513, 1975.

Levin W, Blair RN: Clinical experiences with combined whole body hyperthermia and medication in Streffer C (ed): *Cancer Therapy by Hyperthermia and Radiation.* Baltimore, MD, Urban and Schwartzenberg, 1978, pp 322–325.

Lu T, Macasaet MA, Nelson JH: The barrel-shaped cervical carcinoma. *Am J Obstet Gynecol* 124:596–600, 1976.

Malkasian GD Jr: Gynecological chemotherapy in Sciarra J (ed): *Gynecology and Obstetrics.* Hagerstown, MD, Harper and Row, 1977, pp 1–18.

Marcial VA, Bosch A: Radiation-induced tumor regression in carcinoma of the uterine cervix: Prognostic significance. *Am J Roent* 108:113–123, 1970.

Marcial VA: Carcinoma of the cervix. Present status and future. *Cancer* 39:945–958, 1977.

Marcial-Rojas RA, Meigs JV: Cancer of the cervix uteri. A review of 169 necropsied cases. *Am J Pathol* 31:1077–1082, 1955.

Maruyama Y: Indirect effects of radiation upon tumor response in vivo. *Radiology* 91:657–668, 1968.

Maruyama Y, Wrede DE, Sowell G, et al: Probe check of computer dosimetry for gynecological implant therapy. *Acta Radiol* 13:49–56, 1974.

Maruyama Y, van Nagell JR, Wrede DE, et al: Approaches to optimization of dose in radiation therapy of cervix carcinoma. *Radiology* 120:389–398, 1976.

Maruyama Y: Evidence for reinitiation of proliferative activity following alkylation or radiation. *Int J Rad Oncol Biol Phys* 1:903–909, 1976.

Maruyama Y, Feola J: Changes in cell age cohort composition of tumors and normal tissues by radiation and chemotherapy. *Rev Int Am de Radiol* 1:1–7, 1976.

Maruyama Y, van Nagell JR, Martin A, et al: Method for localizing and calculating vaginal dose in brachytherapy. *Radiology* 124:507–517, 1977.

Maruyama Y (ed): *New Methods in Tumor Localization.* Lexington, KY, University of Kentucky, 1977.

Maruyama Y: Radiation-induced cycling activity and chemosensitivity of normal tissues. *Rev Int Am de Radiol* 3:79–87, 1978.

Maruyama Y, Feola J, Tai D, et al: Californium Cf-252 for pelvic radiotherapy. *Oncology* 35:172-178, 1978.

Maruyama Y, van Nagell JR, Utley J, et al: Radiation and small bowel complications in cervical carcinoma therapy. *Radiology* 12:699-703, 1974.

Maruyama Y, Paig C, Yoneda J, et al: Experiences with an alternative method of anesthesia for intracavitary therapy of pelvic carcinoma. *Radiology* 13:216-217, 1979.

Maruyama Y: Rapid clearance of advanced pelvic carcinomas by californium Cf-252 Therapy. *Radiology* 133:473-475, 1979.

Maruyama Y, Yoneda J, Krolikiewicz H, et al: Report on early responses in a clinical trial for advanced cervico-vaginal carcinomas using californium Cf-252 fast neutron therapy. *Int J Rad Oncol Phys Biol* 6:1629-1637, 1980.

Maruyama Y, Beach JL, Feola J: Scheduling of hypoxic tumor therapy using neutron brachytherapy. *Radiology* 137:755-781, 1980.

Maruyama Y, Yoneda J, van Nagell JR, et al: Tumor regression and histological clearance after neutron brachytherapy for large localized cervical carcinomas by combined radiation and surgery. *Cancer.* Accepted for Publication.

Mason GR, Dietrich P, Friedland GW, et al: The radiological findings in radiation-induced enteritis and colitis. A review of 30 cases. *Clin Radiol* 21:232-247, 1970.

Mathe G: Study of the efficacy of bleomycin in human cancer. *Br Med J* 2:643-645, 1970.

Mendecki J, Friedenthal E, Botstein L: Introduction of hyperthermia in deep seated tumors by a special microwave applicator, in Streffer C (ed): *Cancer Therapy in Hyperthermia and Radiation.* Baltimore, MD, Urban and Schwarzerberg. 1977, pp 125-127.

Mickal A, Torres JE, Schlosser JV: Complications of therapy for carcinoma of the cervix. *Am J Obstet Gynecol* 112:556-565, 1972.

Michsche M, Luger T, Michalica W, et al: Investigations on general immune reactivity in untreated cervical cancer patients. *Oncology* 35:206-209, 1978.

Miller CW: Recent developments in linear accelerators for therapy. *Br J Radiol* 35:182-185, 1962.

Miller CW: Cancer of the Uterine Cervix, in Kaplan HS, Tsuchitani PJ (eds): *Cancer in China.* New York, A.R. Liss, 1978, pp 140-143.

Miyamoto T: A sequential combination of bleomycin and mitomycin C (B-M) in the treatment of metastatic cervical cancer, in Carter SK, Crooley ST, Umezawa H (eds): *An Overview of Clinical Studies in the United States on Bleomycin: Current Status and New Developments.* New York, Academic Press, 1978, pp 185-190.

Moller C, Mellin L: Radiation proctocolitis. Incidence and clinical features. *Ann Chir Gynaecol* 59:94-100, 1970.

Morales A, Steyn J: Late development of vesical fistulas following radiotherapy for carcinoma of the cervix. *Arch Surg* 104:836-837, 1972.

Nelson JH, Macasaet MA, Lu T, et al: The incidence and significance of para-aortic lymph node metastases in late invasive carcinoma of the cervix. *Am J Obstet Gynecol* 118:749-756, 1974.

Nelson AJ, Fletcher GH, Wharton JJ: Indications for adjunctive conservative extrafascial hysterectomy in selected cases of carcinoma of the uterine cervix. *Am J Roent* 123:91-99, 1975.

Nieminen U, Pollanen L, Forss M: Vaginal fistulae following radiotherapy for carcinoma of the cervix uteri. *Ann Chir Gynaecol* 59:90-93, 1970.

Nolan JF, DuSault L: Optimum dosage studies for radiation therapy of carcinoma of uterine cervix. *Radiology* 62:862-867, 1954.

NCRP Report No. 39: *Basic Radiation Protection Criteria.* Washington, DC, 1971.

Onai Y, Tomaru T, Ififuna T, et al: Construction of storage, remote afterloader and treatment facility for californium-252 medical sources and radiation protection survey. *Nippon Acta Radiol* 38:642–653, 1978.

Orton CG, Ellis F: A simplification in the use of the NSD concept in practical radiotherapy. *Br J Radiol* 46:529–532, 1973.

Palmer Saunders, J: The cancer center: Its coordinating role. *Hosp Pract* 11:16, 1978.

Papavisiliou C, Angelakis P, Gouvalis P, et al: Treatment of cervical carcinoma by methotrexate combined with cyclophosphamide. *Cancer Chemother Rep* 53:255–261, 1969.

Paterson R: *Treatment of Malignant Disease by Radium and X-rays.* Baltimore, MD, William and Wilkins, 1948.

Paterson R: Clinical trials in malignant disease — part I. Principles of random selection. *J Fac Radiologists* 9:80–85, 1957.

Paterson R, Russell MH: Clinical trials in malignant disease. VI. Cancer of the cervix. Is x-ray therapy more effective given before or after radium? *Clin Radiol* 13:313–315, 1962.

Paterson R, Russell MH: Clinical trials in malignant disease. VII. Cancer of the cervix uteri. Evaluation of adjuvant x-ray therapy in Stages 1 and 2 — interim report. *Clin Radiol* 14:17–19, 1963.

Paunier JP, Delclos L, Fletcher GH: Causes, time of death and sites of failure in squamous cell carcinoma on the uterine cervix on intact uterus. *Radiology* 88:555–562, 1967.

Peckham BM, Kline HC, Schultz AE, et al: Radiation dosage and complications in cervical cancer therapy. *Am J Obstet Gynecol* 104:485–494, 1969.

Perez CA, Vnuska Z, Askin F, et al: Prognostic significance of endometrial extension from primary carcinoma of the uterine cervix. *Cancer* 35:1493–1504, 1975.

Perez CA, Breaux S, Madoc-Jones J, et al: Correlation between radiation dose and tumor recurrence and complications in carcinoma of the uterine cervix: Stages I and II. *Int J Rad Oncol Biol Physics* 5:373–383, 1979.

Peters LJ, Hussey DH, Fletcher GH, et al: Preliminary report of the M.D. Anderson Hospital Texas A & M variable energy cyclotron fast neutron therapy pilot study. *Am J Roent* 132:637–642, 1979.

Phillips TL: The interaction of drug and radiation effects on normal tissue. *Int J Rad Oncol Biol Physics* 4:59–64, 1978.

Peirquin B: The destiny of brachytherapy in oncology. *Am J Roent* 123:495–499, 1976.

Piver MS, Barlow JJ: Para-aortic lymphadenectomy, aortic node biopsy lymphangiograph in staging patients with advanced cancer. *Cancer* 32:367–370, 1973.

Piver MS, Chung WS: Prognostic significance of cervical lesion size and pelvic node metastases in cervical carcinoma. *Obstet Gynecol* 46:507–512, 1975.

Piver MS, Vongtama V, Barlow JJ: Para-aortic lymph node irradiation for carcinoma of the uterine cervix using split course technique. *Gynecol Oncol* 3:168–175, 1975.

Piver MS, Barlow JJ: High dose irradiation to biopsy confirmed aortic node metastases from carcinoma of the uterine cervix. *Cancer* 38:1234–1246, 1977.

Pomp H: Clinical applications of hyperthermia in gynecological malignant tumors, in Streffer C (ed): *Cancer Therapy by Hyperthermia and Radiation.* Baltimore, MD, Urban and Schwarzenberg, 1978, pp 326–327.

Pride GL, Buchler DA: Carcinoma of the vagina 10 or more years following pelvic irradiation therapy. *Am J Obstet Gynecol* 127:513–517, 1977.

156

Punnonen R, Gronroos M, Rauramo L: Complications following radiotherapy in gynaecological carcinoma—comparison between x-ray and megavoltage therapy. *Ann Chir Gynaecol* 65:62-67, 1976.

Quimby E, Glasser D, Taylor LS, et al (eds): *Physical Foundations of Radiology.* NY, Hubler, 1959.

Reagan JW, Harmonic MJ, Wentz WB: Analytical study of cells in cervical squamous cell cancer. *Lab Invest* 5:241-250, 1957.

Regaud C, Fernoux R: Discordance, des effets des rayons X, d'une part dans lapeau, d'autre part dans le testicule, par le fractionnement de la dose: Dimution de l'efficacite dans le peau, maintein de l'efficacite dans le testicule. *CR Soc Biol* 97:431-434, 1927.

Roddick JW, Greenlaw RH: Treatment of Cervical Cancer. *Am J Obstet Gynecol* 109:754-764, 1971.

Rousseau J, Fenton J, Debertrand PH, et al: Carcinoma of the cervix. A 7 year study on 1,212 cases treated at Foundation Curie, Paris. *Radiology* 103:413-418, 1972.

Rutledge FN: Can irradiation destroy metastatic pelvic lymph nodes? *JAMA* 193:1102-1103, 1965.

Rutledge FN, Gutierrez AG, Fletcher GH: Management of Stage I and II adenocarcinomas of the uterine cervix on intact uterus. *Am J Roent* 102:161-164, 1968.

Rutledge FN, Galakatos AE, Wharton JT, et al: Adenocarcinoma of the uterine cervix. *Am J Obstet Gynecol* 122:236-243, 1975.

Rutledge FN, Wharton JT, Fletcher GH: Clinical studies with adjunctive surgery and irradiation therapy in the treatment of carcinoma of the cervix. *Cancer* 38:596-602, 1976.

Saunders JE: Analysis of dose, dose-rate and treatment time in the production of injuries by radium treatment for cancer of the uterine cervix. Letter. *Br J Radiol* 50:151, 1977.

Schabel FM: Experimental basis for adjuvant chemotherapy, in Salmon SS, Jones SE (eds): *Adjuvant Therapy of Cancer.* New York, Elsevier, 1977, pp 3-14.

Schellhas H: Extraperitoneal para-aortic node dissection through an uppor abdominal incision. *Obstet Gynecol* 46:444-447, 1975.

Schmitt EH, Symmonds RE: Intestinal radiation injuries: resection *vs* bypass. *Obstet Gynecol* (In press).

Schmitz RL, Chao JH, Bartolome JS: Intestinal injuries incidental to irradiation of carcinoma of the cervix of the uterus. *Surg Gynecol Obstet* 138:29-32, 1974.

Schwarz G: An evaluation of the Manchester system of treatment of carcinoma of the cervix. *Am J Roent* 105:579-585, 1969.

Sheline GE, Phillips TL, Field SB, et al: Effects of fast neutrons on human skin. *Am J Roent* 111:31, 1971.

Shierholz JD, Buchsbaum HJ, Lipshitz S, et al: Pyometra complicating radiation therapy of uterine malignancy. *J Reprod Med* 19:100-102, 1977.

Shingleton HM, Fowler WC, Pepper FD, et al: Ureteral strictures following therapy for carcinoma of the cervix. *Cancer* 24:77-83, 1969.

Shukovsky LJ: Dose-time volume relationships in squamous cell carcinoma of the supraglottic larynx. *Am J Roent* 108:27-29, 1970.

Silberstein AB, Aaron BS, Alexander LL: Para-aortic lymph node irradiation in cervical carcinoma. *Radiology* 95:181-184, 1970.

Slater JM, Fletcher GH: Ureteral stricture after radiation therapy for carcinoma of the uterine cervix. *Am J Roent* 111:269-272, 1971.

Smith JP, Rutledge FN, Burns BC, et al: Systemic chemotherapy for carcinoma of the cervix. *Am J Obstet Gynecol* 97:800-807, 1967.

Stone RS: Neutron therapy and specific ionization. *Am J Roent* 59:771–785, 1948.

Strandquist M: Studien uben die kumulative wirkung der rontgen strahlen bei fraktionierung. *Acta Radiol* (suppl) 55:1–300, 1944.

Streffer C (ed): *Cancer Therapy by Hyperthermia and Radiation*. Baltimore, MD, Urban and Schwartzenberg, 1978.

Strockbine MF, Hancock JE, Fletcher GH: Complications in 831 patients with squamous cell carcinoma of the intact uterine cervix treated with 3,000 rad or more whole pelvis irradiation. *Am J Roent* 108:293–304, 1970.

Suit HD, Moore EB, Fletcher GH, et al: Modification of Fletcher ovoid system for afterloading, using standard-sized radium tubes. *Radiology* 81:126, 1963.

Suzuki M, Watanabe M, Sato A: Effect of bleomycin on gynecological carcinomas in Gann monograph on cancer research #19. *Fundamental and Clinical Study of Bleomycin*. Tokyo, University Park Press. 1976, pp 221–230.

Swan DS, Roddick JW: A clinical-pathological correlation of cell type classification of cervical cancer. *Am J Obstet Gynecol* 116:666–670, 1973.

Tai D, Maruyama Y: Assessment of neutron/gamma ray ratios in californium Cf-252 pelvic therapy. *Radiology* 128:795–797, 1978.

Tai D, Maruyama Y: Application of linear programming to dose optimization in intracavitary therapy. *Acta Radiol* 18:337–366, 1979.

Thomlinson RH, Gray LH: The histological structure of some human cancers and possible implications for radiotherapy. *Br J Cancer* 9:539–549, 1959.

Thomson JM, Spratt JS: Factors affecting survival in over 500 patients with Stage II carcinoma of the cervix. *Radiology* 123:181–183, 1977.

Thompson SG, Street K Jr, Ghiorso A, et al: The new element californium (atomic no. 198), *Phys Rev* 80:790–796, 1950.

Tod MC: Optimum dosage in the treatment of cancer of the cervix by radiation. *Acta Radiol* 28:564–575, 1957.

Tod MC, Meredith WJ: A dosage system for use in the treatment of cancer of the uterine cervix. *Br J Radiol* 11:809–823, 1938.

Tod MC, Meredith WJ: Treatment of cancer of the cervix uteri. A revised "Manchester Method". *Br J Radiol* 25:252–257, 1953.

Tsuya A, Kaneta K, Onai Y, et al: Clinical experience with californium-252 (first report). *Nippon Acta Radiol* 37:238–247, 1977.

UcMakli A, Bonney WA: Retroperitoneal lymph node metastases in untreated cancer of the uterine cervix. *Radiology* 113:173–175, 1974.

Underwood PB, Lutz MH, Smoak DL: Ureteral injury following irradiation therapy for carcinoma of the cervix. *Obstet Gynecol* 49:663–669, 1977.

Urtasun RC, Bard PR, Chapman JD, et al: Radiation and high dose metronidazole in supratentorial glioblastoma. *N Engl J Med* 294:1364–1367, 1976.

Vaeth JM: Combined effects of chemotherapy and radiotherapy on normal tissue tolerance, in *Frontiers of Radiation Therapy and Oncology*, vol 13. Baltimore, MD, University Park Press, 1978.

Van Dyke AH, van Nagell JR: The prognostic significance of ureteral obstruction in patients with recurrent carcinoma of the cervix uteri. *Surg Gynecol Obstet* 141:371–373, 1975.

van Nagell JR, Parker JC, Maruyama Y, et al: Bladder or rectal injury following radiation therapy for cervical cancer. *Am J Obstet Gynecol* 119:727–733, 1974.

van Nagell JR, Maruyama Y, Parker JC, et al: Small bowel injury following radiation therapy for cervical cancer. *Am J Obstet Gynecol* 118:163–167, 1974.

van Nagell JR, Donaldson ES, Wood EG, et al: Small cell carcinoma of the uterine cervix. *Cancer* 40:2243–2249, 1977.

158

van Nagell JR, Parker JC, Maruyama Y, et al: The effect of pelvic inflammatory disease on enteric complications following radiation therapy for cervical cancer. *Am J Obstet Gynecol* 128:767–771, 1977.

van Nagell JR, Kielar R, Donaldson ES, et al: Correlation between retinal and pelvic vascular status: a determinant factor in patients undergoing pelvic irradiation for gynecologic malignancy. *Am J Obstet Gynecol* 134:551–555, 1979.

van Nagell JR, Rayburn W, Donaldson ES, et al: Therapeutic implications of patterns of recurrence in cancer of the uterine cervix. *Cancer* 44:2354–2361, 1979.

Vider M, Maruyama Y, Narvaez R, et al: Significance of the vertebral venous (Batson's) plexus in metastatic spread of colorectal carcinoma. *Cancer* 40:67–71, 1976.

Villasanta U: Complications of radiotherapy for carcinoma of the uterine cervix. *Am J Obstet Gynecol* 114:717–726, 1972.

Vongtama V, Piver MS, Tsukada Y, et al: Para-aortic node irradiation in carcinoma. *Cancer* 34:169–174, 1974.

Wall JA, Collins VP, Hudgins PT, et al: Carcinoma of the cervix: Review of clinical experience during a 20-year period (1946–1965). *Am J Obstet Gynecol* 96:57–63, 1966.

Walter LH, Cherry CP, Glucksmanns A: Serial biopsies, in Deeley TJ (ed): *Gynecological Neoplasms.* New York, Appleton-Century-Crofts, 1974, p 114.

Wasserman TH: Bleomycin and radiotherapy, in Carter SK, Crooly ST, Umezawa H (eds): *An Overview of Clinical Studies in the United States on Bleomycin: Current Status and New Development.* New York, Academic Press, 1978, pp 253–265.

Watson ER, Halnow KE, Dische S, et al: Hyperbaric oxygen and radiotherapy: A medical research council trial in carcinoma of the cervix. *Br J Radiol* 51:879–887, 1978.

Wentz WB, Reagan JW: Survival in cervical cancer with respect to cell type. *Cancer* 12:384–388, 1959.

Wentz, WB: Histologic grade and survival in cervical cancer. *Obstet Gynecol* 18:412–416, 1961.

Wentz WB, Lewis GC: Correlation of histologic morphology and survival in cervical cancer following radiation therapy. *Obstet Gynecol* 26:229–232, 1965.

Wharton JT: Pretreatment evaluation and therapy selection for patients with invasive carcinoma of the cervix, in Rutledge F, Boronow RC, Wharton JT (eds): *Gynecologic Oncology* New York, J. Wiley and Sons, 1976, pp 21–25.

Wheeless CR: Small bowel bypass for complications related to pelvic malignancy. *Obstet Gynecol* 42:661, 1973.

Wilson LC, Maruyama Y: Safety considerations in radioactive implant therapy. *Appl Radiol* 3:57–59, 1974.

Zippin C, Bailar JC, Kohn HJ, et al: Radiation therapy for cervical cancer. Late effects on life span on leukemia incidence. *Cancer* 28:937–942, 1971.

Zornoza J, Wallace S, Goldstein JM, et al: Transperitoneal percutaneous retroperitoneal lymph node aspiration *Biopsy Rad* 122:111–115, 1977.

Zornoza J, Lukeman JM, Jing BS, et al: Percutaneous retroperitoneal lymph node biopsy in carcinoma of the cervix. *Gynecol Oncol* 5:43–51, 1977.

6 Recurrent Cervical Cancer

Hugh R. K. Barber

The problem of recurrent or persistent cancer of the cervix after an attempted cure by some modality of therapy, usually radiation, is a serious problem, one that taxes the ingenuity of the responsible physician and the resources of the hospital. The fact remains that the majority of patients with cancer of the cervix given primary treatment, usually radiation, are still dying of the disease.

During the past three decades at least two important contributions have been made to the management of gynecologic oncology in cervical cancer: 1) The cytologic screening test adapted to the early detection of malignant changes in the cervix by Papanicolaou. This also serves as an aid to early diagnosis of a recurrence following primary treatment of cancer of the cervix. 2) The treatment, as well as the rehabilitation, of patients with advanced cancer of the cervix, as described by Brunschwig. This investigator also demonstrated that, following radiation therapy failure recurrence, an appreciable degree of salvage of these patients is made possible by appropriate surgery if extrapelvic metastases have not occurred. Desultory, intensive palliation by means of renewed radiation therapy and sedation as needed had heretofore been the lot of these unfortunate patients.

HOST RESISTANCE AND TYPE OF TUMOR

It is important to digress for a moment and search for an explanation to throw light upon the apparent response of certain tumors to treatment, and lack of response by others. There are two intangibles that are under investigation, which as yet have not been resolved, namely, the type of tumor and host resistance. Brunschwig et al (1964), as well as others, have reported on the problem of host resistance, with particular reference to gynecologic cancer, but the problem of type of tumor has received less attention. Green (1952) has directed attention to the tumor by evaluating its potential for growth and differentiation after implantation into the anterior chamber of the rabbit's eye. A study demonstrated that one group was heterotransplantable and associated with a rapidly fatal course, while the other group was not heterotransplantable, and the patients lived for considerable periods of time. While the tumors appeared to be the same histologically, there was a marked difference in growth potential among them. Employing this observation for evaluating tumor growth in humans, an argument can be advanced for the existence of pseudotumor having a histologic appearance similar to that seen in rapidly growing tumors, but characterized by a weak growth potential. The impression that true as well as pseudo cancer exists offers an explanation for certain peculiarities in tumor behavior. It is not inconceivable that pseudo cancers constitute the greatest number of malignancies of the cervix and account for the cures, whereas true cancers resist all efforts at cure.

Undoubtedly, sufficient facts have accumulated, and only new approaches and application of this information within the overall framework of the interrelationship between the type of tumor and host resistance are needed. This concept is based on the presupposition that biological phenomena and the molecular approach to the problem eventually can be evaluated in terms of physical and chemical principles.

CANCER TREATMENT

Surgery

Today, surgery offers patients with many types of cancer more chance for a cure than any other known treatment. For this reason, surgery is the most widely used form of cancer therapy. Surgical procedures have inherent limitations in the total cure of the cancer patient, but their great importance in the management of early cancer now and in the foreseeable future makes it imperative that all areas of possible improvement be exploited. The defense of this statement is that cancer in situ of the uterine cervix accounts for over 45,000 new cases annually. It is obvious that most of these are treated surgically.

Curative surgery   To cure cancer by surgery, treatment must take place before the cancer has spread and become established beyond the tissues that can be removed. During the past century, increasingly extensive operations for cancer were devised and evaluated, and such procedures are now carried out wherever good cancer care is practiced.

Despite the increasing extent of the procedures, the risk of surgical operations for cancer has been and still is being progressively reduced. This has permitted application of surgical methods to more and more patients whose cardiovascular status, kidney function, or general metabolism is seriously impaired. Such concomitant handicaps are, of course, frequent in the older age groups. This reduction in operative risk is absolutely crucial to the application of preventive surgery, the removal of suspicious tumors or ulcerations, or the removal of certain pathologic areas which predispose to cancer.

Recent attempts to establish even more extensive surgical procedures have not resulted in increased rates of cure, and there now appears to be relatively little prospect of major advances from more extensive removal of tissues.

Importance of Early Diagnosis

Good surgical treatment is now able to cure, using the five-year criterion, at least 95% of patients with skin cancer, about 60% of women with breast cancer (virtually all of those in which the disease remains localized), about 40% of patients with cancer of the colon and rectum, and 70% of women with cancer of the uterus. In virtually every category there is a striking difference in cure rates between patients with localized cancer, whose regional lymph nodes have not become involved, and patients in whom regional lymph node involvement is present. (Such involvement is indicative of probable further spread of disease.)

Clearly, one of the reasons why surgery is not universally more successful, is the continued failure to diagnose cancer early. By the time the surgeon sees the patient, the cancer has often metastasized and is beyond his reach. This failure is due to several factors, including a natural biologic behavior of certain cancers which do not cause symptoms until they have spread; fear, indifference, or lack of alertness on the part of the patient; insufficient knowledge, training, and equipment of some physicians; and the overwork or carelessness of competent physicians. Almost all of these reasons reflect in some way the shortage of properly trained doctors and health educators.

Cancer Detection

If cancers are discovered when they are still localized, the majority can be cured by surgery and radiotherapy. Early detection, followed by prompt, appropriate treatment, is presently the most effective method of reducing the mortality from cancer.

It is the capacity of the cancer to grow and disseminate that makes early detection so important. A cancerous tumor of 1 cc (approximately $\frac{1}{16}$ cubic inch) in size, weighing about 1 g (approximately $\frac{1}{30}$ ounce) is about the smallest that can be detected by palpation or by x-ray, yet it contains about one billion cancer cells, each perhaps capable of originating a new focus of disease. Discovery of cancers when they are considerably smaller — microscopic in size — should materially increase cure rates. The past decade has witnessed startling innovations in the development of methods and instruments for cancer detection, as well as the perfection of established procedures. It is as important to make an early diagnosis of a recurrence as it is to make the diagnosis initially, if successful treatment is anticipated.

Palliative Surgery

In addition to the role of surgery in saving lives by eradicating cancer, the surgeon is also frequently called upon to improve the remaining months or years of a patient whose cancer cannot be eradicated. Much judgment must be exercised, however, because the objective is to prolong an enjoyable and productive life — not to prolong agony.

For those patients in whom the growth of the tumor leads to pain, the neurosurgeon can often bring great relief by dividing the nerve pathways which carry the painful sensations. In the lower two thirds of the body, this can usually be done with minimal impairment of other functions. Numerous other surgical procedures, which can be categorized under the general designation of palliative surgery, are of great help to the patient. They often contribute significantly to longevity and, if they can bring comfort and usefulness back to the patient, they are worth the considerable effort which is often involved.

The long-term future may belong to the immunologist and the geneticist, the intermediate future to the chemotherapist, but the present and immediate future belong in the main to the surgeon, and, to some extent, to the radiologist.

More specifically, to the extent that curative chemotherapy is developed first, surgery will be needed less. But in those fields in which early detection is developed first, it will be mainly surgery which will convert these gains and cure patients by extirpation of the cancer before it has spread. It therefore becomes a vital part of the attack on cancer to provide outstanding physical facilities, incentives to attract able persons, educational programs to prepare excellent surgeons, and the means to achieve a broad delivery of services to all who require them.

Radiation Therapy

Radiation therapy is second in importance only to surgery as a means for the curative treatment of a wide range of cancer. In addition, it has an important role in palliative treatment for patients who are too far advanced for cure. It makes use of ionizing radiation — x-rays and electrons, produced by man-made machines, and gamma rays, which emanate from naturally or artificially radioactive elements — to destroy cells by injuring their capacity to divide. Since the central attribute of cancer cells is their sustained, uncontrolled, lawless proliferation, injury to this property is precisely what is desired. Although some rapidly dividing normal cells are also killed during radiotherapeutic eradication of the cancer, the large reservoir of similar normal cells outside the irradiated field in most instances is readily able to replenish the supply and repair the irradiated tissues. Thus, in favorable cases, when the cancer gradually disappears completely during treatment, the acute radiation reaction in normal tissue slowly subsides and, one or more years later, the patients may have no external evidence of radiation reaction. Currently, radiation therapy is used either for cure or palliation, and an estimated 50% to 60% of all cervical cancer cases receive radiation therapy at some stage in their evolution. However, the development of radiation therapy in the United States has been hampered by a serious shortage of medical and paramedical manpower, lack of research and capital funds for major equipment and facilities, and ineffective organizational relationships.

RECURRENT CANCER OF THE CERVIX

The treatment of recurrent cancer to the cervix can be divided into two main categories, definitive and curative, and palliative. The definitive and curative approach will be discussed first. Almost one half of the patients with cancer of the cervix seen on the gynecologic service of most large medical centers are instances of recurrent or persistent disease after one or more attempts to cure by radiation. There have been comparatively few reports about recurrent cancer of the cervix and its treatment. It is assumed that about 55% to 60% of patients treated by radiation, which is the treatment usually chosen for the country as a whole, fail to be cured. Since there is a tendency for cancer of the cervix to remain localized in the pelvis for relatively long periods of time, there must be an appreciable number of patients constituting radiation failures who live for a relatively long time with the disease confined to the pelvis. These patients are suitable for further treatment of their disease. Reradiation has little to offer in terms of cure, and is accompanied by a high complication rate and augmentation of symptoms. If certain limits are exceeded in applying radiation, tissue necrosis may develop, which often proves as distressing to the patient as the advancing neoplasm itself. Although certain investigators have reported a certain measure of success in employing reradiation, a perusal of their reports indicates that the diagnosis of recurrence may be questioned because of the lack of biopsy in these patients. Reliance upon clinical findings in making a diagnosis of recurrence introduces an appreciable degree of error.

The tendency of cancer of the cervix to remain localized to the pelvis, despite the fact that it is advanced, provides an opportunity to attack the disease by a surgical approach. These patients are operated upon just as though they represented primary cases, and the procedure which is carried out is tailored to the extent of the disease and the needs of the patient. The results of this approach, which will be reviewed later, would indicate that an updating of our management of these patients is needed. The principle that, if radiation has failed, there is no further hope for cure, must now be abandoned.

Nodal involvement is an index of prognosis which should not deter the responsible physician from carrying out planned therapy in the face of otherwise localized disease. Positive nodes are found in only slightly more than one half of patients who require pelvic exenteration to encompass their disease. The salvage rate in patients with positive nodes appears to vary inversely with the size of the local lesion. A feature to emphasize is that, in general, cancer of the cervix does not spread rapidly outside the pelvis, but apparently remains localized for relatively long periods of time. It has been shown that, even in patients dying of cervical cancer, 50% have no gross disease beyond the pelvis at the time of death. This observation provides an explanation for the significant survival rate after an extended surgical attack in patients with advanced and recurrent cancer of the cervix.

SURGICAL PATHOLOGIC CLASSIFICATION

In 1952, Meigs and Brunschwig proposed a surgical pathologic classification based upon gross microscopic examination of the specimen after it has been excised. This fulfilled a real need in classifying the extent of disease in patients presenting with a recurrence or persistence of disease. This classification affords an opportunity for an accurate evaluation, and, at the same time, serves to document the natural history of the disease. The correlation of clinical as well as cytopathologic findings permits a standard to compare results among clinics carrying out a surgical program. Class and alphabet are used instead of stage and numerals to avoid confusion with the FIGO classification.

The surgical-pathologic classification is as follows.

Class O — Carcinoma in situ, microcarcinoma.

Class A — Carcinoma limited to the cervix.

Class Ao — No tumor in the cervix in the surgical specimen after positive biopsy specimen of infiltrating carcinoma.

Class B — Extension of the carcinoma from the cervix to involve the vagina, except the lower third; extension into the corpus, possibly involving the upper vagina and corpus; vaginal or uterine extension, or both; may be by direct or metastatic spread.

Class C — Involvement of the paracervical or paravaginal tissue, or both, by direct extension or by lymphatic vessels, or in nodes within such tissues, or direct extension or both, in the lower third of the vagina.

Class D — Lymph vessel and node involvement beyond the paracervical and paravaginal regions, including all lymphatic vessels or nodes, or both, in the true pelvis, except as described in Class C; metastases to the ovary or tube.

Class E — Penetration to the serosa, musculature, or mucosa of the bladder, colon, rectum, or some combination of these.

Class F — Involvement of the pelvic wall (fascia, muscle, bone, or sacral plexus, or some combination).

Combinations are used; for example, *DC* — node at the periphery of the pelvis, and parametrial or paracervical extension. *CN* — parametrial or paracervical extension, as well as a positive node, in the parametrial or paracervical area. *D* — reserved for positive nodes at the periphery of the pelvis. *PR* — Preoperative irradiation. *R* — Curative irradiation followed by failure. *S* — Surgical attempt at cure prior to recurrence. *RS* — Irradiation and surgery employed curatively, but further surgery required for persistence or recurrence of disease.

Carcinoma of the cervical stump is classified in the same manner as cervical cancer with the uterus intact.

Adenocarcinoma of the cervix is classified in the same manner as epidermoid cancer.

Although the classification is long, it supplies a real need, and permits a study of the natural history of disease as well as serving to anticipate prognosis.

DIAGNOSIS OF RECURRENCE

The problem of diagnosing a recurrence is often a very difficult one. In the early stages of recurrence the patient characteristically has no symptoms and few objective signs. A high index of suspicion is paramount in making the diagnosis, and is reinforced by the realization that one half or more of patients receiving radiation as primary treatment, will present themselves at a later date with a recurrence. The possibility of detecting and diagnosing recurrence in an early stage is increased by evaluating the problem from three approaches, namely, symptoms, physical examination, and laboratory data. Usually there are no symptoms, but any new developments which appear in a patient who has received treatment for cancer of the cervix merits careful evaluation. At the time of examination, any mass, thickening, or nodularity should arouse suspicion, and a biopsy must be carried out. Particularly important is the development of any asymmetry in the pelvic organs, especially if there has been none previously. A Pap smear, biopsy, and an intravenous pyelogram are helpful in evaluating the problem. Progressive deterioration in the pyelogram following irradiation therapy for cancer of the cervix usually indicates the presence of a recurrence in the pelvis.

JUSTIFICATION FOR SURGERY FOR RECURRENCE

The question, "What justification is there for carrying out procedures of the magnitude of an exenteration with its inherent morbidity and mortality?" The most convincing answer is supplied by equating the five-year survival rate that ranges from 20% to about 40% against the thorough studies of Truelsen (1949). In his review there were no five-year survivors in either the group with persistence of disease after irradiation, or those found to have recurrence of disease after apparent healing. The true test for the justification of pelvic exenteration are the results that have been achieved.

Added proof is offered by comparing the five-year salvage rate for cancer of the cervix with results following a surgical attack on all other visceral lesions except those of the colon. The five-year results obtained by surgical treatment of recurrent cancer of the cervix are considerably better than the results obtained for several sites (both operable and inoperable), namely, bladder, kidney, stomach, lungs, esophagus, and gallbladder.

The criticism directed against the surgical approach in treating recurrent cancer of the cervix is not justified. Criticism occasionally may be directed against the indications in a particular patient, but the intangibles of surgical judgment, training, and knowledge of the natural history of the disease, undoubtedly influence the course in any given case.

The evidence advanced in support of justification for a surgical attack on recurrent cancer of the cervix is self-revealing. Perusal of the literature discloses widespread acceptance for the surgical approach as a form of accepted treatment of recurrent cancer of the female pelvis.

TYPE OF OPERATIONS

When Meigs reintroduced radical surgery for cancer of the cervix in 1939, an additional useful modality became available. In order to follow a surgical program, it is necessary to employ a wide range of operations, from radical hysterectomy to pelvic exenteration. The surgical procedures used for the treatment of cancer of the cervix are: 1) total hysterectomy and bilateral salpingo-oophorectomy, 2) Wertheim hysterectomy, 3) radical hysterectomy, salpingo-oophorectomy, and pelvic node dissection, 4) excision of cervical stump with pelvic lymph node dissection, 5) radical resection of cervical stump, 6) radical vaginal hysterectomy (Schauta operation), 7) anterior pelvic exenteration, 8) posterior pelvic exenteration, and 9) total pelvic exenteration.

Preoperative Orders, Outlined in Steps

1. CBC and urinalysis.
2. SMA 12.
3. Electrolytes.
4. Chest x-ray and intravenous pyelogram.
5. Barium enema, skeletal survey, lymphangiogram, ultrasound, as indicated.
6. Electrocardiogram.
7. Blood volume.
8. Regular diet.
9. Out of bed.
10. pHiso Hex shower each day prior to surgery.
11. A triple-sulfa vaginal cream each day.
12. Thirty ml of 50% magnesium sulfate solution × 3 days.
13. Castor oil (45 ml) the day before surgery.
14. Neomycin (1 g) every hour for 6 doses.
15. An appropriate antibiotic the day prior to surgery, if considered necessary.
16. Nothing by mouth after midnight.
17. Abdominal perineal prep.
18. Secobarbital (100 mg) at bedtime, repeated once if necessary.
19. Atropine (0.4 mg)—on-call to the operating room.
20. Meperidine hydrochloride (50 mg) or hydroxyzine pamoate (50 mg). In elderly patients, some anesthetists prefer not to use preoperative narcotics because of the respiratory acidosis that is produced.
21. Cut-down with large needle or intracatheter should be placed in a large vein prior to going into the operating room.

Postoperative Management

The postoperative management for all types of radical treatment is extremely important, and is as follows:

1. Nothing by mouth.
2. Blood pressure, pulse, and respiration are noted and recorded at 15-minute intervals until the patient has fully recovered from the immediate effects of the operation.
3. Measure and record intake and output.
4. Pain-relieving medication is given, in smaller doses than usual.
5. Urinary output is recorded hourly. This is a good indication of the success of ureteral transplantation, as well as the status of tissue perfusion.
6. Inspection of the perineal and abdominal dressing to detect any increase in the amount of bleeding.
7. Weigh the patient daily.
8. There are four signs of alarm during the immediate postoperative period: hypotension, respiratory obstruction, excessive depression of respiration, and the excitement stage. The cause may be determined and measures instituted to correct the problem.
9. Insertion of nasogastric tube as needed.
10. Appropriate broad-spectrum antibiotic therapy: ampicillin, 2 g every 6 hours in the Volutrol, and/or gentamicin, up to 1.6 mg/kg IM, or IV 3 times a day. If anaerobes are present, add clindamycin, 300 mg IM 3 times a day.
11. Since respiratory complications are frequent, particularly in the elderly, the patient should be taught how to use the IPPB apparatus preoperatively. In the postoperative period, the patient's trachea should be carefully aspirated.
12. In the presence of a denuded pelvis, the following fluids and electrolyte intake are necessary to secure an adequate urinary output: 1000 ml of 5% glucose and water; 1000 ml of 5% glucose and saline; another 1000 ml of 5% glucose and water; and 250 to 500 ml of plasma per day. Potassium is given as needed. The minimum daily requirement after postoperative day one is 40 mEq of potassium chloride. Transfusion of whole blood is given as needed.
13. The patient is not given anything by mouth until bowel sounds have been normal for at least two days. They are usually very feeble for the first three days after radical surgery, particularly after pelvic exenteration. When fluids are started by mouth, tea or water, 60 ml every hour as desired, is given as a test during the first day. If this is tolerated, the amount can be increased.
14. The pack should be removed within 48 to 72 hours postoperatively.
15. Oxytetracyline suppositories should be inserted into the pelvic

cavity each day after the pack is removed. A minimum of six should be used on the first day.

16. Ileus is the most common problem after radical surgery, particularly after pelvic exenteration. It can be handled as any case of ileus, and usually responds after three or four days. It is generally secondary to a low-grade pelvic infection complicated by the presence of the pelvic pack. In most instances, a nasogastric tube is indicated; careful management of fluids and electrolytes is life-saving. The daily baseline requirement as outlined in step 12 must be supplied. All fluids lost from the nasogastric tube and the denuded pelvis must be replaced in kind and in the amount lost.

17. If there is urinary abdominal stoma, a bag should be applied immediately to protect the skin after surgery. Disposable Bongart bags can be used right after surgery. At the end of ten days, the patient should be fitted with a permanent bag. The Perma bag has been the one we have used most frequently.

18. Urea nitrogen, potassium, chlorides, CO_2, hemoglobin, hematocrit, and protein are carefully followed during the first week.

19. An intravenous pyelogram should be made before the patient leaves the hospital.

20. Four major complications especially associated with pelvic exenteration are: 1) urinary tract obstruction of the fistula, 2) sepsis, 3) major rupture of a large vessel, and 4) intestinal fistula. The patient should be evaluated each day.

21. The miniheparin which was started the day before surgery should be continued for at least the first week following surgery.

Role of Pelvic Exenteration in the
Treatment of Recurrences Following Radical
Surgical Excision as Initial Treatment

Of 222 patients presenting with recurrence following radical surgery, only 35 were treated by pelvic exenteration. Comparison of the surgical pathologic classification at the time of initial surgery, and at the time of treatment for recurrence, revealed that there was marked progression of disease. Of the 35 patients, eight survived five or more years, indicating that fewer patients are suitable for pelvic exenteration after primary surgery then after primary irradiation. However, when it is technically possible to carry out pelvic exenteration, the results are about the same.

Pelvic Exenteration and
Untreated Cancer of the Cervix

Since the patient loses her bladder and/or rectum with pelvic exenteration, there is little enthusiasm for exenteration as a primary form of treatment. In general, pelvic exenteration should be reserved for patients who have no chance for cure by any other modality.

Incomplete Excision of Cancer

Unless all macroscopic disease can be excised, pelvic exenteration is contraindicated. In patients with disease still remaining in the pelvis, the mean survival rate was slightly over three months, and there was little, if any, palliation. These patients do poorly in the postoperative period, have ileus, low-grade fever, and gradually deteriorate. Patients in whom all macroscopic disease has been removed from the pelvis, but in whom the tumor is reported still present in the paraaortic nodes (usually after negative frozen section report), usually have a similar period of survival, but the postoperative course generally is not as stormy.

Extensive Radiation Necrosis

Occasionally patients with radiation necrosis will require pelvic exenteration or radical excision of the lesion by a radical hysterectomy. In each instance, the clinical picture is complicated by severe pain, urinary and/or intestinal fistula, bleeding, copious foul discharge, and physical deterioration of the patient. It is clinically difficult to differentiate recurrent cancer from radiation reaction and damage, but, with proper selection of patients, pelvic exenteration is justified even though only radiation necrosis is found. The fact that cancer is not always found at the time of pelvic exenteration does not mean that cancer is not present. In one series, three of seven patients died of cancer within five years, without cancer having been detected at the time of surgery. This confirms the natural history of cervical cancer, and also reinforces the observation that it is difficult to differentiate clinically between persistent cancer and radiation necrosis, even in the presence of a negative biopsy. Patients treated by pelvic exenteration for visceral necrosis are labile, and constant supervision is essential. The operative results achieved in terms of physical welfare appear to justify the procedure since, before surgery, the patient's existence was hardly bearable in most instances. It appears that pelvic exenteration is indicated in selected patients for radiation necrosis and other damage which produces severe symptoms.

It is indeed difficult to differentiate between visceral radiation necrosis and recurrent cancer. The symptoms and clinical findings are similar. Furthermore, the suspicion that cancer may be present is reinforced by reports that in about 50% of the patients receiving primary therapy, usually radiation for cancer of the cervix, will present at a later date with persistent or recurrent cancer.

Philosophy and orientation have changed from a radical to a conservative approach for the management of radiation necrosis. It must be emphasized that the smallest procedure that will control this complication should be employed. When large, necrotic sloughs produce vesicovaginal or rectovaginal fistulas accompanied by pain, bleeding, foul discharge, and overall deterioration, there may be no alternative other than to carry out a pelvic exenteration. In general, however, a more conservative approach is advocated. Diversions, control of infections, and improvement of nutrition should be tried before exenteration is considered for definitive treatment. Pelvic exenteration is usually restricted to those patients in whom a positive biopsy for cancer is obtained. There are certain patients, however, in whom the operation is undertaken with negative biopsies in order to control the severe pain, malnutrition, cachexia, and progressive deterioration associated with urinary and large bowel fistulas. The results achieved justify the operation, since life was anything but bearable in most instances. As pointed out previously, a conservative approach for management is first pursued and, if this fails, a more aggressive plan of treatment must be adopted.

Complications

After pelvic exenteration, the most important factor in the patient's survival (aside from the question of recurrence, and disregarding complications common to any major pelvic and intraabdominal operation) is the preservation of the urinary tract.

The prognostic significance of obstruction by tumor resulting in a nonfunctioning kidney can be summarized by stating that, if the recurrence obstructs the ureter at the ureterovesical junction, the results are approximately the same as though it were a central recurrence. However, the results are dramatically less impressive if the obstruction occurs in the deep, posterolateral part of the pelvis.

Urinary tract fistula following pelvic exenteration occurs in about 5% of patients. A combination of altered metabolism (secondary to operation) and local infection contributes to the development of urinary fistula as a complication of pelvic exenteration.

A meticulous surgical technique must be employed in the construction of the urinary diversion. When fistula occurs after pelvic exenteration, the patient is in a highly critical condition. Because of the wide variety of conditions for which pelvic exenteration is performed, there is no single method to manage this complication.

Although urinary tract complications are the most frequent and most important considerations in the patient's survival, the patient may be subject to any complication encountered in any surgical procedure. Surgical shock, peritonitis, sepsis, uremia, and intestinal fistula account for the major postoperative causes of death.

Criteria for Judging the Time of Discharge From the Hospital

Criteria have been established for the patient's discharge from the hospital. The patient must: 1) feel well physically and mentally; 2) tolerate a normal diet; 3) have no fever for at least five days; 4) walk without difficulty; 5) show interest in being discharged from the hospital; 6) start to resume interest in her previous work or hobbies; 7) demonstrate that she can take care of herself at home; 8) have skill and confidence in managing her stomal bags; 9) have stable or increasing weight; 10) have minimal drug requirements; 11) understand the labile nature of her condition and accept responsibility for reporting any complications immediately; 12) understand the importance of continued follow-up examinations; 13) have immediate family members who understand the nature of the problem; and 14) be able to return to home surroundings where the problems of the patient are accepted.

Success of Treatment

The result of treatment and the chances for a long survival are difficult to predict. The operation is of considerable magnitude, and the patient has less resistance to any physical insult than the nonexenterative patient, who is prone to develop infections. A high percentage of patients require additional surgery, usually for complications of the bowel or urinary tract.

The success of treatment may be evaluated by the following: 1) At the time of operation, planes of dissection were developed with relative ease; 2) the recurrence was confined to the midline with minimal lateral spread; 3) there is relative certainty that all macroscopic disease has been removed; 4) technically, the urinary and bowel anastamoses were carried out with little trauma and no tension; 5) there was a reasonable, uncomplicated postoperative course; 6) hospital stay did not exceed one month; 7) postoperative pyelograms were within normal limits; 8) there were no attacks of pyelonephritis; 9) no fever occurred beyond the first five or six postoperative days; 10) there has been suggestive improvement in association with a marked decrease in requirements of analgesic or narcotic drugs; 11) the clinical appearance correlates with the laboratory findings, indicating progressive improvement; 12) there has been a leveling off or reversal of the downward weight curve; 13) performance status of the patient has improved; 14) there has been an emotional adjustment to the operation; 15) blood chemistry and x-ray findings remain within normal limits; 16) all of the above are met and maintained for at least 12 months.

Contraindications to Pelvic Exenteration

Pelvic exenteration is contraindicated when considered only for relief of pain. In cases where all macroscopic evidence of disease was not excised, survival was brief, and the incidence of postoperative complications so high that the procedure was indeed not worthwhile. Other contraindications to exenteration for cure include metastases outside the pelvis, lower extremity edema with increasing sciatic pain, psychosis, cancer spread outside the pelvis or fixed to the pelvic wall, and ureteral obstruction by the cancer in the deep, posterolateral part of the pelvis. For a more extensive review of contraindications to pelvic exenteration, see *Surgical Clinics of North America* 49:431, 1969.

Survival

The results in terms of long-range survival in patients with respect to previous radiation, status of lymph nodes, preoperative nonfunctioning kidneys, small bowel involvement, or diabetes, are definitely poorer than those found in the overall exenteration series. A comparison of the five-year survival in those patients with negative nodes and no previous radiation (35.3%), and those with positive nodes and previous radiation (5.8%), is revealing.

In the continued pursuit of an optimal surgical program for advanced pelvic cancer (mostly cancer of the cervix), a review of the results relative to preoperative findings has been made to determine if "sharpening" of the indications might lead to a better selection of patients for surgery. The review has served to give some impression as to whether the symptoms and size of the lesion may prognosticate good or poor results for prolonged survival. For example, it has become apparent that, if the preoperative intravenous pyelogram shows one kidney nonvisualized, the prognosis for five-year survival (10%) is only one half as good as when both kidneys are visualized preoperatively (22%). If the obstruction to the ureter causing a nonfunctioning kidney is posterior and deep in the pelvis along the pelvic wall, there is little chance for long-term survival. In contrast, obstruction at the urethrovesical junction or along the ureter with a free space posteriorly, lends itself to an aggressive surgical attack, and an appreciable period of survival is anticipated. The explanation is that the extent of disease is less in the latter group, and the chances for cure are increased. There is an important lesson to be learned here, namely, patients should be given the benefit of an exploratory laparotomy, and, only under unusual circumstances, should they be declared nonresectable without benefit of an exploratory laparotomy. The difference between inoperable and nonresectable is obvious.

Early in these experiences it was learned that in pelvic exenteration performed for relief of pain, but in which all macroscopic evidence of disease was not excised from the pelvis, postoperative survival was generally so brief and the incidence of postoperative complications so great, that it was not considered worthwhile. Also, it should be made clear that similar results would follow if paraaortic lymph nodes were left behind, despite the excision of all macroscopic cancer from the pelvis. However, in this group the survival was more prolonged and the morbidity less than in those patients in whom disease was not fully removed (macroscopically) from the pelvis.

A series of patients who received pelvic exenteration in which a loop of small bowel was entrapped in the cancerous pelvic mass, have been reviewed. None of the survivors had pelvic lymph node metastases. The worst sign in this group of patients was the finding of actual invasion by cancer of a loop of small bowel, especially on the mesenteric side, plus the presence of pelvic lymph node metastases. In this group of recurrent cancers, the increased complication rate as well as the poor survival rate can be anticipated and accepted, since the only hope for survival is offered by extensive, radical surgery.

RADIOTHERAPY

If a patient has received a full course of radiotherapy and the tumor persists, further irradiation would appear to be futile. Although it is true that tumors partially controlled by 5000 rad may occasionally be fully controlled by 6000 to 7000 rad, this occurs infrequently.

At Roswell Park Memorial Institute, Murphy adopted a policy of reradiating patients with recurrence, giving additional radiation or nearly a full course for a second time. Among a selected series of 46 patients, 9 (19%) were living and well at the end of five years. Seven of these had a positive biopsy before treatment, so that the final, five-year cure rate for those with proved recurrences is 16% (7 of 44). Interestingly enough, all the surviving patients except one had a central lesion. The one exception had induration of the broad ligaments, but not to the pelvic wall. Of the total number of 32 patients with central recurrence, 9 (28%) survived five years, free of disease. It must be remembered that there must be a great deal of selection in both recurrent and persistent cases that are retreated.

A histologic diagnosis of recurrence must be established in all cases before giving definitive treatment. Cytologic criteria of tumor cells on needle aspirate are an acceptable substitute for biopsy. Although an exception to this rule is made from time to time, one frequently has cause to regret it. Radiotherapy or radical surgery for signs erroneously diagnosed as cancer may lead to disastrous complications. The vaginal smear has come to be a standard part of the follow-up procedure in most clinics. It can detect recurrence before it is evident clinically. However, aggressive treatment should not be carried out on the positive findings of one Pap smear.

Reradiation of Recurrent Cancer
of the Cervix After Surgical Resection

Recurrent carcinoma of the cervix after surgical resection, localized in the pelvis and the vagina, is given as follows:

External pelvic irradiation (4000 rad) to the pelvis through opposing anterior and posterior portals, over a period of four weeks. Following this, an additional 2000 rad in a two-week period, using multiple field technique (four-field), is given.

PALLIATIVE TREATMENT

Patients with recurrent and nonresectable cancer of the cervix often develop complications that require treatment. Among these are bowel necrosis, ureterocutaneous fistula, ureterovaginal and vesicovaginal fistulas, pelvic hematoma, abscess formation, bowel obstruction, and hemorrhage. Surgery is carried out only to relieve obstructed ureters, if there is hope to provide additional therapy. However, if the disease is nonresectable and beyond treatment, nothing is done to relieve ureteral obstruction.

There are cases where a ureterovaginal or vesicovaginal fistula occurs and causes the patient great discomfort. If the patient is terminal and the anticipated life expectancy is very short, nothing is done. However, some of these patients look surprisingly well and are actively conducting their duties each day. In these cases it is felt that some sort of therapy should be offered so that they may be comfortable for whatever time remains for them to live. There is usually little hope of repairing these fistulas, so that a type of urinary diversion is usually carried out. The same situation applies to patients with a rectovaginal fistula. A colostomy usually controls the complication and allows the patient to be comfortable during the remainder of her life.

The problem relative to hemorrhage is a difficult one, particularly in the presence of recurrent and nonresectable cancer. Unless the hemorrhage is a fatal one, laparotomy is usually carried out with the hope of controlling it. In many of these patients the disease is located along the hypogastric vessels, and, indeed, it is very often difficult to ligate these vessels. Having ligated the hypogastric to reduce the head of pressure in the vessels, it is still necessary to search for the vessel that is bleeding and tie it off. Otherwise, the patient will continue to bleed because of the numerous collaterals among the vessels in the pelvis. Abscess formation often makes these patients miserable, weak, and saps them of their energy. Unless death is imminent, there is an obligation to drain the abscess, and try and correct whatever situation started the lesion. Bowel obstructions, both large and small, are handled as if the patient had no malignant disease. Constant vomiting is associated with a loss of dignity, and even the therapeutic nihilist accepts the fact that this is not an easy way to die.

Rarely, patients will develop metastases to bone which causes pain, or to the supraclavicular or inguinal areas. To control pain and reduce the incidence of a fungating lesion, these areas can be managed with spot irradiation. The philosophy should not be to prolong agony, but to improve the quality of whatever life remains.

CHEMOTHERAPY

Chemotherapy has been tried for palliation in cancer of the cervix. Both single agents and combination therapy have been used. The degree of success has not been great. However, some of these patients do get relief from some of their symptoms after chemotherapy is given. Most single agents and combinations of them have been given to carefully selected patients. Bleomycin gave great promise for being the drug of choice, because of its ability to be concentrated in squamous cells. However, for a variety of reasons, it has not lived up to expectations. In addition, there are a great number of complications from this drug, including pulmonary fibrosis, very marked dermatitis, a flu-like syndrome, vomiting, and fever.

Recently, mitomycin (20 mg intravenously as a bolus, followed by 1.5 g fluorouracil intravenously over a 24-hour period each day for four to five days) has given promise as a potentially hopeful addition to the physician's armamentarium.

Intraaortic chemotherapy has been given to about 40 patients by the author. After a catheter is inserted in the aorta through the femoral or brachial artery and placed at any level desired, anticancer drugs are infused. Some of these patients lived for surprisingly long periods of time, and one is clinically free of disease. All other patients presented with far advanced and/or recurrent cancer of the cervix, and had previously received multiple forms of treatment. The original plan was to deliver the drugs in sequence, hopefully to attack the cells by using a drug most likely to damage them in a given phase of their cycle. However, treatment has been altered and a standard plan is now employed. Epidermoid carcinomas of the cervix, vagina, and vulva are given cyclophosphamide (200 mg a day for two days), actinomycin D (1 mg in 8 hours), bleomycin (15 units a day for two days), vincristine (1 mg in 6 hours), and, recently, doxorubicin (50 mg in 24 hours) has been added. In the early part of the project methotrexate (50 mg) was given in 24 hours, and repeated. Later, the dosage was reduced to 30 mg. From time to time, methotrexate is still included as part of the regimen.

Before therapy is begun, the blood count, platelets, blood chemistries, and bone marrow must be evaluated. The blood count and chemistries are studied approximately three times a week during treatment.

Each series of treatments is interrupted for 48 hours, or until the blood count and chemistries return to normal, and then the regimen is repeated. The average time for giving treatment is six weeks. One patient received therapy for about five months, and is now free of disease. The primary lesion was squamous cell cancer of the cervix. Patients presenting with pain were almost universally free of pain within a short time after starting therapy, and some have remained comfortable for extended periods of time. Most had a sense of well being and were improved. Unfortunately, the response is usually short-lived. This may be the direct result of the natural history of the disease, or it may be due to a present lack of understanding of the optimal dosages and methods of administration of the anticancer drugs.

BIBLIOGRAPHY

Barber HRK, Roberts S, Brunschwig A: Prognostic significance of the preoperative non-visualizing kidney in patients receiving pelvic exenteration. *Cancer* 16:1674, 1963.

Barber HRK, Brunschwig A: Pelvic exenteration for extensive necrosis following radiation therapy for gynecologic cancer. *Obstet Gynecol* 25:575, 1965.

Barber HRK, Brunschwig A: Pelvic exenteration for advanced and recurrent ovarian cancer. *Surgery,* 58:935, 1965.

Barber HRK, Brunschwig A: Results of the surgical treatment of recurrent cancer of the cervix, in Lewis CG, Jr, Wentz WB, Jaffe RM (eds): *New Concepts in Gynecological Oncology.* Philadelphia, F.A. Davis Co, 1966, p 145.

Barber HRK, Brunschwig A: Excision of major blood vessels at the periphery of the pelvis in major surgery. *Surgery* 62:426, 1967.

Barber HRK, Brunschwig A: The role of radical surgery in gynecological cancer. *Acad Med NJ Bull* 16:102, 1970.

Barber HRK: Relative prognostic significance of preoperative and operative findings in pelvic exenteration. *Surg Clin North Am* 49:431, 1969.

Barber HRK, Graber EA: Treatment of advanced cancer of the cervix by pelvic exenteration. *Bull NY Acad Med* 40:870, 1973.

Barber HRK: Results of surgical treatment of cancer of the cervix at the Memorial-James Ewing Hospitals, New York, in Marcus S, Marcus C, (eds): *Advances in Obstetrics and Gynecology.* Baltimore, The Williams & Wilkins Co, 1967, vol 1, p 622.

Barber HRK, Brunschwig A, Mangioni C: Advanced cancer of the vulva and vagina, treated by anterior and total pelvic exenteration 1947-1962 at the Memorial-James Ewing Hospitals. *Cancer* 22:949, 1968.

Barber HRK, Brunschwig A: Treatment of recurrent corpus cancer by anterior and total pelvic exenteration at the Memorial-James Ewing Hospitals, 1947 through 1962. *Ann Obstet Gynec* 4:219, 1968.

Bricker EM, Modlin J: Role of pelvic exenteration. *Surgery* 30:76, 1951.

Brunschwig A: Complete excision of pelvic viscera for advanced carcinoma. *Cancer* 1:177, 1948.

Brunschwig A, Barber HRK: Extended pelvic exenteration for advanced cancer of the cervix. Long survivals following added resection of involved small bowel. *Cancer* 17:1267, 1964.

Brunschwig A: What are the indications and results of pelvic exenteration? *JAMA* 194:274, 1965.

Brunschwig A: Surgical treatment of carcinoma of the cervix, recurrent after irradiation or combination of irradiation and surgery. *Am J Roentgenol* 99:365, 1967.

Brunschwig A, Barber HRK: Pelvic exenteration combined with resection of segments of bony pelvis. *Surgery* 65:417, 1969.

Brunschwig A: L'Exenteration pelvienne. Paris, Masson et Cie, 1964, p 55.

Brunschwig A, Southam CM, Levin AG: Host resistance to cancer. Clinical experiments by homotransplants, autotransplants, and admixture of autologous leukocytes. *Am Surg* 162:416, 1965.

Cherry CP, Glucksmann A: Lymphatic embolism and lymph node metastases in cancers of the vulva and uterine cervix. *Cancer* 8:564, 1955.

Cox EF, Ketchum AS, Villa Santa U, et al: Patient evaluation for pelvic exenteration. *Am Surg* 30:574, 1964.

Dearing R: A study of the renal tract in carcinoma of the cervix. *J Obstet Gynaecol Brit Emp* 60:165–174, 1953.

Ellis F: The dose-time relationship of radiotherapy. *Brit J Radiol* 36:153, 1963.

Fletcher GH, Rutledge FN, Chan PM: Policies of treatment in cancer of the cervix uteri. *Am J Roentgenol* 87:6, 1962.

Friedell GH, Graham JB: Regional lymph node involvement in small carcinoma of the cervix. *Surg Gynecol Obstet* 108:513, 1959.

Friedell GH, Cesare F, Parsons L: Surgical treatment of cancer of the cervix recurring after primary irradiation therapy. *N Engl J Med* 264:781, 1961.

Friedell GH, Parsons L: The spread of cancer of the uterine cervix as seen in giant histological sections. *Cancer* 14:42, 1961.

Friedell GH, Parsons L: Blood vessel invasion in cancer of the cervix. *Cancer* 15:1269, 1962.

Friedell GH: Cancer of the cervix — A selection review, in Sommers SC (ed): *Pathology Annual 1966.* New York, Appleton-Century-Crofts Division of Meredith Publishing Co, p 48.

Graham JB, Graham RM: The curability of regional lymph node metastases in cancer of the uterine cervix. *Surg Gynecol Obstet* 100:149–155, 1955.

Graham JB, Sotto LS, Paloncek FP: *Carcinoma of the Cervix.* Philadelphia, W.B. Saunders Co, 1962.

Green HSN: Significance of heterologous transplantability of human cancer. *Cancer* 5:24, 1952.

Gusberg SB, Fisk SA, Ym-Ying Wang: Growth pattern of cervical cancer. *Obstet Gynec* 2:557, 1953.

Herovici CA: Polychrome stain for differentiating precollagen from collagen. *Stain Techn* 38:204, 1963.

Herovici CA: Study of reaction of connective tissue in malignant tumors of the uterine cervix. *Neoplasm (Bratisl)* 11:225, 1964.

Ingersoll FM, Ulfelder H: Pelvic exenteration for carcinoma of the cervix. *N Engl J Med* 274:648, 1966.

Ingersoll FM: Pelvic exenteration for carcinoma of the cervix. *Obstet Gynecol Digest* 10:49, 1968.

Inguilla W, Cosmi EV: Pelvic exenteration for advanced carcinoma of the cervix. *Am J Obstet Gynecol* 99:1083, 1968.

Jones HW, Jr: Surgical treatment of carcinoma of the cervix recurrent after irradiation or combination of irradiation and surgery (editorial comment). *Obstet Gynecol Survey* 22:674, 1967.

Jones HW, Jr: Pelvic lymphadenectomy as an adjunct to radiation therapy in the treatment for cancer of the cervix (editorial comment) *Obstet Gynecol Survey* 20:840, 1965.

Kelly JWM, Parsons L, Friedell GH, et al: A pathologic study in 55 autopsies after radical surgery for cancer of the cervix. *Surg Gynecol Obstet* 110:423, 1960.

Kiselow M, Butcher HR, Jr, Bricker EM: Results of the radical surgical treatment of advanced pelvic cancer: A 15 year study. *Ann Surg* 166:428, 1967.

Lange P: Clinical and histological studies on cervical carcinoma. *Acta Path Microbiol Scand* 50(suppl 14):143, 1960.

Mattingly RF: Indications, contraindications and method of total pelvic exenteration. *Oncology* 21:241–259, 1967.

Mattingly RF: Total pelvic evisceration. *Clin Obstet Gynecol* 8:705, 1965.

McClure-Brown JC: Pathology and treatment of malignant glandular metastases of the lateral pelvic wall (discussion). *J Obstet Gynaecol Brit Emp* 67:724, 1960.

Meigs JV, Brunschwig A: Proposed classification for cases of cancer of the cervix treated by surgery. *Am J Obstet Gynecol* 64:413, 1952.

Mikuta JJ: Pelvic exenteration in carcinoma of the cervix, a review of the literature. *Am J Med Sci* 236:797, 1958.

Munnell E: Can recurrent cervical carcinoma be successfully managed? *JAMA* 194:275, 1965.

Murphy WT, Schmitz A: The results of reirradiation in cancer of the cervix. *Radiology* 67:378, 1956.

Murphy WT: *Radiation Therapy.* Philadelphia, WB Saunders, 1959.

Nelson JH: *Atlas of Radical Pelvic Surgery.* New York, Appleton-Century-Crofts, 1969, p 1.

O'Leary JA, Symmonds RE: Radical pelvic operations in the geriatric patient. A 15 year review of 133 cases. *Obstet Gynecol* 28:745, 1966.

Parsons L, Bell JW: Evaluation of pelvic exenteration operation. *Cancer* 3:205, 1950.

Parsons L: Pelvic exenteration. *Clin Obstet Gynecol* 2:1151, 1959.

Parsons L, Cesare F, Friedell GH: Primary surgical treatment of invasive cancer of the cervix. *Surg Gynecol Obstet* 109:279, 1959.

Parsons L, Friedell G: The evaluation of pelvic lymphadenectomy in the treatment of cervical cancer, in Meigs J, Sturgis S (eds): *Progress in Gynecology.* New York, Grune & Stratton Inc, vol IV, 1963, p 445.

Reagan JW, Hamonic MJ, Wentz WB: Analytical study of the cells in cervical squamous cell cancer. *Lab Invest* 6:241, 1957.

Rutledge F, Burns B: Pelvic exenteration. *Am J Obstet Gynecol* 91:692, 1965.

Schewe EJ, Sala JM: Bilateral ureteral obstruction complicating the treatment of cancer of the cervix. *Am J Roentgenol* 81:125–129, 1959.

Stallworthy J: Radical surgery following radiation treatment. *Ann Roy Coll Surg* 34:161, 1964.

Truelsen F: *Cancer of the Uterine Cervix, A Report of 2918 Cases.* London, H.D. Lewis & Co, Ltd, 1949.

Ulfelder H: Extended radical surgery for recurrent and advanced cervical cancer. *Clin Obstet Gynecol* 10:940, 1967.

Wentz WB: Histologic grade and survival in cervical cancer. *Obstet Gynecol* 18:412, 1961.

7 Cancer of the Vagina

John R. van Nagell, Jr.
Deborah F. Powell
E. C. Gay

Primary cancer of the vagina is quite rare, comprising only 1% to 2% of gynecologic malignancies. There is, however, a great variety of histologic types of vaginal cancer which affect females of all ages. Characteristically, embryonal rhabdomyosarcomas occur in infants, diethylstilbestrol-induced clear-cell adenocarcinomas in teenage girls, and squamous cell carcinoma, melanoma, sarcoma, and adenocarcinoma in adult women. The diagnosis of these lesions may be delayed due to the lack of symptoms in early stage disease, the reticence of young girls to undergo pelvic examination, or the misconception that vaginal cytologic screening is no longer necessary in women who have had prior hysterectomy. The biologic behavior of many of these tumors is quite different, often requiring varying combinations of therapy. It is only by a thorough understanding of these histologic and biologic variables, as well as the anatomic pathways of spread of these neoplasms, that proper treatment can be individualized to the needs of each patient.

ETIOLOGY AND EPIDEMIOLOGY

The established criteria for the designation of vaginal carcinoma are that: 1) the growth is in the vagina, 2) the cervix is intact, and 3) there is no evidence of a primary tumor in another site (Rutledge 1967). The incidence of vaginal carcinoma varies from one per 200,000 in the United States to one per 280,000 in Sweden. In a review of 2102 cases of vaginal cancer, Plentyl and Friedman (1971) reported that squamous cell carcinomas occurred in 93.5% of patients. The age distribution of patients with squamous cell carcinoma of the vagina is presented in Figure 7-1. The peak incidence of this cancer occurs in the seventh and eighth decades of life, with vaginal carcinoma in situ occurring most commonly during the sixth decade.

Epidemiologic studies have indicated no clear etiology for squamous cell carcinoma of the vagina. Several investigators have suggested the possible role of chronic irritation in the genesis of vaginal carcinoma. Kaiser and colleagues (1952) reported that 9 of 55 patients with squamous cell carcinoma of the vagina (16%) had worn a pessary or had severe procidentia. Likewise, Rutledge (1967) noted pessary use in over 10% of these patients.

A second reported etiologic agent in vaginal cancer is ionizing radiation, particularly in the intermediate dose range. Pride and Buchler (1977), for example, concluded that a significant, but low risk of radiation-induced malignancy in the vagina exists in patients receiving radiation therapy for uterine or cervical cancer. This risk was highest in those tissues exposed to an intermediate (nontumoricidal) radiation dose.

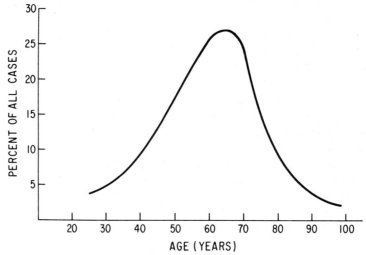

Figure 7-1 Age distribution of patients with invasive squamous cell carcinoma of the vagina (from Herbst et al 1963, Hilgers 1978, Perez et al 1973, Pride et al 1979, and Rutledge 1967).

The mean time interval from primary radiation exposure to the diagnosis of a potentially radiation-induced malignancy was over 18 years.

There is also evidence to support the concept that squamous cell carcinoma of the vagina may occur as part of a "field cancer" involving the entire lower genital tract. Woodruff and Williams (1963), Rutledge (1967), and Ostergard and Morton (1967) reported relatively large series of patients with multiple simultaneous cancers of the lower female genital tract including the vagina. The implication of these observations was that there is a multifocal response of a susceptible field of epithelium to a carcinogenic stimulus. This theory would help explain the increased incidence of carcinoma in situ of the vagina in women previously treated for intraepithelial neoplasia of the cervix (Barclay 1979). With respect to invasive vaginal carcinoma, the carcinogenic stimulus might well be exposure to genital herpesvirus or papovavirus. For this hypothesis to be valid, however, one would have to postulate a greater susceptibility of cervical epithelium to this oncogenic stimulus than vaginal epithelium, since vaginal carcinoma occurs significantly later in life then cervical carcinoma.

The role of maternal ingestion of diethylstilbestrol (DES) during the first trimester of pregnancy in the genesis of vaginal adenocarcinoma in young women has been clearly established. The vagina is derived embryologically from the lower, fused portion of the Müllerian ducts and the urogenital sinus. Characteristically, the urogenital sinus invaginates toward the Müllerian tubercle in a cephalad direction, and then canalizes to form the distal vagina. This process is complete by the fifth month of gestation, and results in squamous epithelium lining the majority of the vaginal canal. Columnar epithelium, derived from the Müllerian ducts, is usually confined to the area surrounding the external cervical os. Present evidence suggests that stilbestrol and other nonsteroidal estrogens taken during the first trimester of human pregnancy inhibit replacement of Müllerian epithelium by squamous epithelium. This results in the persistence of glandular epithelium in the vagina (adenosis) which, after exposure to carcinogenic stimuli, can undergo malignant transformation. Further support for this concept comes from experimental animal models. Administration of estrogen to the pregnant rat has been reported to arrest development of the urogenital sinus and to induce an increase in glandular epithelial mitotic activity in female offspring.

It has been estimated that between 10,000 and 16,000 females were exposed in utero to DES each year in the United States from 1960 to 1970. Drugs ingested included DES, dienestrol, or hexestrol. A progestational agent, in addition to estrogen, was used in 7% of cases. The daily dose of maternally ingested nonsteroidal estrogen varied from 1.5 mg to over 300 mg. In order for there to be a significant risk for the subsequent development of clear-cell adenocarcinoma, DES had to be taken during the first trimester of pregnancy. Data from the Registry for Clear-Cell Adenocarcinoma indicates that the size of the at-risk female population for this cancer is between 500,000 and 2 million. The risk for development of vaginal cancer in women whose mothers took DES is currently estimated to be 0.14 to 1.4 per 1000 exposed cases. Over 90% of the patients who have developed vaginal clear-cell cancer have been over 14 years of age, with a mean age of 19 years (Herbst 1976). The youngest reported patient with DES-related clear-cell carcinoma in the Registry is seven years of age, whereas the oldest is 29 years of age (Herbst et al 1979).

At the present time, there seems to be no clear theory as to the genesis of vaginal rhabdomyosarcomas. Hilgers and co-workers (1970) reviewed the prenatal and obstetric histories of over 80 patients with pelvic embryonal rhabdomyosarcomas, and could find no apparent etiologic agent for this tumor. Furthermore, no pattern of familial vaginal sarcoma or associated congenital anomalies could be detected. Growth and development of these children appeared to be normal. A history of prior pelvic radiation has been strongly implicated in the pathogenesis of uterine sarcomas (Norris and Taylor 1965, Aaro et al 1966), and theoretically could apply to vaginal leiomyosarcomas since these lesions occur in older patients. However, the latent period between radiation and the clinical observation of sarcomas has been in excess of ten years, and the number of reported cases of vaginal sarcomas following radiation has been small.

Theories as to the pathogenesis of vaginal melanomas are essentially the same as for melanomas of other sites. Intraepithelial melanoblasts have been observed in approximately 3% of vaginas (Nigogosyan et al 1964), and could serve as a precursor cell for malignant melanomas. The exact origin of these melanoblasts is unknown. Migration of melanoblasts from the neural crest to the basal cells of the vaginal epithelium has been proposed (Norris and Taylor 1966). This theory might explain the common occurrence of melanomas in the lower third of the vagina, since this portion of the vagina is anatomically formed from the ectodermally derived urogenital sinus. Other investigators (Ragni and Tobon 1973) have reported that vaginal melanocytes may arise from the mutation of active junctional cells. There is very little evidence that vaginal melanomas arise as a result of trauma or from the malignant transformation of preexisting nevi. The importance of genetic factors in the development of malignant melanoma has been emphasized by Anderson et al (1967). These investigators reported a kindred in which 15 of 250 descendants of three sisters developed malignant melanoma. This was significantly greater than the incidence of this tumor in the control group. This and other studies indicate that there is a hereditary basis for the genesis of melanoma in some patients and their relatives. Interestingly, melanomas occurring in kindreds have been shown to occur at an earlier age than would normally be expected, and to present in multiple sites relatively early in the biology of the disease.

EVALUATION

One of the most common misconceptions on the part of the public is that vaginal cytologic examinations are no longer necessary following hysterectomy. Although the incidence of vaginal epithelial abnormalities is significantly less than abnormalities of the cervical epithelium (Petrilli et al 1980), periodic cytologic sampling of the vagina should be performed. The frequency of this sampling depends upon a number of factors, including a history of cervical neoplasia, previous pelvic irradiation including the vagina, and in utero exposure to nonsteroidal estrogens. It should be emphasized that approximately 20% of patients with invasive vaginal cancer are asymptomatic. Generally, cytologic screening of the vagina in asymptomatic patients who have had a hysterectomy should be performed at least every two years.

The major symptoms of vaginal carcinoma are vaginal bleeding, vaginal discharge, and pelvic pain. The most common symptom is vaginal bleeding, which has been reported to occur in 40% to 50% of all patients (Perticucci 1972, Pride et al 1979). This bleeding is characteristically painless and occurs each day, or after sexual intercourse. Vaginal discharge occurs in approximately 20% of patients with vaginal cancer. An additional 10% of patients with vaginal cancer present with the complaint of pelvic pain. The description of this pain depends upon the location of the lesion. Anterior vaginal tumors often produce bladder pain, dysuria, and frequency, whereas carcinomas of the posterior vagina may be associated with constipation and pain with defecation. Any patient experiencing these symptoms should have a pelvic examination, including a vaginal cytologic sample, whether or not hysterectomy has been performed. In this regard, it is important to emphasize the necessity of careful inspection of all areas of the vagina. Vaginal epithelial abnormalities are often obscured by the speculum, and proper sampling is not performed. Every patient who presents with abnormal vaginal cytology should have a thorough pelvic examination, including colposcopy and iodine staining of the vagina. Appropriate biopsies of suspicious areas should be taken, and the dimensions, location, and clinical type of the lesion should be described. If the lesion is fully visible and well localized, every attempt should be made to excise it. In this way, the histologic characteristics of the lesion, as well as the extent of stromal invasion, can be more accurately evaluated. Although the concept of microinvasive carcinoma of the cervix has been clinically useful, no such data are available for vaginal epithelial lesions. Until the clinical significance of microinvasive carcinoma in the vagina has been evaluated in a sufficiently large number of patients, all vaginal lesions with stromal invasion should be treated as frankly invasive carcinoma.

Once the diagnosis of invasive vaginal carcinoma has been established,

186

all lesions should be classified histologically as squamous cell carcinoma, adenocarcinoma, sarcoma, or melanoma. The location of each tumor within the vaginal canal is particularly important since the pattern of spread depends directly on the lymphatic drainage of the area involved. In a review of over 700 cases, Plentyl and Friedman (1971) reported that the most common location of vaginal tumors was in the posterior wall of the upper vagina. Over 50% of squamous cell cancer occurred in the upper third of the vagina, as compared to 19% in the middle third, and 30% in the lower third. In general, lymphatics from the anterior wall of the upper and middle portions of the vagina anastomose with the pericervical and vesical lymphatics. These lymphatics then cross laterally over the ureter and empty into the internal iliac and external iliac lymph nodes (Figure 7-2). The anterior vaginal wall is relatively fixed so that tumors located in this area often penetrate into the urethra and bladder base. The posterior vaginal lymphatics drain to the obturator, pararectal, and aortic lymph nodes. The posterior vaginal wall is usually more pliable than the anterior vaginal wall, and a rapidly enlarging tumor can expand by direct extension without involving subvaginal tissues. Lymphatics in the lower third

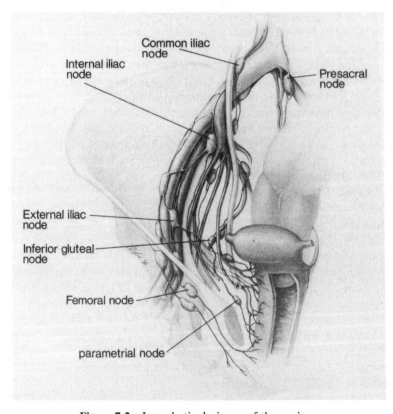

Figure 7-2 Lymphatic drainage of the vagina.

of the vagina drain primarily into the femoral nodes. In a collected series of 604 patients with vaginal cancer, Hilgers (1978) reported that 72 (11%) had palpably enlarged or histologically confirmed inguinal lymph node metastases. The majority of patients with spread to these lymph nodes had primary lesions in the lower third of the vagina. However, selected cases of upper vaginal cancer also demonstrated inguinal lymph node metastases. Perticucci (1972) reported histologically confirmed inguinal lymph node metastases in 6 of 16 patients with carcinoma in the lower vagina. Therefore, an essential part of the evaluation process for vaginal cancer includes careful palpation of both inguinal areas for the presence of enlarged lymph nodes. Such nodes should be biopsied and the presence of metastatic disease confirmed histologically.

Although it has been estimated that approximately 20% of patients with vaginal cancer have metastatic disease present in pelvic lymph nodes, the incidence of extrapelvic lymph node spread is unknown. Recently, Hughes and colleagues (1980) reported a five-year survival of 20% in patients with extrapelvic lymph nodal metastases from cervical cancer who were treated with extended field irradiation. Therefore, patients with bulky vaginal cancers (particularly those located in the upper vagina) should have routine pretherapy evaluation of both pelvic and paraaortic lymph nodes. Methods for lymph node evaluation include lymphangiography, selected lymph node biopsy, and CAT scanning with fine needle biopsy. The major methods utilized to evaluate extrapelvic lymph nodes have been discussed in Chapter 2. Briefly, the accuracy of lymphangiography in the evaluation of lymph node metastases from pelvic cancer has been reported to be quite variable. Piver and Barlow (1973), for example, noted that 23 of 24 patients with positive lymphangiographic findings actually had histologic evidence of disease. In contrast, Lagasse and coworkers (1979) reported only 67% agreement between lymphangiographic and lymph node biopsy findings. These authors concluded that extraperitoneal lymph node biopsies could provide information, not available by lymphangiography, which would be helpful in treatment planning.

The final method for evaluation of extrapelvic lymph nodal metastases is computer-assisted tomography (CAT) scanning followed by percutaneous fine needle biopsy. The technique has been reported to be quite accurate in the evaluation of lymph node metastases from cervical cancer, and has been associated with very few complications (Zornoza et al 1977). This method is the technique presently advocated by the authors in the evaluation of metastatic disease to the pelvic and paraaortic lymph nodes.

Finally, it should be emphasized that the anatomic proximity of the vagina to other normal structures such as the bladder, urethra, and rectum allows for direct spread to these organs at a relatively early stage in the biologic progression of these tumors (Figure 7-3). Evaluation of

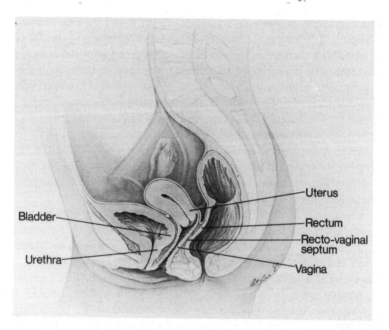

Figure 7-3 Anatomic proximity of normal pelvic structures such as the bladder, urethra, and rectum to the vagina.

patients with anterior vaginal tumors should include cystoscopic examination of the bladder and urethra. In addition, a urine sample should be submitted for cytologic examination. Patients with posterior vaginal lesions should have a sigmoidoscopic examination with biopsy of any suspicious areas. All patients should have an intravenous pyelogram, chest x-ray, and careful inspection of the introitus to rule out any areas of direct extension to the vulva.

Although the correlation between clinical estimation of extent of vaginal tumor involvement and histologic confirmation of spread is often poor, every attempt should be made to stage each lesion. Staging is not only of prognostic importance but allows for comparison of different treatment modalities in the therapy of similar vaginal tumors. Several different staging systems for vaginal cancer have been proposed (Palmer and Biback 1954, Smith 1955). However, the most recent staging system proposed by the Cancer Committee of the International Federation of Gynecology and Obstetrics (Table 7-1) is most useful. This staging system is based entirely upon clinical examination and cannot be changed at the time of surgery.

A special comment should be made concerning the evaluation of patients at risk to develop clear-cell carcinoma of the vagina. Although a very small number of exposed females will develop vaginal clear-cell cancer, approximately 85% of them will have other benign abnormalities,

Table 7-1
International Federation of Gynecology and Obstetrics
Staging System for Vaginal Cancer

Stage 0	Carcinoma in situ; intraepithelial carcinoma.
Stage I	The carcinoma is limited to the vaginal wall.
Stage II	The carcinoma has involved the subvaginal tissue, but has not extended to the pelvic wall.
Stage III	The carcinoma has extended to the pelvic wall.
Stage IV	The carcinoma has extended beyond the true pelvis or has involved the mucosa of the bladder or rectum. Bullous edema as such does not permit a case to be allotted to Stage IV.
Stage IVa	Spread of the growth to adjacent organs.
Stage IVb	Spread to distant organs.

including vaginal adenosis, cervical ectropion, and transverse vaginal and cervical ridges. It is obvious that any premenarchal patient who has vaginal bleeding or discharge should have a complete pelvic examination, including cytology and colposcopy of the cervix and vagina. Cytology has been reported to be abnormal in approximately 70% of patients with adenocarcinoma of the vagina when proper sampling of the anterior, posterior, and lateral vaginal wall is obtained (Herbst et al 1974). Such an examination should be performed even if a general anesthetic is required. Since only 10% of patients with DES-related vaginal carcinoma are under the age of 12, pelvic examination is not recommended in asymptomatic patients until menarche or the age of 14.

Recent studies have indicated that there is an increased risk of vaginal squamous epithelial abnormalities developing in areas of adenosis undergoing active metaplasia. The prevalence of squamous cell dysplasia, carcinoma in situ, and invasive squamous cell carcinoma in DES-exposed females is illustrated in Table 7-2. Squamous epithelial abnormalities occurring in areas of adenosis varied from 2.1% to over 20%. However, only 20 cases of severe dysplasia or carcinoma in situ were reported in over 1000 cases followed. In the majority of reported series, the most severe squamous epithelial abnormalities were noted in areas of cervical rather than vaginal adenosis. The occurrence of squamous abnormalities in areas of glandular epithelium undergoing metaplasia does emphasize the need for periodic examinations of these patients. Most investigators recommend yearly pelvic examination, including cytology and colposcopy, for DES-exposed patients.

Once the diagnosis of invasive clear-cell adenocarcinoma of the vagina has been made, several steps in the evaluation process should be made in addition to those previously mentioned for patients with squamous cell carcinoma of the vagina. First, an accurate history of maternal drug intake in pregnancy should be obtained. This includes the

Table 7-2
Prevalence of Squamous Neoplasia in Cervicovaginal Adenosis

Investigator	No. of Patients	Mild-Moderate Dysplasia	Severe Dysplasia Carcinoma in situ	Total
Stafl and Mattingly (1974)	131	3	4	7 (5.3%)
Fetherston (1975)	43	4	3	7 (15.2%)
Bibbo et al (1977)	229	8	0	8 (3.5%)
Ng et al (1977)	140	2	1	3 (2.1%)
Veridiano et al (1978)	203	15	4	19 (9.3%)
Burke et al (1978)	250	15	0	15 (6.0%)
Fowler and Edelman (1978)	199	36	8	44 (22%)
Total	1195	83	20	103 (8.6%)

specific dose and duration of each drug ingested, as well as the time during pregnancy when drug usage was begun. Preliminary evidence suggests that the risk for clear-cell carcinoma is inversely related to the time in pregnancy that DES was started. Also, any history of oral contraceptive usage by patients with vaginal adenocarcinoma should be recorded. Herbst and co-workers (1979) have reported that patients in the Registry who took oral contraceptives had a significantly greater survival than patients with vaginal adenocarcinoma not taking contraceptives. Possible reasons given for this improved survival include: 1) better medical surveillance in patients taking oral contraceptives leading to earlier diagnosis, and 2) a direct effect of the oral contraceptive on the tumor itself (Herbst 1979). Finally, it should be noted that vaginal adenocarcinomas have high propensity to spread to expelvic sites, and specifically to the lung and lymph nodes. Therefore, careful examination of both these areas is mandatory in the evaluation of these patients.

Evaluation of patients with vaginal sarcomas is complicated by the fact that the majority of these lesions occur in children. The most common vaginal sarcoma, embryonal rhabdomyosarcoma, usually presents in the form of a grape-like mass protruding from the vagina (sarcoma botryoides). Examination under anesthesia is usually necessary to define the size and stage of these lesions accurately. Cystoscopy should be performed at the time of examination under anesthesia to rule out occult bladder spread, since these tumors have been shown to have a high incidence of urinary tract involvement. Biopsies should be taken from different areas of the tumor so that representative sections can be analyzed histologically. Part of the evaluation of children with this lesion should include psychosocial analysis of both the patient and her family. Therapy for this lesion often involves a rather pronounced change in the lifestyle of these patients, and every effort should be made to insure a supportive environment during and after therapy. Similarly, nutritional evaluation of these children should be undertaken so that total nutritional and hormonal requirements for growth can be provided during a time of intensive chemotherapy and radical surgery.

Vaginal melanomas are quite rare, with fewer than 100 cases being reported in the recent literature. In a study from the Memorial Sloan-Kettering Cancer Center, Chung and co-workers (1980) reported that melanoma of the vagina comprised 2.8% of all vaginal tumors and 0.8% of all malignant melanomas treated at that institution. The age distribution of patients with vaginal melanoma is not unlike that of patients having squamous cell carcinoma of the vagina, with a majority of patients being over 50 years of age. In a review of vaginal malignant melanomas seen at the Armed Forces Institute of Pathology (Norris and Taylor 1965) the mean age of these patients was 62 years (range 47–72 years). Vaginal discharge and bleeding remain the most common presenting symptoms and the majority of patients have a visible, pigmented vaginal lesion. The most common site of origin of melanomas is the lower third of the vagina, and the anterior vaginal wall is more commonly involved than the posterior wall (Laufe and Bernstein 1971). Complete histologic evaluation of each melanotic lesion is extremely important since the method of treatment is influenced by the depth of tumor invasion, which should be determined in all cases according to the method of Breslow (1975). Pigmented lesions of the vagina should be excised, including a 1 to 2 cm margin of normal tissue, so that all pertinent histologic parameters can be examined. Finally, it should be emphasized that vaginal melanomas tend to metastasize early to regional pelvic lymph nodes. Spread to the groin nodes has been reported to occur in over 30% of patients with vaginal melanoma (Chung et al 1980). Therefore, the status of the inguinal, pelvic, and paraaortic lymph nodes should be thoroughly evaluated in all patients with this lesion.

PATHOLOGY

Vaginal Intraepithelial Neoplasia

The histologic changes characteristic of vaginal intraepithelial neoplasia are essentially the same as those previously described for cervical intraepithelial neoplasia. Intraepithelial lesions can be found at any location in the vagina, but occur most frequently in the upper vaginal vault. It should be noted that carcinoma in situ of the vagina has been described as multifocal in at least 50% of the cases, and may be associated with invasive carcinoma. Therefore, adequate excisional biopsies of all colposcopically abnormal areas should be submitted for examination.

Squamous dysplasia of the vagina may be separated into three grades—mild, moderate, and severe—according to the degree of cellular atypia and epithelial architecture.

Mild dysplasia   Loss of polarity and regular stratification is minimal. The nuclei are always enlarged, often irregular, and are darkly stained. Mitoses are often found, and are occasionally abnormal; they are confined to the lower third of the epithelium. The cytoplasm is generally well preserved and keratinization of single cells or of the epithelial surface is a common feature.

Moderate dysplasia   The degree of epithelial abnormality is intermediate between mild and severe dysplasia.

Severe dysplasia   Atypia is very pronounced. There is loss of polarity, and the crowded cells have large, darkly stained nuclei. Mitoses, occasionally including atypical forms, are seen. The abnormal cells tend to be present in the upper third, as well as the middle and lower thirds, of the epithelium. The superficial cells show a degree of maturation. A layer of flattened cells may form the surface.

Carcinoma in situ   A lesion in which all or most of the epithelium shows the cellular features of carcinoma. There is no invasion of the underlying vaginal stroma.

Squamous Cell Carcinoma

As previously stated, the prognostic implications of microinvasive carcinoma of the vagina are unknown. Until a sufficiently large number of patients with microinvasive cancer has been studied, all patients with any degree of stromal invasion should be classified as having invasive vaginal cancer. Invasive squamous cell carcinoma of the vagina (Figure 7-4) should be classified according to the histologic criteria proposed initially by Reagan et al (1957) for squamous cell carcinoma of the cervix:

Large-cell nonkeratinizing cancer   This tumor is characterized by large cells with a high nuclear-cytoplasmic ratio, coarse granular nuclear chromatin, basophilic cytoplasm, and limited pleomorphism.

Keratinizing squamous cell carcinoma   This tumor contains large cells with a high degree of pleomorphism. The production of structured keratin material (eg, keratin pearls) is essential for inclusion into this category.

Small-cell carcinoma   This tumor is identified by the presence of small primitive cells with dark, coarsely granular nuclei. These cells are remarkably uniform in size and have the highest nuclear cytoplasmic ratio of all cervical squamous carcinomas.

In addition to cell type, histologic specimens of invasive squamous cell carcinoma of the vagina should be examined for the presence of lymph-vascular space invasion by tumor cells. This finding has been shown to be of prognostic significance in squamous cell carcinoma of the

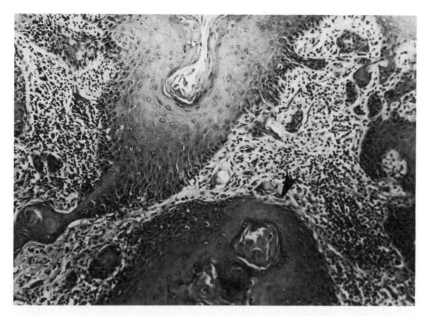

Figure 7-4 Squamous cell carcinoma of the vagina. The tumor is of the large-cell keratinizing type, characterized by formation of keratin "pearls" (arrow). Hematoxylin and eosin stain. Magnification 120×.

cervix, and may well be related to patient survival in vaginal squamous cancer as well.

Adenocarcinoma

A histologic classification of adenocarcinoma of the vagina has been proposed by Herbst et al (1979). According to these investigators, clear-cut adenocarcinoma should be divided into three cell types depending on the predominant pattern of the tumor: tubulocystic, papillary, and solid. The latter two patterns are characterized by cysts with an epithelial lining (Figure 7-5). In the tubulocystic pattern, these cysts and tubules are lined by "hobnail" cells with a single layer of prominent protruding nuclei. In contrast, the cysts of the papillary pattern are lined by delicate, epithelial papillary projections. In the solid pattern, the tumor cells are arranged in sheets of vacuolated "clear" cells with glycogen-rich cytoplasm. It should be emphasized that any or all of these patterns can be seen in the same tumor, and that the tumor is classified by the predominant pattern.

Sarcoma

Sarcomas comprise approximately 2% of malignant vaginal neo-plasms. The most common vaginal sarcomas are embryonal rhabdomyo-

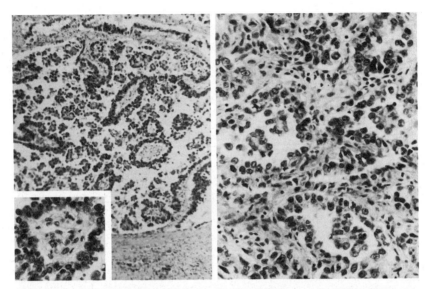

Figure 7-5 Patterns of vaginal clear-cell adenocarcinoma. (Left) Papillary pattern with tumor cells arranged around fibrous connective tissue cores. Hematoxylin and eosin stain. Magnification 40×. (Insert) Higher magnification of tumor cells with prominent nuclei. Hematoxylin and eosin stain. Magnification 300×. (Right) Tubulocystic pattern with cystic spaces lined by "hobnail" cells. Hematoxylin and eosin stain. Magnification 300 ×.

sarcomas which occur in infants and young girls, and leiomyosarcomas which occur usually in adults.

Embryonal rhabdomyosarcoma   The botryoid variety of embryonal rhabdomyosarcoma commonly occurs in hollow viscera such as the vagina. These tumors usually consist of edematous polypoid masses which give the impression of grape-like clusters protruding into the lumen of the vagina. Microscopically, these tumors often contain small polygonal and spindle-shaped cells with hyperchromatic nuclei and numerous mitotic figures (Figure 7-6). Rhabdomyoblasts are characteristically elongated and contain cross-striations easily demonstrable by special stains such as Mason's trichrome and phosphotungstic acid hematoxylin.

Leiomyosarcoma   Leiomyosarcomas present as firm bulky tumors, often with central areas of necrosis and hemorrhage. Tumor cells may destroy the overlying vaginal epithelium or remain confined to the stroma. Microscopically, these tumors contain interlacing bundles of round or elongated cells with large, hyperchromatic nuclei. Multinucleated tumor giant cells occasionally occur in pleomorphic sarcomas.

Although several investigators have attempted to classify sarcomas on the basis of cellular atypism (Spiro and Koss 1965) tumor grade, or pattern of growth (Silverberg 1971), we believe that the most important prognostic histomorphologic factor is the number of mitotic figures per ten high-power fields (HPF) of tumor tissue. Tumors containing more than five mitoses per ten HPF are definitely malignant, and tumors with high mitotic activity (> 50 mitoses per ten HPF) are associated with a high recurrence rate and poor prognosis.

Malignant Melanoma

Malignant melanomas of the vagina characteristically present as pigmented lesions slightly elevated above the vaginal mucosa (Figure 7-7). Lesions usually vary from 0.5 cm to 10.0 cm in diameter, and occur most frequently in the lower third of the vagina (Chung et al 1980). Malignant melanomas of the vagina should be classified histologically as superficial spreading melanoma, or lentigo maligna melanoma, according to the criteria of Clark and co-workers (1969). Briefly, superficial spreading melanoma is an elevated lesion which usually has an arcuate outline, whereas lentigo maligna melanoma is a flattened lesion with an irregular border. Nodular melanoma is an elevated nodular lesion which is quite regular in outline but which may have an ulcerated surface. Microscopically, these tumors are classified according to predominant cell type

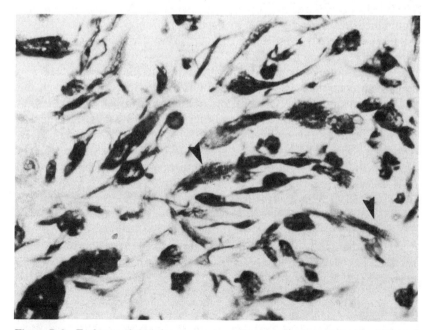

Figure 7-6 Embryonal rhabdomyosarcoma. Tumor cells are small with elongated cytoplasm and cytoplasmic cross-striations (arrows). Phosphotungstic acid hematoxylin (PTAH) stain. Magnification 780×.

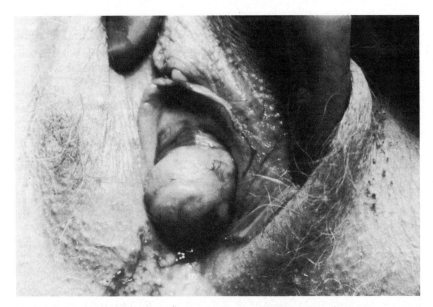

Figure 7-7 Malignant melanoma of vagina. This lesion has both pigmented and nonpigmented (amelanotic) areas, and presents as a slightly elevated lesion in the lower third of the vagina.

as epithelioid, spindle cell, or small cell (Figure 7-8). Spindle cell predominance has been reported to occur commonly in lentigo maligna melanoma, whereas epithelioid cells are most frequently observed in superficial spreading melanomas.

The histomorphologic criteria of greatest prognostic significance in malignant melanomas is the depth of tumor invasion. In 1969, Clark and colleagues proposed a classification of tumor invasion for malignant melanomas of the skin. They defined four levels of invasion of the dermis and subcutaneous fat, and demonstrated that prognosis, independent of treatment, was inversely related to the level of invasion. In vaginal melanomas, however, the anatomic structures used to differentiate levels of invasion are less clear, and the authors favor the system proposed by Breslow (1975). This system is based on accurate measurement of the maximal thickness of each lesion using an ocular micrometer (Figure 7-9). The incidence of lymph node metastases has been shown to be directly related to the depth of invasion (Wanebo et al 1975). Likewise, patient survival has varied inversely with the depth of invasion of vaginal melanomas (Chung et al 1980).

THERAPY

Carcinoma in situ of the vagina may be treated by local excision, topical 5-fluorouracil (5-FU), cryotherapy, laser therapy, or radiation.

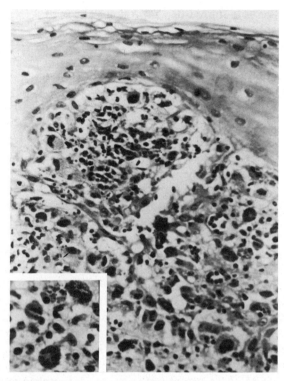

Figure 7-8 Malignant melanoma of the vagina. Nests of melanoma cells involve the squamous mucosa and extend into the submucosal tissue. Hematoxylin and eosin stain. Magnification 300×. (Insert) Tumor cells containing granular melanin pigment. Hematoxylin and eosin stain. Magnification 480×.

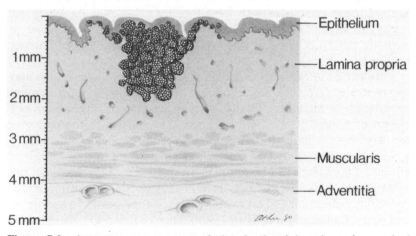

Figure 7-9 Accurate measurement of the depth of invasion of a vaginal melanoma using the system proposed by Breslow (1975). The maximal thickness of the lesion is measured with an ocular micrometer.

The type of therapy utilized depends upon the size and location of the lesion, the histologic severity of the epithelial abnormality, whether the lesion is unifocal or multifocal, and the age of the patient. Therapy should be individualized, and every effort should be made to maintain normal vaginal function, particularly in the younger patient. The anatomic extent of each epithelial lesion should be defined, using colposcopy and staining with Lugol's solution or toluidine blue. Although unifocal areas of mild and moderate vaginal dysplasia can be treated by cryotherapy, more severe histologic grades of vaginal intraepithelial neoplasia should be surgically excised. In that way, pathologic examination of the full extent of the epithelial abnormality can be performed, thereby ruling out any possible areas of microinvasive cancer.

In multifocal vaginal intraepithelial neoplasms, colposcopically-directed laser therapy offers the theoretical advantage of destroying sites of abnormal epithelium while preserving intervening areas of normal vaginal mucosa. The use of the carbon dioxide laser in the treatment of patients with vaginal intraepithelial neoplasia has been reported by Petrilli and co-workers (1980). Laser therapy was performed at a power setting of 20 watts, and all areas of epithelial abnormality were treated, as well as a 3 mm margin of normal vaginal tissue. The estimated depth of treatment was 3 to 4 mm below the epithelial surface. All ten of the lesions treated were located at the vaginal apex, and seven were multifocal. Seven patients were treated without analgesia, whereas three required general anesthesia because of the extent of the lesion. A complete response, defined as the total disappearance of the lesion, was achieved in nine of the patients (90%). No complications from this procedure were noted other than the pain experienced when patients were treated on an outpatient basis. It should be pointed out, however, that relatively few centers have had sufficient experience with laser therapy to warrant its use in the therapy of vaginal neoplasia. Like many other sophisticated treatment methods, the efficacy of laser therapy is only as good as the physician who is using it.

Multifocal intraepithelial neoplasia limited to the upper vagina may also be treated by partial vaginectomy. The area of vagina excised should be sufficient to encompass all sites of epithelial abnormality, as well as a margin of normal tissue. Split-thickness skin grafting to the operative site may be necessary to preserve normal vaginal depth and function.

In 1975, Woodruff and co-workers reported the successful use of topical 5-fluorouracil (5-FU) cream in the treatment of carcinoma in situ of the vagina. This drug interacts directly with the RNA in the tumor cell, preventing replication and eventually producing cell death. In a more recent study, Ballon and colleagues (1979) reported that 5-FU was effective in eradicating vaginal intraepithelial neoplasia in 12 patients. The topical preparation used consisted of 5% 5-fluorouracil in a white petrolatum base (Efudex). Topical 5-FU was applied intravaginally twice daily for a period of two weeks, and the normal vulvar skin was protected with a barrier ointment. Eight weeks were allowed for healing, and a second course of therapy was given only if a cytologic smear suggested persistent vaginal neoplasia. Conversely, if vaginal cytology was normal, the patient was considered to be in remission, and was followed with repeat cytologic smears every three months. Using this protocol, five patients were cured after one course of therapy, six patients required two courses of treatment, and one patient was cured after three courses of treatment. Three of these patients developed recurrent vaginal intraepithelial neoplasia 11 to 16 months after therapy, and all were successfully retreated with topical 5-FU. Vaginal irritation occurred in all patients during the period of drug application, but no serious complications were noted.

A second treatment regimen using 5-FU has been suggested by Petrilli and colleagues (1980). These investigators first gave a 5-ml test dose of 5-FU intravaginally, and the patient was examined four days later. If no changes in the vaginal epithelium were noted, the patient was instructed to insert 5 ml of 5-FU cream twice daily for five days. If the test dose caused ulceration of the lesion, a modified dose of 5 ml once daily was initiated. In postmenopausal women, the duration of the treatment course was reduced to four days. Each course of treatment was repeated every three months if indicated on the basis of cytologic or colposcopic abnormalities. This therapeutic regimen was effective in eradicating various degrees of vaginal intraepithelial neoplasia in 12 of 15 patients treated.

In the past, the most common method of treating multifocal vaginal carcinoma in situ was radiation therapy. Radiotherapy is given usually from one of a variety of intravaginal applicators which provide approximately 6000 to 7000 rad to the vaginal surface (Figure 7-10). The advantage of intracavitary radiation is that a maximal dose can be given to the abnormal epithelium without significantly affecting normal submucosal tissues. For lesions involving the upper vagina, an applicator which combines ovoids and a vaginal cylinder is useful. The size of the ovoids and the cylinder can be varied according to the anatomical dimensions of the individual patient. For lesions involving the middle and lower vaginal canal, a vaginal cylinder alone may be sufficient. These applicators are loaded in such a way as to maximize the dose to the area of epithelial abnormality, and to spare adjacent normal tissues.

Using these techniques, the treatment of vaginal carcinoma in situ is highly effective. Rutledge (1967) reported that there were no recurrences noted in 31 patients treated for vaginal carcinoma in situ. Twenty-seven of these patients were treated primarily by radiation therapy. Similarly, Brown and colleagues (1971) noted only four recurrences in 34 patients with vaginal carcinoma in situ treated with radiotherapy. All of the recurrences were located in the vaginal vault. These vault failures were presumably due to "cold" spots of inadequate radiation caused by vaginal ridges or dimples preventing proper contact of all the mucosa with ap-

200

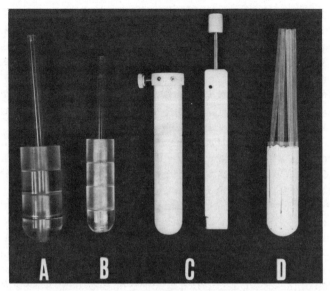

Figure 7-10 After-loading Kentucky applicators used in the treatment of vaginal carcinoma. **(A)** Vaginal cylinder for large vaginal vault (central tandem). **(B)** Vaginal cylinder for narrow vaginal vault (central tandem). **(C)** Vaginal cylinder with crossing sources at vault. Central tandem for surface core (right) inserts into cylinder (left). **(D)** Surface cylinder for small vaginal lesions. Needles inserted into tubes as determined by lesion size. Variable leading of central tendem and peripheral tubes. (Courtesy of Maruyama Y, Beach JL, Mendiondo O, Department of Radiation Medicine, University of Kentucky Medical Center.)

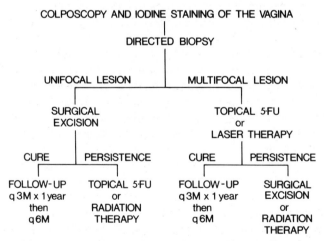

Figure 7-11 Schematic proposal for diagnosis and management of vaginal intra-epithelial neoplasia.

plicator. The major complication of this treatment method is vaginal fibrosis and subsequent stenosis. For this reason, every effort should be made to limit the treatment field to those areas of epithelial abnormality, and to spare as much of the normal vagina as possible.

A general approach to the therapy of vaginal intraepithelial neoplasia is presented in Figure 7-11. It is recommended that small unifocal lesions be treated initially by surgical excision, whereas multifocal disease can first be treated by topical 5-FU or the carbon dioxide laser. More extensive surgical procedures or radiation therapy should be reserved for patients with multifocal lesions which do not respond to initial methods of therapy. Following therapy for vaginal intraepithelial neoplasia, patients should be examined every three months for two years, and every six months thereafter. A vaginal cytologic specimen should be obtained at the time of these regular clinical examinations.

Invasive Cancer

The therapy of invasive vaginal cancer must be individualized according to the cell type, stage, and anatomic location of the lesion. Therapy is made more difficult by the anatomic proximity of the rectum, bladder, and urethra to the vagina. In certain cases, it is impossible to give tumoricidal doses of radiation without exceeding the normal tissue tolerance of these adjacent structures. Likewise, it is often surgically difficult to excise carcinoma involving the anterior vaginal wall without damaging bladder and urethral function.

Small Stage I squamous cell carcinomas involving the upper 3 cm of the vagina can be treated with radical hysterectomy, upper vaginectomy, and pelvic lymphadenectomy, particularly in younger patients. Split-thickness skin grafting may be required to maintain vaginal function in selected cases in which a significant amount of vaginal tissue is excised. However, ovarian function is preserved and the complications of radiation therapy, including vaginal fibrosis, are avoided. Radiation therapy can also be used as a treatment method in patients with squamous cell carcinoma of the upper vagina. In Stage I and II lesions of the vaginal vault with an intact uterus, radiation is given in the form of 4000 rad external therapy followed by an intracavitary implant. In most cases, intracavitary therapy can be given by an intrauterine tandem plus ovoids. A total of 8000 rad is delivered to the surface of the vaginal lesion in one or two implants, using this technique. If the uterus is absent, intracavitary therapy is usually given from a Bloedorn-type applicator or a vaginal cylinder.

Radiation therapy is the preferred treatment method in carcinomas involving the lower two thirds of the vagina. The pelvis is usually given 4000 rad external therapy at a rate of 180 to 200 rad per day. The parametrial and lateral pelvic wall lymph nodes are then given a boost of

1000 to 1500 rad through reduced fields with midline shielding. This is usually followed by intralesional therapy using radium or iridium needles. Carcinomas involving the distal one third of the vagina or the introitus often spread to the inguinal lymph nodes (Plentyl and Friedman 1971). Consequently, the addition of bilateral inguinal lymphadenectomy is necessary in the treatment of these lesions. Advanced stage lesions are treated with 5000 rad external therapy to the pelvis, 1000 to 2000 rad to a reduced field including the tumor, and interstitial needles delivering 2000 to 3000 rad to the lesion itself. Large central lesions involving the rectum or bladder often require anterior or posterior exenteration. Likewise, exenterative surgery is indicated in selected cases of central recurrent vaginal carcinoma after primary irradiation.

There have been very few reports concerning the efficacy of various chemotherapeutic agents in the treatment of widely metastatic primary or recurrent squamous cell carcinoma of the vagina. Piver and co-workers (1978) reported the response rate of 100 patients with squamous cell carcinoma of the cervix or vagina to a variety of chemotherapeutic agents. The highest response rate (57%) occurred in patients treated with a combination of doxorubicin, cyclophosphamide and 5-fluorouracil. There were no differences noted in the response rate of cervical and vaginal carcinomas. Therefore, it is quite likely that chemotherapeutic agents effective in the therapy of squamous cell carcinomas of the cervix will also be useful in vaginal squamous cancers. The overall five-year survival of patients treated for invasive squamous cell carcinoma of the vagina is presented in Table 7-3.

Table 7-3
Five-Year Survival of Patients
with Squamous Cell Carcinoma of the Vagina

Stage	No. of Patients	5-Year Survival
I	64	49 (77%)
II	166	81 (48%)
III	60	15 (25%)
IV	37	2 (5%)

Data from Brown et al (1971), Herbst et al (1963), Perez et al (1974), Prempree et al (1977), and Pride et al (1979).

The same therapeutic considerations previously discussed in patients with squamous cell vaginal cancers are also applicable in patients with clear-cell carcinomas of the vagina. Initial treatment results (Herbst et al 1979) have indicated that radical surgery is quite effective in early stage tumors. The five-year survival of patients with Stage I disease was 87% and the lowest recurrence rate occurred in patients who were treated by radical hysterectomy, vaginectomy, and pelvic lymphadenectomy (Table

7-4). Wharton and colleagues (1975), however, reported the effective treatment of Stage I and II vaginal carcinomas using a combination of radiotherapeutic modalities. Stage I tumors were treated with a 4 to 5 cm transvaginal cone from an orthovoltage (140 KV) source. The diameter of the cone encompassed the cancer and 1 to 2 cm of surrounding normal tissue. The radiation dose ranged from 5000 to 6000 rad and often followed local excision of tumor. Stage II lesions were treated by whole pelvis external radiation followed by intracavitary therapy with a Bloedorn applicator or iridium needles. There were no recurrences noted in eight patients treated using this technique. However, vaginal stenosis was commonly observed following completion of therapy.

Table 7-4
Five-Year Survival of Patients with Clear-Cell Carcinoma of the Vagina

Stage	No. of Patients	5-Year Survival
I	142	87%
II	39	76%
III	27*	40%
IV	5*	0%

*May include clear-cell carcinoma of both the cervix and vagina since it is impossible to determine the primary site of origin in selected cases.
Modified from Herbst et al (1978) and Herbst (personal communication, 1980).

A variety of chemotherapeutic agents have been used in the treatment of metastatic clear-cell carcinoma of the vagina. However, the number of patients studied is small and the response rate has been disappointing. Doxorubicin, actinomycin D, and cyclophosphamide have all been somewhat effective in the treatment of these tumors with approximately one third of patients achieving objective remissions (Herbst 1979). No patients have responded to progesterone therapy alone.

The therapy for vaginal sarcomas and, specifically, embryonal rhabdomyosarcomas has undergone marked change during the past decade. Prior to 1970, these lesions were treated by radical surgery, radiation therapy, or a combination thereof. The anatomic extension of these tumors into the bladder or rectum often necessitated primary exenterative surgery which was associated with a high complication rate and poor survival, as well as severe psychologic trauma to many of the children with this disease. Exelby (1974), for example, reported that the two-year survival of 108 children with embryonal rhabdomyosarcoma treated at New York's Memorial-Sloan Kettering Hospital from 1960 to 1966 was only 18%. More recently, the use of combination chemotherapy with vincristine, actinomycin D, and cyclophospamide (VAC) with or without doxorubicin has markedly improved the survival of patients with these tumors. Kumar and co-workers (1976) reported the successful use of primary combination chemotherapy (VAC) and low dose radiation prior to surgery in three girls with vaginal rhabdomyosarcoma. Pelvic exenteration was avoided in every case, and all patients were surviving without evidence of recurrent disease 32 to 54 months following therapy. Similarly, Rivard and colleagues (1975) noted that radical surgical procedures could often be avoided entirely if intensive combination chemotherapy (VAC) was combined with low-dose radiation to the primary tumor as the initial method of therapy. It would appear, therefore, that vaginal rhabdomyosarcomas should be treated primarily with combination chemotherapy (VAC), and that the extent of surgery or radiation therapy should depend upon the response rate of the tumor to chemotherapy. It is quite likely that radical surgery and even radiation therapy can be avoided in selected patients whose tumors respond completely to chemotherapy. The present two-year survival of these lesions using combined therapeutic modalities is approximately 80% (Exelby 1974). The treatment of leiomyosarcomas and reticulum cell sarcomas of the vagina involves surgical excision followed by irradiation. Additional combination chemotherapy is indicated in patients with advanced-stage disease or in tumors with a high mitotic index (> 20 mitoses/10 HPF).

Malignant melanoma of the vagina is best treated by radical excision of the lesion and regional lymphadenectomy. For lesions in the upper and middle vagina, the surgical procedure of choice is radical hysterectomy and subtotal vaginectomy with pelvic lymphadenectomy. Melanomas confined to the lower third of the vagina should be treated by radical partial vaginectomy, vulvectomy, and inguinal lymphadenectomy. To date, radiation therapy has been ineffective in the treatment of these lesions. Chung and co-workers (1980) reported that only one of eight patients with vaginal melanomas treated primarily by irradiation showed evidence of local disease control, and that one patient eventually died of metastatic tumor. Methyl CCNU, dacarbazine, and triethylenemelamine have all been used in the chemotherapeutic management of vaginal melanoma, but with limited success. The overall five-year survival of the largest reported series of malignant melanoma of the vagina was only 21% (Chung et al 1980). This limited survival is related, at least in part, to the tendency of vaginal melanomas to have penetrated deeply into the submucosal tissue by the time they are first diagnosed. For this reason, any melanotic lesion of the vagina should be excised and sent for histologic examination as soon as possible.

Major complications of therapy have been reported in 10% to 15% of patients treated for primary vaginal cancer (Marcus et al 1978, Brown et al 1971). This unusually high complication rate is related to the fact that the vagina is adjacent to the bladder, urethra, rectum, and sometimes even the small bowel (Figure 7-12). These normal pelvic structures are often damaged as a result of radical surgery or radiation therapy necessary to eradicate primary vaginal tumors. Pride and co-workers

(1979) reported major complications in 8 of 43 patients treated for vaginal cancer. Rectovaginal fistulae occurred in four patients and vesico-vaginal fistulae were noted in two patients. The most common complication in patients treated by radiation therapy is vaginal stenosis. Patients should be encouraged to maintain vaginal function following completion of irradiation, and may even require the periodic use of a vaginal dilator. The incidence of complications in patients treated by radiation therapy is directly related to the dose delivered to the vaginal mucosa. Marcus and colleagues (1978), for example, reported that all major complications occurred in patients who received in excess of 10,000 rad to the vaginal surface. Likewise, no complications were noted in patients who received less than 4000 rad from interstitial implants.

RECURRENCE AND FOLLOW-UP

Approximately 40% of patients with vaginal cancer will develop recurrence following primary therapy. Available data suggest that the pattern of recurrence of squamous cell carcinoma of the vagina closely resembles that of cervical carcinoma. The majority of recurrences occur within two years of primary treatment, and most commonly are confined

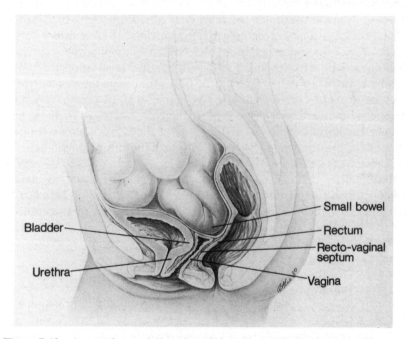

Figure 7-12 Anatomic proximity of small bowel to upper vagina in patient who has previously undergone a hysterectomy. This proximity may limit the radiation dose given to a carcinoma of the vaginal apex.

to the pelvis. Herbst and colleagues (1970) reported that 16 of 18 recurrences of primary vaginal squamous cancers were limited to pelvic structures, with the vagina being the most common site involved. Similarly, recurrences of clear-cell carcinoma of the vagina have been located within the pelvis in 60% of reported cases. The majority of these recurrences have been diagnosed within three years of initial therapy (Herbst et al 1978). Following treatment of invasive vaginal cancer, it is recommended that follow-up pelvic examinations including vaginal cytology be performed at monthly intervals for one year, every two months for two years, and every six months thereafter. Other common sites of recurrence include the bladder and ureters in all cell types of vaginal cancer, and the supraclavicular lymph nodes and lungs in clear-cell carcinomas. Therefore, it is suggested that an intravenous pyelogram and a chest x-ray be performed at yearly intervals following therapy, and that careful palpation of the supraclavicular area be performed at the time of clinical examinations.

The treatment of recurrent vaginal cancer depends upon a number of factors including the method of therapy used to treat the primary tumor, the site of recurrence, and the size or extent of the recurrent tumor. Radiation therapy can be used effectively in patients whose tumors were treated initially by radical surgery. However, the majority of patients with invasive vaginal carcinoma are treated primarily by irradiation and thus have received the maximum tolerable dose of radiotherapy. In these patients, radical surgery is the only effective method to treat tumor recurrence. Radical surgical excision with inguinal lymphadenectomy can occasionally be effective in the treatment of small recurrences located in the distal vagina, but the vast majority of postradiation tumor recurrence must be treated by pelvic exenteration (Figure 7-13). In a recent review of 296 pelvic exenterations performed at the MD Anderson Hospital and Tumor Institute (Rutledge et al 1967), 37 of these procedures were performed for recurrent vaginal cancer. Although this operation can be quite effective in the treatment of vaginal cancer, it is a formidable surgical procedure which is associated with a significant incidence of major postoperative complications. Therefore, every effort should be made to select those patients who are the best candidates for this operation. Generally, pelvic exenteration should *not* be performed in patients with recurrent vaginal cancer who have the following findings:

1. Unilateral leg edema with associated sciatic pain
2. Extrapelvic metastatic disease
3. Metastases to a large number of lateral pelvic wall lymph nodes
4. Metastatic tumor in the small bowel
5. Ureteral obstruction on intravenous pyelography.

Rutledge and colleagues (1977) reported that only 2 of 30 patients undergoing pelvic exenteration for recurrent cervical or vaginal carcinoma who had metastatic disease in the pelvic lymph nodes survived without cancer. Similarly, Barber and colleagues (1963) reported a five-year survival rate of only 10% following pelvic exenteration in patients with unilateral nonfunction of the kidney. If ureteral obstruction was associated with positive pelvic lymph nodes, the overall survival rate declined even further to 3%. It should be pointed out that there have been numerous technical improvements in the operation of pelvic exenteration since it was initially described. Notable among these improvements are the use of the ileum as a urinary conduit (Bricker et al 1960), reconstruction of the pelvic floor using the omentum (Buchsbaum and White 1973), and the use of skin and myocutaneous grafts to construct a neovagina

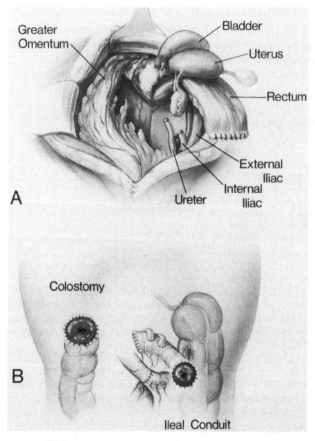

Figure 7-13 Total pelvic exenteration performed for recurrent vaginal cancer. Note the vaginal tumor is extending anteriorly to involve the bladder and posteriorly to involve the rectum.

(Morley et al 1973). Most importantly, the five-year survival of patients with recurrent vaginal carcinoma treated by pelvic exenteration is in excess of 40% when the aforementioned criteria are used for patient selection (Rutledge et al 1977).

Chemotherapy is required when recurrent vaginal cancer is diagnosed in extrapelvic sites. The specific chemotherapeutic agents utilized depend largely upon the cell type of the primary tumor. As has been previously mentioned, combination chemotherapy with doxorubicin, cyclophosphamide, and 5-fluorouracil has been shown to be reasonably effective in metastatic squamous cell carcinoma of the vagina (Piver et al 1978). Likewise, doxorubicin, actinomycin D, and cyclophosphamide have all produced responses in patients with metastatic clear-cell carcinomas. At the present time, however, the duration of chemotherapeutically-induced responses has been somewhat limited in patients with both squamous cell carcinomas and clear-cell carcinomas, and patient survival has been only minimally prolonged. The best response of vaginal tumors to chemotherapy has been observed in patients with rhabdomyosarcomas treated by a combination of vincristine, actinomycin D, and cyclophosphamide (VAC). Present data would suggest that the use of combination chemotherapy has been the most important therapeutic factor in the recently observed increase in two-year survival of patients with these tumors from approximately 20% 15 years ago to over 70% at the present time (Exelby 1974, Kumar et al 1976).

BIBLIOGRAPHY

Aaro LA, Symmonds RE, Dockerty MB: Sarcoma of the uterus. *Am J Obstet Gynecol* 94:101–104, 1966.

Anderson DE, Smith JL, McBride CM: Hereditary aspects of malignant melanoma. *JAMA* 200:741–746, 1967.

Balch CM, Murad TM, Song SJ, et al: Tumor thickness as a guide to surgical management of clinical Stage I melanoma patients. *Cancer* 43:883–888, 1979.

Ballon SC, Roberts JA, Lagasse LD: Topical 5-fluorouracil in the treatment of intraepithelial neoplasia of the vagina. *Obstet Gynecol* 54:163–165, 1979.

Barber HRK, Roberts S, Brauchwig A: Prognostic significance of the preoperative non-visualizing kidney in patients receiving pelvic exenteration. *Cancer* 16:1674–1678, 1963.

Barclay DL: Carcinoma of the vagina after hysterectomy for severe dysplasia or carcinoma in situ of the cervix. *Gynecol Oncol* 8:1–11, 1979.

Bibbo M, Gill WB, Azizi F, et al: Follow-up study of male and female offspring of DES exposed mothers. *Obstet Gynecol* 49:1–8, 1977.

Breslow A: Tumor thickness, level of invasion and node dissection in Stage I cutaneous melanoma. *Ann Surg* 182:572–575, 1975.

Bricker EM, Butcher HR, Lawlor WH: Surgical treatment of advanced and recurrent cancer of the pelvic viscera. *Ann Surg* 152:388–402, 1960.

Brown GR, Fletcher GH, Rutledge RN: Irradiation of "in-situ" and invasive squamous cell carcinoma of the vagina. *Cancer* 28:1278–1283, 1971.

Buchsbaum HJ, White AJ: Omental sling for management of the pelvic floor following exenteration. *Am J Obstet Gynecol* 117:407–412, 1973.

Burke A, Antonioli D, Rosen S: Vaginal and cervical squamous cell dysplasia in women exposed to diethylstilbestrol in utero. *Am J Obstet Gynecol* 132:537–544, 1978.

Chung AF, Casey MJ, Flannery JT, et al: Malignant melanoma of the vagina — Report of 19 cases. *Obstet Gynecol* 55:720–727, 1980.

Clark WH, Fram L, Bernadino EA, et al: The histogenesis and biologic behavior of primary human malignant melanomas of the skin. *Cancer Res* 29:705–726, 1969.

Clatworthy HW, Braren V, Smith JP: Surgery of bladder and prostatic neoplasms in children. *Cancer* 32:1157–1160, 1973.

Clement PB, Benedet JL: Adenocarcinoma in situ of the vagina. A case report. *Cancer* 43:2479–2485, 1979.

Collantes TM, Pratt JH, Dockerty MB: Primary malignant melanoma of the vagina. *Gynecol* 29:508–514, 1967.

Creasman WT, Rutledge F: Carcinoma in situ of the cervix. An analysis of 861 patients. *Obstet Gynecol* 39:373–380, 1971.

Daw E: Primary melanoma of the vagina. *Am J Obstet Gynecol* 112:307–308, 1972.

Devos I, Abell MR: Sarcomas of the vagina. *Obstet Gynecol* 47:342–350, 1975.

Douglas GW: Observations on the pathology of primary carcinoma of the vagina and its relation to therapy. *Surg Gynecol Obstet* 98:456–459, 1954.

Exelby PR: Management of embryonal rhabdomyosarcoma in children. *Surg Clin North Am* 54:849–857, 1974.

Fehr PE, Prem KA: Post-irradiation sarcoma of the pelvic girdle following therapy for squamous cell carcinoma of the cervix. *Am J Obstet Gynecol* 116:192–200, 1973.

Fenn ME, Abell MR: Melanomas of vulva and vagina. *Obstet Gynecol* 41:902–911, 1973.

Fetherston WC: Squamous neoplasia of the vagina related to the DES syndrome. *Am J Obstet Gynecol* 122:176–181, 1975.

Fowler WC, Edelman DA: In utero exposure to DES. Evaluation and follow-up of 199 women. *Obstet Gynecol* 51:459–463, 1978.

Fu Yao-Shi, Robboy SJ, Pratt L: Nuclear DNA study of vaginal and cervical squamous cell abnormalities in DES exposed progeny. *Obstet Gynecol* 52:129–137, 1978.

Grosfeld JL, Smith JP, Clatworthy HW: Pelvic rhabdomyosarcoma in infants and children. *J Urol* 107:673–675, 1972.

Henson D, Tarone R: A epidemiologic study of cancer of the cervix, vagina, and vulva based on the Third National Cancer Survey in the United States. *Am J Obstet Gynecol* 129:525–532, 1977.

Herbst AL, Green TH, Ulfelder H: Primary carcinoma of the vagina. *Am J Obstet Gynecol* 106:210–218, 1963.

Herbst AL, Kurman RJ, Scully RE, et al: Clear-cell adenocarcinoma of the genital tract in young females. Registry report. *N Engl J Med* 287:1259–1264, 1972.

Herbst AL, Robboy SJ, Scully RE, et al: Clear-cell adenocarcinoma of the vagina and cervix in girls: Analysis of 170 registry cases. *Am J Obstet Gynecol* 119:713–724, 1974.

Herbst AL, Scully RE, Robboy SJ, et al: Stilbestrol-induced abnormalities of the genital tract in young women. *Prog Gynecol* 6:647–668, 1975.

210

Herbst AL: Summary of the changes in the human female genital tract as a consequence of maternal diethystilbestrol therapy. *J Toxicol Environ Health [Suppl]*1:13–20, 1976.

Herbst AL, Norusis MJ, Rosenow PJ, et al: An analysis of 346 cases of clear cell adenocarcinoma of the vagina and cervix with emphasis on recurrence and survival. *Gynecol Oncol* 7:111–112, 1979.

Herbst AL, Cole P, Norusis MJ, et al: Epidemiologic aspects and factors related to survival in 384 registry cases of clear cell adenocarcinoma of the vagina and cervix. *Am J Obstet Gynecol* 135:876–883, 1979.

Hernadez W, DiSaia PJ, Morrow CP, et al: Mixed mesodermal sarcoma of the ovary. *Obstet Gynecol* 49:59s–63s, 1977.

Hilgers RD, Malkasian GD, Soule SH: Embryonal rhabdomyosarcoma (botryoid type) of the vagina. *Am J Obstet Gynecol* 107:484–502, 1970.

Hilgers RD: Squamous cell carcinoma of the vagina. *Surg Clin North Am* 58:25–38, 1978.

Horn RC, Enterline HT: Rhabdomyosarcoma: A clinico-pathological study and classification of 39 cases. *Cancer* 11:181–199, 1957.

Hughes R, Brewington K, Hanjani P, et al: Extended field irradiation for cervical cancer based on surgical staging. *Gynecol Oncol* 9:153–161, 1980.

Kanbour AI, Klionsky B, Murphy AI: Carcinoma of the vagina following cervical cancer. *Cancer* 34:1838–1841, 1974.

Kumar APM, Wrenn EL, Fleming ID, et al: Combined therapy to prevent complete pelvic exenteration for rhabdomyosarcoma of the vagina or uterus. *Cancer* 37:118–122, 1976.

Kurman RJ: Abnormalities of the genital tract following stilbestrol exposure in utero. Recent results. *Cancer Res* 66:161–174, 1979.

Lagasse LD, Ballon SC, Berman ML, et al: Pre-treatment lymphangiography and operative evaluation in carcinoma of the cervix. *Am J Obstet Gynecol* 134:219–224, 1979.

Laufe LE, Bernstein ED: Primary malignant melanoma of the vagina. *Obstet Gynecol* 37:148–154, 1971.

Marcus RV, Million RR, Daly JW: Carcinoma of the vagina. *Cancer* 42:2507–2512, 1978.

Morley GW, Lindenauer SM, Young D: Vaginal reconstruction following pelvic exenteration. *Am J Obstet Gynecol* 116:996–1002, 1973.

Morrow CP, Townsend DE: Management of adenosis and clear-cell adenocarcinoma of vagina and cervix. *J Reprod Med* 15:25–27, 1975.

Ng AB, Reagan, JW, Nadji M, et al: Natural history of vaginal adenosis in women exposed to diethylstilbestrol in utero. *J Reprod Med* 18:1–8, 1977.

Nigogosyan G, DeLa Pava S, Pickren JW: Melanoblasts in vaginal mucosa. *Cancer* 17:912–913, 1964.

Norris HJ, Taylor HB: Post-irradiation sarcomas of the uterus. *Obstet Gynecol* 26:689–694, 1965.

Norris HJ, Taylor HB: Melanomas of the vagina. *Am J Clin Path* 46:420–426, 1966.

Ostergard DR, Morton DG: Multifocal carcinoma of the female genitals. *Am J Obstet Gynecol* 99:1006–1015, 1967.

Palmer JP, Biback SM: Primary cancer of the vagina. *Am J Obstet Gynecol* 67:377–385, 1954.

Perez CA, Arneson AN, Galakatos A, et al: Malignant tumors of the vagina. *Cancer* 31:36–44, 1973.

Perez CA, Arneson AN, Dehner LP, et al: Radiation therapy in carcinoma of the vagina. *Obstet Gynecol* 44:862–872, 1974.

Perticucci S: Diagnostic, prognostic, and therapeutic considerations in invasive carcinoma of the vagina. *Obstet Gynecol* 40:843–850, 1972.

Petrilli ES, Townsend DE, Morrow CP, et al: Vaginal intraepithelial neoplasia: Biologic aspects and treatment with topical 5-fluorouracil and the carbon dioxide laser. *Am J Obstet Gynecol* 138:321–327, 1980.

Piver MS, Barlow JJ: Para-aortic lymphadenectomy, aortic node biopsy, and aortic lymphangiography in staging patients with advanced cervical cancer. *Cancer* 32:367–370, 1973.

Piver MS, Barlow JJ, Exynos FP: Adriamycin alone or in combination in 100 patients with carcinoma of the cervix or vagina. *Am J Obstet Gynecol* 131:311–313, 1978.

Plentyl A, Friedman E: *Lymphatic System of the Female Gentialia.* Philadelphia, W.B. Saunders, 1971, pp 57–74.

Pratt CB, Hustu HO, Fleming I, et al: Coordinated treatment of childhood rhabdomyosarcoma with surgery, radiotherapy, and combination chemotherapy. *Cancer Res* 32:606–610, 1972.

Prempree T, Viravalthana T, Slawson R, et al: Radiation management of primary carcinoma of the vagina. *Cancer* 40:109–118, 1977.

Pride GL, Buchler DA: Carcinoma of vagina 10 or more years following pelvic irradiation therapy. *Am J Obstet Gynecol* 127:513–517, 1977.

Pride GL, Schultz AE, Chuprevich TW, et al: Primary invasive squamous carcinoma of the vagina. *Obstet Gynecol* 53:218–225, 1979.

Ragni MV, Tobon H: Primary malignant melanoma of the vagina and vulva. *Obstet Gynecol* 43:658–664, 1973.

Reagan JW, Hamonic MS, Wentz WB: Analytical study of the cells in cervical squamous cell cancer. *Lab Invest* 6:241–250, 1957.

Rivard G, Ortega J, Hittle R, et al: Intensive chemotherapy as primary treatment of rhabdomyosarcoma of the pelvis. *Cancer* 36:1593–1597, 1975.

Robboy SJ, Herbst AL, Scully RE: Clear cell adenocarcinoma of the vagina and cervix in young females: Analysis of 37 tumors that persisted or recurred after primary therapy. *Cancer* 34:606–614, 1974.

Robboy SJ, Keh PC, Nickerson RJ, et al: Squamous cell dysplasia and carcinoma in situ of the cervix and vagina after prenatal exposure to diethylstilbestrol. *Obstet Gynecol* 51:528–535, 1978.

Rutledge F: Cancer of the vagina. *Am J Obstet Gynecol* 97:635–655, 1967.

Sheets JL, Dockerty MG, Decker DG, et al: Primary epithelial malignancy in the vagina. *Am J Obstet Gynecol* 89:121–129, 1964.

Silverberg SG: Leiomyosarcoma of the uterus. *Obstet Gynecol* 38:613–627, 1971.

Silverberg SG, DeGiorgi L: Clear cell carcinoma of the vagina. *Cancer* 29:1680–1689, 1977.

Smith FR: Primary carcinoma of the vagina. *Am J Obstet Gynecol* 69:525–531, 1955.

Spiro RH, Koss LG: Myosarcoma of the uterus: A clinico-pathological study. *Cancer* 18:571–588, 1965.

Stafl A, Mattingly RF: Vaginal adenosis: A precancerous lesion. *Am J Obstet Gynecol* 120:666–677, 1974.

Valdecasas RG, Rico LR, Linares, J, et al: Malignant melanoma of the vagina. A case diagnosed cytologically. *Acta Cytol* 18:535–537, 1974.

van Nagell JR, Parker JC, Hicks LP, et al: Diagnostic and therapeutic efficacy of cervical conization. *Am J Obstet Gynecol* 124:134–139, 1976.

van Nagell JR, Donaldson ES, Wood EG, et al: The significance of vascular invasion and lymphocytic infiltration in invasive cervical cancer. *Cancer* 41:228–234, 1978.

Veridiano NR, Tancer ML, Weiner EA: Squamous cell carcinoma in situ of the vagina and cervix after intrauterine DES exposure. *Obstet Gynecol* 52(suppl): 30–33, 1978.

Wanebo HJ, Woodruff J, Fortrer JG: Malignant melanoma of the extremities: A clinicopathologic study using levels of invasion (microstage). *Cancer* 35: 666–676, 1975.

Wharton JT, Rutledge FN, Gallager HS, et al: Treatment of clear cell adenocarcinoma in young females. *Obstet Gynecol* 45:365–368, 1975.

Wilkinson TS, Paletta FX: Malignant melanoma: Current concepts. *Am Surg* 35:301–309, 1969.

Woodruff JD, Parmley TH, Julian CG: Topical 5-fluorouracil in the treatment of vaginal carcinoma-in-situ. *Gynecol Oncol* 3:124–128, 1975.

Woodruff JD, Williams TJ: Multiple sites of anaplasia in the lower genital tract. *Am J Obstet Gynecol* 85:724–743, 1963.

Zornoza J, Lukeman JM, Jing BS, et al: Percutaneous retroperitoneal lymph node biopsy in carcinoma of the cervix. *Gynecol Oncol* 5:43–51, 1977.

8 Cancer of the Endometrium

Hugh R. K. Barber

Cancer of the endometrium is on the increase. There were 27,000 new cases reported in 1978, and the projected figure for 1981 is 38,000 new cases. It is interesting that, although the number of cases has increased dramatically in number, the projected number of deaths for 1981 declined only slightly, from 3200 in 1979 to 3100 in 1981. On the basis of the incidence of cancer reported in the Third National Cancer Survey and the U.S. Lifetables for 1970, the probability for developing endometrial cancer has been reported. About 2.2% of newborn girls (one of 45), will develop endometrial cancer at some time in their lives. Cancer of the endometrium is a disease of suburbia, and is found more frequently among affluent women.

The increased frequency of endometrial cancer has been due in large part to the emergence of a neoplasm having more malignant glandular and squamous components, in contrast to endometrial adenocarcinoma. The adenosquamous cancers are more readily detected by cellular methods, occur in older age groups, have a shorter symptomatic period, are associated with less differentiated glandular components, are more advanced at the time of detection, and have a poor five-year survival rate. The overall survival rate for this group of tumors is only 20%.

213

Cancer of the endometrium in its early stages can be successfully treated with relatively unsophisticated techniques, and is cured more easily and frequently than malignant disease of any other organ except the skin. It is to be emphasized that this applies only to cancer of the endometrium in its early stages. Endometrial cancer is generally considered to have a high rate of cure, but survival figures do not bear this out. Gusberg has reported a five-year survival rate of only 55.9%, and Frick reported an overall survival rate of 66.1%. Perhaps it is time for the concept of cancer of the endometrium being a relatively benign type of malignancy to be reevaluated. The question must be raised as to whether an increased survival rate can be achieved by reevaluation of current methods of treatment and adherence to more rigid control protocols.

One of the problems in evaluating any series of patients with cancer of the endometrium is that it is often difficult to interpret the pathological specimen. Adenocarcinoma of the endometrium constitutes about 95% of all endometrial neoplasms. The term carcinoma of the endometrium is selected for the condition which arises in the endometrial *epithelium*. The characteristics of a tumor depend, to some extent, on the site of origin. Terms describing the extent of the lesion, such as carcinoma of the corpus and carcinoma of the colli, are excellent for describing the clinical lesion, but they do not suggest the basic nature of the lesion. Ng and Reagan (1970) have shown that there has been a shift from the classical type of adenocarcinoma of the endometrium to a mixed adenosquamous or adenoepidermoid type. An endometrial cancer which extends into the cervix is a different tumor than the adenocarcinoma which originates in the endocervix and extends into the endometrial cavity or myometrium. The former is treated as a cancer of the endometrium, and the latter as cancer of the cervix. Apparently, there is no evidence that has been advanced which distinguishes the epithelium of the lower section of the endometrial cavity from that of the main cavity. If a cancer extends from the corpus into the cervix, it is staged as endometrial cancer.

It is often difficult to make a diagnosis of early invasion. The problem of differentiating adenomatous hyperplasia of the endometrium from carcinoma in situ often is difficult. Preoperatively, the invasive cancer of the endometrium must be judged by malignant epithelial cells, since it is unlikely that myometrial tissue will be obtained on curettage, thus making a histologic diagnosis often a matter of subjective decision on the part of the pathologist. In addition, different criteria are employed to interpret the results of fractional curettage in Stage II cancer of the endometrium. The FIGO (International Federation of Gynecology and Obstetrics) classification is specific in spelling out the criteria, but the interpretation by different investigators may make a comparison of results a difficult problem.

MEDIAN SURVIVAL TIME BY AGE, 1960 TO 1973

The overall five-year survival rates increased from 72% in 1950–1954 to 75% in 1965 for white women, and 48% to 52% for black women, respectively. There was a strong, observed gradient when survival by specific age groups was examined; the survival rate decreased markedly as the age of the patient increased. This gradient was even stronger in blacks than in white women with endometrial cancer, who were, on the average, about 11 years older than those with cervical cancer. Less than 2% of the tumors of the corpus uteri were diagnosed when the patient was 45 years of age, and about 40% were diagnosed in patients 65 years of age and over.

The median survival time, by age, for white patients in all ages is more than ten years; under 45, more than 10 years; 45 to 54, more than 10 years; 55 to 64, over 10 years; 65 to 74, 5.8 years; and 75 and over, 2.1 years.

One half of black women have localized endometrial cancer at the time of diagnosis, 23% have extension to regional nodes, and 27% have distant metastases. There is an apparent increase in the incidence of endometrial cancer among older women. The five-year survival rate for blacks is considerably poorer than that for whites, 52% and 75%, respectively.

Although there has always been a great number of obese black women, the incidence of cancer of the endometrium did not parallel that observed among white women. This may be related to the diet of black women, which was high in carbohydrates. As their socioeconomic status has improved, they have begun to include more fats in their diet. Conceivably, this may be a contributing factor to the increase in the incidence of endometrial cancer.

The observed median survival time for black patients with cancer of the endometrium is 1.7 years for all ages; under age 45, over 10 years; 45 to 54, 5.2 years; 55 to 64, 1.8 years; 65 to 74, 1.2 years; and 75 and over, 0.9 years.

PREDISPOSING FACTORS

It is obvious that the degree of success of treatment of any cancer, and particularly cancer of the endometrium, is related to early diagnosis. Therefore, attention must be focused on early diagnosis, and, to this end, a plan is presented for isolating the high-risk group of patients who are candidates for developing endometrial cancer. This is made possible by the knowledge that is currently available to identify clinically the group at high risk for the development of endometrial cancer.

Garnet (1958) suggested that abnormal pituitary function may be a prime etiologic factor. He suggested that several parameters frequently are associated with endometrial cancer. These include obesity, nulliparity, reduced glucose tolerance, hypertension, hyperestrogenism, continuous uninterrupted stimulation, menses continuing beyond age 50, history of dysfunctional uterine bleeding, a history of anovulation, and a history of prolonged amenorrhea.

It has been reported that there is an increased incidence in endometrial cancer in the United States, Great Britain, and Israel, in the age group between ages 30 and 39. In populations with a relatively high level of nutrition and, perhaps, some increase in cholesterol and fatty acid levels or some unknown factor, more endometrial cancer is being seen at an earlier age. The indigent patient is often identified as being obese, but with a much lower rate of endometrial cancer than that seen in more affluent patients. Obesity in the indigent patient is often due to an increased intake of carbohydrates. In patients from suburbia and the more affluent sections of society, the diet is high in fats, and, therefore, has more cholesterol and fatty acids. Hormone-associated tumors such as breast, endometrium, and ovary have occurred more frequently since diet has progressively changed to one containing more fat. Although this observation is under intensive study, there are no convincing data in humans.

Cutler et al (1972) reported two definite and one probable cases of endometrial carcinoma in women who had gonadal dysgenesis and were treated with stilbestrol. The treatment had been given for five or more years. There are similar cases in the recent literature. The question is raised, and rightfully so, whether stilbestrol fed to cattle and chickens has contributed to the increase in incidence of endometrial cancer. Although the government has stopped the feeding of stilbestrol to chickens, the cattle industry is still permitted to give this substance up until one day prior to slaughter. Can this drug in some way be contributing to the incidence of epithelial "unrest" in the uterus, and perhaps even in the breasts of women who consume these products?

It is obvious that the problem is more complicated. Recent genetic studies in man have revealed an extraordinarily high association between certain HL-A phenotypes in human disease. For example, virtually every patient with the disease called ankylosing spondylitis expresses HL-A B 27 antigen in her cells. The major histocompatibility complex (MHC) includes several different kinds of genes: those that encode for histocompatibility antigens which are important in allograft immunity, those that govern the amount of antibody produced in response to antigenic challenge (IR genes), and genes governing susceptibility to oncogenic viruses. It is conceivable that some patients have a predisposition to develop malignancy through the major histocompatibility complex, and that the insult from continuous, uninterrupted estrogen stimulation brings about changes in the major histocompatibility complex leading to invasive cancer of the endometrium.

Garnet (1958) reported that a combination of at least five of the following factors is required to define hyperestrogenism: early menarche, delayed onset of ovulation, cessation of ovulation later in reproductive life, dysfunction of uterine bleeding, amenorrhea, involuntary sterility, endometrial polyps and hyperplasia, habitual abortion, severe cystic disease of the breast, and other findings associated with unopposed estrogen stimulation of the endometrium. All these parameters help to identify the clinically high-risk patient, but screening methods employing cytologic studies have been more elusive.

Cytologic screening programs, carried out to identify early changes in cervical abnormalities, have not yielded the same results in identifying patients with early changes in the endometrium, who will be at risk. Pathologists state that it is often difficult to make a firm diagnosis with the tissue available. Therefore, it is often impossible for them to make a diagnosis on cytologic examination. In most instances, the obviously benign lesion and the obviously malignant one can be identified on cytologic examination. However, the precursors are usually more difficult for the pathologist to report. Therefore, it is highly unlikely that screening programs directed at detecting cancer in the endometrium will have a major impact on lowering the morbidity and mortality rates in the foreseeable future. The cytologist can ascertain whether the endometrium is benign or malignant, but he has trouble in detecting the in-between groups with adenomatous hyperplasia, dysplasia, or cancer in situ. However, this can be done with a high degree of accuracy if tissue is obtained for paraffin-block histologic examination.

RISK FACTORS FOR ENDOMETRIAL CANCER

Family Tendency

Sommers (1973) has reported that there is evidence in some families of an autosomal-dominant inheritance of susceptibility to endometrial cancer. Worthin's famous cancer family G, studied since 1895, now comprises over 650 blood relatives recently reviewed by Lynch and Krush (1971). Eighteen members over 40 years of age have had endometrial adenocarcinoma and 53, colonic carcinomas. In general, the association is not strong, and, since endometrial cancer is much less common than cancer of the breast (38,000 versus 108,000 new cases each year in the United States), it does not seem useful to regard women with a family history of endometrial cancer as a high-risk group in the same sense that women with familial history of breast cancer are at high risk for that disease. The question naturally raised is whether there is a cancer-susceptible genome interacting with an oncogenic virus. This has been alluded to above as part of the major histocompatibility complex. The counterargument to this is that families tend to have the same diets, and frequently are exposed to the same carcinogens. It is suggestive, but not conclusive, that, by controlling the diet and environment, approximately 80% of malignancies could be eliminated.

Race

Cancer of the endometrium is rare among the Japanese; it is common among Jewesses. It is on the increase in the United States and is the most common genital cancer reported today. Since the incidence has risen sharply over the past ten years while the mortality has remained stationary, it is logical to ask whether the diagnostic acumen has increased or whether it represents overdiagnosis.

Endometrial Hyperplasia

The significance of this condition in the postmenopausal patient is greater than reported in premenopausal women. In the postmenopausal patient it may be a precursor of cancer, particularly if it is related to a feminizing ovarian tumor or if there is continuous stimulation from exogenous estrogen.

Endometrial Polyps

The association between endometrial polyps and carcinoma of the endometrium has been observed. Way (1961) has focused attention on the potential danger of an endometrial polyp in the postmenopausal patient. This is particularly so in the woman who is high risk by the criteria listed earlier in this chapter.

Leiomyomas, Fibroids, and Endometrial Cancer

These are found together in approximately 35% of the patients. However, this is the incidence of fibroids normally occurring in this age group. The significance of fibroids may be in accepting the abnormal bleeding as being secondary to the fibroids, and this causes delay in making the diagnosis of endometrial cancer. Benign and malignant tumors often occur simultaneously.

Menstrual Disturbances

Cancer of the endometrium is being reported in increasing frequency among young girls with a long history of anovulation and amenorrhea. These girls are markedly obese and often have a Stein-Leventhal syndrome. There have been several case reports and one series of 16 patients with this syndrome. The Stein-Leventhal syndrome usually manifests itself in the decade or two after puberty, and most of the reported endometrial cancers have been in patients under 40 years of age, when endometrial cancer is not common. Dockerty (1951) suggested that clinical evidence of the syndrome is found in 20% of patients with endometrial cancer under 40 years of age.

Other Diseases

There is little doubt that cancers of the endometrium and breast, and of the endometrium and ovary, tend to occur in the same women more frequently than would be expected by chance. The associations are not strong, and the possibility cannot be ruled out that they result simply from demographic and personal factors that are common to women with the three diseases. Association of cancers of the endometrium and bowel has also been reported.

PRECURSORS OF ENDOMETRIAL CANCER

Adenomatous hyperplasia, a typical precancerous lesion, may be a focal or a general change, with the greatest problems being in women of perimenopausal age with dysfunctional bleeding. Characteristically, histologic examination of curettings show the glands to be crowded together and frequently back-to-back; there is pseudostratification of the glandular epithelium and, in the most intense form, a characteristic pallor or eosinophilic stain reaction of these glands with intense proliferation of glandular epithelium, forming buds and islands within the gland lumen. Adenomatous hyperplasia is the preferred term for this group of patients, rather than carcinoma in situ. The term carcinoma in situ has been reserved by many pathologists for those lesions with undoubted invasions of the stroma, high differentiation, and confinement to a local area of the endometrium. In the past, this lesion was called adenoma malignum. Gusberg (1973) considers adenomatous hyperplasia as a clear cancer precursor. In a nontreated group of about 100 patients followed prospectively between five and ten years, approximately 12% developed a cancer. It is estimated that approximately 25% would develop cancer if left untreated for a 20-year period. The importance of treatment for this group of patients is obvious.

New Symptoms

The first and most important symptom is abnormal vaginal bleeding. It is related not only to the peri- and postmenopausal patient, but is the most common and important symptom in all age groups. Lawless, abnormal bleeding at any age should be explored and diagnosed without delay.

Just because a benign lesion such as a cervical polyp is found does not mean that a malignant lesion has been ruled out. The patient may have both. The point to emphasize is that abnormal vaginal bleeding in any age group should be given special attention. The practice of giving hormones to women with abnormal bleeding, particularly after the time of the menopause when there has been no previous study of endometrial histology, is to be condemned. A safe rule to follow is "when in doubt, scrape it out."

Diagnosis

Attention must be focused on early diagnosis. Knowledge available to us provides the opportunity to identify clinically the patient at high risk of developing endometrial cancer. For a variety of reasons, an early diagnosis may be delayed when cancer is present in the endometrium, among them being the old wives' tale that abnormal bleeding is a normal sequence of menopause. Abnormal bleeding is to be studied by fractional curettage, and even a negative Pap smear or endometrial aspiration is not sufficient for making the diagnosis. Cancer may be present in the corpus, but unable to escape through a stenosed cervix. The percentage pickup ranges from 50% for the vaginal pool to 93% for the procedures that invade the uterine cavity. It is to be reemphasized that a curettage (fractional) should be carried out in every postmenopausal patient with a bleeding problem.

Pathology

A historic landmark in the pathology of uterine cancer is Cullen's monograph of 1900. Under adenocarcinoma of the body of the uterus, endometrial cancer is described grossly and microscopically by stages, and has been well illustrated by Max Brödel.

The morphology of endometrial carcinoma, also called carcinoma of the corpus or fundus, has thus been defined for over 70 years. Grossly invasive endometrial cancer is localized or diffused. The localized type may arise in a polyp, particularly in women over 65 years of age, but usually presents as a flattened, pyramidal thickening of the endometrium. The diffuse type involves most of the lining of the upper part of the uterus with a rough, protrusive, granular growth. Carcinomatous tissue is typically dry, friable, yellow-tan in color, and sufficiently characteristic to be recognized grossly from curettings. In contrast, the curretings of endometrial hyperplasia are wet, mucoid, smooth, soft, and resilient.

Endometrial carcinoma of the lower uterine segment involves part or all of the mucosal circumference just above the internal os, while sparing the fundus. Grossly and microscopically, it often resembles a cross between endocervical and fundal adenocarcinoma.

Histology

Endometrial cancer is not the most obvious and easily recognized neoplasm. Unless the myometrium has clearly been invaded, experience is needed to establish the correct diagnosis. Two characteristics of endometrial cancer not shared by hyperplasia are glands that grow back-to-back without any wisp of intervening endometrial stroma, and secondary glands formed within the larger glands, producing a cribriform pattern. Distinctive foci like this, found in regions of cystic, adenomatous, or atypical hyperplasia, constitute early endometrial cancer. From the degree and extent of compression and infiltration of the adjacent uninvolved endometrial stroma, myometrium, or both, invasive cancer is recognized. The stroma of endometrial cancer may contain nests of foam cells.

Histologic grading of endometrial cancer is helpful in establishing statistically valid, prognostic information. The best differentiated type is typically composed of medium-sized tortuous glands of columnar epithelial cells with acidophilic cytoplasm and normal chromatic nuclei, closely packed together. Grade 1 adenocarcinoma, once called adenoma malignum, exhibits sluggish growth activity. Another variant of Grade 1 endometrial carcinoma is the secretory or clear-cell type, with many subnuclear and supranuclear glycogen-filled cytoplasmic vacuoles, imitating the postovulatory secretory phase. Traditionally, this is the most curable of all endometrial carcinomas. Grade 2 endometrial carcinoma is the most familiar type. It has intermingled small and large glands with moderately variable nuclear size and chromatin content, and some areas where strips of neoplastic epithelium appear between the glands.

Grade 3 tumors are undifferentiated carcinomas which grow in solid sheets and cell cords, recognizable as epithelial cuboidal shapes, occasionally with small, poorly formed glands. These carcinomas grossly are often bulky, and at times have a slick, pale gray cut surface. They may not be easily distinguishable, grossly or microscopically, from endometrial stromal carcinoma. Grade 4 lesions are included with Grade 3, according to Ewing's grading, a modification of Bröder's classification.

ADENOSQUAMOUS CARCINOMA

The adenoacanthoma is a adenocarcinoma with acanthomatous elements, differing not at all from the usual adenocarcinoma in virulence or prognosis. Reagan has described an adenosquamous carcinoma or adenoepidermoid carcinoma which is increasing in incidence, and is a more virulent tumor than the adenocarcinoma. Over three decades there has been a progressive decreased detection in the number of cervical squamous cell cancers, and an increase in the number of precancerous changes. Over this period of time there was a progressive increase in the

222

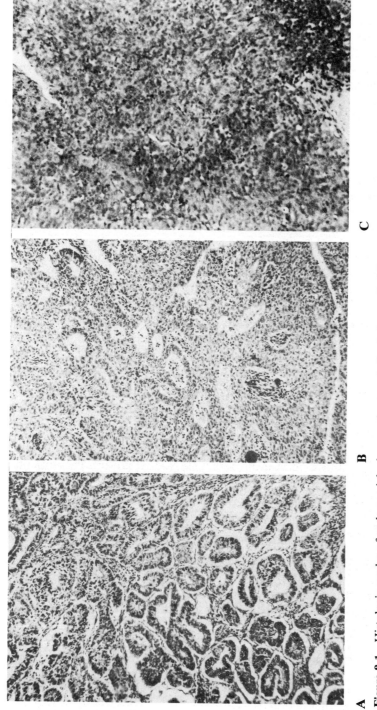

Figure 8-1 Histologic grades of endometrial adenocarcinoma. **A** Grade I or well-differentiated adenocarcinoma is characterized by well-formed glands. **B** Grade II or moderately differentiated adenocarcinoma is characterized by less well-formed but still identifiable gland formation. C Grade III or poorly differentiated adenocarcinoma is characterized by sheets of malignant epithelial cells.

number of glandular neoplasms detected in the uterus. Endometrial cancer accounted for most of the increase. One type of endometrial cancer, the adenosquamous cancer, has been detected more commonly in the last decade. The emergence of this neoplasm is of some importance because of the short duration of symptoms and the poor response to ionizing radiation. In Reagan's series, the number of such tumors includes one third of his material. Mixed adenosquamous carcinomas are very aggressive, and metastasize early. About 50% are blood-borne, and one-third have been found going through the Fallopian tube into the peritoneal cavity. Examination with an electron microscope demonstrates keratohyalin-like granules, desmosomes with tonofilaments, structures regarded as characteristic of squamous cells. The overall prognosis is very poor, and is reported for Stages I through IV as 20%.

Natural History and Direction of Spread

Adenocarcinoma of the endometrium is either localized or diffuse. Cancer arising in the endometrium tends to remain within the uterus for a long period of time, spreading by local extension within the endo-

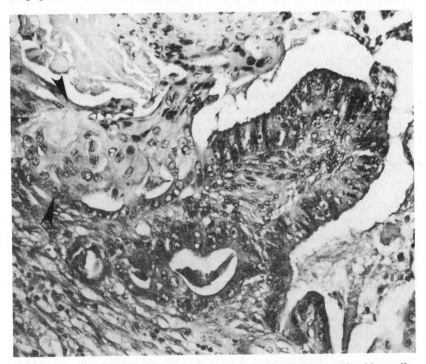

Figure 8-2 Endometrial adenoacanthoma. This tumor is characterized by malignant glands which are usually well or moderately differentiated and nests of benign metaplastic squamous epithelium (arrows).

metrium. As it grows, it invades the myometrium and advances toward the isthmus and endocervix; from there it spreads to the paravaginal and paracervical areas, or may invade directly through the myometrium to the serosa and peritoneal cavity. Since the lymphatic vessels increase in number as the serosa of the uterus is approached, deep penetration of the myometrium is associated with an increased incidence of positive node involvement. Since the myometrium in the postmenopausal woman is much thinner than in the premenopausal woman, relatively minor penetration in the myometrium may bring the cancer into contact with the lymphatics, thus accounting for the greater danger of endometrial cancer among postmenopausal women. Free transplantation of malignant endometrial cells may account for implants on the ovary and surface of the tube and broad ligament. This mode of spread also has been considered by some as the means by which some vaginal metastases occur. This is difficult to accept, since the cells have been dropping into the vagina for a long period of time, and not all patients have metastases to this organ.

The lymphatic drainage of the upper part of the body of the uterus occurs along the course of the infundibular ligament. In view of this anatomic type of drainage, the metastasis should involve the aortic, caval, lumbar, and high common iliac nodes. This is obviously not common in the early stages of endometrial cancer, and occurs only after there has been deep infiltration of the cancer involving the lymphatics of the myometrium close to the serosa of the uterus. From the cervical area, the spread of cancer parallels that seen in cancer of the cervix. Anastamosis of the lymphatics between the body of the uterus and the round ligament may be responsible for the rare metastases occurring in the inguinal area.

Cancer of the endometrium not only grows locally but spreads to the lymphatic system. Reports indicate that metastases within the pelvis are associated with the disease outside the pelvis in a high percentage of cases. If this were so, the salvage rate would not be increased by treating the pelvic nodes, and it would be difficult to achieve a 70% five-year survival rate.

Approximately 10% to 15% of patients with Stage I cancer of the endometrium, and 40% of those with Stage II tumors will have lymph node metastases to the pelvis. The depth of myometrial invasion is also directly related to the percentage of lymph node metastases. Lewis (1970) reported that, when there was no myometrial invasion or less than 2 mm of invasion, none of his patients exhibited pelvic node metastases. However, when the invasion extended within 2 mm of the serosa, 36% had metastases to the pelvic nodes. The depth of invasion correlates well with the incidence of positive nodes.

Extension of endometrial cancer to the cervix creates a more serious problem. Surely, retrograde lymphatic extension to the vagina must occur in some cases, since all metastases cannot be explained as being due to operative implantation. The problem of cervical involvement is associated with a very poor prognosis (Stage II). Stage II cancer of the endometrium accounts for 10% to 15% of cases, and at least 40% will have positive nodes. In addition, endometrial cancer invades the myometrium; there is extension into the cervix, and from there into the parametrial tissues. The poorly differentiated cancers have a propensity for deep penetration in the myometrium, with spread to the cervix and involvement of the pelvic nodes. Documentation of the involvement of the cervix is very important, not only for staging the extent of the cancer, but for the management of these patients.

Histologic and Nuclear Grading

Histologic grading serves as one more parameter for evaluating the incidence of pelvic node metastases and the depth of myometrial invasion. Although such grading does not correlate with the incidence of nodal involvement as well as the depth of myometrial invasion, it should be carried out. Reports indicate that cytologic grading of endometrial cancer, particularly by measuring nucleoli and their RNA content, has demonstrated that the higher grade carcinomas have larger single nucleoli, and, in more advanced or more undifferentiated tumors, there are larger numbers of multiple nucleoli with greater variation in nuclear and nucleolar structure.

Nuclear grading may be considered an adjunct to and refinement of histologic grading of cancers. There are three nuclear grades. Nuclear Grade 1 is the most abnormal, with wide variation in nuclear size, chromatin content, and appearance. Nuclear Grade 2 has definite, but less severe, nuclear and nucleolar atypism. Grade 3 comprises differentiated cancer cells whose nuclei closely resemble those of adjacent non-neoplastic cells.

It is evident that a test is needed that will help in selecting those patients who will be benefited by a node dissection. Perhaps, in the future, those patients showing good cell-mediated immunity and no enhancing or blocking antibodies, and in whom the nodes grossly appear normal, may best be treated by leaving the nodes in situ, while those with poor cellular immunity and a high blocking antibody may be candidates for eradicating the pelvic nodes, either by surgery or radiation.

It can be stated that patients at high risk for extrauterine spread are those with: 1) involvement with the lower uterus or cervix, 2) histologic Grade 3 lesions, and 3) myometrial invasion.

EXOGENOUS ESTROGENS AND ENDOMETRIAL CANCER

Estrogen is a drug, and should be used with all the indications and contraindications of any drug. It should be given when needed and indicated, and should be withheld when there is a contraindication to its use. There have been several recent papers in the literature which have attempted to identify a relationship between the use of estrogen and endometrial cancer. There are as many investigators who disagree with the findings of these groups. They advance information and statistics to show that there is no presently recognized correlation.

Currently, there are 27 million women in the United States who are undergoing the menopause. A great number of these are on estrogen replacement therapy. Although the number of endometrial cancers has risen steadily in the last few years, the death rate has remained constant at about 3300 per year. It can be concluded that endometrial cancer is either being overdiagnosed, or that the use of estrogens helps to unmask the lesion at an earlier stage. Another explanation is that the patients are more inclined to have careful supervision by their physicians, with routine scheduled pelvic examinations and endometrial aspirations.

The quality of life is an important consideration in making a decision as to the use of estrogens. Literally, millions of women today are taking estrogens because it brings them relief from many of the symptoms of the menopause—hot flushes, fatigue, insomnia, marked sweating, and atrophic vaginitis. To be effective as prophylaxis against the development of osteoporosis, estrogen replacement must be started promptly after cessation of ovarian function. Estrogen therapy will usually arrest progression of osteoporosis but will not reverse it, and the duration of the beneficial effect appears to be limited to two or three years. Morris has shown that a number of statistical papers have described an increased incidence of endometrial cancer in the United States. Among other sources he cited the Connecticut State Tumor Registry. The entire increase in endometrial cancer in the Connecticut Cancer Registry has been in the earlier stages of the disease. The incidence of carcinoma in situ of the endometrium in Connecticut during the years 1970–1974 (1.8 per 100,000 women) was double that for 1960–1964, and that of localized invasive disease (19.6 per 100,000) was nearly 20% greater, while the occurrence of nonlocalized invasive disease (3.2 per 100,000) remained essentially unchanged in this period.

Perhaps the most significant figure for the Connecticut Registry is the change in the death rate of uterine cancer. The age-adjusted mortality rate from corpus carcinoma per 100,000 women has dropped from 8.2 in the five-year period from 1940–1944, to 4.6 in 1960–1964, and to 4.1 during 1970–1974.

BENEFITS OF HORMONAL REPLACEMENT

Symptoms that are most often controlled by estrogen replacement are flushes, flashes, sweats, insomnia, and atrophic vaginitis. What the patient does not notice until it is too late is the calcium loss. Bone loss with age is well documented. The loss of bone in women is more severe than in men, from 1% to 3% at menopause. Significant osteoporosis is estimated to occur in about 25% of postmenopausal women.

This condition is usually discovered when x-rays are taken because of fractures or chronic back pain. While the ratio of fractures in youth and middle-age in women and men are essentially the same, in the older age groups the female-to-male ratio of fractures of the hip is approximately 3:1, of the spine 4:1, and the wrist 10:1. The problem is a serious one, since the risk of hip fractures may reach 20% or more in older women.

Various studies have shown that approximately 80% of hip fractures occur in patients over age 60, and that 85% of this group are women. The mortality rate for hip fractures ranges from 4% to 32%. In 30 reported series of cases totalling 10,978 fractures, the combined mortality was 13.2%. Of the 1114 cases reported from Sweden, 9% of the patients were dead in one month, and 15% died within three months of the injury.

Morris (1978) reported that there were 294 hip fractures treated in New Haven in one year commencing July 1, 1975, as compared with 68 cases of endometrial cancer during that period. The National Center for Health Statistics estimated that there were 184,000 hip fractures in the United States in 1975, of which more than 132,000 occurred in women. While the estimated annual death rate for hip fractures is considerably greater than that for endometrial cancer, broken bones do not seem to strike the terror elicited by the word cancer, which to some is synonymous with death.

All patients on estrogen replacement should be seen regularly at 6- to 12-month intervals. At these examinations, blood pressure should be taken, breasts examined, and rectovaginal examination should be carried out. Routine Pap smears as well as endometrial aspiration or biopsy should be done at yearly intervals for patients on replacement estrogen therapy. The estrogen should be interrupted for at least one week of each month, and, after 18 months of therapy, the treatment should be discontinued temporarily or permanently, and the patient evaluated for any of the marked signs and symptoms of estrogen withdrawal.

Some women for whom substitutional estrogen replacement is contraindicated may have severe menopausal symptoms. Such patients have occasionally been helped by the use of sedatives, pharmacologic agents such as Bellergal, androgens, or progesterones. However, these therapeutic regimens are not as effective as estrogen replacement therapy. Injectable progestational compounds such as medroxyprogesterone acetate suspension have been used to relieve some of the vasomotor instability symptoms. However, they are of no value in treating the problems of atrophic vaginitis or urethritis.

CYTOGENETIC FACTORS IN CANCER OF THE ENDOMETRIUM

The accumulated data show that the majority of cases of cancer of the endometrium have near-diploid, modal chromosomal numbers; the lowest substantial number have model numbers in the triploid-tetraploid range. Cancers of the endometrium in the low-ploidy group tend to be better differentiated than tumors in the high-ploidy group. It follows that the prognosis is better for the low-ploidy group. The frequent occurrence of diploid modes is contrary to observations in most other types of invasive cancers. In other human epithelial tumors there is a considerable variation in chromosomal numbers within the tumors, and a variety of modes have been observed. A specific karyotype pattern has not been found in endometrial cancers, although overrepresentation of group C chromosomes seems to be a common feature. In view of the exceptionally high incidence of pseudodiploid and diploid cells in endometrial carcinoma, it seems that complete karyotype analysis of seemingly normal cells is essential in the cytoplasmic investigation of these lesions. It has been reported that diploid cells are common in cancers of the endometrium, and the number decreases with progression of this disease. It is important that representative sections of tissue be examined so that there will be no more bias in the findings.

HORMONE RECEPTORS

With the discovery that breast cancer cells retain the ability to incorporate and retain estrogens, both in vitro and in vivo, a new era was started in cancer endocrinology. The road has been uphill, progressing from outmoded to sophisticated methodology. A great deal of information is now available to us. The concept of utilizing the available data on hormone receptors in clinical oncology serves to eliminate much of the guesswork in spotting the high risk patient, to supply a more logical selection in monitoring of therapy, and also to provide a method for selecting and controlling the management of recurrent endometrial cancer.

It has been confirmed that cells which depend on hormones for optimal growth and function contain specific steroid-binding proteins, the so-called hormone receptors. Jensen's work (1968) in the selective binding of estradiol by the rat uterus opened this field of research. The mechanism for the interaction of hormone with target cells takes place by at least a two-step, and, perhaps, by an undetermined number of steps. Although the first observation was made on the endometrium of the rat uterus, the application of the concept to breast cancer has advanced more rapidly and extensively than to the endometrium.

Estrogen receptor assays make it possible to predict with a greater degree of confidence than was previously possible, the response of a given tumor to endocrine treatment. Estrogens, whether administered pharmacologically or secreted by an endocrine-active tissue, are carried in the blood, bound to a plasma transport protein. The steroid hormone enters the cell, presumably by passive diffusion, and combines with a specific receptor protein. This reaction is labeled *uptake*. The steroid hormone receptor complex is next activated so that it can enter the nucleus. Entrance of the activated complex into the nucleus is labeled *translocation*. Once inside the nucleus, the steroid hormone-receptor complex associates with nuclear chromatin, and this is labeled *retention*. The interaction of steroid hormone with nuclear chromatin stimulates RNA synthesis, which in turn leads to the synthesis of certain cell proteins. It is these new proteins which lead to the induced effects of the steroid hormone.

From current knowledge of hormone-receptor interactions it is obvious that a cell will not respond to a specific steroid unless it contains specific receptors. In the absence of specific receptors, the cell will not respond to the hormone. This is true of neoplastic as well as normal cells.

The assay for hormone receptors usually requires a minimum of 500 mg of tumor tissue. The tumor must be frozen within 15 minutes after removal from the uterus. It is better to perform the assay on a biopsy specimen rather than a hysterectomy specimen. The lengthy surgical procedure required for the hysterectomy may injure the tissue, and there will be unavoidable delay in processing the specimen. The best results require a close working relationship between the clinician and the pathologist. Once alerted that the specimen is being sent to the laboratory, the pathologist will then be able to prepare the specimen by trimming off normal tissue and by being certain that the specimen is truly neoplastic.

Endometrial tissue contains receptors for estradiol and progesterone. The concentrations of these receptors vary throughout the menstrual cycle. During the follicular phase, in which estradiol is secreted by developing follicles, the concentration of estradiol receptors in the proliferative endometrium is high. During the luteal phase, after the formation of the corpus luteum and the onset of significant ovarian secretion of progesterone, and while estradiol secretion continues, the concentration of estradiol receptors in the secretory endometrium diminishes drastically. There is a reduction of the total number of estradiol receptors as determined by simultaneous measurements in the cytosol and nuclei, or by analysis of nuclei alone after cytoplasmic receptors have been translocated to the nucleus during incubation with an excess of estradiol.

There are few progesterone receptors in early proliferative endometrium, but they increase to a maximum with ovulation, most likely as a result of estrogen stimulation. Control studies show nuclear uptake of estradiol and progesterone both by glandular epithelium and stroma in human endometrium. The results of these studies indicate that receptors are present in both cell types as expected from morphologic evidence of changes during the cycle.

Hyperplastic endometrium from postmenopausal women has an estradiol-receptor concentration comparable to that found in proliferative endometrium. Specimens of well-differentiated adenocarcinoma from postmenopausal women show a large variability in estradiol-receptor content. On the average, the values are higher than those seen in secretory normal endometrium, but lower than those in proliferative tissue. However, it is interesting that some endometrial carcinomas contain low levels of estradiol receptors, as is the case in some breast tumors. Since only a small number of specimens have been analyzed, a wide variety of methodologies has been used. The specimens themselves show a large degree of cellular heterogeneity, and it is difficult to propose intrinsic differences in estradiol concentrations that could characterize endometrial hyperplasia or carcinoma of various degrees of differentiation. Concentrations of progesterone receptors have been reported to decline, with loss of differentiation in endometrial cancer. Several reports support the concept that patients whose uteri are exposed over long periods of time to estrogen in the absence of progesterone, are at high risk for the development of hyperplasia and cancer. This situation is found, for instance, in postmenopausal women and in those with estrogen-secreting tumors.

Hausknecht and Gusberg (1969) measured the urinary metabolites of estradiol in normal postmenopausal women and postmenopausal women with endometrial carcinoma. They found no statistical difference in the excretion of classic estrogen or in the estriol quotient. It has been suggested that there is an increased peripheral conversion (two or three times normal) of estrogen precursors, namely, androstenedione in the postmenopausal woman that produces an excess amount of estrone. This, in turn, may produce endometrial hyperplasia in older women. Gusberg showed that there is a higher ratio of estrone to estradiol in the blood of postmenopausal women with endometrial cancer. He did not find that postmenopausal women with endometrial cancer secrete less total estriol glucuronide (as compared to estrone glucuronide) than normal postmenopausal women, and suggested that the protective effect of estriol had been lost. He has also reported a significantly higher conversion rate of 4-androstenedione to estrone in these postmenopausal women with endometrial cancer.

Rubin (1972), measuring the circulating estrone and estradiol concentrations, showed the mean ratio once again to be significantly higher than in those women who have cancer. Gusberg reported that it appears that the postmenopausal pre-hormone is androstenedione, and the notable postmenopausal estrogen is estrone. It must be pointed out that circulating estrone is converted to some extent to blood-borne estradiol, and that estradiol is taken up by the tissues. This has been confirmed in in vitro experiments. It raises the question of which of the two estrogens is actually responsible for the estrogenic action. Estradiol, not estrone, is found to be bound to the nuclear chromatin. This indicates that estrone is not estrogenic per se, but rather exerts its effect after conversion to estradiol, both peripherally and in the target tissue.

Estriol, a metabolite of secreted estradiol, has recently received special attention in regard to its possible physiological role as an anti-estrogen. It has been shown that estriol, when administered in a single pharmacologic dose, can compete with estradiol for binding to the receptor, but is not retained in the nucleus long enough to exert a full estrogenic effect. It has been shown that estriol is capable of competing with estradiol in the human endometrium, and such a direct competition has been shown in in vitro studies with proliferative tissue.

The modulating effects of progesterone on estrogen action have been known for a long time, but only very recently have specific mechanisms for the anti-estrogenic action of progesterone been proposed. One of the suggested mechanisms involves the regulation of estradiol-receptor concentrations, and another is related to the induction of the enzyme that converts estradiol to estrone, ie, estradiol-17-β-dehydrogenase.

The depressant effect of progesterone on levels of estradiol receptors, suggested by the low concentrations of receptors in secretory endometrium, has been demonstrated experimentally by oral or intrauterine administration of progestational agents to women in the follicular phase of the menstrual cycle. After two to four days of treatment, the concentrations of estradiol receptors declined to one half of the control values. During the same experimental period, the activity of estradiol-17-β-dehydrogenase increased markedly.

A reasonable goal for studies on endometrial cancer presently is to establish a relationship between progesterone-receptor concentrations, therapeutic effectiveness of progesterone, and responsiveness of the neoplastic tissue, evaluated morphologically or by biochemical measures such as induction of estradiol-17-β-dehydrogenase, in vitro or in vivo.

PREOPERATIVE EVALUATION

Based on our study of a review of the literature, a protocol is presented for pretreatment evaluation and for therapy. The preoperative workup consists of:

1. Routine history and physical examination
2. Complete blood count
3. Urinalysis
4. SMA-12
5. Chest x-ray
6. Intravenous pyelogram
7. Metastatic x-ray studies

8. Proctoscopy
9. Barium enema
10. Cystoscopy
11. Bone scan
12. Lymphangiogram

Each patient should be examined under anesthesia, and a fractional curettage with sounding of the uterus should be carried out.

THERAPY

There are several modalities of therapy used in the management of carcinoma of the endometrium. However, there are two that have been uniformly accepted as the treatment of choice. One group of investigators has reported that any cancer beyond Stage IaG1 should receive preoperative, external x-ray therapy followed by surgery, and then, in the postoperative period, a vaginal applicator. The advantages to this mode of therapy are that the tumor cells are often damaged, the lymphatics are closed, and even the blood vessels have an obliterated endarteritis. Theoretically, this is advantageous in that the tumor is not spread with manipulation during surgery. Another group has advocated the use of primary surgery and, depending upon the histologic findings, the addition of external x-ray therapy as well as a vaginal applicator. The advantage to this approach is that the patient can be evaluated more accurately, particularly those suspected of having Stage III cancer. An accurate determination can be made, whether it be a metastasis or a separate, primary lesion. The specimen is fresh and the extent of invasion of the myometrium can be determined, as well as whether the endocervix is involved. It does not help in staging except after the fact, but if cancer is found in the endocervix, external x-ray and vaginal radiation therapy are indicated.

Therapy includes the preoperative use of x-ray treatment. However, when indicated, postoperative x-ray therapy is given, using the same fields and dosage regimen.

Stage O The management of carcinoma in situ should be guided by the definition established by the pathology department of a given hospital, and should be tailored to fit the needs of the patient, her age, and her desire for future childbearing. In selected, young patients with minimal disease, an alternative to hysterectomy may be repeat curettage in three or four months after a course of progestational agents or induction of ovulation followed by repeat curettage.

Stage IaG1 Total hysterectomy and bilateral salpingo-oophorectomy should be followed by postoperative vaginal radiation. Some oncologists may elect a random study, employing a type of radical hysterectomy.

In patients in whom the histologic grade is G2 or G3, external pelvic radiation should be given preoperatively, followed by total hysterectomy, bilateral salpingo-oophorectomy, and vaginal radiation postoperatively.

If preoperative external radiation has not been given and the surgical specimen reveals moderate or extensive myometrial invasion (one third or more of myometrial penetration), postoperative external radiation should be given. In those patients in whom the histologic grade is found to be G2 or G3 instead of G1, external x-ray therapy should be given postoperatively.

Stage Ib Preoperative external pelvic radiation is followed by total hysterectomy and bilateral salpingo-oophorectomy six weeks later. Postoperative vaginal radiation is indicated. The alternative to total hysterectomy may be a randomized selection of a type of radical hysterectomy.

Stage II Preoperative external pelvic radiation is followed in six weeks by a modified radical hysterectomy and pelvic node dissection. Postoperative vaginal radiation should be given. Since there is an increased incidence of pelvic nodes (up to 37%) in this group, careful biopsies should be taken of the paraaortic nodes.

Stage III If the lesion involves only the adnexal structures, preoperative x-ray therapy followed by total hysterectomy and bilateral salpingo-oophorectomy should be the treatment of choice. Postoperatively, vaginal radiation is given. An alternative plan to total hysterectomy is to substitute a modified radical hysterectomy.

Stage IV If the spread is limited to the pelvis with bladder and/or rectal involvement, the patient should be treated with external x-ray treatment, as well as intravaginal and intrauterine radium insertion. In four to six weeks the patient may qualify for a radical surgical procedure, and, if the disease is limited to the midline, pelvic exenteration should be considered as a modality of treatment. Boronow has challenged many of the old traditions and outlines new methods of approach to cancer of the endometrium.

Distant metastases Primary progestational therapy is indicated. Localized disease without response to progestational therapy should be treated with radiation. In the presence of widespread disease and no response, chemotherapy should be tried. However, in general, cancer of the endometrium does not respond to chemotherapy.

Recurrent adenocarcinoma of the endometrium Primary therapy is started with progestational agents. Localized symptomatic cancer should be treated with radiation. Selected patients may be candidates for pelvic exenteration.

Recurrent Cancer of the Endometrium

Although there are fewer indications for pelvic exenteration in patients with cancer of the endometrium than in those with cervical cancer, there is a place for pelvic exenterations among the methods of treatment used as definitive therapy for this cancer. Barber and Brunschwig (1968) reported on the results of treatment for recurrent cancer of the endometrium. There were 36 patients receiving pelvic exenterations, seven received their initial treatment less than one year prior to treatment for recurrence, and none survived more than 15 months. Of 29 patients who were free of disease for at least one year after initial treatment before receiving pelvic exenteration for recurrence, five lived five or more years. Although the results are not spectacular, pelvic exenteration may be considered in highly selected patients.

Radiation Therapy

Radiation therapy has improved the five-year survival rate from cancer of the endometrium. It has been shown that adjunctive radiotherapy in a patient with Stage IaG1 disease does little to improve survival. However, in disease beyond this stage, there is no doubt that adjunctive radiotherapy does add to the number of women surviving at five years. This is particularly true as far as controlling vaginal recurrence is concerned.

There is still controversy about the relative effectiveness of preoperative, as opposed to postoperative, external x-ray therapy. The advantages and disadvantages of each have been reviewed earlier in this chapter.

The use of intracavitary radium, cesium, or cobalt implant has been phased out by many services in the United States. Gusberg (1973) has shown that it is extremely difficult to calculate the dose inside the uterus when multiple Heyman capsules are used. In calculating the optimum dose, this investigation recommends the basic plan of delivering 3000 gamma roentgens to a point 1 cm from the uterine cavity, and 1800 gamma roentgens at a point 1 cm below the vaginal mucous membrane. This amount of irradiation is not considered a cancericidal dose. If the tumor has spread beyond the uterus, the results are poor with this plan of treatment. External therapy is the preferred method of giving radiation therapy.

The external fields to which therapy is administered extend from the midpoint of L-5 down to the pubis, and laterally to the head of the acetabulum (*not* the head of the femur). This includes the node-bearing areas, and uniformly radiates the entire pelvis. Although the use of radiation therapy is given for each stage in the protocol, a more detailed plan is presented for guidance and actual management of the patient. In Stage IaG1, with a well-differentiated tumor of 8 cm or less in the uterine cavity, no preoperative radiation is used. However, postoperative radiation, cesium, or cobalt delivering a dose of 3000 to 4000 rad at 1 cm below the mucous membrane by means of a Burnet applicator, is recommended. If the tumor is found to have invaded more than one third of the myometrium, external therapy should be added, delivering 4000 rad in four weeks to the pelvis. In Stage IaG2 or G3 and Stages IbG1, G2 or G3, with a uterine cavity of less than 8 cm and a moderately undifferentiated tumor or uterus of greater than 8 cm (particularly in postmenopausal patients), preoperative external therapy delivering 4000 rad in four weeks is followed by the postoperative use of vaginal radiation, 3000 to 4000 rad at 1 cm as outlined above.

In Stage II, when there is involvement of the cervix, preoperative external therapy delivering 4000 rad in four weeks is followed by a radical hysterectomy and node dissection, as well as the use of vaginal application as outlined above. Stage III, which indicates spread to the adenexa, is treated preoperatively by 4000 rad in four weeks to the entire pelvis, followed postoperatively with vaginal radiation as described above. In all other instances of Stage III, primary radiation is generally recommended, but being limited in Stage IV to the pelvis. With bladder or rectal involvement, primary radiation therapy is generally recommended as outlined above. When distant metastases are present, primary x-ray therapy should be given to the pelvis, and progestational agents administered to control the metastatic cancer. The external therapy administered to the pelvis should include the lymph nodes in the area.

For those given postoperative x-ray therapy, the therapy is administered in exactly the same way, except that it is given in the postoperative period. Vaginal radiation is given in the same manner.

Pyometra

The management of endometrial carcinoma associated with pyometra is somewhat different from that of patients who do not have this complication. The triad of symptoms consisting of vaginal spotting, vaginal discharge, and/or rectal and suprapubic pain should alert the physician to the possibility of pyometra. The diagnosis is made by passing a sound. One should be very aware of the possibility of perforation, since the wall of the extended uterine cavity, particularly in postmenopausal women, is extremely thin. The discharge has a foul odor. Anaerobic organisms are found in about 90% of cases, the most frequent being anaerobic streptococci. One should not do a D&C at the time of the original drainage, but should dilate the cervix daily or insert a catheter. After the discharge has ceased, a diagnostic D&C should be done. Based upon the findings, treatment is administered as previously outlined.

Chemotherapy

Chemotherapy includes the usual anticancer drugs as well as hormones. Hormones have played an important role in the control of metastatic disease, particularly to the lungs. The ideal patient for hormone therapy is one whose disease recurs a few years after the original therapy, particularly when the lesion is well differentiated. Bone lesions have also responded fairly well to the progestational agents. Localized disease in the pelvis has not responded as well as has metastatic disease. One of the problems in using hormonal therapy is that the doses are often below an optimal level. It is recommended that a loading dose (400 mg) of medroxyprogesterone acetate suspension be given intramuscularly every day for at least two weeks, followed by megestrol acetate (40 mg by mouth) three times a day and medroxyprogesterone acetate suspension (400 mg) once a week or once every two weeks. The same plan is followed when hydroxyprogesterone caproate is used. A daily dose of 1250 mg is given intramuscularly for ten days to two weeks, followed by megestrol acetate (40 mg by mouth) three times a day, and hydroxyprogesterone caproate (1250 mg) once a week or once every two weeks for an indefinite period of time. Some patients whose tumors have recurred promptly, as well as those with a tumor that is not well differentiated, have also responded to this regimen.

Chemotherapy in the form of anticancer drugs has not been as effective as anticipated. Combinations of cyclophosphamide, actinomycin D and 5-FU have been used in the past. Recently doxorubicin has given some encouraging results. With the addition of cis-platinum and cyclophosphamide to the doxorubicin, preliminary studies indicate that these drugs may be effective in controlling cancer of the endometrium that is advanced or recurrent. An alternate plan includes 20 mg of mitomycin given intravenously as a bolus, and followed by 1500 of 5-FU intravenously over a 24-hour period and continued daily for five days.

BIBLIOGRAPHY

Aikawa M, Ng ABP: Mixed (adenosquamous) carcinoma of the endometrium: electron microscopic observations. *Cancer* 31:385, 1973.

Barber HRK, Brunschwig A: Treatment and results of recurrent cancer of the corpus uteri in patients receiving anterior and total pelvic exenteration. *Cancer* 22:949, 1968.

Barber HRK: Cancer of the endometrium, in Barber HRK, Fields DH, Kaufman SA (eds): *Quick Reference to Ob-Gyn Procedures,* ed 2. Philadelphia, J.B. Lippincott Company, 1979.

Barber HRK, Graber EA, Sommers SC, et al: Cancer of the endometrium. *Rhode Island Med J* 58:257, 1975.

Barber HRK, Kwon TH: The endometrium, in Nealon TF, Jr (ed): *The Management of the Patient with Cancer,* ed 2. Philadelphia, W.B. Saunders Company, 1976, p 641.

Broder AC: Grading and practical application. *Arch Pathol* 2:376, 1926.

Cancer Facts and Figures. New York, American Cancer Society 1979.

Charles D: Endometrial adenoacanthoma: A clinicopathological study of 55 cases. *Cancer* 18:737, 1965.

Cullen TS: *Cancer of the Uterus. Pathology, Symptomatology, Diagnosis, and Treatment.* New York, Appleton & Co, 1900.

Cutler BS, Forbes AP, Ingersoll FM, et al: Endometrial carcinoma after stilbestrol therapy in gonadal dysgenesis. *N Engl J Med* 287:628, 1972.

Dockerty MB, Mussie E: Malignant lesions of the uterus associated with estrogen producing ovarian tumors. *Am J Obstet Gynecol* 61:147, 1951.

Ewing J: *Neoplastic Disease.* Philadelphia, W.B. Saunders, 1928.

Frick HC II, Munnell EW, Richart RM, et al: Carcinoma of the endometrium. *Am J Obstet Gynecol* 115:663, 1973.

Garnet JD: Constitutional stigmas associated with endometrial carcinoma. *Am J Obstet Gynecol* 76:11, 1958.

Gusberg SB: *An Approach to the Control of Cancer of the Endometrium.* New York, American Cancer Society, 1973.

Hausknecht RV, Gusberg SB: Estrogen metabolism in patients at high risk for endometrial cancer. *Am J Obstet Gynecol* 105:1161, 1969.

Hertig AT, Sommers SC, Bengloff H: Genesis of endometrial carcinoma III. Carcinoma in situ. *Cancer* 2:964, 1949.

Hertig AT, Sommers SC: Genesis of endometrial carcinoma. I. Study of prior biopsies. *Cancer* 2:946, 1949.

Jensen EV, Suzuki J, DeSombre ER: A two-step mechanism for the interaction of estradiol with rat uterus. *Proc Nat Acad Sci USA* 59:632, 1968.

King RJB: Clinical relevance of steroid-receptor measurements in tumors. *Cancer Treat Rev* 2:273, 1975.

Kirk ME: Gynecology. *Prog Hum Path* 5:253, 1974.

Koss LG: Diagnosis of early endometrial cancer and precancerous states. *Ann Clin Lab Sci* 9:189, 1979.

Lewis BV, Stallworthy J, Cowdell R: Adenocarcinoma of the body of the uterus. *J Obstet Gynecol Br Commw* 77:343, 1970.

Lynch HT, Krush AJ: Cancer family "G" revisited: 1895–1970. *Cancer* 27:1505, 1971.

MacMahon B: Risk factors for endometrial cancer. *Gynecol Oncol* 2:122, 1974.

Marin WJ Jr, Mortel R, Ward SP, et al: Concomitant existence of carcinoma and secretory endometrium. *Gynecol Oncol* 6:275, 1978.

Morris JM: Hormone therapy for the menopause. *The Female Patient* 3:29, 1978.

Morrow CP, DiSaia PJ, Townsend DE: Current management of endometrial cancer. *Obstet Gynecol* 42:399, 1973.

Nachtigall L, Natchtigall R, Beckman M: Letter. *N Engl J Med* 294:848, 1976.

Ng ABP, Reagan JW: Incidence and prognosis of endometrial carcinoma by histologic grade and extent. *Obstet Gynecol* 35:437, 1970.

Pollow K, Lübert H, Boquoi E, et al: Characterization and comparison of receptors for 17 β-estradiol and progesterone in human proliferative endometrium and endometrial carcinoma. *Endocrinology* 96:319, 1975.

Rubin BL, Gussberg SB, Butterly J et al: Screening test for estrogen dependence of endometrial carcinoma. *Am J Obstet Gynecol* 114:660, 1972.

Sitteri PK, Schwarz B, MacDonald P: Estrogen receptors and the estrone hypothesis in relation to endometrial and breast cancer. *Gynecol Oncol* 2:228, 1974.

Smith DC, Prentice R, Thompson DJ, et al: Association of exogenous estrogen and endometrial carcinoma. *N Engl J Med* 293:1164, 1975.

Sommers SC: Carcinoma of the endometrium. Reprinted from the *Uterus International Academy of Pathology Monograph No. 14.* Baltimore, Williams and Wilkins Co, 1973, p 276.

238

Sommers SC, Hertig AT, Bengloff H: Genesis of endometrial carcinoma. II. Cases 19 to 35 years old. *Cancer* 2:957, 1949.

Tseng L, Gurpide E: Effects of progestins on estradiol receptor levels in human endometrium. *J Clin Endocrinol Metab* 41:402, 1975.

United States Department of Health, Education and Welfare. *Cancer Patient Survival, Report, Number 5.* Bethesda, National Institutes of Health, 1976.

VanBogaert L-J, Maldague P, Staquet JP: Endometrial biopsy interpretation: Shortcomings and problems in current gynecologic practice. *Obstet Gynecol* 51(1):25, 1978.

Vellios F: Endometrial hyperplasia and carcinoma in-situ. *Gynecol Oncol* 2:152, 1974.

Wakonig-Vaartaja T, Auersperz N: Cytogenetics and gynecologic neoplasms. *Clin Obstet Gynecol* 13:813, 1970.

Way S: *Malignant Disease of the Female Genital Tract.* Philadelphia, Blakiston Co, 1951.

Ziel HK, Finkle WD: Increased risk of endometrial carcinoma among users of conjugated estrogens. *N Engl J Med* 293:1167, 1975.

9 Cancer of the Ovary

Hugh R. K. Barber

Deaths from cancer of the ovary have slowly increased over the last 40 years, and the rate is now two and one-half times that of 1930. It is now anticipated that 1.4% or one of every 70 newborn girls will develop cancer of the ovary at some time during their lives. In 1981, the projected figure for new cases of cancer of the ovary is 18,000. The age-specific incidence rate for ovarian cancer shows a steady rise up to age 80, where the incidence drops off slightly.

Cancer of the ovary is the leading cause of death from gynecologic cancer in the United States. Approximately 11,400 deaths are estimated for 1981. The dramatic figure is that ovarian cancer constitutes about 25% of gynecologic cancers, but accounts for 47% of all deaths from cancers of the female genital tract.

Unfortunately, progress in curing ovarian cancer has been disappointingly slow. More than 100,000 women have died of this disease in the past decade, and ovarian cancer continues to increase as a major gynecologic disease in the United States. Currently, the optimal treatment for each stage of the disease is not even known. The results of therapy were no better in 1980 than had been achieved in the previous two decades. Current methods of management are helping these women to live longer and, probably, more comfortably, but at present the dismal five-year survival rate has not changed.

The incidence of ovarian cancers starts to rise at age 40 with an annual rate of 10 per 100,000 women, increases to a peak at about age 77 where the rate is about 52 per 100,000, and then drops after age 80 when there is a rate of about 45 per 100,000. The incidence plateaus and stabilizes for the remainder of life. It is obvious that the ovary gets too old to function, but never gets too old to develop a cancer. It is essential that these figures and the distribution of the incidence be kept in mind when making the decision whether to retain the ovaries at the time of hysterectomy in women over age 40. Since the incidence of ovarian cancer is on the increase in highly industrialized nations, an effort must be made to achieve earlier diagnosis than has been possible in the past, or to practice prophylaxis by removing ovaries at the time of surgery in women over age 40.

Ovarian cancer is one of the most frustrating problems in gynecology. For those patients not cured, death is often prolonged, with repeated bouts of intestinal obstruction. The cancer spreads over the surface of the bowel, and, although the lumen of the bowel is not obstructed, the end result is the same as though it were. Segments of the bowel are so coated with cancer that the gut is paralyzed and, like a sewer pipe, has no peristalsis. Therefore, it is not able to propel its contents along the lumen. Patients develop inanition and malnutrition, and literally vomit themselves to death. It is unfortunate that these individuals remain alert up until the very moment of death. They often become ravenously hungry, and, after ingesting food or liquids, begin to vomit. It is a dismal clinical picture of a woman who not only is terminally ill, but also is being tormented by her hunger and thirst. The pathology described as carcinomatosis ileus is one of the few indications for the intermittent use of the nasogastric tube as definitive therapy to decompress the bowel. Responsible physicians should be well versed in gastroenterology and surgery for gastroenterologic disorders. Those therapeutic nihilists who plead that the patient should be left to die with dignity, must face a dilemma when forced to apply their philosophy to the case of a woman dying with advanced ovarian cancer.

EPIDEMIOLOGY

Cancer epidemiology seeks to correlate differences in the incidence of various types of cancer with differences in the external or internal environment of persons developing these cancers. The correlation between cigarette smoking and lung cancer is an established example of cancer epidemiology.

Recent investigations have raised some intriguing questions that call for further study. These include the sevenfold higher incidence of breast cancer and ovarian cancer among Americans as compared to Japanese women; the much greater incidence of colon cancer in the United States than in certain areas of Africa; and the spotty geographic distribution of esophageal cancer throughout Africa.

So far, the results of epidemiologic research strongly suggest that variations in social practices and exposure to environmental agents are largely responsible for variations in the incidence of cancer among different groups of people. Therefore, if such environmental exposures and social practices could be identified and eliminated, most cancers in man might be prevented. Because of the complexity of the relationship between man and his environment, and the long latent period of cancer development, the identification of particular cancer-inducing factors is extremely difficult. But, there is no other area of cancer research that holds more promise for cancer prevention.

The epidemiology of ovarian cancer depends primarily on accurate diagnosis. For example, a specific tumor, a specific histologic type within a single organ, may point to a particular causal factor. When accurate diagnosis is not possible, epidemiologic work is handicapped. Berg and Baylor (1973) have disclosed just such a situation in ovarian cancer. Nowhere is accurate diagnosis more important than with ovarian cancer. These tumors are difficult to manage and have a high mortality rate. Moreover, ovarian cancers differ from country to country, and it is from these differences that important etiologic factors may emerge. The Danes have a high incidence of ovarian cancer, whereas the Japanese women in their homeland have relatively low rates. The Danes eat a high, dairy-product diet, and, therefore, a high cholesterol diet, while the Japanese diet is low in cholesterol. Studies in nutrition and hormones among those two groups have contributed little towards finding an etiologic factor. The descendants of the Japanese who have moved to the United States have an increased rate of ovarian cancer, and some investigators have reported it is higher in their offspring than in native American women. In our highly industrialized nation, more people than ever are eating high-fat diets.

A number of epidemologic factors are suspected of being linked with ovarian cancer. Among these are nulliparity, endometriosis, infertility, marked premenstrual tension, abnormal breast swelling, marked amenorrhea, increased spontaneous abortions, early menopause, adenocarcinoma of the endometrium, group A blood type, irradiation of pelvic organs, environmental factors, industrial products such as asbestos and talc, higher socioeconomic status, celibacy, breast cancer, and resistance to mumps parotitis. A family history of ovarian cancer has occasionally been identified. The role of stress is once again receiving attention, and should be investigated in more detail.

There are seven major demographic leads:

1. Ovarian cancer, particularly in postmenopausal women, is less common in Japan than in the Western world. Compared with Caucasian women, Oriental women, who have a low incidence of breast and ovarian cancer, have a high estriol titer between ages 15 and 19. It is now recognized that estriol acts as an antagonist of carcinogenic activity of estriol-estrone. As each group moves toward age 40, the difference decreases until it is negligible. Because there is little difference at the time the cancer in these organs begins to develop, it must be concluded that estriol was protecting the immature cell.
2. Among first generation Japanese women in the United States, ovarian cancer occurs more commonly than in Japan.
3. Not only has there been an increase in the incidence of ovarian cancer in the Western world, there has also been some increase in Japan as this nation has become more industrialized.
4. Cancer of the ovary tends to be somewhat more common in upper than in lower income groups in the West.
5. Ovarian cancer in New York City is more common among Jews than other religious groups, particularly in postmenopausal women.
6. There is a positive correlation between the pattern of incidence of ovarian, mammary, and endometrial cancers.
7. In several studies, ovarian cancer has been reported to be more common among single and nulliparous women.

CLINICAL MANIFESTATIONS

It is usually stated that there are no early manifestations of ovarian cancer. This in itself is considered a major contributing factor to the poor therapeutic results. The usual manifestations of abdominal swelling, pain, and a mass, as recorded in hospital charts, are associated with an advanced stage of the disease.

The earliest manifestations are usually insidious, and include vague abdominal discomfort, dyspepsia, indigestion, gas with concomitant distention, flatulence, gastrointestinal unrest, feeling of fullness after a light meal, slight loss of appetite, and other mild digestive disturbances. Although the "specific" manifestations are certainly not specific, such gastrointestinal complaints are not uncommon. They are suggestive of ovarian cancer and may signal difficulty. Unfortunately, such complaints are usually not considered important.

The gastrointestinal manifestations may precede other symptoms by months. It is imperative to rule out ovarian cancer in women over age 40 who present with gastrointestinal symptoms that cannot be definitely diagnosed. Elderly women without pelvic complaints, but with complaints referable to the intestinal tract, are more apt to consult their internist or family doctor for their extrapelvic complaints. Such clinicians have a great opportunity to diagnose ovarian cancer in an early stage.

The following triad may be an aid in the diagnosis of ovarian cancer: 1) A woman 35 years of age or over has a significant risk because of her age. With advancing age, the ovary ceases to function, but remains a risk for development of ovarian cancer; 2) In a patient over 40 years of age, persistent gastrointestinal symptoms which cannot be definitely diagnosed; 3) A long history of ovarian imbalance or malfunction, including increased premenstrual tension, heavy menstruation with marked breast tenderness, dysfunctional bleeding, a tendency for spontaneous abortion, infertility, nulliparity, as well as an early menopause, should alert the clinician to the possibility that ovarian cancer may be developing. The ovary is like a cam running off center.

When the triad is present, it is important to consider the possibility of ovarian cancer, and systematically carry out all diagnostic measures as outlined below. Unfortunately, there are no specific diagnostic measures for early ovarian cancer, but a high index of suspicion and education of the public will achieve an earlier diagnosis, and occasionally an *early* diagnosis.

DIAGNOSIS

The early diagnosis of ovarian cancer is a matter of chance and not a triumph of the scientific approach. Means of early detection are extremely limited. In the majorty of cases, the findings of a pelvic mass is the only available diagnostic sign, with the exception of functional tumors, which may manifest endocrine activity with minimal ovarian enlargement. In some cases, pelvic findings may be uncertain, even late in the disease. Pain in the early stages is associated with a complication, such as torsion or a rupture. Later, pain occurs when adjacent organs or nerve sheaths are infiltrated by tumor.

Menstrual disorders may result from hormone-producing tumors. In the menopausal patient, vaginal bleeding may occur. This has been attributed to the functioning stroma in the malignant ovary. Ascites with malignant cells is a sign of advanced disease.

In terms of function, it must also be emphasized that a variety of endocrine effects, such as hypercalcemia, hypoglycemia, and Cushing's syndrome, as well as disorders such as hemolytic anemia, may occasionally be related to the presence of an ovarian tumor.

The pelvic findings are often inconclusive, even late in the disease. The tumor may be deep in the pelvis, the patient may be obese, heavy muscled, and uncooperative. The elderly patient may have an inelastic conical vagina, complicated by marked atrophy. Occasionally, there may be widespread metastases with minimal pelvic findings. The usual signs and symptoms, as well as the physical findings associated with ovarian cancer, all represent an advanced cancer of the ovary. The abdominal mass or distention, or both, are the most common diagnostic features reported in most hospital charts. However, ovarian cancers seldom give symptoms until they grow to a size of 15 cm. They cannot be palpated abdominally until they achieve this size. Pain in the early stages is usually associated with a complication such as torsion, perforation, or hemorrhage. Ascites with positive cells is a sign of advanced disease, and the five-year survival rate is reported to be less than 8% in these patients.

Pelvic Examination

Routine pelvic examination will detect about one cancer in 10,000 examinations of asymptomatic women. Pelvic findings are often minimal, and are not helpful in making a diagnosis, even in patients with advanced disease. However, combined with a high index of suspicion, the findings on pelvic examination may help alert the physician to the diagnosis. The most helpful pelvic findings in suggesting the presence of an ovarian cancer are: 1) a mass in the ovarian area; 2) relative immobility due to fixation and adhesions; 3) irregularity of the tumor, particularly a difference in consistency; one area may be cystic, another rubbery, another soft. This difference is due to the rapid growth of the tumor, resulting in ischemic areas; 4) a shotty consistency with increased firmness; 5) tumors in the cul-de-sac, described as a "handful of knuckles"; 6) relative insensitivity of the mass; 7) increasing size under observation; 8) bilaterality (70% of ovarian cancer vs 5% of benign cases); and 9) in late disease, common findings of nodular hepatomegaly, ascites, and palpation of an omental mass.

Other Diagnostic Procedures

The Pap smear has been reported to be positive in 40% of patients with advanced disease. Positive cells in cul-de-sac caps have been reported in 90% of patients; the author's results are very poor when compared with these figures. Ultrasound and the CAT scan have added little to the early diagnosis of ovarian cancer. They do help in monitoring treatment, and often confirm the diagnosis. The value of laparoscopy appears to be in staging of ovarian cancers, and, perhaps, in monitoring their response to treatment, but has not contributed significantly to early diagnosis.

Carcinoembryonic antigens, (CEA), alpha fetoprotein (AFP), lactic dehydrogenase (LDH), and chorionic gonadotropin (CG), are of no help in making the diagnosis, but, if elevated, serve to monitor the patient's response to therapy.

One of the most exciting areas of gynecologic oncology is the present effort to diagnose ovarian cancers by means of immunologic techniques. The laboratory at Lenox Hill Hospital, as well as others, have identified what appears to be an antigen that is specific to human, common epithelial tumor. The antigen has been used to produce a heterologous antiserum in rabbits. The antigen is identified by double diffusion or agar gel, as well as by immunofluorescent tests.

An antigen-antibody complex has been identified in ascitic fluid. The peritoneal effusions of patients with ovarian cancer contain sizeable amounts of free and complex immunoglobulins. Antibodies can be recovered by salt precipitation procedures; after purification and concentration, they display a high degree of specificity against ovarian carcinoma cells. The autologous antibody has been polymerized to form a column for the identification and, hopefully, isolation of an antigen that is purer than those previously identified. By combining the autologous antibody with a protein-A matrix, a new blocking technique has been prepared that gives promise of greater specificity and sensitivity.

The use of 8M urea as a chemotactic agent for the dissociation of immune complexes has advantages over the acid dissociation method. The low pH levels necessary to effect dissociation of complexes (pH 2.8 to 3.0) and their subsequent neutralization, represent relatively harsh conditions which may result in significant levels of irreversible denaturation of some IgG molecules, rendering them unfit for use in certain procedures, such as complement fixation. However, even such extremes of pH have been found to be ineffective in the separation of antigen from antibody in complexes recovered from the sera of animals with experimental tumors. It is often difficult to separate immune complexes with high-binding affinities.

Solutions of 8M urea are highly effective chemotactic agents, yielding almost complete dissociation of immune complexes. The denaturation of antibodies produced by 8M urea is reversible, and the removal of urea by dialysis allows the quantitative recovery of antibody and antigen whose physical properties and immunologic reactivities are unaltered. In addition, since urea is non-ionic, it does not interfere with the separation of dissociated antibody from antigen by ion exchange chromatography. Chromatography of serum proteins or immune complexes on anion exchange resins yield pure IgG, as determined by agar gel electrophoresis, with subsequent elution of other proteins by high salt solutions. This agent is currently in use in our laboratory at Lenox Hill Hospital, and is providing us with clean, highly reproducible preparations with substantial tumor-related reactivity.

Laser nephelometry is being used in the evaluation of tumor-related activity of antibody preparations. Each new antibody preparation is first tested by nephelometry, over a wide range of dilutions, against a pool of soluble antigen from ovarian cancers, to determine its level of reactivity. Those showing reaction curves indicative of substantial levels of activity are screened at an appropriate dilution against a group of soluble antigen extracts from a variety of normal, benign, and malignant tissues.

Hopefully, these findings can be converted to a radioimmunoassay for the detection of early ovarian carcinoma.

EARLY DETECTION AND PREVENTION

In the last five years, ovarian cancer has become the leading cause of death among gynecologic cancers. There are only two methods available to lower the mortality rate: 1) early diagnosis; and 2) prophylaxis.

Unfortunately, there is no method presently available for making an early diagnosis, and there is a strong resistance to prophylaxis on the part of the patient as well as the physician. However, when a hysterectomy is indicated in a patient over 40 years of age, it is important to explain to her that ovarian cancer is on the increase, that it is the leading cause of death from gynecologic cancer, and that most cases are in Stages III and IV when the diagnosis is made. Bilateral salpingo-oophorectomy should also be advised.

In evaluating patients admitted with the diagnosis of ovarian cancer, it was found that the incidence of cancer in the retained ovary of patients who had previous pelvic surgery was reported as approximately 3% 30 years ago. In 1962, it was reported as 7%; in 1967 as 8.9%; and in 1971 as 20% by Gibbs. Since the incidence of ovarian cancer is increasing and is the leading cause of death from gynecologic cancer, it would be interesting to know what the figure is today. There is no indication that the risk of ovarian cancer is lessened by removing one ovary. Currently, more than 800,000 hysterectomies are performed each year, and most of these are done in women over 40 years of age. These are the patients at risk to develop ovarian cancer.

INDICATIONS FOR EXPLORATORY LAPAROTOMY

Exploratory laparotomy is indicated for the following findings:

1. Any pelvic mass that has appeared after menopause, particularly an adnexal mass.
2. An adnexal mass in a woman of any age that progressively enlarges beyond 5 cm while under observation. This is particularly so if the patient is on oral contraceptives, or has had one or two menstrual periods without a change in the size of the mass.

3. An adnexal mass of 10 cm or more in size. Follicle cysts, corpus luteum cysts, and even endometrial cysts are seldom larger than 10 cm in diameter.
4. A mass which cannot be definit'ly diagnosed as either a fibroid or a carcinoma.
5. The presence of an ovary which is of normal size in the premenopausal woman is abnormal in the postmenopausal period.

The complete workup for a patient suspected of having an ovarian cancer includes:

1. Careful history
2. Physical examination
3. Pelvic examination and Pap smear
4. Proctosigmoidoscopy, as indicated
5. CBC and urinalysis
6. SMA-12 (blood chemistries)
7. Chest x-ray
8. Intravenous pyelogram
9. GI series
10. Barium enema
11. Paracentesis, laparoscopy, and lymphangiogram (optional)

This workup documents the extent of disease and determines whether the cancer is primary or metastatic. About 5% to 10% are metastatic.

OCCURRENCE OF OVARIAN TUMORS BY AGE GROUPS

Age is an important consideration in the evaluation and management of a patient with an adnexal mass. Therefore, it is important to divide patients into three age groups, namely, birth to age 20, 20 to 40 years, and over 40 years. An adnexal mass in pregnancy is a separate category.

A mass in the very young and the very old is presumed to be abnormal. The best management consists of a careful workup, a knowledge of the type of tumor that commonly occurs in that age group, and exploratory laparotomy. There is no time or place for observation and procrastination in patients before puberty or after the menopause. Management of an adnexal mass diagnosed during pregnancy or in patients between ages 20 to 40 may arouse controversy.

Birth to Age 20

The most common tumor diagnosed in the birth-to-age-20 group is the germ-cell tumor, followed by the gonadal-stroma tumor. Although ovarian tumors account for only about 1% of new growths in children under age 16, they still remain the most frequent genital neoplasm of childhood and adolescence. They give rise to a great deal of confusion about diagnosis and management, and this is compounded by a marked emotional problem that involves the patient, her family, and the doctor.

If a graph of tumor incidence is drawn for these age groups, it appears to be bell-shaped with a peak at about puberty. This has led to conjecture that some control mechanism may be activated, or that pituitary stimulation of an ovarian factor may be the triggering mechanism.

The most common tumors in infants and young children are cystic teratomas (dermoids). They have been found soon after birth as well as later. Among all the ovarian tumors that occur during this age group, only about one in ten are malignant. Prior to puberty, most of these tumors present as abdominal masses. It is not until puberty, or after, that the female pelvic organs descend into the pelvis. Therefore, any mass in the pelvis in the prepubertal patient has to be viewed with suspicion.

Ovarian tumors in children may produce few symptoms. They are related to the rapidity of growth, position, degree of malignancy, as well as to the tumor's ability to secrete hormones. The complications

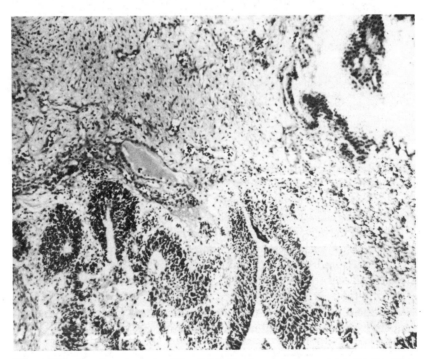

Figure 9-1 Ovarian teratoma: Histologically these ovarian germ cell tumors are characterized by varying proportions of mature and immature tissues, and are graded histologically by the amount of immature tissue. The dark staining tubular structures in this photomicrograph represent immature neural elements.

associated with tumors, such as twisting, rupture, infection, and hemorrhage focus attention on them.

Diagnostic procedures should include a blood count, urinalysis, chest x-ray, intravenous pyelogram, and, if indicated, x-ray studies of the gastrointestinal tract. In patients suspected of having a hormone-producing tumor, hormone assays may have some value. X-ray studies of the epiphyses may be even more helpful. The role of ultrasonography and laparoscopy at this age remains to be clarified. The alpha fetoprotein may be significantly elevated if the patient has an extraembryonal tumor, such as an endodermal sinus tumor. An elevated chorionic gonadotropin titer may be present in extraembryonal tumors, especially when chorionic elements are found, such as choriocarcinoma.

The key to treatment in this age group is conservatism. However, any spread beyond the ovary demands a more aggressive approach. Treatment should be outlined by groups of tumors within a given classification. Although the common, epithelial ovarian tumors are rare in this age group, the physician may occasionally encounter a mucinous or serous cystadenocarcinoma. If the tumor is unilateral and encapsulated, if there is negative pelvic cytology, and if the opposite ovary is negative on biopsy, unilateral salpingo-oophorectomy is acceptable therapy. But, if there is evidence of spread of disease beyond the ovary, total hysterectomy, bilateral salpingo-oophorectomy, and omentectomy (if an omentum has developed) is indicated.

Germ-cell tumors vary a great deal in their response to treatment. The extraembryonal tumors, such as endodermal sinus tumor and choriocarcinoma, are highly malignant. They are usually unilateral, and, until the advent of treatment by triple and quadruple chemotherapy, few patients survived longer than two years. With the newer forms of chemotherapy, the results are surprisingly good.

The most common germ-cell tumor is the dysgerminoma, which is a highly radiosensitive tumor with a bilaterality rate of 10%. The treatment of choice, although controversial, is unilateral salpingo-oophorectomy. This is based on the assumption that there are no positive cells present in the pelvis. The value of pelvic cytology in dysgerminoma has not been established. The opposite ovary must be free of tumor on biopsy. If there is spread beyond the ovary in which the tumor arises, total hysterectomy and bilateral salpingo-oophorectomy should be carried out. X-ray therapy should be employed as the disease spreads to the pelvis and/or upper abdomen. The necessity for immediate paraaortic and supraclavicular node therapy with x-rays has not been determined for this age group.

Gonadal-stromal tumors include tumors that have the potential to produce either a feminizing or masculinizing effect, although they do so in only 25% of the patients. Approximately 25% of these tumors are malignant, and about 10% are bilateral. Of the female type, the only important malignant tumor is the granulosa cell tumor. It is usually

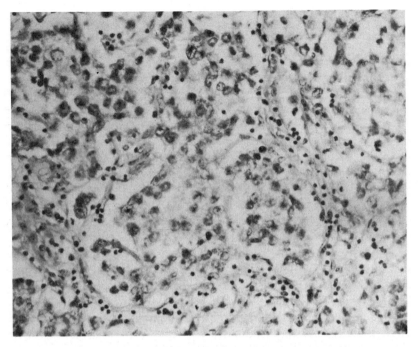

Figure 9-2 Dysgerminoma: This germ cell tumor, histologically analogous to the testicular seminoma, is composed of loose aggregated or primitive tumor cells interspersed with delicate fibrous stroma containing varying numbers of lymphocytes, seen in this photomicrograph as small darkly staining cells.

unilateral, and late recurrence is frequently encountered, often beyond five years. Typically, spread is local, and recurrence is confined to the pelvis. Since the tumor has a low grade malignancy and is seldom bilateral, unilateral oophorectomy is indicated when the tumor is encapsulated and the other ovary is normal. The same principles are followed in managing Sertoli-Leydig cell tumors.

Gonadoblastoma is composed of germ cells and gonadal-stromal cells in nearly equal proportion. Its malignant potential is determined by the type of germ cell present. The gonadoblastoma is usually found in the intersexual patients, and, since these patients cannot menstruate or reproduce, treatment consists of bilateral oophorectomy.

In this age group, metastatic ovarian cancer is treated as in the adult. As much tumor as possible is removed, including the primary cancer. Adjunctive therapy is chosen, depending upon the type of tumor.

Ages 20 to 40

Controversy may arise over management of an adnexal mass as the patient approaches age 20. A careful history is of prime importance, followed by a thorough pelvic examination to include the vaginal, rectal, and rectovaginal areas. The ideal time to examine the patient is after she has been given an enema. There are other explanations for an adnexal mass other than ovarian pathology. In the 40-year-old group, diverticulitis must be considered, whereas ectopic pregnancy is more common when the patient is in her twenties. The preoperative workup must be thorough so that the primary site of the metastatic tumor, if it happens to be metastatic, is not overlooked. This has already been discussed.

If the patient is in her twenties and the mass is cystic, smooth, and unilateral, it is acceptable medical practice to reevaluate her after one or two menstrual periods. A functional cyst should start to regress during this time. Some investigators have advocated use of an estrogen-progesterone combination to inhibit pituitary stimulation of the ovary. If it is a functional cyst, it should promptly begin to regress. But, even a short period of observation is not justified if the patient is taking oral contraceptives.

At the time of laparotomy, management of the adnexal mass of the patient in her twenties is similar to that described for tumors in childhood. It is important to individualize treatment, not only according to histologic classification, but also according to stage of the disease. In general, the conservative approach is justified if the tumor is unilateral, well-differentiated,

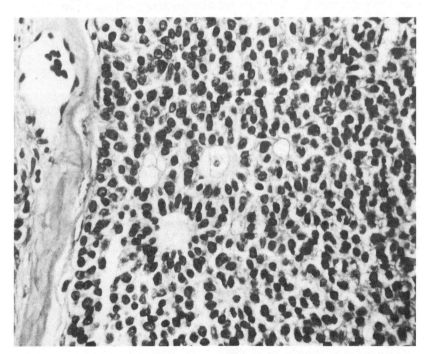

Figure 9-3 Granulosa cell tumor: Well-differentiated granulosa cell tumors form characteristic rosette-like spaces known as Call-Exner bodies.

and encapsulated, with negative cytology. Germ-cell and gonadal-stromal tumors lend themselves more often to a conservative approach than do the common epithelial ovarian tumors. The patient should be of low parity or nulliparous with a negative biopsy in the opposite ovary, as well as with negative omentum, and negative pelvic and aortic node biopsies. Any evidence of spread beyond the ovary in which the tumor arose, demands aggressive surgical treatment as described above.

Ages 40 and Older

Patients 40 years of age and older compose the high-risk group because they are either perimenopausal or postmenopausal. The same diagnostic workups and differential diagnosis are followed as in the 20-to-40-age group. Metastatic cancers of the ovary are probably more common in this high-risk group. Since the chances of malignancy are higher in this group, there is no indication for observation, especially if the mass is larger than 5 cm, adherent, and gives the impression that there are solid as well as cystic, soft, and rubbery areas present. Although the treatment will be discussed by stages later in this chapter, the treatment should generally consist of a total hysterectomy, bilateral salpingo-oophorectomy, appendectomy, omentectomy, and the option for instillation of phosphorus-32. The epithelial ovarian tumor is the most commonly encountered ovarian tumor in this age group. About 8% occur before age 40, and the incidence peaks at 52 to 55 years.

UNILATERAL MASS IN PREGNANCY

The adnexal mass in pregnancy is always cause for concern. Approximately 1 in 1000 pregnancies is complicated by an ovarian tumor. If the mass is unilateral, less than 10 cm in size, well encapsulated, and freely movable, observation is justified until the patient is in the second trimester. If the mass increases or persists in its size, then it cannot be considered a corpus luteum cyst, and exploratory laparotomy is indicated. On the other hand, if the mass is bilateral, hard, knobby, and has a variegated consistency, exploratory laparotomy is indicated without the usual period of observation.

THE POSTMENOPAUSAL
PALPABLE OVARY SYNDROME (PMPO)

With the present state of diagnostic development, diagnosis of an ovarian tumor is a matter of chance rather than a scientific method. By the time it has been diagnosed, ovarian cancer has, in more than 60% to 70% of patients, spread beyond the ovary. The hard fact remains that a pelvic mass found during pelvic examination is the only practical and consistent clinical method presently available to detect ovarian tumor. Certain functional or dysontogenetic tumors with hormonal activity are the exception. However, there are only a few such tumors compared to the common epithelial ovarian cancers, which compose the main group of "killers." It has been reported that the chances of detecting an ovarian neoplasm during routine pelvic examination in an asymptomatic woman is 1 in 10,000.

One diagnostic sign of early ovarian cancer in the postmenopausal patient has proved to be both valuable and consistent in our hands. Simply, it is the palpation of what is interpreted as a normal-sized ovary in the premenopausal woman, represents an ovarian tumor in the postmenopausal woman. This may appear to be insignificant in terms of the total problem, but it has been the author's experience that all such palpable findings proved to be a new growth; they were not all necessarily malignant, but none were functional or dysfunctional. It is my opinion that a postmenopausal palpable ovary is a most significant finding, and gynecologists should be alert to its importance.

The designation "postmenopausal palpable ovary syndrome" is a misnomer, and it is unfortunate that a more descriptive term was not chosen. It does not mean that anything that is palpated in the adnexa is abnormal. Every gynecologist has been able to feel an ovary that measures 2 cm in a very thin, relaxed patient with an elastic and distensible vagina. It is to be reemphasized that the PMPO syndrome is simply that the palpation of what is interpreted as a *normal sized ovary in the premenopausal woman represents an ovarian tumor in the postmenopausal woman.*

MANAGEMENT

Tumors of the common epithelial variety make up approximately 80% to 90% of ovarian cancers. Only about 8% occur in women under age 40; most occur in women after age 40. In the latter group, conservative therapy is not indicated, even for tumors of low-grade malignancy. Treatment consists of curettage, exploratory laparotomy, total hysterectomy, bilateral salpingo-oophorectomy, omentectomy, appendectomy, and the option for the instillation of phosphorus-32, and, possibly, prophylactic chemotherapy. The use of prophylactic chemotherapy remains to be evaluated. This will require treatment of a large number of cases.

Technique

The surgical technique will not be discussed in detail. However, certain pertinent principles will be reviewed. Upon opening the abdomen,

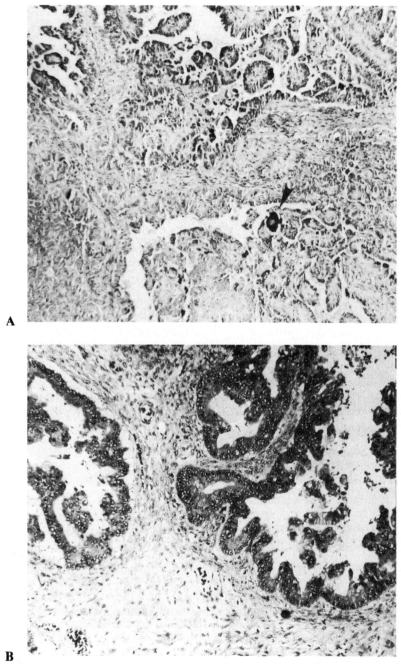

A

B

Figure 9-4 Ovarian epithelial tumors: **A** Serous cystadenocarcinoma is characterized by cystic spaces lined by papillary projections of malignant columnar epithelial cells resembling tubal epithelium plus occasional calcified psammoma bodies (arrow). **B** Endometrioid carcinoma exhibits an invasive growth of glands

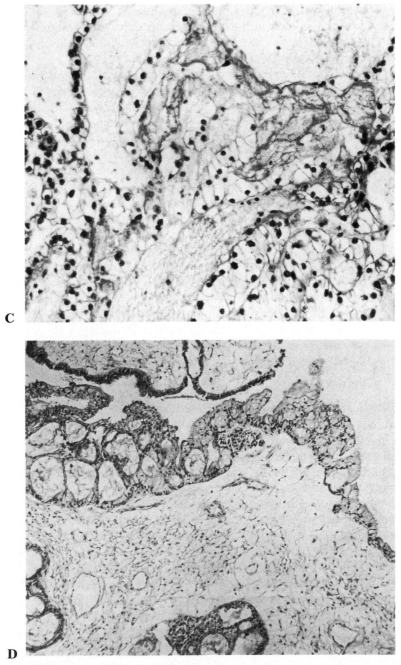

C

D

histologically similar to endometrial carcinoma. **C** Clear cell carcinoma exhibits solid and cystic areas with characteristic clear and hobnail cells. **D** Mucinous adenocarcinoma of the ovary. The tumor cells retain their goblet-cell appearance, but show stratification of nuclei and atypia.

any fluid present should be aspirated and examined for cells. If none are present, saline should be instilled into the upper abdomen and retrieved, and then saline instilled into the pelvis and retrieved, and both should be sent to the laboratory for cytologic examination.

The incision, of course, should be a vertical one, and should extend beyond the upper limits of the tumor. There is no place for a transverse incision in the treatment of common epithelial ovarian cancer. Once the abdomen is open and the fluid has been aspirated, it is important to explore the upper abdomen very carefully, including the large and small bowel, the retroperitoneal area, the area between the liver and the diaphragm, and the posterior peritoneum. The ovarian cancer itself should not be handled at this point because of the possibility of starting a hemorrhage. Having explored the upper abdomen carefully, it is important to identify the infundibulopelvic ligament on both sides, size the peritoneum lateral to the ligament, and identify the ureter. Having done this on both sides, the infundibulopelvic ligaments should be clamped, cut, suture-ligated, and doubly secured with a free tie. These vessels are often very large, even in the elderly patient. This procedure will reduce the blood supply to the ovary, and the operation can then be carried out with less blood loss. The actual procedures for each stage will be discussed later. On closing the abdominal cavity, it is important to use retention sutures on all ovarian cancer patients. Their metabolism and nutrition is less than optimal, and the use of retention sutures insures a more secure type of closure.

Management of the Common Epithelial Ovarian Cancers

Stages Ia, Ib, and Ic Exporatory laparotomy, total hysterectomy, bilateral salpingo-oophorectomy, omentectomy, appendectomy, and the option for the instillation of phosphorus-32 constitute the recommended treatment. All patients should have any free fluid aspirated, and, if none is present, the pelvis and abdomen should be irrigated with saline and the fluid submitted to the laboratory for cytologic examination according to the Papanicolaou technique. There is considerable controversy over the value of omentectomy. Occasionally, islands of tumor cells will be found in the omentum, advancing the disease to Stage III, assuming that the initial diagnosis was a lesser stage. In addition, the omentum interferes with the even distribution of phosphorus-32, and is, therefore, best removed if instillation of phosphorus-32 is contemplated.

Ovarian cancer is the only genital cancer that can be staged during and after surgery. Metastatic disease may be found in a normal-appearing ovary. Reports in the literature indicate that approximately 10% of patients with apparent clinical Stage I ovarian cancer will be found to have metastatic disease between the liver and the diaphragm along the posterior wall of the abdominal cavity. The cancer is then considered a

Stage III. In view of this, our regimen has been revised to include pro-phylactic chemotherapy in Stage I cancers of the ovary.

Stage IIa and IIb   The treatment recommended is exploratory laparotomy, total hysterectomy, bilateral salpingo-oophorectomy, omentectomy, appendectomy, and instillation of phosphorus-32. All adhesions surrounding the ovarian cancer should be biopsied to docu-ment the extent of disease. Chemotherapy is also given prophylactically and/or therapeutically for all Stage II cancers of the ovary.

Stage III   The surgical approach, if possible, is the same as for Stages I and II, and should consist of exploratory laparotomy, total hysterectomy, bilateral salpingo-oophorectomy, appendectomy, and omentectomy. Total abdominal radiation is no longer employed as a definitive method of treatment for common epithelial ovarian cancer. Since it is necessary to shield the kidneys and liver, it is felt that these pa-tients are selected for failure. The results of the use of radiation therapy, using orthovoltage, kilovoltage, and then megavoltage has not improved the survival rate over the past 30 or 40 years, and it is felt that other methods should be explored. Chemotherapy, therefore, is given in Stage III cancer of the ovary.

Stage IV   The ideal management consists of removal of as much cancer as possible, including total hysterectomy, bilateral salpingo-oophorectomy, appendectomy, and omentectomy. Chemotherapy is given as the definitive treatment, and radiation is reserved for control of the disease in the supraclavicular and/or inguinal areas.

Management of Nonepithelial Ovarian Cancer

Nonepithelial lesions comprise 10% of all ovarian tumors, and are the most common gynecologic tumor in children and adolescents. The cancer progresses rapidly, and is susceptible to torsion due to the long infundibulopelvic ligament found in the adolescent child.

Germ-Cell Tumors

Germ-cell tumors occur almost exclusively in children and adolescents. Such tumors vary a great deal in response to treatment; therefore, the treatment depends on the type of tumor found. The dysger-minomas resemble sexually undifferentiated germ cells of the early gonad. Some patients have subnormal gonadal development and pseudo-hermaphroditism, but these findings are not caused by the tumor, and the patient's ambiguous sexual status is not altered after removal of the le-sion. In a patient over the age of 35 years with a dysgerminoma which has spread beyond the ovary, or in those with testicular feminization, the ideal treatment is exploratory laparotomy, total hysterectomy, bilateral salpingo-oophorectomy, omentectomy, appendectomy, and biopsy of the paraaortic nodes with postoperative irradiation to the pelvis and para-aortic nodes as indicated. It is recommended that cytologic examination of aspirated fluid be carried out, although some investigators challenge its value in patients with germ-cell tumors.

In the young patient who has evidence of spread, or in patients with gonadal dysgenesis, testicular feminization, or other evidence of intersex problems, this is also the type of treatment that is chosen. However, in the young patient with a unilateral, encapsulated dysgerminoma, who wants to have a family, there is controversy about the ideal treatment. Since the chance of the tumor being bilateral is 5% to 10%, and the survival rate is high, there is justification for conservative surgery. The treatment, then, is exploratory laparotomy, unilateral salpingo-oophorectomy, bisection and biopsy of the opposite ovary, with exploration of the paraaortic areas; any nodes encountered are examined by frozen section. The pelvis is always aspirated and/or washed with saline, and the fluid is sent for cytologic examination and cell block. This has not been very productive in finding malignant cells, because germ-cell tumors appear to shed cells less often than do epithelial tumors. These tumors should be followed carefully with routine rectovaginal examination and chest x-ray studies. Consideration should be given for a second-look operation at approximately 8 to 12 months following the initial surgery.

The role of a second-look operation merits discussion. If the mass was greater than 15 cm in diameter at the time of the original operation; if the pathology report indicated a triad or anaplasia, medullary structure, and numerous mitoses; and if residual tumor is left, a second look is definitely indicated after postoperative x-ray therapy and/or combination chemotherapy has been given. A five-year survival rate of up to 90% can be expected from this treatment. The dysgerminomas are highly radiosensitive, and recurrent tumors respond well to radiation treatment. These patients are advised to have a hysterectomy and removal of the remaining ovary following the completion of their family.

Teratomas

Embryonal A highly malignant form of germ-cell tumor is the embryonal (immature) teratoma. They are usually solid, and are composed of mixtures of embryonal and mature tissues derived from all three germ layers. Judgment of the degree of malignancy can be made only by microscopic examination. According to Teilum, the term "embryonal carcinoma" should be restricted to tumors composed of undifferentiated neoplastic cells. These are often classified with other forms of germ-cell tumors. Some have used the terms "malignant embryonal teratoma" and "embryonal carcinoma" interchangeably. The prognosis of the embryonal carcinoma depends upon the predominant type of cell present, ie, a tumor containing abundant neural tissue carries a much better prognosis than does one containing choriocarcinoma or other extraembryonal components. Approximately 10% occur bilaterally. In those instances in which the tumor occurs unilaterally and is encapsulated, radical surgery has not been shown to have any advantage over unilateral oophorectomy. However, in the presence of spread, excision of the uterus, tubes, ovaries, appendix, and omentum should be performed.

There are increasing amounts of data to support the treatment of recurrence with a regimen of triple-agent chemotherapy. Prophylactic chemotherapy is being evaluated and, although the results appear promising, it is too early to make any positive statement. Radiation therapy has not been helpful in the management of these tumors.

Extraembryonal   The endodermal sinus tumors and the choriocarcinomas are considered extraembryonal tumors. They are highly malignant. Management generally consists of exploratory laparotomy, total hysterectomy, and bilateral salpingo-oophorectomy. No strong argument can be made for a radical approach over a more conservative one, since the survival rate from each is near zero unless multiple-drug chemotherapy is used. These tumors are not radiosensitive. Triple and quadruple chemotherapy have shown some promising and encouraging results. A second-look operation is recommended in patients surviving more than six months on a three-drug regimen.

Adult (mature)   More than one third of ovarian tumors in children are benign cystic teratomas (dermoids). These tumors are composed of all three germinal layers, although epithelial structures predominate. Studies of nuclear, sex chromatin, and ovarian teratomas have uniformly shown a female pattern. The teratomas are chromatin-positive, indicative of the presence of XX chromosomes; this has been confirmed by chromosomal studies. The presence of nuclear sex chromatin denotes that these cells are diploid, rather than haploid.

The solid adult teratoma is a benign lesion, commonly occurring in patients over 35 years of age. Conservative treatment is not indicated in this age group, despite the fact that the lesion is benign. The cystic teratoma, which accounts for 50% of ovarian tumors in childhood has a malignant rate below the 2% reported in adults, and is bilateral in less than 10% of the patients. Conservative management *is* recommended in children and adolescents.

Gonadal-Stromal Tumors

The female gonadal-stromal (formerly called sex cord tumors) lesions are often referred to as feminizing tumors, although most are nonfunctioning. The granulosa cell tumor, the most important in this category, is bilateral in 5% of patients. Diagnosis is frequently made following rupture with the development of a hemoperitoneum. In women over 35 years of age, treatment involves total hysterectomy and bilateral salpingo-oophorectomy. In children and adolescents the tumor is usually unilateral and encapsulated, and unilateral salpingo-oophorectomy is usually sufficient treatment.

Male sex cord lesions, formerly grouped together as arrheno-blastomas are now termed Sertoli-Leydig-cell tumors. The designation, arrhenoblastoma, has been abandoned since not all of these tumors produce masculinization. When these tumors function they first produce defeminization and then masculinization. They are managed in the same manner as the granulosa cell tumors. Since both are characterized by late recurrence, total hysterectomy and removal of the remaining ovary is recommended when a patient has completed her family.

Gonadoblastoma (Mixed Cell Type)

Gonadoblastoma, a rare ovarian tumor, is composed of germ cells (dysgerminoma) and gonadal-stromal cells (granulosa or Sertoli-Leydig). Sex chromatin studies usually show a negative nuclear pattern (46 XY) or a sex chromosome mosaicism (XO/XY). Most patients are intersexual, with a phenotype female habitus, amenorrheic, and possibly virilized. The malignancy rate is near zero, but the gonads are useless and both ovaries should be removed. All streaks should be removed. Hormone therapy in the form of estrogen and progesterone should be given.

Gynandroblastoma

Gynandroblastomas contain typical aggregates of granulosa cells with Call-Exner bodies and either hollow tubules or Leydig cells containing crystalloids of Reinke. There are no reports of this tumor in childhood; there is no reason to believe that it would differ in its behavior from granulosa cell or Sertoli cell tumors.

Sarcoma

Ovarian sarcoma occur more frequently in children than in adults. It is extremely rare. It is usually primary, but may be the result of secondary malignant change in a fibroma or a teratoma. Grossly, these tumors are solid, lobulated, or soft growths. The most common symptoms reported are abdominal pain and swelling. The survival rate is poor. In patients with unilateral encapsulated disease, unilateral salpingo-oophorectomy has been effective, as has more radical surgery. The role of triple-agent chemotherapy or treatment with doxorubicin remains to be determined. Since the results from surgery and/or x-ray therapy have been so dismal, chemotherapy in combinations should be employed, either prophylactically or therapeutically.

Pregnancy in Ovarian Cancer

The incidence of carcinoma and ovarian tumors during pregnancy has been reported at 2.5% to 5%. The disease is most common in women over 30 years of age. The incidence, insofar as all pregnancies are concerned, is 1 in 8000 to 20,000. It should be remembered that these figures include abortions.

The treatment is the same as in the nonpregnant state. The surgeon finds an ovarian malignancy at the time of abdominal exploration. He should immediately stage the disease, collect peritoneal fluid for cell block diagnosis, and remove the lesion for immediate frozen section for definitive diagnosis and documentation. This is followed by whatever surgery is indicated, depending upon the type of tumor, its histologic grading, and degree of anatomic spread. Biopsies of the omentum, peritoneum, or any other intraabdominal area where one suspects tumors, are indicated.

The survival rate of ovarian cancer in pregnant patients is no different from that in the nonpregnant group. The type of tumor and its anatomic spread determines the five-year survival rate. Pregnancy has no effect on the tumor, and interruption of the pregnancy has no beneficial effect on the future course of this disease.

At the time of any cesarean section, routine inspection of the tubes and ovaries is mandatory.

Metastatic Ovarian Cancer

Approximately 10% of ovarian cancers are metastatic (excluding metastases found at prophylactic oophorectomy for breast cancer), and the survival rate is very low. Most metastatic lesions for the ovary arise in the large bowel. Krukenberg tumors usually occur bilaterally, are kidney-shaped, and are characterized by signet-ring histology at the time of histologic examination. Among patients having prophylactic oophorectomy for metastatic breast cancer, approximately 40% are found to have metastases, many of which are not evident on gross examination. Since cancer of the colon is on the increase among women, and is the second most common cancer, the incidence of metastases in the ovary from colon cancer is also increasing. On careful sectioning of the ovaries, it has been found that approximately 25% of colon cancer patients had metastases to the ovary.

The same plan of management should be followed in treating metastatic disease as is employed for primary ovarian cancer; as much tumor as possible should be removed.

Radiation Therapy

External x-ray therapy for the treatment of the common epithelial ovarian cancer has been phased out. There are many reasons for this, including the inability of the radiation therapist to radiate nodules greater than 2 cm. The cells in the center of the nodules develop anoxia, sicken, but they do not die, and later start to grow. It takes three times the amount of radiation to kill these cells as compared to cells in a well-oxygenated field. It is obvious that this amount of radiation would damage the bowel in Stage III cancers of the ovary. In addition, it is necessary to protect the liver and the kidneys with lead shields, and it is impossible to deliver a cancericidal dose with this method. Therefore, by the use of radiation therapy, these patients in effect are selected out for failure.

Radiation therapy has a very important role in the treatment of germ-cell tumors and gonadal-stromal tumors. These tumors appear to be more radiosensitive than the common epithelial ovarian cancer and, unlike it, have an entirely different natural history. The common epithelial ovarian cancer spreads over the surfaces of the peritoneum and bowel, kidney, and liver, on up to the level of the diaphragm. The dysgerminoma spreads along the paraaortic area and the retroperitoneal space, while the gonadal-stromal tumor remains in the pelvis for long periods of time. Even at the time of recurrence, it is found in the pelvis. It is obvious that they lend themselves to radiation therapy without the anticipated morbidity and mortality associated with the treatment of the common epithelial ovarian cancer.

Chemotherapy

Whether chemotherapy will increase the overall five-year survival is difficult to estimate at this time. These patients are living longer and more comfortably as a result of the judicious use of chemotherapy. Although the subject of chemotherapy in general will be discussed in Chapter 20, certain principles will be pointed out at this time. Each center has its own criteria, but, in general, patients with metastases and ascites have been chosen for chemotherapy. Chemotherapy given in a well-controlled manner does not produce as much morbidity as does radiation therapy delivered to the upper abdomen. Following response, and in the absence of palpable disease, a second-look operation may be undertaken to determine whether the patient is a candidate for excision of any remaining tumor, continued chemotherapy, or a change of chemotherapy.

Single-agent chemotherapy with the alkylating group of agents has proved very valuable for the treatment of the common epithelial ovarian cancer. An increasing number of reports are appearing in the literature that indicate combination chemotherapy has given excellent results, particularly in the recurrent cancer patient. Although single-agent chemotherapy with the alkylating agents has proved very valuable for the treatment of common epithelial ovarian cancer, multiple-drug chemotherapy should be given for the treatment of germ-cell or gonadal-stromal tumors. Young et al have reported a randomized trial comparing a four-drug combination—hexamethylmelamine, cyclophosphamide, methotrexate and 5-fluorouracil (Hexa-CAF), with the oral alkylating agent melphalan. Treatment with the four-drug combination was associated with a significantly increased overall response rate (75% vs 54%), more complete remission (33% vs 16%), and longer median survival (29 vs 17 months), but more severe toxicity than occurred with melphalan. Patients with minimal residual disease had a significantly higher overall response rate than patients with extensive residual disease (84% vs 53%).

There are two methods most often selected for the administration of chemotherapeutic drugs, ie, the continuous (maintenance) method or the intermittent method. The drugs commonly chosen for the treatment of ovarian cancer are cyclophosphamide, melphalan, hexamethylmelamine, cis-platinum, and doxorubicin. These drugs will be discussed in detail in Chapter 20.

BIBLIOGRAPHY

Azoury RS, Woodruff JD: Primary ovarian sarcoma: Report of 47 cases from the Emil Novak Ovarian Cancer Registry. *Obstet Gynecol* 37:920, 1971.

Bagley CM Jr, Young RC, Canellos GP, et al: Treatment of ovarian carcinoma: Possibilities for progress. *N Engl J Med* 287:856, 1972.

Bagley CM, Young RC, Chabuer BA, et al: Ovarian carcinoma metastatic to the diaphragm frequently undiagnosed at laparotomy. *Am J Obstet Gynecol* 116:397, 1973.

Barber HRK: *Ovarian Carcinoma: Etiology, Diagnosis and Treatment.* New York, Masson Publishing USA, Inc, 1978.

Barber HRK: Ovarian cancer, part I. *Ca-A Cancer Journal for Clinicians.* 29:341, 1979.

Barber HRK: Ovarian cancer, Part II. *Ca-A Cancer Journal for Clinicians.* 30:2, 1980.

Barber HRK, Buterman I, Kakarla R: Cancer of the ovary, in *Practice of Surgery, Volume on Gynecology.* Hagerstown, MD, Harper & Row, Publishers, Inc, 1979.

Barber HRK, Graber EA: The PMPO syndrome (postmenopausal palpable ovary syndrome). *Obstet Gynecol* 38:921, 1971.

Barber HRK: The postmenopausal palpable ovary syndrome. *Comprehensive Therapy* 5:58, 1979.

Barber HRK, Graber EA: Gynecological tumors in childhood and adolescence. *Obstet Gynecol Surv* 28:357, 1973.

Barlow JJ, Piver MS: Single agent vs. combination chemotherapy in the treatment of ovarian cancer. *Obstet Gynecol* 49:609, 1977.

Berg JW, Baylor SM: The epidemiologic pathology of ovarian cancer. *Hum Pathol* 4:537, 1973.

Blom J, Park R, Blessing J: Treatment of women with disseminated and recurrent ovarian carcinoma with a single and multichemotherapeutic agents. *Proc Am Assoc Cancer Res* 19:338, 1978.

Bush RS, Allt WEC, Beale FA, et al: Treatment of epithelial carcinoma of the ovary: Surgery, irradiation and chemotherapy. *Am J Obstet Gynecol* 127:692, 1977.

Cancer Facts and Figures 1980. American Cancer Society, New York, 1979.

Gibbs EK: Suggested prophylaxis for ovarian cancer. *Am J Obstet Gynecol* 111:756, 1971.

Krükenberg F: Fibrosarcoma ovarii mucocellulare. *Arch Gynakol* 1:287, 1896.

Krükenberg F: Uber das fibrosarcoma ovarii mucocellulare (carcinomatodes). *Arch Gynakol* 30:287, 1896.

Lingeman CH: Etiology of cancer of the human ovary. *J Natl Cancer Inst* 53:1603, 1974.

McGowan L, Davis RH: Peritoneal fluid cellular patterns in obstetrics and gynecology. *Am J Obstet Gynecol* 106:979, 1970.

McGowan L: A morphologic classification of peritoneal fluid cytology in women. *Int J Gynecol Obstet* 11:173, 1973.

McGowan L, Davis RH, Bunnag B: The biochemical diagnosis of ovarian cancer. *Am J Obstet Gynecol* 116:760, 1973.

McGowan L: *Cancer in Pregnancy.* Springfield, Ill, Charles C Thomas, 1967, p 84.

McGowan L: *Gynecologic Oncology.* New York, Appleton-Century-Crofts, 1978.

Morris JM, Scully R: *Endocrine Pathology of the Ovary.* St Louis, Mosby 1958, p 65.

Rosenberg B, van Camp L: Inhibition of cell division in Escherichia coli by electrolysis products from a platinum electrode. *Nature* 205:698, 1965.

Rosenoff SH, Young RC, Anderson T, et al: Peritoneoscopy: A valuable staging tool in ovarian carcinoma. *Ann Int Med* 83:37, 1975.

Scully R: Recent progress in ovarian cancer. *Human Path* 1:73, 1970.

Smith JO, Rutledge F, Wharton JT: Chemotherapy of ovarian cancer: New approaches to treatment. *Cancer* 30:1565, 1972.

Teilum G: Tumors of germinal origin, in *Ovarian Cancer.* International Union Against Cancer Monograph Series, vol 11. New York, Springer Verlag, 1968, p 58.

Tobias JS, Griffiths CT: Management of ovarian carcinoma. Current concepts and future prospects. *N Engl J Med* 294:818; 294:877, 1976.

West RO: Epidemiologic study of malignancies of the ovaries. *Cancer* 19:1001, 1966.

Wynder EL, Dodo H, Barber HRK: Epidemiology of cancer of the ovary. *Cancer* 23:352, 1969.

Young RC: Acute leukemia after alkylating agent of ovarian cancer. *N Engl J Med* 297:177, 1977.

Young RC: Advanced ovarian adenocarcinoma. *N Engl J Med* 299(23):1261, 1978.

Young RC, Hubbard SP, DeVita VT: The chemotherapy of ovarian carcinoma. *Treat Rev* 1:99, 1974.

Young RC: Chemotherapy of ovarian cancer: Past and present. *Semin Oncol* 2:267, 1975.

10 Cancer of the Fallopian Tube

Hugh R. K. Barber

Cancer of the Fallopian tubes is the rarest carcinoma of the female genital tract. It is part of the upper genital tract that includes the endometrium and breast. It is interesting to speculate why the breast and the endometrium are so often involved in the neoplastic process, whereas the Fallopian tube is not. The Fallopian tubes are peculiar among genital organs for the ease with which they succumb to infection, and their almost total resistance to malignant change. The average gynecologist may expect to see perhaps one case of primary carcinoma of the Fallopian tube in a professional lifetime.

BASIC PRINCIPLES

Carcinoma of the Fallopian tube accounts for less than 0.1% of cancers of the genital tract. The incidence of this disease among all abdominal gynecologic surgical cases is about one in a thousand. It may occur at any age (19 through 80); the mean age is 52. The most frequent occurrence is in patients in the same age group as those with endometrial carcinoma. Since both arise from Müllerian tissue, it is not surprising that the mean age of occurrence is the same, but the incidence of endometrial cancer is much greater.

The most common form of cancer of the Fallopian tube arises from the mucosa, forming papillary or medullary anaplastic lesions. The metastatic pattern is similar to that for ovarian cancer. The Fallopian tube is commonly involved secondarily in advanced cases of endometrial and ovarian cancer. A preliminary review of ovarian cancers at Lenox Hill Hospital indicates that a certain percentage of previously listed ovarian cancers are indeed Fallopian tube cancers.

Primary sarcomas arising from the muscularis portion of the tube are very rare and, among the reported cases, are uniformly fatal. Choriocarcinoma has also been reported in the Fallopian tube.

SYMPTOMS

There are usually no, or only slight, symptoms until the disease is well advanced. The patient is usually perimenopausal or postmenopausal. Most patients present with symptoms of vaginal bleeding or discharge, pain, abdominal distention, and pressure. The symptoms may occur singly or in combination. Vaginal or uterine bleeding is the most common symptom in one half of the patients. Irregular vaginal bleeding raises the suspicion of cancer of the endometrium.

Pain is the next most common symptom. Colicky pain may be present early, but later there is a sensation of heaviness and pelvic pressure. The pain may result from the fact that the tumor and the discharge from the mass are enclosed in a cavity which, when distended, causes tension in the wall and pain. Although the pain is usually intermittent and cramp-like, located unilaterally in either lower quadrant, it is referred down the thigh or into the back, and may present as a persistent backache or a continuous nagging, dragging type of pelvic pain. From time to time there is sudden relief of the pain, accompanied by a profuse vaginal discharge, and this is suggestive, but not conclusive, of cancer of the Fallopian tube.

Pain, in combination with a profuse watery vaginal discharge, constitutes the syndrome of hydrops tubae profluens. There is usually relief from pain after an episode of profuse vaginal discharge. This has been considered as pathognomic of cancer of the tube.

Enlargement of the abdomen has been the presenting symptom in a number of cases. In order to be palpated above the pelvic brim, the tumor must be at least 12 cm to 15 cm in diameter. Like any fast-growing tumor, cancer of the Fallopian tube may grow so rapidly that it has a deficient blood supply with resultant necrosis and rupture.

A positive Pap smear in the presence of a negative curettage should alert the clinician to this diagnosis. Although an adnexal mass is present on pelvic examination, with the corpus and cervix seemingly normal, nevertheless, the exact diagnosis is rarely made preoperatively. Reports indicate that a correct preoperative diagnosis is made in only 2% of the recorded cases.

DIAGNOSIS

A pelvic tumor is palpable in over 50% of the cases. The tumor may be palpated in the characteristic adnexal location, or it may be ill-defined, and may even present as a midline mass. In advanced cases there may be enlargement of the abdomen with ascites. There is little in the family history, marital history, or menstrual history that can contribute to the diagnosis of this disease. Parity has been reported as low among this group of patients.

A series of events directs the attention to the diagnosis of cancer of the tube:

1. A triad of pain, menorrhagia, and leukorrhea.
2. Pelvic mass and hydrops tubae profluens.
3. History of unexplained metrorrhagia with no evidence of malignancy in endometrial curettings.
4. Persistent positive Pap smears with no evidence of malignancy in cervical biopsies or endometrial curettings.
5. The differential diagnosis includes carcinoma of the corpus, salpingitis, pedunculated and intraligamentous fibroid, and ovarian tumor.

Laboratory Findings

Cytologic examination of cervical vaginal smears or of a vaginal tampon yields malignant cells in well over 50% of the patients reported.

A flat plate of the abdomen may show a mass, as may ultrasonography. At present, too few cases have been reported to make a firm statement. However, with the increased use of ultrasonography, more cases may be reported.

Hysterosalpingography, performed when the diagnosis is suspected, has not been popular in the United States because of fear that the cancer may be spread by the examination.

Cul-de-sac taps have been used as a diagnostic measure. This technique has not had wide acceptance.

EPIDEMIOLOGY AND ETIOLOGY

A review of the medical literature reveals that there are many single case reports of carcinoma of the Fallopian tube. There are very few comprehensive reviews on this disease and, therefore, it is difficult to develop an understanding of its natural history, clinical manifestations, and evaluation of factors that influence survival.

Chronic inflammation of the tube has been suggested as an important predisposing factor. However, the high frequency of this lesion, in contrast to the rarity of tubal carcinoma, casts doubt on this relationship. Tubal tuberculosis has been proposed as a factor, but the same counter-argument as stated for chronic inflammation applies here. It has been found to coexist with cancer of the tube in a number of instances. In at least some of these cases, the combination is incorrectly interpreted because the adenocarcinoma-like picture is seen in some cases of tuberculosis salpingitis.

LOCATION OF THE PRIMARY LESION

The mass is located in the distal third of the tube in most cases. It is unilateral in 95% of the patients and, for unexplained reasons, is predominantly on the right side. In a review, 70% occurred in the ampullar portion, in contrast to 30% in the isthmic portion. The significance of location is incompletely understood at this time. However, it is reasonable to assume that proximal lesions will more likely invade toward the myometrium and endometrium, whereas lateral lesions tend to travel toward the ovaries and aortic nodes.

As a recipient of metastatic cancer, the tube is often the site of secondary lesions arising from either the uterus or the ovaries. Such tumors are readily recognized as such and easily differentiated from primary tubal cancer by their location, generally within the lymphatics. As they invade the tubal wall, they project into the lumen by eroding the tubal epithelium. Primary lesions arise from the tubal epithelium and tend to remain intralumenal for long periods of time, making differentiation more or less apparent. The tangential aspect of secondary tumors supports the hypothesis that lymphatic dissemination may occur centrifugally and centripetally to the tube, and perhaps from the tube as well.

Although 95% of these tumors are unilateral, bilaterality has been reported, suggesting either a multicentric origin or metastasis. The proponents of the theory of multicentric origin of cancer draw attention to the relative frequency with which such tumors arise bilaterally in the absence of other metastases, particularly implants in the endometrium or on the peritoneal cavity. Woodruff argues that bilateral involvement almost certainly does not result from simultaneous development of the lesion in each tube, except perhaps in rare instances. He believes that the situation arises either by direct mucosal extension, or as a process analogous to transmigration of the ovum. He also raises the possibility of lymphatic extension across the pelvis, acknowledging that the extensive mucosal involvement and relative absence of muscular wall invasion favors direct extension. Few data are available at present.

PATHOLOGY

Gross clinical findings may vary. The mass is located in the distal third of the tube in most cases. The majority of tubal carcinoma cases present as an unexpected operative finding, and the surgeon may be confronted for the first time with its unfamiliar pathology at the operating table. In an early stage of this malignancy, the pathologic changes consist of enlargement of the Fallopian tube caused by the tumor located in the mucosa of the lumen. The common picture is of an enormously enlarged, sausage-shaped structure which gives the impression of a huge pyosalpinx, except that, and like the latter, it usually presents few or no adhesions to the surrounding structures. The external surface is usually quite smooth.

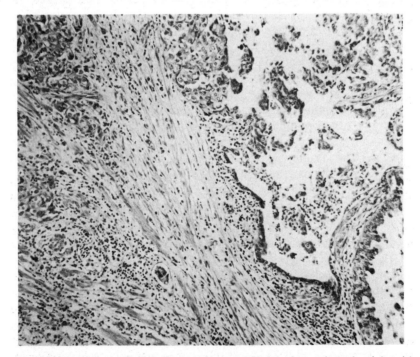

Figure 10-1 Fallopian tube adenocarcinoma. The tube lumen is to the right with papillary growth of malignant cells. The smooth muscle of the wall is to the left.

Early cancer of the tube is highly suggestive of hydrosalpinx but, if this occurs in the postmenopausal patient, it should arouse suspicion of a malignancy. A hematosalpinx or bloody effusion in the lumen of the tube frequently accompanies the carcinoma. After accumulating within the lumen of the tube, the blood may spill into the peritoneal cavity through the abdominal osteum of the tube, causing hemoperitoneum.

The lack of invasion of the tubal muscularis is very characteristic, although extensive intratubal disease protrudes from the fimbriated end. Sites of metastases, in order of frequency, are peritoneum, ovaries, uterus, intestines, vagina, lymph nodes, liver, and generalized carcinomatosis.

The microscopic pattern is that of a typical carcinoma composed of tall, abnormal, tubal epithelial cells. They may assume either a papillary pattern or an alveolar appearance because of fused papillae. An admixture is frequent. Histologic examination of the aveolar-papillary pattern is not very helpful for differentiation from ovarian cancer because certain cases of serous cystadenocarcinoma of the ovary may present a very similar histologic pattern.

The criteria for identification of a primary tubal carcinoma as stated by Finn and Javert (1949) are:

1. The epithelium of the endosalpinx is replaced in whole or in part by adenocarcinoma.
2. The histologic character of the cells resembles the epithelium of the endosalpinx.
3. The endometrium and ovaries are:
   a. normal
   b. affected by a benign lesion, or
   c. contain a malignant lesion that, by its small size, distribution, and histologic characteristics appears to be metastatic to the tube.
4. The prime involvement is in the endosalpinx and perisalpinx; the lymphatics of the muscularis and mesosalpinx are rarely involved.
5. Tuberculosis should be carefully excluded.

The microscopic classifications of tubal carcinoma vary little. These tumors are classified into three groups: papillary, Grade 1; papillary-alveolar, Grade 2; alveolar-medullary, Grade 3. Some classifications divide the latter grade into two, alveolar and medullary.

Johnson et al (1978) reported on the ultrastructure of Fallopian tube carcinoma. They report that this tumor is one of the rarest primary gynecologic malignancies. Normal tubal epithelium is composed of secretory, ciliated, and interciliary cells. To determine the cellular composition and ultrastructural details of this rare neoplasm, a moderately well-differentiated tubal carcinoma was studied with the electron microscope. A prominent feature was the formation of numerous ultramicro-alveolar spaces lined by cell surface microvilli. The nuclei of the neoplastic cell demonstrated a variety of fine structural abnormalities. Based on cell size and shape, a possible dual tumor cell population was suggested. However, no cilia were seen in any of the tumor cells, and almost all were devoid of secretory granules. These latter observations suggest that this tumor was primarily a proliferation of interciliary cells.

DIFFERENTIAL DIAGNOSIS OF
PRIMARY *vs* METASTATIC CANCER

Metastatic tumors from other organs, particularly the ovary, breast, and gastrointestinal tract, are most commonly found in the tube. The four most common methods of spread from the primary carcinoma are: 1) lymphatic and/or blood vessel permeation, 2) direct extension, 3) implantation, and 4) drop metastasis.

The carcinomas may be unilateral or bilateral; when unilateral, they tend to involve either tube. The size of the metastases varies from that of a microscopic lesion to a large mass involving neighboring tissues with extensive adhesions.

A standard for differentiation of secondary tubal carcinoma suggested by Finn and Javert (1949) is:

1. The tube may be normal, may show evidence of salpingitis, or may be extremely involved by cancer.
2. Extensive cancer is found elsewhere on the endometrium, the ovary, or in an extragenital location such as the sigmoid colon.
3. Histologically, the carcinomas are identical with the primary carcinomas from which the metastases arose. The criteria are:
    a. The endosalpinx is normal, shows chronic salpingitis, or may contain cancer. Extensive carcinomatous involvement suggests a primary cancer of the tube, unless the gross examination shows otherwise.
    b. The carcinomatous cells resemble those of the primary lesion in the endometrium, ovary, or intestine.
    c. The surface of the tube and the lymphatics of the muscularis and mesosalpinx are usually involved. The lymphatics of the endosalpinx and the endosalpinx itself are involved more rarely.

Treatment is that of the primary carcinoma with excision of the metastatic disease. The prognosis is that of the primary disease with metastasis, and is poor.

274

CLINICAL STAGING

There is no official staging classification for cancer of the Fallopian tube. Tubal carcinoma has usually been staged by the FIGO staging system used for ovarian cancer because the anatomic location and modal spread are similar in both tumors. In addition, they are Müllerian in origin and share a common blood supply as well as lymphatic drainage.

The International Federation of Gynecology and Obstetrics (FIGO) Staging

Stage Ia   Growth limited to one tube; no ascites.
1. No tumor on the external surface; capsule intact.
2. Tumor present on the external surface, capsule(s) ruptured, or both.
Stage Ib   Growth limited to both tubes; no ascites.
1. No tumor on the external surface; capsule intact.
2. Tumor present on the external surface, capsule(s) ruptured, or both.
Stage Ic   Tumor either Stage Ia or Stage Ib, but with ascites present, or with positive peritoneal washings.
Stage II   Growth involving one or both tubes with pelvic extension.
Stage IIa   Extension and/or metastases to the uterus and/or ovaries.
Stage IIb   Extension to other pelvic tissues.
Stage IIc   Tumor either Stage IIa or Stage IIb, but with ascites and positive peritoneal washings.
Stage III   Growth involving one or both tubes with intraperitoneal nodes, or both. Tumor limited to the true pelvis with histologically proven malignant extension to small bowel or omentum.
Stage IV   Growth involving one or both tubes with distant metastases. If pleural effusion is present, there must be positive cytology to allot a case to Stage IV. Parenchymal liver metastases indicate Stage IV.

TREATMENT

The treatment for cancer of the tube is essentially the same as that carried out for cancer of the ovary. It is important to select the correct incision. It should be vertical and long enough to permit a careful exploration. A Pfannenstiel incision should not be used in the treatment of ovarian or tubal carcinoma. It is not only impossible to stage the cancer accurately, but there is also an increased risk of rupturing the tumor. Ovarian and tubal cancers are all too often understaged, and therefore are inadequately treated.

When the abdomen is opened, the pelvis and abdomen should be aspirated or washed, or both, to obtain cells for cytologic examination. The abdomen and pelvis should be carefully explored. Special attention should be paid to the area between the liver and diaphragm on the posterior peritoneum.

Treatment should be tailored both to the needs of the patient and the extent of the disease. Total hysterectomy, bilateral salpingo-oophorectomy, omentectomy, appendectomy with the instillation of phosphorus-32 (optional), is the treatment that should be chosen. The author's preference is to give chemotherapy prophylactically, but this is debatable at present.

Surgery is considered the keystone of treatment. If it is not possible to remove all of the cancer, an attempt should be made to reduce the tumor burden to a minimum. Because tubal carcinoma is a surface spreader, much like ovarian cancer, radiation therapy is not used. It spreads over the liver and kidneys, and, if radiation is to be used, a lead shield has to be placed over the liver and kidneys in order to protect them. This all too often selects the patients for failure of treatment. High radiation doses damage vital organs, particularly the bowel. Therefore, chemotherapy has been selected as the treatment for Fallopian tube carcinoma following surgical removal or debulking.

The treatment of recurrent tubal cancers is by combination chemotherapy. Currently, the regimen selected includes cyclophosphamide, cis-platinum, and doxorubicin. There is one case of success on record following pelvic exenteration, but this is rare.

Using the FIGO staging system, a number of cases with tubal carcinomas were staged retrospectively by Sedlis (1978) on the basis of the description of operative findings. He calculated three-year survival figures by stage as follows: Stage I, 60%, Stage II, 40%, Stage III, 10%, Stage IV, 0%. The effect of therapeutic modality on survival is even more difficult to evaluate because no series of patients was treated in a consistent manner.

OTHER TUMORS OF THE FALLOPIAN TUBE

The literature reports a variety of different types of neoplasms associated with the Fallopian tube.

Sarcoma

There are a few sarcomas recorded in the literature. They usually include a wide range of varieties including undifferentiated sarcoma, reticular sarcoma, leiomyosarcoma, carcinosarcoma, and lymphoma. About one-third are bilateral when discovered; the prognosis is very poor.

Grossly, the tumor appears not to have any predilection for either tube, being bilateral in about one third of the cases. In about one half, the tumor fills the lumen of the tube, and sometimes even protrudes beyond the fimbriated end. The microscopic appearance is similar to that of sarcoma elsewhere.

The tumor may spread by direct extension to the pelvic tissues and by lymphatic or blood stream metastasis. Metastases to the lung are very common. The treatment is total hysterectomy and bilateral salpingo-oophorectomy. Combination chemotherapy is suggested as adjuvant therapy.

Choriocarcinoma

Choriocarcinoma of the Fallopian tube is extremely rare. It may follow an ectopic or intrauterine pregnancy. Hematogenous dissemination, particularly to the lungs, is common, being analogous to that generally seen in association with intrauterine carcinomas. The presence of chorionic gonadotropins provides a method to judge the success of treatment accurately. The treatment is total hysterectomy and bilateral salpingo-oophorectomy, followed by combination chemotherapy.

BIBLIOGRAPHY

Barber HRK: *Manual of Gynecologic Oncology*. Philadelphia, J.B. Lippincott Co, 1980.

Barber HRK, Fields DH, Kaufman SA: *Quick Reference to Ob-Gyn Procedures,* ed 2. Philadelphia, J.B. Lippincott Co, 1979.

Benson PA: Cytologic diagnosis in primary carcinoma of fallopian tube. *Acta Cytolog* 18:429, 1976.

Carapeto R, Nogales FF Jr, Matella A: Ectopic pregnancy coexisting with a primary carcinoma of the fallopian tube: A case report. *Int J Gynaecol Obstet* 16(3):263, 1978.

Falk E: Ueber primare epitheliale Nenbildungen der Eileiter (Eileiterkrebs). *Klin Wochenschr* 35:554, 1898.

Finn WF, Javert CT: Primary and metastatic cancer of the fallopian tubes. *Cancer* 2:803, 1949.

Frick HC, II: Cancer of the Fallopian tube, in Gusburg SB, Frick HC, II (eds). *Corscaden's Gynecologic Cancer,* ed 5: Baltimore, Williams & Wilkins, 1978.

Hapfel-Kreimer I, Mikuz G: Accidental cytological findings in routine vaginal smear in primary carcinoma of the fallopian tube. *Pathol Res Proct* 163(2):163, 1978.

Henderson SR, Harper RC, Salazar OM, et al: Carcinoma of the fallopian tube: Difficulties of diagnosis and treatment. *Gynecol Oncol* 5:168, 1977.

Hertig AT, Gore H: *Atlas of Tumor Pathology. Section IX—Fascicle 33. Tumors of the Female Sex Organs. Part 3. Tumors of the Ovary and Fallopian Tube.* Washington, Armed Forces Institute of Pathology, 1961.

Johnson L, Diamond I, Jolly G: Ultrastructure of fallopian tube carcinoma. *Cancer* 42:1291, 1978.

Manes JL, Taylor HB: Carcinosarcoma and mixed Müllerian tumors of the fallopian tube. Report of four cases. *Cancer* 38:1687, 1976.

Panerstein CP: *The Fallopian Tube: Reappraisal.* Philadelphia, Febiger, 1974.

Park RC, Parmley TH: Fallopian tube cancer, in McGowan L (ed):*Gynecologic Oncology.* New York, Appleton-Century-Crofts, 1978.

Sedlis A: Carcinoma of the fallopian tube. *Surg Clin North Am* 58:121, 1978.

Sedlis A: Primary carcinoma of the fallopian tube. *Obstet Gynecol Surv* 16:209, 1961.

Segal S, Adoni A, Schenker J: Choriocarcinoma of the fallopian tube. *Gynecol Oncol* 3:40, 1975.

Vinall PS, Buxton N, Cowen PN: Primary carcinoma of the fallopian tube associated with tuberculous salpingitis: A case report. *Br J Obstet Gynaecol* 86:984, 1979.

Weiss PD, MacDougall MK, Reagan JW, et al: Primary adenosquamous carcinoma of the fallopian tube. *Obstet Gynecol* 55(3):885, 1980.

Yoonessi M: Carcinoma of the fallopian tube. *Obstet Gynecol Surv* 34:257, 1979.

11 Cancer of the Vulva

Elvis S. Donaldson
Deborah F. Powell

Carcinoma of the vulva accounts for 3% to 5% of all gynecologic cancer. Although the majority of vulvar cancers occur on the surface epithelium, there usually is significant patient delay in seeking medical attention. Furthermore, the primary physician may fail to recognize the significance of vulvar symptoms and attempt extended medical therapy without histologic examination.

During the past two decades, improvement in the survival of patients with invasive vulvar cancer has been achieved by an aggressive surgical approach utilizing radical vulvectomy with bilateral inguinal and pelvic lymphadenectomy. More recently, however, attempts have been made to individualize therapy according to the extent of the lesion. This has necessitated a more thorough evaluative process, including an accurate description of 1) the anatomic size and location of each tumor, 2) predominant cell type, and 3) histomorphologic criteria, ie, the presence of vascular or perineural invasion. Also, new classification systems for the vulvar dystrophies have been proposed, thereby facilitating the systematic medical treatment of these lesions.

In the present review, specific sections will be devoted to etiology and epidemiology, evaluation, pathology, treatment, and follow-up. In each section, variation according to the primary cell type of the lesion will be emphasized.

ETIOLOGY AND EPIDEMIOLOGY

Squamous cell cancer of the vulva is typically a disease of the elderly female with its peak incidence occurring in the seventh and eighth decades of life. Franklin and Rutledge (1972) reported that the mean age of patients with invasive vulvar cancer was 63 years, which was approximately 15 years greater than that of patients with intraepithelial carcinoma. Over 35% of these patients were over 70 years of age, whereas only 15% were younger than 40 years of age. In contrast, 40% of patients with carcinoma in situ of the vulva are under 40 years of age (Buscema et al 1980).

The similarity between patients at risk to develop endometrial cancer and those most likely to develop vulvar cancer has been noted. The incidence of obesity, hypertensive cardiovascular disease, diabetes mellitus, and nulliparity is significantly higher in patients with vulvar cancer than in age-matched control populations. However, no hypothesis as to the etiologic relationship between these clinical correlates and vulvar cancer has been substantiated.

An increased incidence of venereal disease, including syphilis, granuloma inguinale, and lymphopathia venereum, has been reported in patients with vulvar cancer (Franklin and Rutledge 1972, Friedrich et al 1980). Chronic granulomatous disease was noted to precede squamous carcinoma in over 60% of Jamaican patients with vulvar cancer (Hay and Cole 1969). Syphilis was present in 50% of these patients. It is interesting to note that vulvar cancer tended to occur at an earlier age and to be more aggressive biologically in patients having previously diagnosed granulomatous disease.

There is presently some controversy concerning the risk of subsequent invasive vulvar cancer in patients with vulvar dystrophies. It was once estimated that carcinoma would develop in up to 50% of patients with vulvar dystrophies (Taussig 1930). More recent evidence, however, seems to suggest that the risk of developing invasive cancer in patients with vulvar dystrophies is less than 5% (Jeffcoate 1966, Franklin and Rutledge 1972). This risk increases in the presence of progressive degrees of cellular atypia.

Although all of the factors involved in the genesis of squamous cell carcinoma of the vulva are unknown, there is considerable indirect evidence to suggest a possible viral etiology for this disease. The association of genital herpes (HSV-2) with cervical neoplasia is well known and has been established on the basis of seroepidemiologic studies, and the detection of virus-related antigens in cervical cancer cells (Aurelian et al 1973). It is highly likely, therefore, that HSV-2 could also have an oncogenic potential in lower genital tract sites, ie, the vagina and vulva. Cervical or vaginal carcinoma has been observed in 10% to 20% of patients with vulvar cancer, and a number of cases of multifocal carcinoma in all three sites have been reported. This suggests a field response to a common etiologic agent. In addition, intraepithelial vulvar neoplasia has been reported following herpes vulvitis in pregnancy (Friedrich 1972).

There is even more evidence implicating the papovavirus in the genesis of vulvar cancer. The association between condyloma accuminata and carcinoma of the vulva is well documented (Josey et al 1976) and papovavirus particles can be detected by electron microscopy in approximately 50% of condylomas (zur Hausen 1976). Also, papovaviruses have recently been propagated in tissue culture, and viral DNA has been detected in infected human cells. Carcinoma often arises directly within condylomatous lesions, and histologic transition from papillomatous epithelium to invasive vulvar cancer has been observed (Kovi et al 1974). An additional finding suggestive of an etiologic relationship between papovavirus infection and vulvar carcinoma is the relatively young age at which vulvar cancer occurs in patients having condylomata. Josey and colleagues (1976) reported that the average age at diagnosis of vulvar cancer patients following treatment of condyloma was 42 years. In contrast, the average age of the total group of patients with squamous carcinoma of the vulva was 58 years. Similarly, vulvar carcinoma has been reported in several teenage girls following papovavirus infection (Lister and Akinla 1972, Boutselis 1972).

Melanoma is the second most common malignancy of the vulva, and accounts for 5% to 10% of vulvar cancers. The peak incidence of vulvar melanoma occurs in the sixth, and seventh decades, with approximately 30% diagnosed in premenopausal patients (Chung et al 1975). Melanoma is most frequently observed in fair-complexioned individuals and is reported to be two to four times as common among Caucasians as Negroes (Pack et al 1963). The association between pregnancy and vulvar melanoma has frequently been made. Certain investigators believe that the pigmentary changes in pregnancy predispose to the initiation of malignant change in nevi (Karlen et al 1975). Similarly, familial predisposition to the development of malignant melanoma has been reported (Miller and Pack 1962). Although the vulva occupies no more than 2% of the body surface area in the adult female, it produces over 5% of all melanomas in women (Morrow and DiSaia 1976). This may be due to the fact that a very high percent of vulvar nevi have junctional activity.

It is generally recognized that melanomas may arise primarily from junctional nevi or the junctional component of compound nevi. The cell of origin of the malignant melanoma is the melanocyte. Primitive melanocytes migrate peripherally during embryonic life often in direct association with nerve fibers, and biopsies of the normal vulva show melanocytes and their dendritic processes interspersed along the basal layer of epithelium. The designation, junctional nevus, refers to those lesions in which there is localization of melanocytes at the dermis-epidermis junction. Neoplastic transformation of these melanocytes results in the formation of malignant melanoma. The presence of a high incidence of junctional activity in vulvar nevi has led many investigators to recommend that every pigmented lesion of the vulva be surgically excised.

Vulvar sarcomas are rare tumors comprising approximately 2% to 3% of vulvar cancer. The age range of patients with these tumors is related to the specific histologic type of sarcoma, but generally varies between 30 and 50 years (Davos and Abell 1975). The most common cell type of vulva sarcoma is leiomyosarcoma, followed by rhabdomyosarcoma and neurofibrosarcoma (DiSaia et al 1971). There is no clear theory as to the genesis of these tumors. Hilgers and colleagues (1970) reviewed the obstetric histories of over 80 patients with pelvic rhabdomyosarcomas, including those of the vulva, and could find no etiologic agent for these lesions. Pelvic radiation, particularly in the low and intermediate dose ranges, has been implicated in the causation of uterine sarcomas. However, there are so few reported cases of vulvar sarcoma in patients having received prior pelvic radiation that a significant etiologic role of radiation in these tumors seems quite unlikely.

Adenocarcinoma of the vulva consists primarily of Bartholin gland carcinoma. These tumors are quite rare and account for less than one percent of vulvar cancer. Bartholin gland adenocarcinoma occurs most frequently in the fifth and sixth decades of life. The etiology of this lesion is unknown. Chronic inflammation of the Bartholin gland tissue has been observed in many cases of carcinoma (Dodson et al 1970), but the etiologic significance of this observation has not been established. Apocrine gland carcinoma has been noted almost exclusively in the presence of vulvar Paget's disease (Boehm and Morris 1971). Patients with apocrine gland carcinoma have a similar age distribution to those with Bartholin's gland carcinoma, and the majority of patients are between 50 and 70 years of age at the time of initial diagnosis. Because of the association between Paget's disease of the vulva and apocrine gland carcinoma, every attempt should be made to evaluate histologically the apocrine glands in surgical specimens from patients treated for vulvar Paget's disease.

EVALUATION AND DIAGNOSIS

In almost every major series of patients with vulvar cancer, there is significant delay between the onset of symptoms and histologic diagnosis.

Magrina and co-workers (1979) for example, noted that 62% of patients with invasive vulvar cancer had been symptomatic for more than 12 months before seeking medical attention. This delay is due to 1) patient reticence to seek medical evaluation of vulvar symptoms, and 2) improper medical therapy without obtaining histologic verification of a vulvar epithelial abnormality. The most common symptoms of vulvar neoplasia are persistent vulvar pruritis or pain often associated with an ulcerative lesion or a mass. Buscema and colleagues (1980) reported that pruritis was present in 45% of patients with vulvar intraepithelial carcinoma, and that approximately one third of these patients noted some visible or palpable abnormality of the vulva. Public education is imperative to encourage patients with these symptoms to obtain prompt medical attention.

In patients with vulvar symptoms, careful surveillance of the vulvar skin with a magnifying glass and satisfactory lighting is essential. Although the patient is often unaware of a discrete lesion, thorough inspection often will delineate the full anatomic extent of the abnormality. Friedrich and co-workers (1980) reported that 90% of patients with intraepithelial carcinoma of the vulva has a lesion with a raised surface elevated above the level of the surrounding skin. The size, elevation, consistency, and color of each lesion should be described. Also, the presence of an associated erosion or ulceration should be noted.

In patients who are symptomatic but without a clinically apparent vulvar lesion, toluidine blue staining may be helpful. A 1% solution of toluidine is applied to the vulvar skin and allowed to remain in place for approximately two minutes. The area is then rinsed with a solution of 1% acetic acid. Toluidine blue is a nuclear stain, which is preferentially taken up by metabolically active areas of epithelium. The most superficial layer of normal stratified squamous epithelium has no nuclei and, therefore, does not take up the stain. In contrast, areas of epithelial abnormality containing neoplastic cells with increased nuclear size usually stain prominently (Collins et al 1966). It should be noted that there are false negative and false positive staining reactions using this method. For example, abrasions of the vulvar skin may take up the stain in the absence of an epithelial abnormality due to exposure of the underlying nuclei. In contrast, foci of increased keratinization overlying an area of vulvar neoplasia may prevent proper absorption of the dye by abnormal cells. Available data suggests that approximately 60% of neoplastic vulvar lesions take up toluidine blue (Friedrich et al 1980). It has been emphasized that nearly 70 percent of epithelial lesions of the vulva are multifocal in origin. Therefore, the entire vulvar area including the perianal skin should be evaluated.

All vulvar lesions not obviously of infectious origin should be biopsied. Excisional biopsy is indicated in small, localized lesions. The biopsy should be deep enough to establish the presence of stromal invasion, and should contain a margin of normal tissue. In large multifocal lesions, selected biopsies can be obtained using a Keys dermal punch. Toluidine blue staining will often be helpful in identifying the area of greatest metabolic activity.

Although there have been numerous systems for the classification of vulvar dystrophies, the one recently proposed by the International Society for the Study of Vulvar Disease (1976) is most appropriate. According to this classification (Table 11-1), vulvar dystrophies should be designated as either hyperplastic or lichen slcerosus with or without atypia. In general, the prognosis of these lesions varies according to the degree of associated cellular atypia, and therapy is based upon histologic assessment of each case.

Table 11-1
Classification of Vulvar Dystrophy

I. Hyperplastic dystrophy
   A. Without atypia
   B. With atypia
II. Lichen sclerosus
III. Mixed dystrophy (lichen sclerosus, foci of epithelial hyperplasia)
   A. Without atypia
   B. With atypia

Intraepithelial neoplasia of the vulva is classified in a manner similar to that for cervical intraepithelial neoplasia (see Pathology section). In addition, specific histologic types of vulvar intraepithelial carcinoma, ie, Bowen's disease or Paget's disease, should be distinguished since these lesions have specific prognostic implications. The association between Paget's disease of the vulva and underlying apocrine gland carcinoma necessitates careful evaluation of the vulvar subcutaneous tissue in these patients. Recent reports have indicated that up to 30% of patients with carcinoma in situ of the vulva will demonstrate multifocal disease of the lower genital tract (Buscema et al 1980). The most commonly associated neoplasm is carcinoma of the cervix. Friedrich and co-workers (1980), eg, reported that 26% of patients with vulvar intraepithelial carcinoma demonstrated either carcinoma in situ or invasive carcinoma of the cervix. For this reason, every patient with carcinoma in situ of the vulva should have a thorough evaluation of the cervix and vagina. This evaluation should include cytology, colposcopy, Schiller staining, and biopsy if indicated.

Once the diagnosis of stromal invasion has been confirmed, the lesion is designated as invasive vulvar cancer. Unlike cervical cancer, there are no universally accepted histologic criteria that define microinvasive cancer of the vulva. Several investigators have indicated that the incidence of lymph nodal metastases is extremely low with stromal invasion of less than 5 mm.

Wharton and co-workers (1974), eg, noted no lymph nodal metastases in 25 patients with vulvar carcinomas invading the stroma to a depth of 5 mm or less. None of these patients developed tumor recurrence and none died of cancer. Similarly, DiSaia and colleagues (1979) reported no nodal metastases in 18 patients with invasive vulvar cancer limited to 5 mm in depth. Other investigators, however, have reported lymph nodal metastases in patients with less than 3 mm stromal invasion (Barnes et al 1980). DiPaola and co-workers (1975) reported lymph nodal metastases in three of 11 vulvar cancer patients with stromal invasion of less than 5 mm. For this reason, the potential for lymph nodal metastases must be considered in every patient with histologic verification of invasive vulvar cancer.

The importance of lymph-vascular space invasion in early invasive vulvar cancer has been emphasized by Donaldson and co-workers (1981). These investigators reported that lymph nodal metastases were not observed in 25 cases having less than 5 mm stromal invasion and no evidence of lymph-vascular space invasion. In contrast, 11 of 13 early invasive lesions, in which there was lymphatic or vascular space invasion, had regional lymph node metastases.

The exact location of the primary lesion should be recorded in each case since the manner of spread varies according to the anatomic structures involved. The most common location of squamous cell carcinoma of the vulva is on the labia (Table 11-2). Approximately 70% of all invasive vulvar lesions are confined to the labia, with the labia majora being involved approximately two times more frequently than the labia minora. Likewise, squamous cell carcinoma originates primarily on the anterior portion of the vulva (Green et al 1978). For unknown reasons, these tumors are reported to occur more commonly on the right side of the vulva than on the left (Figge 1974, Magrina et al 1979). The clitoris is involved in about 15% of the cases, followed in order by the perineum and urethra. It should be noted that up to 20% of squamous cell carcinomas are multi-

Table 11-2
Location of Squamous Cell Carcinomas of the Vulva

Site	Patients
Labia majora	407 (39%)
Labia minora	279 (26%)
Clitoris	114 (11%)
Perineum	136 (13%)
Urethra	38 (4%)
Vaginal introitus	63 (6%)
Anus	12 (1%)

Data from Franklin and Rutledge (1971), Franklin (1972), Japaze et al (1977), Smith and Pollack (1947), and Tompkins et al (1961).

centric in origin, and that there is continuing and free communication between the vulvar lymphatics (Way 1960). Therefore, a full evaluation of the entire vulvar epithelium and regional lymph nodes is essential in all cases.

In order to appreciate the pattern of lymph node metastases in vulvar cancer, the lymphatic drainage of the vulva must be understood. The anterior portion of the labia minora is drained by lymphatic trunks, which bypass the clitoris, and course anteriorly toward the mons veneris (Figure 11-1). Within the fatty tissue of the mons veneris, the lymphatics change to a lateral direction and terminate in the upper medial nodes of the femoral group. The lymphatics of the posterior labia minora extend laterally to join those of the labia majora. The lymphatics of the labia majora drain laterally into a number of collecting trunks in the labial-crural fold, which turn cephalad and empty laterally into the superior group of femoral lymph nodes. The posterior aspects of the labia majora drain laterally into the lymphatic trunks of the crural fold, which progress anteriorly and, at the aponeurosis of the gracilis and adductor longus muscles, turn laterally to terminate in the central group of femoral lymph nodes.

The posterior fourchette and perineum are drained by lymphatic channels that originate medially and extend posteriorly and laterally to the perianal area. These lymphatic trunks then turn and course anteriorly to the labial-crural fold. At this point, they join the lymphatics from the labia majora to terminate in the superficial femoral lymph nodes.

The lymphatic drainage of the clitoris can be divided into two major pathways. A presymphysial plexus draining the glans clitoris extends cephalad into the tissue of the mons veneris. These lymphatics then empty laterally into collecting channels, which drain into the superficial femoral nodes, and secondarily through the cribriform fascia to the deep femoral nodes. A second group of different lymphatics from the clitoris extend retropubically parallel to the urethra and empty into lymphatics on the anterior surface of the bladder, or directly into the obturator and iliac lymph nodes (Figure 11-2). Therefore, some investigators believe that the lymphatic drainage of the clitoris can bypass the femoral lymph nodes and extend directly into the deep pelvic nodes (Collins et al 1971, Krupp and Bohm 1976). However, other studies (Morley 1976, Piver 1977, Green 1978) have failed to demonstrate pelvic lymph nodal disease in the absence of metastases to the superficial or deep femoral lymph nodes.

Available data concerning the lymphatic drainage of the Bartholin gland is somewhat incomplete. However, present information indicates that lymphatics draining the Bartholin gland course laterally to communicate with lymphatic channels from the labia majora and then terminate in the superficial femoral nodes. Preliminary but unconfirmed observations have also suggested that there is an alternate pathway of efferent lymphatic drainage from the Bartholin gland (Plentyl and Fried-

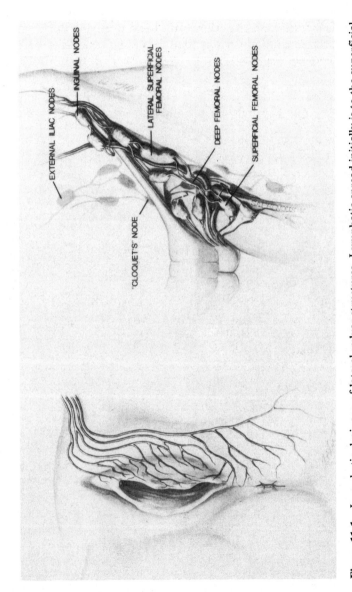

Figure 11-1 Lymphatic drainage of lateral vulvar structures. Lymphatic spread initially is to the superficial femoral nodes above the cribriform fascia and secondarily to the deep femoral nodes. Cloquet's node is the most proximal of the deep femoral nodes.

288

man 1971). These lymphatics reportedly course along the lateral margins of the vagina and rectum to empty into the inferior gluteal and internal ilial nodes (Figure 11-2).

It is apparent, therefore, that most of the primary lymphatic drainage of the vulva is to the superficial femoral nodes, which lie between Camper's fascia and the cribriform fascia overlying the femoral vessels. The deep femoral nodes surround the vessels beneath this layer.

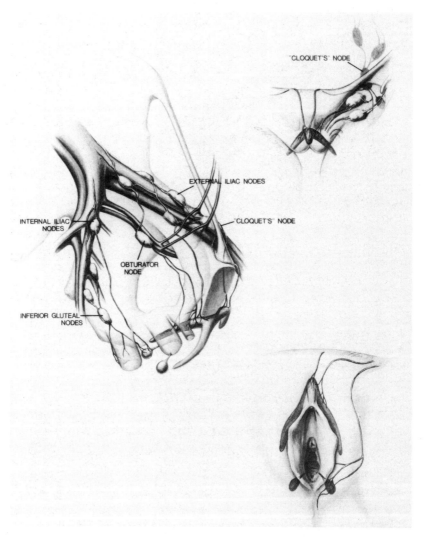

Figure 11-2 Lymphatic drainage of the central vulvar structures including the clitoris, urethra, and Bartholin glands. The sagittal section demonstrates efferent lymphatics from both the clitoris and the Bartholin glands to the deep pelvic nodes without intervening spread to the inguinal nodes.

The lateral superficial femoral nodes penetrate the external oblique aponeurosis to drain directly into the external iliac nodes. The deep femoral nodes usually are involved secondarily as a result of spread from the superficial inguinal nodes. The most proximal lymph node in the deep femoral chain is Cloquet's node, which is located in the femoral canal beneath Poupart's ligament (Figure 11-1). If the superficial or deep femoral lymph nodes are free of tumor metastases, then it is unlikely that vulvar cancer has spread to involve the internal or external iliac nodes within the pelvis.

Three factors of prognostic significance, which should be evaluated in all vulvar cancer patients, are: 1) the presence of lymph nodal metastases, 2) lesion size, and 3) histologic differentiation of the tumor. Approximately 35% of patients with vulvar cancer have femoral lymph node metastases at the time of diagnosis and 8% have pelvic lymph nodal disease (Table 11-3). There is some evidence, however, that with the trend toward earlier diagnosis, the incidence of lymph nodal metastases may be decreasing. For example, Green (1978) reported that the frequency of lymph node metastases in vulvar cancer patients treated at the Massachusetts General and Pondville Hospitals decreased from 55% during the years 1927 to 1950 to 38% in the 1951 to 1976 time period. Similarly, the incidence of inguinal lymph node metastases in patients with invasive carcinoma of the vulva treated at Charity Hospital in New Orleans has decreased from 27% to 20% in consecutive series (Collins et al 1971, Krupp and Bohm 1979). The prognostic effect of lymph node metastases is illustrated in Table 11-4.

In a collected series from the recent literature, the presence of inguinal lymph node metastases decreased the five-year survival from 89%

Table 11-3
Incidence of Inguinal and Pelvic Lymph Nodal Metastases in Patients with Vulvar Cancer

Author	Patients	Inguinal Node Metastases	Pelvic Node Metastases
Taussig (1938)	65	25 (38%)	5 (8%)
Way (1960)	143	60 (42%)	23 (16%)
Merrill and Ross (1961)	25	8 (32%)	2 (8%)
Collins et al (1963)	71	22 (31%)	6 (8%)
Rutledge et al (1970)	101	48 (48%)	11 (11%)
Morley (1976)	205	74 (36%)	6 (3%)
Krupp and Bohm (1978)	195	40 (20%)	9 (4%)
Green (1978)	142	54 (38%)	18 (13%)
TOTAL	947	331 (35%)	80 (8%)

Table 11-4
Five-Year Survival Related to Inguinal Lymph Node Status in Patients
with Squamous Cell Carcinoma of the Vulva

Author	Patients	Five-Year Survival	
		Negative Nodes	Positive Nodes
Way (1960)	81	28/36 (78%)	19/45 (42%)
Merrill and Ross (1961)	13	7/8 (88%)	2/5 (40%)
Collins et al (1963)	51	22/32 (69%)	4/19 (21%)
Krupp et al (1975)	76	51/55 (93%)	5/21 (24%)
Morley (1976)	153	100/105 (95%)	16/48 (33%)
Green (1978)	107	58/61 (95%)	28/46 (61%)
Curry et al (1980)	191	117/134 (87%)	22/57 (38%)
TOTAL	672	383/431 (89%)	96/241 (40%)

to 40%. The number of inguinal lymph nodes containing tumor metastases is also important. Green (1978), for example, reported that 89% of patients with fewer than four positive nodes were cured by radical surgery as opposed to only 12% in patients with four or more positive nodes. Likewise, Curry and co-workers (1980) noted that there were no patients with three or less unilaterally positive groin nodes who had positive deep pelvic nodes. The five-year survival of patients having less than four positive nodes was 68% as opposed to no survivors in the group having four or more positive inguinal nodes.

It is important to emphasize the relative inaccuracy of clinical estimation of lymph node status. Way (1960) reported that 22 of 51 patients (43%) whose inguinal lymph nodes were not palpably enlarged had histologic evidence of lymph nodal metastases. Conversely, approximately 15% of lymph nodes thought by clinical examination to contain tumor metastases were normal. This data has been confirmed by other investigators (Rutledge et al 1970, Green et al 1978). In recent series (Morley 1976, Krupp and Bohm 1978), pelvic lymph nodes have been involved by tumor metastases in 3% to 4% of the cases. The most common pelvic lymph nodes involved are the obturator nodes followed by the external iliac and common iliac groups. Since it is practically impossible to clinically ascertain the status of these nodes, it is recommended that any patient with palpably enlarged inguinal nodes have an intravenous pyelogram, and either lymphangiography or CT scanning in order to evaluate more completely the presence of pelvic lymph nodal metastases.

Lesion size is directly related to the incidence of lymph nodal metastases in patients with vulvar cancer. Franklin and Rutledge (1972) reported that only 1 of 18 patients with a vulvar lesion less than 1 cm in diameter had inguinal lymph node metastases. In 48 patients whose lesions were less than 2 cm in diameter, lymph node metastases were present in seven cases (15%). The frequency of lymph nodal metastases increased to 34% in patients with lesions 2 to 8 cm in diameter and to 50% in lesions greater than 8 cm in diameter. Similarly, Collins and co-workers (1963) reported that five of 30 vulvar cancer patients whose lesions were less than 3 cm in diameter had lymph nodal metastases. Pelvic nodal disease was present in only one of these patients. In contrast, lesions larger than 3 cm were associated with lymph nodal spread in 41% of the cases. In a subsequent report from the same institution, Krupp and Bohm (1979) reported that bilateral inguinal lymph node metastases almost never occurred in lesions less than 3 cm in diameter.

The histologic grade of each vulvar tumor is also of prognostic significance and should be evaluated in all cases. Way (1960) reported that the incidence of positive lymph nodes was 62% in anaplastic tumors, as opposed to only 35% in well-differentiated vulvar lesions. The frequency of bilateral lymph nodal metastases was nearly three times more common in undifferentiated tumors than in well-differentiated lesions. These findings were confirmed by Krupp and Bohm (1978). Similarly, Franklin and Rutledge (1971) noted that there were no lymph nodal metastases in well-differentiated tumors less than 2 cm in diameter. The prognostic effect of histologic differentiation seemed to lessen somewhat with the increasing size of the primary tumor. In a more recent study, Donaldson and colleagues (1981) reported that the frequency of lymph nodal metastases increased from 33% in well-differentiated vulvar tumors to 75% in poorly differentiated tumors.

Although there have been numerous staging systems proposed for the evaluation of patients with invasive vulvar cancer (Taussig 1949, McKelvey 1970), the International Federation of Gynecology and Obstetrics (FIGO) Staging Classification initially adopted in 1971 is the most suitable. This system is based on the size and location of the primary tumor (T), clinical assessment of the regional lymph nodes (N), and the presence of distant metastases (M), as determined by pelvic examination and radiologic techniques (Table 11-5).

The exact definition of each clinical stage is presented in Table 11-6. Stage I consists of lesions confined to the vulva less than 2 cm in diameter with no associated lymphadenopathy. Stage II lesions are also confined to the vulva but are in excess of 2 cm in diameter. The prognostic difference between these two stages has been emphasized by Franklin (1972) who reported that the incidence of inguinal lymph metastases increased from 14% in patients with Stage I disease to 38% in patients with Stage II disease. The location of the primary lesion was unrelated to prognosis provided that it did not involve a mucosal surface ie, the vagina or urethra. Lesions of any size confined to the vulva but with suspicious groin nodes, or lesions extending beyond the vulva in the presence of

Table 11-5
TNM Classification for Vulvar Cancer

T Primary Tumor

T1	Tumor confined to the vulva — 2 cm or less in largest diameter.
T2	Tumor confined to the vulva — more than 2 cm in diameter.
T3	Tumor of any size with adjacent spread to the urethra and/or vagina and/or perineum and/or to the anus.
T4	Tumor of any size infiltrating the bladder mucosa and/or the rectal mucosa or both, including the upper part of the urethral mucosa and/or fixed to the bone.

N Regional Lymph Nodes

N0	No nodes palpable.
N1	Nodes palpable in either groin, not enlarged, mobile (not clinically suspicious of neoplasm).
N2	Nodes palpable in either one or both groins, enlarged, firm and mobile (clinically suspicious of neoplasm).
N3	Fixed or ulcerated nodes.

M Distant Metastases

M0	No clinical metastases.
M1a	Palpable deep pelvic lymph nodes.
M1b	Other distant metastases.

clinically normal groin nodes, are included in Stage III. Finally, Stage IV includes: 1) lesions of any size with grossly positive groin nodes, 2) tumors involving mucosa of the bladder, urethra, or rectum, and 3) pelvic, bony, or distant metastases. Tumors present in the vulva as secondary growth from either a genital or extragenital site are excluded, and malignant melanomas are separately reported (American Joint Committee for Cancer Staging 1978). In order for proper staging to be performed, all patients with vulvar cancer should have a thorough physical examination, including careful palpation of regional and supraclavicular lymph nodes. Intravenous pyelography, lymphangiography, CT scanning, chest x-ray, cystoscopy, and sigmoidoscopy can be helpful in determining the extent of disease in advanced lesions.

Recently, new staging systems have been proposed utilizing postoperative histologic assessment rather than clinical estimation of nodal metastases. Krupp and co-workers (1975) advocated the use of a 3 cm-diameter lesion size to differentiate between Stage I and Stage II disease. This classification was further modified by Friedrich and DiPaola (1977) to include specific sites of tumor metastases and to further subdivide cases according to the presence of bilateral or unilateral lymph nodal involvement (Table 11-7). Using this classification, it was found that patients with

Table 11-6
International Federation of Gynecology and Obstetrics Staging System for Vulvar Cancer

---

Stage I

T1 N0 M0	Tumor confined to the vulva−2 cm or less in the larger
T1 N0 M0	diameter. Nodes are not palpable, or are palpable in either groin, not enlarged, mobile (not clinically suspicious of neoplasm).

Stage II

T2 N0 M0	Tumor confined to the vulva−more than 2 cm in diameter.
T2 N1 M0	Nodes are not palpable, or are palpable, in either groin, not enlarged, mobile (not clinically suspicious of neoplasm).

Stage III

T3 N0 M0	Tumor of any size with 1) adjacent spread to the lower urethra
T3 N1 M0	and/or the vagina, the perineum, and the anus, and/or 2) nodes
T3 N2 M0	mobile, not fixed (but clinically suspicious of neoplasm).
T1 N2 M0	
T2 N2 M0	

Stage IV

T4 N0 M0	Tumor of any size 1) infiltrating the bladder mucosa, or the
T4 N1 M0	rectal mucosa, or both, including the upper part of the urethral
T4 N2 M0	mucosa, and/or 2) fixed to the bone or other distant metastases.
T1 N3 M0	Fixed or ulcerated nodes in either one or both groins.
T2 N3 M0	
T3 N3 M0	
T4 N3 M0	

All other conditions containing M1a or M1b.

Stage I and II disease involving lateral vulvar structures had a 100% five-year survival as opposed to only 72% when the clitoris was involved. Likewise, 50% of patients with unilateral lymph nodal metastases survived versus no survivors in the group having bilateral lymph nodal metastases. Therefore, the value of both preoperative and postoperative staging is evident in defining those patients requiring further therapy.

The evaluation of patients with malignant melanoma of the vulva is similar to that for patients with vulvar squamous cell carcinoma. There are certain biologic differences, however, between the two tumors that must be taken into consideration in the evaluation process. As has been previously mentioned, all pigmented lesions of the vulva should be surgically excised. This recommendation is based largely on the high frequency of junctional activity in nevi occurring on the vulvar skin. Presumptive signs of malignant activity in a nevus include: change in color, rapid increase in size, development of irregular margins or satellite lesions, and change in surface characteristics ie, ulceration or bleeding. Also, the onset of itching or burning in a pigmented vulvar lesion in-

Table 11-7
Postoperative Staging System for Carcinoma of the Vulva*

Stage 0 — Carcinoma in situ
  A. Unifocal
  B. Multifocal
  C. Clitoral

Stage I — Invasive cancer, confined to vulva, < 3 cm in diameter, negative nodes
  A. Unifocal
  B. Multifocal
  C. Clitoral

Stage II — Invasive cancer, confined to vulva, ≥ 3 cm in diameter, negative nodes
  A. Unifocal
  B. Multifocal
  C. Clitoral

Stage III — Invasive cancer, any size
  A. Involves distal ⅓ of urethra; distal ⅓ of vagina and/or anus
  B. Histologically (+) nodes, unilateral
  C. Histologically (+) nodes, bilateral

Stage IV — Invasive cancer, any size
  A. Involves proximal urethra, bladder, and/or upper vagina
  B. Histologically positive nodes
  C. Distant metastases

*Reprinted with permission from Friedrich EG, DiPaola GR: Postoperative stage of vulvar carcinoma: A retrospective study. *Int Gynecol Obstet* 15:220-224, 1977.

dicates the need for immediate evaluation. The most common symptoms of patients with vulvar melanoma are bleeding, pruritis, or burning associated with an enlarging mole. Morrow and Rutledge (1972) reported that pruritis or bleeding were present in over one third of patients with vulvar melanomas, but that 60% of these patients delayed seeing a physician longer than three months after the onset of symptoms. In addition, a vulvar or groin mass is present in half of the patients with malignant melanoma.

The specific location of malignant melanomas of the vulva is illustrated in Table 11-8. Over 60% of melanomas arise from central vulvar structures including the labia minora, clitoris, and vaginal introitus. This is in contrast to squamous cell carcinomas of the vulva, which occur most

The central location and biologic aggressiveness of vulvar melanomas increase the potential of these lesions to spread to inguinal and pelvic lymph nodes. For example, Chung and co-workers (1975) reported that nearly 50% of patients with vulvar melanomas had lymph nodal metastases. Also, 30% of patients undergoing lymph node dissections for melanoma have been shown to have pelvic lymph nodal metastases. For this reason, most investigators favor radical vulvectomy with combined inguinal and pelvic lymphadenectomy as the treatment of choice for this lesion. As in squamous cell carcinoma of the vulva, prognosis was directly related to lymph nodal metastases. For example, Yackel and co-workers (1970) noted that 44% of patients without lymph nodal metastases survived five years. In contrast, there were no survivors in the group of patients having lymph nodal metastases. It should be noted that there is a relatively high incidence of extrapelvic metastases in vulvar melanoma, particularly to the liver, lung, and brain (Morrow and DiSaia 1976). Therefore, a chest x-ray and radionuclide or CT scans of the liver and brain should be performed as part of the initial evaluation of patients with vulvar melanoma. Lesion size is of prognostic significance in malignant melanoma of the vulva and should be accurately recorded in all patients (Morrow and DiSaia 1976). Karlen and co-workers (1975) reported that all patients with vulvar melanomas who survived five years following therapy had lesions smaller than 2 cm in diameter. No patient with a lesion greater than 2 cm in diameter or with clinically positive groin nodes survived.

The clinicopathologic finding of greatest prognostic significance in malignant melanoma is the depth of tumor invasion. Histologic classification systems to define the extent of tumor penetration have been proposed by Clark (1969) and Breslow (1970), and will be presented in the Pathology section. In performing an excisional biopsy of a melanotic lesion, every effort should be made to remove the underlying subcutaneous tissue so that the full extent of tumor invasion can be assessed.

The four criteria commonly mentioned as essential for the diagnosis of primary carcinoma of the Bartholin gland are: 1) correct anatomic position of the tumor on the vulva, 2) location of the tumor deep in the labium, 3) presence of some elements of glandular epithelium, and 4) overlying skin intact (Barclay et al 1964). The most common presenting symptom in these patients is a painful labial swelling or tumor. Bilaterality of primary Bartholin's gland carcinoma has not been reported, although

Table 11-8
Location of Malignant Melanomas of the Vulva

Site	Patients
Labia majora	36 (30%)
Labia minora	41 (34%)
Clitoris	31 (26%)
Urethra	8 (6%)
Perineum	2 (2%)
Vaginal introitus	2 (2%)
TOTAL	120 (100%

Data from Chung et al (1975), Karlen et al (1975), Morrow and Rutledge (1972), and Yackel et al (1970).

involvement of both glands by metastatic tumor has been described (Wharton and Everett 1951). Interestingly, the initial clinical impression is that of a benign cystic or inflammatory lesion in approximately 50% of the cases (Chamlian and Taylor 1972). Consequently, any patient with a persistent labial swelling or a nonhealing lesion in the Bartholin area should be fully evaluated for the presence of malignancy. Included in this evaluation is histologic sampling of the Bartholin gland as well as careful palpation of both groins for the presence of enlarged inguinal lymph nodes. The lymphatic drainage of Bartholin gland carcinoma is essentially the same as that of squamous cell carcinoma of the labia and lower vagina with efferent flow primarily to the superficial and deep inguinal node groups. Eichner (1963), however, has demonstrated additional direct lymphatic channels from the Bartholin gland area to the deep pelvic nodes. Also, Barclay and co-workers (1964) have reported patients who had obturator lymph nodal metastases without involvement of the intervening iliac nodes. For this reason, lymphangiography or CT scanning of the pelvic lymph nodes is indicated in the evaluation of patients with primary carcinoma of the Bartholin gland. Staging of Bartholin gland carcinoma is performed according to the FIGO Staging Classification, and the remainder of the evaluative process essentially is identical to that for squamous cell carcinoma of the vulva.

The evaluation and staging of patients with sarcoma of the vulva essentially is the same as for other vulvar malignancies. The two most important prognostic variables in these tumors are lesion size and the number of mitosis per 10 high power fields (HPF). The propensity of sarcomas for hematogenous spread necessitates careful examination of the lungs and liver to rule out the presence of occult metastases in these organs.

PATHOLOGY

For organizational purposes, the pathology of vulvar epithelial abnormalities will be divided into the vulvar dystrophies, carcinoma in situ, Paget's disease, and the specific histologic types of invasive carcinoma.

Vulvar Dystrophies

Until recently, the nomenclature applied to areas of disordered vulvar epithelial architecture without neoplastic change has been quite confusing. Since many of these lesions were found adjacent to vulvar malignancies, it was erroneously concluded that these lesions were of malignant potential. In 1961, Jeffcoate introduced the term *vulvar dystrophy* to characterize those disorders of epithelial growth and maturation, which often present as white lesions of the vulva. He stated that any keratin-covered epithelium could become thickened and white when constantly exposed to moisture and warmth. Also, he noted that when dystrophic vulvar skin was excised and the area covered with skin from a site not ordinarily subject to such dystrophies, the transplanted epithelium often underwent the same histologic changes. In a subsequent study, he followed 138 women with vulvar dystrophies from 3 to 25 years and noted that carcinoma developed in fewer than 5% of them (Jeffcoate 1966). Similarly, Kaufman and co-workers (1974) reported that invasive carcinoma developed in only one of 110 patients with vulvar dystrophies. Approximately 10% of patients with vulvar dystrophies will demonstrate areas of cellular atypia, and it is these patients who are at highest risk to develop neoplasia (McAdams and Kistner 1958). The importance of performing a biopsy of white lesions of the vulva cannot be overemphasized, since it is impossible to differentiate dystrophic epithelium from intraepithelial neoplasia in the absence of histologic examination.

The International Society for the Study of Vulvar Disease has recently proposed a new classification for the vulvar dystrophies (Table 11-1). According to this classification, there are two basic types of vulvar dystrophy: hyperplastic dystrophy and lichen sclerosus. When both of these histologic types are present in different areas of the same vulva, the lesion is classified as a mixed dystrophy.

Hyperplastic Dystrophy

These lesions are usually white or red and most commonly occur in women between the ages of 40 and 60 (Kaufman et al 1974). They account for approximately one half of all vulvar dystrophies. Histologic characteristics of hyperplastic dystrophy include blunting or widening of the rete ridges with varying degrees of hyperkeratosis. Usually, there is a chronic inflammatory infiltrate within the dermis, and parakeratosis may or may not be present (Figure 11-3). In general, hyperplastic dystrophies respond well to medical therapy, and in the absence of cellular atypia, do not proceed to carcinoma.

Lichen Sclerosus

Lichen sclerosus most commonly occurs in postmenopausal women, but occasionally is found in women of reproductive age and rarely, even in children (Clark and Muller 1967). This lesion often produces flattening and agglutination of the labial folds. The involved area appears white because of a loss of pigment and variable hyperkeratosis (Mann and Cowen 1973). Microscopically, there is thinning of the epithelium and loss

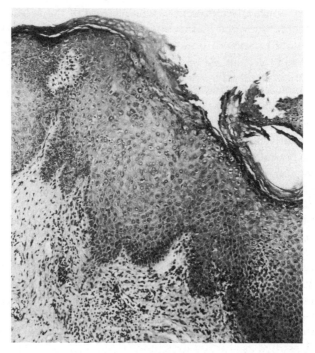

Figure 11-3 Hyperplastic dystrophy. The epidermis is thickened with broadening of the rete ridges. Note hyperkeratosis, parakeratosis, and dermal mononuclear infiltrate. Mild nuclear atypia is present. Hematoxylin and eosin stain, magnification 100 ×.

of the rete ridges. The number of cell layers of the epidermis is reduced, and the basal cell layer is disorganized and hydropic. The dermis just beneath the epithelium is acellular with a very homogenous appearance. Beneath this homogenous zone there are varying degrees of lymphcytic or plasma cell infiltrate (Figure 11-4). In pure lichen sclerosus, atypia does not occur and the risk for carcinomatous transformation is essentially nonexistent. Hart and co-workers (1975) reviewed 107 patients with lichen sclerosus and could find no evidence to substantiate a malignant potential for this lesion. Five patients had coexistent areas of squamous cell carcinoma and lichen sclerosus. However, carcinoma tended to arise in isolated areas of relatively normal vulvar skin.

Mixed Dystrophy

When both types of dystrophy affect different areas of the vulva, the diagnosis of mixed dystrophy is made. Kaufman and colleagues (1974) reported that 18 out of 128 patients with vulvar dystrophy had evidence of a mixed pattern. In spite of their association, it should not be considered that these conditions are different stages of the same abnormality.

Rather, most authorities believe that they represent clones of cells responding differently to the same irritating stimulus (Friedrich 1977). Cellular atypia is usually confined to areas of hyperplastic dystrophy.

Vulvar Epithelial Atypia

Atypical changes within vulvar dystrophy are classified as mild, moderate, or severe, somewhat analogous to the method for defining the various degrees of cervical dysplasia. Atypical cells within the vulvar squamous epithelium often demonstrate a rapid cell turnover rate with increased mitotic activity and a high nuclear/cytoplasmic ratio. Changes present in a variable number of cells include: multinucleation, clumping of nuclear chromatin, and irregularity of the nuclear and cell membranes. Nuclear pyknosis, indicative of accelerated maturation, is often accompanied by a perinuclear halo, forming the so-called corps rond. When these atypical changes are confined to the lower one third of the epithelium and there is normal superficial maturation, the pattern is defined as mild atypia. The presence of cellular atypia in one half to two thirds of the epithelium is indicative of moderate atypia. With severe atypia, there is little epithelial maturation, and cells of the parabasal type

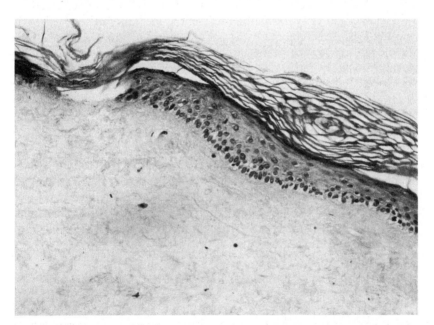

Figure 11-4 Lichen sclerosus. There is marked epidermal atrophy with loss of normal rete ridges. There is some vacuolization of basal cells in the epidermis. The superficial dermis is replaced by an acellular collagenous material. Hematoxylin and eosin stain, magnification 100 ×.

reach almost to the surface. Surface keratinization, however, is still present. Even though it must be assumed that there is a point of irreversibility in vulvar epithelial atypia, many of these lesions undergo spontaneous regression. Likewise, progression rates of vulvar atypia to carcinoma in situ or invasive vulvar carcinoma have not been defined as clearly in the vulva as they have been in the cervix (Friedrich 1977).

Carcinoma in Situ

The gross appearance of carcinoma in situ is quite varied. Lesions may be unifocal or multifocal, and commonly present as white, red, or slightly pigmented macular areas on the vulvar skin or mucous membrane. Papillary lesions are reported in approximately 20% of the patients (Buscema et al 1980).

The histopathology of carcinoma in situ also varies greatly. Lesions are typically characterized by distortion of the epithelial architecture with crowding of the cells and a lack of normal maturation. Cellular abnormalities, including dyskeratosis, increased nuclear/cytoplasmic ratio, multinucleation, and abnormal mitoses, extend throughout the full thickness of the epithelium. An alternative pattern of carcinoma in situ is one in which the surface epithelium appears normal, but atypical maturation and keratin *pearl* formation is present at the tips of the rete ridges. A specific type of carcinoma in situ of the vulva is Bowen's disease. The histologic appearance of this lesion (Figure 11-5) is characterized by parakeratosis, hyperkeratosis, and acanthosis, and by cellular abnormalities including individual cell keratinization, corps ronds, and nuclear clumping (Bowen 1912).

The risk for biologic progression of carcinoma in situ is not known. Friedrich and colleagues (1980) reported that only one of 50 cases of carcinoma in situ progressed to invasive cancer after prolonged observation. Similarly, Buscema and co-workers (1980) noted that only four of 102 patients with carcinoma in situ developed invasive cancer when followed from one to 15 years after treatment. It should also be noted that up to 10% of patients with vulvar carcinoma in situ may experience spontaneous regression of this lesion. Regression occurs most frequently in patients who are young or pregnant (Friedrich 1972).

Paget's Disease of the Vulva

Paget's disease of the vulva has been considered by some authors simply as one type of intraepithelial carcinoma. Because of its unique histologic appearance and clinical behavior, however, it is described herein as a separate entity. Paget's disease of the skin typically occurs at any location from the axilla to the perianal area along the *milk line*. Vulvar disease should not be confused with Paget's disease of the breast, which is associated with underlying intraductal or infiltrating adenocarcinoma. Paget's disease of the vulva occurs characteristically in the fifth and sixth decades of life, and presents as a moist, velvety red lesion with white plaques scattered throughout. The most common symptoms are pruritus or burning, and there is usually an area of excoriation and inflammation surrounding the lesion. In a recent study by Gunn and Gallagher (1980), vulvectomy specimens from patients with Paget's disease were serially sectioned and the extent of histologically evident tumor was mapped. All lesions were multicentric and exceeded the margin of clinically detectable disease in every instance. Although Paget's disease of the vulva is primarily an intraepithelial lesion, a significant number of cases have been reported to have an underlying apocrine gland carcinoma. Tsukada and co-workers (1975) noted an underlying adenocarcinoma in one of eight patients with vulvar Paget's disease, and the frequency of associated apocrine gland carcinoma is even higher in certain

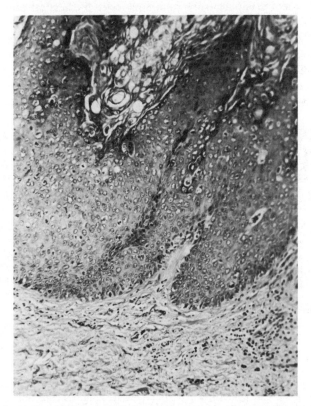

Figure 11-5 Bowen's disease. This form of in situ squamous carcinoma is characterized by hyperkeratosis and parakeratosis as well as dyskeratosis and the formation of corps ronds. Hematoxylin and eosin stain, magnification 100 ×.

302

other investigations (Koss et al 1968, Boehm and Morris 1971). For these reasons, surgical excision of this lesion should include a wide margin of normal skin and be deep enough to adequately evaluate the underlying apocrine glands for the presence of adenocarcinoma. In addition, the incidence of secondary primary carcinomas in such organs as the rectum, bladder, cervix, and breast, is significantly increased in patients with vulvar Paget's disease (Fetherston and Friedrich 1972). Therefore, a thorough evaluation should be undertaken of the common sites of coexistent primary tumors to rule out malignancy in these areas.

Histologically, Paget's disease is characterized by infiltration of epithelium by Paget cells (Figure 11-6). Typically, these are large round cells with a pale clear or granular cytoplasm. The nuclei are usually vesicular, and mitoses are rare. Paget cells contain mucopolysaccharides and stain positively with PAS, mucicarmine, and aldehyde fuchsin. These staining characteristics help differentiate Paget's cells from the large cells occasionally seen in Bowen's disease of the vulva. Ultrastructural studies have indicated that some Paget cells are derived from secretory cells, whereas others originate from squamous cells (Fetherston and Friedrich 1972). It is possible, therefore, that Paget's cells could arise either de novo from cells within the epithelium or migrate to the epithelium from an underlying adenocarcinoma. Parmley and colleagues (1975) point out that the apocrine glands and the squamous epithelium are derived from a common stem cell that may be the origin of these lesions. This would explain the association between Paget's disease and apocrine gland carcinoma.

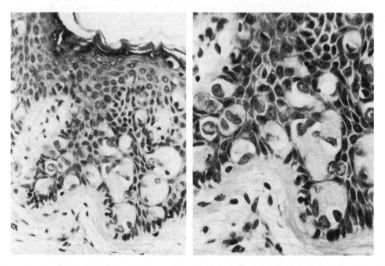

Figure 11-6 Paget's disease of the vulva. *Left,* Paget's cells involve the epidermis, primarily along the epidermal-dermal junction. Hemotoxylin and eosin stain, magnification 250 ×. *Right,* Paget's cells have large atypical nuclei and pale staining cytoplasm, which histochemically contains mucin. Hematoxylin and eosin stain, magnification 400 ×.

Invasive Squamous Cell Carcinoma

Squamous cell carcinoma of the vulva most commonly presents as a raised nodular lesion on the labia majora or minora. Endophytic ulcerated tumors occur in approximately one third of the cases. Histologically, squamous cell carcinomas of the vulva should be classified as well differentiated, moderately differentiated, or poorly differentiated according to the degree of keratin production, nuclear pleomorphism, and nuclear/cytoplasmic ratio. The majority of vulvar squamous cell carcinomas are well-differentiated, keratinizing tumors with minimal nuclear atypicality and few mitoses (Figure 11-7). The incidence of lymph node metastases has been shown to be directly related to the histologic differentiation of the tumor (Way 1960). Therefore, every lesion should be graded histologically at the time of initial evaluation. Verrucous carcinoma is a variant of squamous cell carcinoma with a distinct pattern of biologic behavior. The clinical appearance of these lesions is papillary and resembles that of condyloma accuminata. Microscopically, verrucous carcinomas are well-differentiated and may be difficult to distinquish histologically from condylomas. Stromal invasion in these tumors often is accompanied by an inflammatory response.

The depth of stromal invasion is also prognostically significant and should be measured in every tumor. The incidence of lymph node metastases has been shown to be quite low in those lesions with less than 5 mm stromal invasion. Parker and colleagues (1975) reported that only three of 58 patients (5%) with stromal invasion limited to a depth of 5 mm or less had evidence of lymph node metastases. Similarly, Wharton and col-

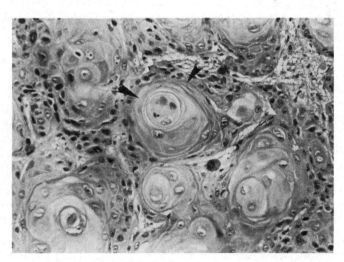

Figure 11-7 Well-differentiated squamous cell carcinoma of the vulva is characterized by mild nuclear atypia and well formed keratin pearls (arrows). Hematoxylin and eosin stain, magnification 250 ×.

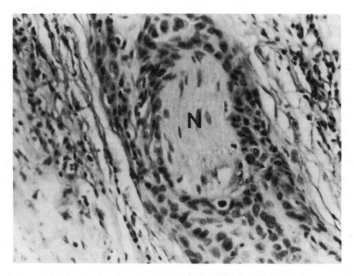

Figure 11-8 Perineural invasion by invasive vulvar carcinoma. Poorly differentiated squamous cells invade lymphatic spaces around a small peripheral nerve (N). Hematoxylin and eosin stain, magnification 250 ×.

leagues (1974) noted that there were no lymph nodal metastases in 25 patients with lesions invading the stroma for a depth of less than 5 mm. The importance of lymph vascular space or perineural invasion by tumor cells recently has been emphasized by Donaldson and colleagues (1981) (Figure 11-8). In patients with early stromal invasion, the frequency of lymph nodal metastases increased from 0% to 84% in the presence of lymph vascular space invasion. For this reason, every effort should be made to examine each tumor for the presence of tumor cells in vascular or perineural spaces.

Malignant Melanoma

The clinical appearance of malignant melanoma of the vulva may be quite varied. These lesions are brown to blue-black in color, and are flat, raised, or polypoid in configuration. The epidermis may be intact, hyperkeratinized, or ulcerated. Melanomas are classified both by tumor growth pattern and cell type. The two major varieties of melanoma that occur on the vulva are the superficial spreading melanoma and the nodular melanoma. Lentigo-maligna melanoma rarely is, if ever, observed on the vulva. The superficial spreading melanoma usually is slightly elevated with variegated coloration. The characteristic histologic feature of this lesion is the presence of malignant melanocytes spreading in the epidermis for a distance of three or more rete pegs lateral to an area of dermal invasion. The nuclei of the melanocytes are typically uniform in size and there is an abundant cytoplasm. Superficial spreading melanomas, as the name implies, tend to spread horizontally at the dermal-epidermal junction, and only late in their course invade vertically into the dermis and subcutaneous tissues. In contrast, nodular melanomas are elevated or polypoid in appearance. Epidermal growth is almost always associated with early dermal invasion and lateral junctional spread is rare.

Prognosis is related generally to the size and location of malignant melanomas and every effort should be made to describe accurately the exact dimensions and site of each lesion. The pathologic finding of greatest prognostic significance in malignant melanoma is the level of tumor penetration. Clark and co-workers (1969) proposed that each melanoma should be classified by its depth of invasion into the various anatomical levels of the skin as follows (Figure 11-9):

Level I   Intraepidermal

Level II   Invasion into the papillary dermis

Level III   Tumor filling the papillary dermis and pressing on the reticular dermis

Level IV   Invasion into the reticular dermis

Level V   Invasion into the subcutis.

Chung and colleagues (1975), using a modification of this classification, reported that vulvar melanoma patients with level I and II lesions all survived, whereas 60% of patients with level III and IV tumors died of recurrent disease. Breslow (1970) proposed a more objective method of measuring tumor thickness using an ocular micrometer. Melanomas less than 0.76 mm in thickness were associated with an excellent prognosis, whereas patients with progressively thicker lesions had a correspondingly poorer survival. Using this system, Balch and co-workers (1979) reported

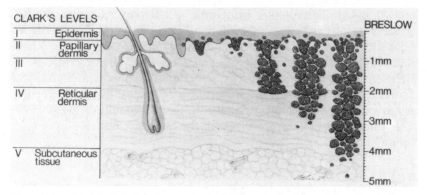

Figure 11-9 Methods of melanoma classification according to depth of invasion. Clark's levels (left) based upon the various anatomic structures involved. Breslow's system (right) measures tumor thickness using an ocular micrometer.

the incidence of regional lymph nodal metastases was 0% in melanomas less than 0.76 mm thick, 25% in lesions with a thickness of 0.76 mm to 1.50 mm, 51% in 1.50 mm to 3.99 mm lesions, and 62% in lesions greater than 4.0 mm in thickness. For this reason, excisional biopsies of melanotic lesions of the vulva should be deep enough so that an accurate measurement of the thickness of each tumor can be made.

Bartholin Gland Carcinoma

Bartholin gland carcinoma typically presents as a swelling in the labial area. The overlying skin is intact and ulceration occurs only in advanced lesions. The Bartholin's duct is lined by squamous epithelium near the vagina, which changes to a transitional type epithelium near the gland. Adenocarcinoma is the most common cell type comprising over 50% of the total cases.

Histologically, this lesion is characterized by poorly formed glands and sheets of cells. Mucin production by the tumor is usually quite abundant.

Approximately one third of Bartholin gland cancers are squamous cell carcinomas. These are similar histologically to squamous carcinomas of the vulva and are classified as well, moderately, and poorly differentiated.

Sarcoma

Sarcomas of the vulva are extremely rare, accounting for 2% to 3% of vulvar cancer. The most common vulvar sarcomas are leiomyosarcomas and rhabdomyosarcomas. Leiomyosarcomas are firm, bulky tumors, which are most commonly located in the labia majora. Usually, they are indolent neoplasms and may remain confined to the vulvar stroma without destroying the overlying epithelium. Microscopically, these tumors contain sheets of round or elongated cells with pleomorphic nuclei and abundant eosinophilic cytoplasm. Rhabdomyosarcomas are aggressive tumors, which consist of small polygonal and spindle-shaped cells with hyperchromatic nuclei and numerous mitotic figures. Rhabdomyoblasts usually are elongated and contain the characteristic cross-striations easily demonstrable by special stains, ie, phyophotungstic-acid hematoxylin (PTAH). As in sarcomas of other sites, the most prognostically important histologic variable is the number of mitoses per 10 HPF. This finding should be recorded with the histologic description of each tumor.

THERAPY

The trend toward individualization of therapy in gynecologic cancer is no more evident than in the treatment of vulvar neoplasms. Separate sections will be devoted to the therapy of vulvar dystrophy, carcinoma in situ, and the various types of invasive vulvar cancer.

Vulvar Dystrophy

The therapy for both hyperplastic dystrophy and lichen sclerosus is medical, and surgery is not required unless these lesions are associated with severe epithelial atypia. Hyperplastic dystrophy is treated best by the topical application of 1% hydrocortisone creme daily for six weeks. This usually produces rapid relief of vulvar pruritis and regression of the lesion. As has been previously mentioned, vulvar epithelial atypia is associated with hyperplastic dystrophy in approximately 10% of the cases. Should this atypia be severe, the involved area is delineated carefully by using toluidine blue staining. This area should be excised surgically and the adjacent skin treated with topical hydrocortisone.

The treatment of choice of lichen sclerosus of the vulva is the topical application of testosterone. Testosterone is readily absorbed through the skin and causes vasodilation, stimulation of the sebaceous glands, and proliferation of the epidermis (Zelle 1971). A 2% ointment of testosterone propionate in a petrolatum base is applied to the vulva, delivering approximately 8 mg to 10 mg of testosterone tid for six weeks or until symptoms are relieved. The dosage is then reduced to bid for four weeks and then to one application daily for four to six months. The area of dystrophic epithelium is then rebiopsied and the treatment stopped if the patient is asymptomatic and the vulvar epithelium appears normal. Using this method, Williams and co-workers (1966) reported symptomatic improvement in virtually every patient treated. In a subsequent study, Zelle (1971) reported that there was a marked improvement in the clinical appearance of the lesion in over 90% of the patients treated. Symptomatic relief was described as excellent in two thirds of the cases and fair in the remaining patients. Histologic changes indicative of resolution of vulvar dystrophy were observed in six of seven patients studied. The vulvar epithelial changes produced by topical testosterone included: diminution or disappearance of hyperkeratosis, thickening of the epithelial layer itself, and restoration of the rete pegs. The side effects of this treatment regimen were minimal and consisted of clitoral hypertrophy and increased libido in approximately 20% of the patients. No abnormalities in 17 ketosteroid or plasma androgen levels were reported. If vulvar pruritis is severe and unresponsive to testosterone, it is recommended that a crotamiton ointment be applied concurrently to the involved area.

Carcinoma In Situ

Therapy for carcinoma in situ of the vulva must be individualated according to the location and extent of the lesion. Treatment is primarily surgical, and varies from local excision to total vulvectomy with skin grafting. In recent years, there has been a trend toward limiting the extent of surgical excision to the site of intraepithelial carcinoma itself. Friedrich and co-workers (1980) reported that wide local excision was just as effective as partial or total vulvectomy in the treatment of carcinoma in situ of the vulva. Three of 17 patients treated by local excision developed recurrence as compared to three of 20 patients who were treated by partial or total vulvectomy. It has been emphasized that up to 70% of vulvar intraepithelial carcinomas are multicentric. Consequently, every effort must be made to define the full extent of each lesion prior to surgical removal. The entire vulvar skin should be carefully observed with a magnifying glass prior to surgery. Also, toluidine blue staining should be performed when possible. In general, the extent of the surgical procedure should be limited to that necessary to remove the involved area and a margin of normal skin. Frozen sections of margins suspect for neoplastic involvement should be performed since the frequency of recurrence is significantly higher when a margin of the surgical specimen contains carcinoma in situ. Other methods, including cryotherapy and the carbon dioxide laser, have been used in the treatment of localized carcinoma in situ. However, they have not been shown as yet to be more effective than local excision. Partial vulvectomy is indicated particularly when there is extensive involvement of the posterior labia and perineum. This procedure allows for preservation of the anterior vulvar structures including the clitoris. In those rare situations in which a vulvectomy is indicated, the *skinning* technique first advocated by Rutledge and Sinclair (1968) is the surgical procedure of choice. This procedure involves skin grafting to the operative site, and is much less deforming than operative methods requiring removal of the underlying subcutaneous tissue of the vulva. Topical 5-fluorouracil has been used in the treatment of multifocal vulvar carcinoma in situ but generally it has been ineffective. Friedrich and co-workers (1980), for example, reported that no response of carcinoma in situ was observed in three patients treated with 5-fluorouracil despite extensive and painful sloughing of the vulva skin.

The therapy for Paget's disease of the vulva depends upon the extent of disease. If the lesion is small and unifocal, wide local excision is sufficient. As has been previously noted, Paget's disease most always extends beyond the limits of a clinically detectable abnormality. Therefore, skin margins must be thoroughly studied in order to rule out evidence of an occult abnormality. Also, the surgical specimen must include the full thickness of the dermis and subcutaneous tissue so that these structures can be examined for the presence of an underlying apocrine gland carcinoma. Should the lesion be more extensive, a total vulvectomy is the surgical procedure of choice. Radical vulvectomy with bilateral inguinal lymph node dissection is reserved for those cases in which an underlying invasive carcinoma is found. Since histologic examination of the vulvectomy specimen often requires significant amounts of time, the procedure is usually staged, and the lymph node dissection performed at a later date.

Invasive Squamous Cell Carcinoma

The standard method of treatment for invasive squamous cell carcinoma of the vulva is radical vulvectomy with bilateral inguinal and femoral lymphadenectomy. Pelvic lymphadenectomy is usually limited to those cases in which there is histologic evidence of metastatic disease in the inguinal nodes, or in which the primary lesion is centrally located. Although there are no universally accepted criteria to define microinvasive vulvar cancer, there is increasing evidence that selected cases of early invasive cancer can be treated with less radical surgery. This is particularly significant in the younger patient in which preservation of sexual function is an important factor.

In order to develop a rational approach toward the treatment of early invasive vulvar cancer, an examination of the pertinent recent literature is essential. Wharton and colleagues (1974) reported that 25 patients with lesions less than 2 cm in diameter and stromal invasion of 5 mm or less had no lymph nodal metastases. None of these patients developed tumor recurrence after treatment, and none died of vulvar cancer. These investigators concluded that patients with early invasive vulvar cancer could be treated by conservative surgery. In a similar study, Parker and co-workers (1975) reported that only three of 58 patients with squamous cancers of the vulva less that 5 mm had pelvic lymph node metastases. Two of the three patients had vascular invasion and one had a poorly differentiated tumor. The prognostic importance of vascular or perineural invasion in early vulvar cancer was confirmed by Donaldson and co-workers (1981). These authors noted no lymph nodal metastases in patients with less than 5 mm stromal invasion and no lymph-vascular space invasion. In a statistical analysis of the benefits of various surgical procedures in the treatment of invasive vulvar cancer, Morris (1977) concluded that contralateral lymph node dissection was not indicated when the ipsilateral lymph nodes draining a unilateral lesion contained no evidence of metastases.

Based on the data presented by these investigators, it would seem that a *good prognosis* group can be defined for patients with early invasive vulvar cancer. This group includes those patients with: 1) well differentiated squamous cell carcinomas, 2) a lesion size of less than 2 cm in diameter involving the labia or perineum, 3) stromal invasion less than 5 mm, and 4) no evidence of perineural or vascular invasion by tumor cells. The appropriate therapy for these lesions has not yet been established. It is reasonable, however, to suggest that hemivulvectomy with preservation of the clitoris would be sufficient. The validity of this approach awaits confirmation by objective data from clinical protocols.

Another approach to the management of early invasive vulvar cancer has been reported by DiSaia and colleagues (1979). Twenty patients with vulvar lesions 1 cm or less in diameter and with focal invasion limited to 5 mm were treated initially with bilateral superficial inguinal lymphadenectomy. Frozen section histologic examinatioin of the removed nodes was then performed with the patient under anesthesia. Eighteen patients had negative superficial inguinal nodes and were treated by wide local excision of the primary lesion including a 3 cm margin of normal skin. Two patients had positive inguinal nodes and were treated by radical vulvectomy with bilateral inguinal and ipsilateral deep pelvic lymphadenectomy. In the 18 patients treated with wide local excision, there was maintenance of normal sexual function. In addition, preservation of the mons veneris and superior vulvar structures resulted in a better cosmetic result than that achieved with radical vulvectomy. Patients were followed from 7 to 74 months following surgery, and none developed tumor recurrence. This approach obviously has been successful, but the need for bilateral inguinal lymphadenectomy in patients with early invasive vulvar cancer remains to be demonstrated. None of the patients in this investigation were shown to have contralateral inguinal lymph node metastases.

The treatment of choice in squamous cell carcinomas invading the stroma in excess of 5 mm or with lymph-vascular space invasion is radical vulvectomy with bilateral inguinal lymphadenectomy. Although there are variations in the operation related to the location and size of the primary lesion, the principle of en bloc resection of the vulva and its regional lymph node drainage is maintained. Prior to surgery the patient is placed in a modified dorsal lithotomy position with the thighs extended such that the abdominal, inguinal, and perineal regions can be operated upon simultaneously without repositioning. A trapezoid incision is utilized (Figure 11-10) including the skin overlying both inguinal areas and the mons veneris. The incision then is extended along the labiocrural folds to cross the perineum above the anus.

The inner incision varies according to the vaginal, urethral, or perineal extension of the primary lesion, but generally follows the hymeneal ring. These incision lines are then carried down to the underlying fascia, thereby removing a full thickness specimen with at least a 1 cm margin of normal tissue. No attempt is made to undermine the skin flaps since this has led to an increased incidence of delayed wound healing. The specific fascial layers, which limit the depth of the vulvar incision, are the rectus abdominis fascia of the abdominal wall, the fascia lata of the thigh, and the inferior fascia of the urogenital diaphragm. The dissection occasionally is extended to include the distal urethra and the paravaginal or pararectal spaces as indicated by tumor location. Inguinal lymphadenectomy is performed by first incising the fascia lata along the border of the sartorius muscle, reflecting the fibroadipose tissue medially, and removing the superficial inguinal nodes anterior to the cribriform fascia. The femoral sheath is incised longitudinally, and all lymph nodal tissue (including Cloquet's node) is removed from the femoral triangle. The fibroadipose tissue immediately inferior to the inguinal ligament also is included in the specimen. The exposed femoral artery and vein are protected, either by closing the femoral sheath or by transposing the sartorius muscle medially.

Frozen section examination is performed on any suspiciously enlarged lymph node. This operation is presently performed by a three-team approach, with individual surgical teams performing each groin dissection

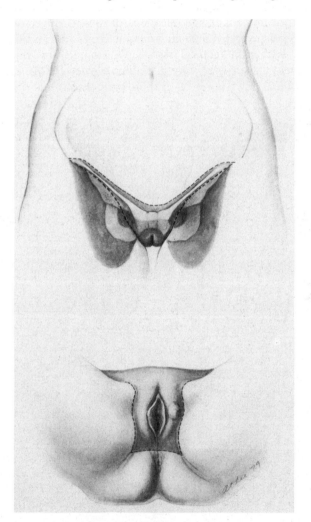

Figure 11-10 Standard trapezoid incision (dotted line) used in radical vulvectomy and bilateral inguinal lymphadenectomy. This incision is modified according to the size and location of the primary lesion and the presence of clinically positive groin nodes.

312

and the vulvar dissection simultaneously. Should pelvic lymphadenectomy be necessary, an incision is made above and parallel to the inguinal ligament and the inferior epigastric artery is ligated. The aponeurosis of the external and internal oblique muscles is transected, and the peritonuem is reflected medially and superiorly. The obturator, external iliac, internal iliac, and common iliac lymph nodes then removed en bloc. The fascial incisions are closed and hemovac drains are placed in both groins. The skin is closed primarily in most cases. However, gracilis myocutaneous pedicle grafts (Figure 11-11) may be required to close the defect produced by resection of a large vulvar tumor (Dinner et al 1979).

The major immediate complications of radical vulvectomy with inguinal lymphadenectomy include: wound necrosis or infection, bleeding from vessels within the femoral triangle, development of lymphocysts in the groin area, and urinary tract infection. Morley (1976), eg, reported that wound breakdown occurred in approximately one half the cases. The

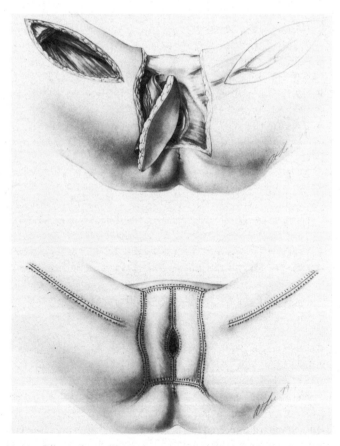

Figure 11-11 Bilateral gracilis myocutaneous pedicle grafts used to close defect produced by radical resection of large vulvar tumor.

significant late complications of the operation are lymphedema of the lower extremities, which occurs in about one third of the patients, and genital prolapse with cystocele or rectocele formation, which is observed in 5% to 10% of cases (Rutledge et al 1970). Additional complications, including difficulty in controlling micturition, thigh and perineal numbness, urethral stenosis, and dyspareunia have also been reported.

In selected cases of advanced Stage IV vulvar cancer, pelvic exenteration is combined with radical vulvectomy and inguinal as well as pelvic lymphadenectomy. This operation was first utilized in the treatment of vulvar cancer by Brunschwig and Daniel (1956), and has been modified by more recent investigators (Thornton and Flanigan 1973, Krupp et al 1975). When vulvar cancer has extended to involve the urethra and base of the bladder, anterior exenteration alone may suffice, whereas posterior exenteration is indicated in vulvar lesions involving the rectum. These operations are usually performed through a transverse incision, and a urinary conduit is constructed from a segment of ileum or colon (Bricker et al 1954). Similarly, a sigmoid colostomy is performed in order to divert the fecal stream following an abdominal-perineal resection of a vulvar cancer involving the posterior vagina and rectum. In a recent literature review, Krupp and colleagues (1975) reported a composite five-year survival of 34.6% in 34 patients undergoing exenterative surgery for advanced vulvar carcinoma.

Radiation therapy generally is of limited use in the treatment of vulvar cancer because the tissue tolerance of normal vulvar structures to irradiation is limited. The vulva is rich in end arteries, and the collateral blood supply is poor. This lack of superficial vascular anastomoses, together with the atrophic moist epithelium present in many patients, explains the limited tissue tolerance of the vulva to radiation. As a result, the incidence of complications is high and the cure rate low when the vulva is treated with therapeutic doses of radiation. Helgason and co-workers (1972), eg, noted that only two of 24 vulvar cancer patients (8.3%) were cured by primary radiation therapy. Frischbier and Thomsen (1975) reported a five-year survival rate of 47% in 118 vulvar cancer patients treated by high energy electrons. However, 24% of these patients developed vulvar induration with persistent ulceration, and 8% experienced extensive tissue necrosis in the inguinal region. For these reasons, the treatment of vulvar cancer by radiation therapy alone is not recommended, and is presently used only in those patients who cannot tolerate major surgery because of severe medical illness.

More recently, several investigators have proposed the use of adjunctive radiation in addition to radical surgery in the treatment of selected patients with invasive vulvar cancer. Daly and Million (1974) advocated the combination of radical excision of the vulva followed by bilateral inguinal and pelvic node irradiation in patients with clinically negative groin nodes. A total dose of approximately 4500 rads was given over a five-week time period. This treatment combination was given to six patients, and there were no lymph nodal recurrences or radiation complication.

Radiation therapy is also being evaluated in the treatment of deep pelvic nodes in patients with vulvar cancer who have metastatic disease in the inguinal nodes (Morley 1976). The established role of radiation therapy in the treatment of pelvic lymph nodal metastases from cervical cancer provides the theoretical basis for its use in vulvar cancer. Initiation of radiation often is delayed significantly, however, because of prolonged wound healing of the vulvar and groin incisions. At the present time, there is no data comparing the efficacy of pelvic radiation *vs* pelvic lymphadenectomy in the treatment of pelvic lymph nodal metastases in vulvar cancer.

Finally, Boronow (1973) has proposed the use of combination preoperative radiation therapy and radical vulvectomy with groin dissection as a therapeutic alternative to primary pelvic exenteration in the treatment of locally advanced vulvovaginal cancer. Generally, patients were treated initially with intracavitary radiation to the vagina followed by external therapy to the inguinal and pelvic nodes. Radical vulvectomy with groin dissection was then performed six to eight weeks later. Nine patients were treated with this therapeutic approach, and five patients were cured of their disease. There was only one major postoperative complication, and all patients has preservation of bowel and bladder function. This format for individualized combination therapy shows promise, but its acceptance awaits further clinical trials in larger numbers of patients.

At the present time, there is very little data concerning the use of chemotherapy in the treatment of squamous cell carcinoma of the vulva. Those chemotherapeutic agents, which have been shown to have a beneficial effect in recurrent or metastatic vulvar cancer, are presented in Table 11-9. The three drugs reported to have activity against squamous cell carcinoma of the vulva are adriamycin, bleomycin, and methotrexate. Likewise, the only combination regimens with demonstrated effectiveness have contained at least two of these drugs. Many patients with squamous cell carcinoma of the vulva are elderly and have a poor performance status. Consequently, physicians have been reticent to enter these patients into experimental chemotherapy protocols. It is quite likely, however, that several drug combinations recently shown to be effective against squamous cell carcinomas in other sites will be equally beneficial in the treatment of vulvar cancers.

Malignant Melanoma of the Vulva

The accepted therapy for malignant melanoma of the vulva includes radical vulvectomy with bilateral inguinal and pelvic lymphadenectomy. In addition, a broader strip of skin is excised from the inguinal regions

Table 11-9
Chemotherapeutic Agents Producing Remission in Squamous
Cell Carcinomas of the Vulva

Chemotherapeutic Agent	Patients	Objective Remission
Single Drug:		
Adriamycin	6	4 (67%)
Bleomycin	32	20 (62%)
Methotrexate	5	2 (40%)
Drug Combination:		
Bleomycin, Methotrexate	1	1 (100%)
Cyclophosphamide, 5-Fluorouracil, Actinomycin D, Vincristine, Cytosine Arabinoside, Methotrexate, and Bleomycin	1	1 (100%)

Data from Barlow et al (1973), Blum et al (1973), Bull et al (1972), Chamoun et al (1974), Deppe et al (1977), Encalada et al (1973), Forney et al (1975), Gorgun et al (1967), Haffner et al (1970), Ichikawa et al (1970), Masterson et al (1965), Mosher et al (1972), Schneider et al (1973), Sirisabya (1974), Srivannaboon et al (1973), Tojo et al (1972), and Vogl et al (1976).

since melanomas tend to produce intracutaneous satellite lesions. Morrow and Rutledge (1972), after reviewing the sites of recurrence in vulvar melanoma, concluded that the weakest point in the operative management of this disease was the vaginal or urethral margin. Consequently, every effort should be made to excise a wide margin of normal vaginal mucosa with the specimen. The aggressive surgical approach advocated by most investigators is warranted because of the propensity of melanomas for lymphatic spread. Also, most melanomas involve the anterior vulva or clitoris, and may spread directly to the deep pelvic nodes. The high incidence of bilateral lymph nodal spread in vulvar melanomas makes unilateral surgical procedures impractical.

Recently, several retrospective studies have related metastatic behavior to the depth of invasion in malignant melanoma. Balch and colleagues (1979) noted no local recurrences or regional lymph nodal metastases in Stage I melanomas less than 0.76 mm thick. Similarly, Bagley and co-workers (1981) reported that no patient with a Clark's level II or III lesion less than 0.76 mm thick died of recurrent melanoma. These investigators concluded that prophylactic regional lymphadenectomy was of no value in these patients, and that lesions invading the stroma less than 0.76 mm should be treated by wide excision alone. A margin of normal tissue of at least two times the diameter of the melanoma minimized the risk of local recurrence. This data concerning minimally invasive melanomas is quite convincing, but has yet to be confirmed in vulvar cases. The therapeutic benefit of regional lymphadenectomy was obvious in more deeply invasive melanomas. The five-year survival of patients treated for melanomas of intermediate (0.77 mm to 3.99 mm) thickness with wide local excision and regional lymphadenectomy was significantly higher (86%) than when these lesions were treated by wide local excision alone (56%). It would seem, therefore, that radical vulvectomy with inguinal and pelvic lymphadenectomy is the treatment of choice in patients with vulvar melanomas more than 0.76 thick. Further clinical trials will be necessary to substantiate the efficacy of wide local excision alone in the treatment of less invasive lesions. Melanomas have been shown to be quite resistant to irradiation (Chung et al 1975), and the use of radiation therapy in the treatment of vulvar melanomas is discouraged.

A variety of chemotherapeutic agents have been shown to have activity against metastatic melanoma. These include: melphalan (Nathanson et al 1967), imidazole carboxamide (Luce et al 1970), and high dose cyclophosphamide (Gotlieb et al 1970). Combination chemotherapy regimens also have been minimally effective in patients with disseminated melanoma. Cohen and co-workers (1972) reported that a combination of vincristine, BCNU, and imidazole carboximide produced objective tumor response in ten of 16 patients (62%). The majority of responses occurred in lymph nodal or cutaneous metastases, and the mean duration of remission was only three months. Two of these patients, however, had a complete response lasting in excess of nine months. Immunologic studies have demonstrated tumor antigens in malignant melanoma, and also, patients with localized melanoma or those undergoing spontaneous regression of disease have been shown to have a higher incidence of antimelanoma antibodies that those with advanced disease (Morton et al 1970). Intralesional injection with BCG has produced disappearance of cutaneous melanoma nodules. Immunotherapy, however, has not produced a significant prolongation of life in these patients.

Bartholin Gland Carcinoma

The recommended treatment of Bartholin gland carcinoma is radical vulvectomy and bilateral inguinal lymphadenectomy with partial resection of the levator muscle and wide vaginal excision on the involved side. As has been previously stated (Barclay et al 1964), there is some evidence that there can be direct spread of Bartholin gland carcinoma to the deep pelvic nodes without involving the intervening inguinal nodes. Therefore, pelvic lymphadenectomy is advocated routinely in the treatment of this disease.

Although there is little data concerning the use of chemotherapy in Bartholin gland cancer, adenocarcinomas of this gland should respond to a number of chemotherapeutic agents, including cisplatin and cyclophosphamide, that have shown activity against mucin-producing adenocarcinomas of other sites. Likewise, metastatic squamous cell tumors of Bartholin gland origin should be sensitive to those drugs proven effective against other squamous carcinomas of the vulva.

Vulvar Sarcomas

The treatment of sarcomas depends partly upon the size, cell type, and mitotic activity of each lesion. As has been previously mentioned, leiomyosarcoma is the most common type of vulvar sarcoma. The majority of these lesions are relatively slow growing and tend to recur locally (Davos and Abell 1975). The appropriate therapy of vulvar leiomyosarcoma is radical vulvectomy with bilateral groin dissection. Pelvic lymphadenectomy is not indicated unless metastatic disease is present in the inguinal lymph nodes. Patients with advanced stage anaplastic sarcomas having high mitotic activity may benefit from adjunctive chemotherapy in addition to radical surgery. The use of combination chemotherapy with vincristine, cyclophosphamide and adriamycin or actinomycin D markedly has improved the survival of children with vulvovaginal sarcomas (Rivard 1975, Kumar et al 1976). Radiation therapy has not been effective in the treatment of vulvar sarcomas (DiSaia et al 1971).

SURVIVAL AND FOLLOW-UP

In recent series of patients with vulvar dystrophies (Kaufman 1974) or intraepithelial neoplasia (Friedrich et al 1980, Iversen 1981), there have been no reported deaths due to recurrent disease. Patients with these abnormalities are usually seen individually as indicated, but should be examined at least every three months for one year and every six months thereafter for a minimum of five years.

The five-year survival of patients with invasive squamous cell carcinoma is presented in Table 11-10. Over 92% of patients with Stage I

Table 11-10
Five-Year Survival Related to Stage in Patients with Invasive Squamous Cell Carcinoma of the Vulva

Stage	Patients	Five-Year Survival
I	400	372 (93%)
II	197	162 (82%)
III	206	147 (71%)
IV	116	25 (22%)

Data from Franklin (1972), Green (1978), Japaze et al (1976), Krupp et al (1975), Magrina et al (1979), Morley (1976), Morris (1977), and Parker et al (1975).

318

Table 11-11
Five-Year Survival of Patients
with Positive Pelvic Nodes Treated Sugically

Investigator	Patients	Five-Year Survival
Way (1960)	9	2 (22.2%)
Rutledge (1970)	12	3 (25.0%)
Collins (1971)	11	1 (9.1%)
Morley (1976)	6	1 (16.7%)
Morris (1977)	3	1 (33.3%)
Green (1978)	18	2 (11.1%)
Curry (1980)	9	2 (22.2%)
TOTAL	68	12 (17.6%)

disease were free of disease five years after therapy as opposed to only 22% of patients with Stage IV disease. The relationship of lymph nodal metastases to prognosis is illustrated in Table 11-4. The presence of inguinal node metastases reduced the five-year survival from 89% to 40%. Only 17% of patients with tumor metastatic to the deep pelvic lymph nodes were alive five years after surgical treatment (Table 11-11).

The majority of recurrences from vulvar squamous cell carconima are located at the site of the previous vulvectomy incision, particularly at the mucosal margins, and in the groins (Rutledge et al 1970). These recurrences commonly are diagnosed within two years of treatment (Lundwall 1961). Approximately 25% of recurrent vulvar carcinomas will present as pelvic or distant metastases (Collins et al 1964) and characteristically occur within three years after initial therapy. Surgical excision of locally recurrent disease occasionally has been successful if performed when the size of the tumor recurrence is minimal. Likewise, pelvic exenteration can be effective in selected cases of advanced recurrent disease (Thornton and Flanagan 1973). Radiation therapy has been successful in treating groin metastases in approximately 15% to 20% of the cases (Linwall 1961). Extrapelvic metastases of squamous cell carcinoma generally have responded poorly to chemotherapy or radiation therapy.

Based on the pattern of tumor recurrence, patients with invasive squamous cell carcinoma of the vulva should be examined monthly during the first year after therapy, every two months for two years, and every six months thereafter.

The five-year survival of patients with malignant melanoma of the vulva is illustrated in Table 11-12. Approximately 34% of patients with vulvar melanoma were alive five years after treatment. It is pertinent to point out that a significant number of patients with melanoma will develop tumor recurrence more than five years following therapy. Karlen and co-workers (1975), eg, noted that 15% of patients with malignant melanoma of the vulva developed recurrences between five and ten years post therapy. Approximately two thirds of recurrent vulvar melanomas will develop locally or regionally. Characteristically, these tumors recur during the first two years after treatment, with the groin and vulva being the most common sites of occurrence. In reviewing the treatment of vulvar melanomas at the M.D. Anderson Hospital, Morrow and Rutledge (1972) reported that recurrences were related to staged procedures, local excision, unilateral surgery, or inadequate margins at the urethra or vagina.

Most commonly, local recurrences of melanoma are treated by wide excision. Various chemotherapeutic regimens have been used to treat metastatic disease, but without appreciable success. The median survival time following recurrent vulvar melanoma is approximately 12 months (Chung et al 1975). Following treatment, the recommended follow-up for patients with vulvar melanoma essentially is the same as that suggested for patients with squamous cell carcinoma of the vulva.

The survival of patients of Bartholin gland carcinoma is presented in Table 11-13. Masterson and Goss (1955) presented a review of the world's

Table 11-12
Five-Year Survival of Malignant Melanoma of the Vulva

Investigator	Patients	Five-year Survival
Das Gupta and D'Urso (1964)	23	7 (30%)
Pack and Oropeza (1967)	20	7 (35%)
Yackel et al (1970)	20	7 (35%)
Morrow and Rutledge (1972)	14	7 (50%)
Karlen et al (1975)	20	5 (25%)
Chung et al (1975)	33	11 (33%)
TOTAL	130	44 (34%)

Table 11-13
Five-Year Survival of Patients with Bartholin Gland Carcinoma

Investigator	Patients	Five-Year Survival
Review: Masterson and Goss (1955)	117	10 (8%)
Recent Series: Sackett (1950)	4	3 (75%)
Barclay et al (1964)	8	5 (62%)
Dodson et al (1970)	4	2 (50%)
Chamlian and Taylor (1972)	24	8 (33%)

literature up to 1955, and reported that the five-year survival of patients with Bartholin's gland cancer was only 8%. More recent investigators, however, have been able to achieve significantly higher survival rates with the use of radical surgery. These tumors characteristically recur locally, and radical surgical excision has been the most effective method of treatment.

Vulvar sarcomas are so rare that an accurate documentation of survival has been difficult. DiSaia and co-workers (1971) reported that five of 12 patients with vulvar sarcomas (42%) were living free of disease five years after therapy. Local recurrence was common, but over 80% of patients with recurrence eventually developed pulmonary metastases.

BIBLIOGRAPHY

Abitol M: Carcinoma of the vulva: Improvements in the surgical approach. *Am J Obstet Gynecol* 117:483–489, 1973.

Acosta A, Given FT, Frazier AB: Preoperative radiation therapy in the management of squamous cell carcinoma of the vulva. Preliminary report. *Am J Obstet Gynecol* 132:198–206, 1978.

Allen AC, Spitz S: Malignant melanoma, A clinicopathological analysis of the criteria for diagnosis and prognosis. *Cancer* 6:1–45, 1953.

Aurelian L, Davis HJ, Julian CJ: Herpesvirus type 2 induced tumor specific antigens in cervical carcinoma. *Am J Epidemiol* 98:1–9, 1973.

Bagley HF, Cady B, Lee A, et al: Changes in clinical presentation and management of malignant melanoma. *Cancer* 47:2126–2134, 1981.

Balch CM, Murad TM, Soong SJ, et al: Tumor thickness as a guide to surgical management of clinical stage I melanoma patients. *Cancer* 43:883–888, 1979.

Barclay DL, Collins CG: Intraepithelial cancer of the vulva. *Am J Obstet Gynecol* 86:95–106, 1963.

Barclay DL, Collins CG, Macey HB: Cancer of the Bartholin gland. A review and report of 8 cases. *Obstet Gynecol* 24:329–336, 1964.

Barlow JJ, Piver MS, Chuang JT, et al: Adriamycin and bleomycin, alone and in combination, in gynecologic cancers. *Cancer* 32:735–743, 1973.

Barnes A, Crissman J, Schellhas H, et al: Microinvasive carcinoma of the vulva: A clinicopathologic evaluation. *Obstet Gynecol* 56:234–238, 1980.

Blum RH, Carter SK, Agre K: A clinical review of bleomycin: A new antineoplastic agent. *Cancer* 31:903–914, 1973.

Boehm F, Morris J: Paget's disease and apocrine gland carcinoma of the vulva. *Obstet Gynecol* 38:185–192, 1971.

Boronow RC: Therapeutic alternative to primary exenteration for advanced vulvovaginal cancer. *Gynecol Oncol* 1:233–255, 1973.

Boutselis JG: Intraepithelial carcinoma of the vulva. *Am J Obstet Gynecol* 113:733–738, 1972.

Bowen JD: Precancerous dermatoses. *J Autan Dis* 30:241–243, 1912.

Boyce CR, Mehram AH: Management of vulvar malignancies. *Am J Obstet Gynecol* 119:48–58, 1974.

Breslow A: Thickness, cross sectional areas and depth of invasion in the prognosis of cutaneous melanoma. *Ann Surg* 11:902–908, 1970.

Breslow A: Tumor thickness, level of invasion and node dissection in stage I cutaneous melanoma. *Ann Surg* 182:572–575, 1975.

Bricker EM, Burcher N, McAffee CA: Late results of bladder substitution with ileal segments. *Surg Gynecol Obstet* 99:469–474, 1954.

Brunschwig A, Daniel W: Pelvic exenterations for advanced carcinoma of the vulva. *Am J Obstet Gynecol* 72:489–496, 1956.

Buchler DA: Multiple primaries and gynecologic malignancies. *Am J Obstet Gynecol* 123:376–381, 1975.

Buchler DA, Kline JC, Tunker JC, et al: Treatment of recurrent carcinoma of the vulva. *Obstet Gynecol Survey* 35:186–188, 1980.

Bull CA, Biggs JC, Newton NC, et al: Bleomycin in squamous cell carcinoma. *Med J Aust* 2:704–707, 1972.

Buscema J, Woodruff JP, Parmley TH, et al: Carcinoma in situ of the vulva. *Obstet Gynecol* 55:225–230, 1980.

Chamlian DL, Taylor HB: Primary carcinoma of Bartholin's gland. A report of 24 patients. *Obstet Gynecol* 39:489–494, 1972.

Chamoun CD, Downing V, Huseby RA: Vulvar carcinoma treated successfully. *Rocky Mt Med J* 71:89–93, 1974.

Chung AF, Woodruff JM, Lewis JL: Malignant melanoma of the vulva. A report of 44 cases. *Obstet Gynecol* 45:638–646, 1975.

Chung CK, Nahhas W, Stryker JA: Analysis of factors contributing to treatment failures in stages Ib and IIa carcinoma of the cervix. *Am J Obstet Gynecol* 138:550–556, 1980.

Clark JA, Muller SA: Lichen slcerosus et atrophicus in children. *Arch Dermatol* 45:638–642, 1967.

Clark WH, From L, Bernadino EA, et al: The histogenesis and biologic behavior of primary human malignant melanoma. *Cancer Res* 29:705–726, 1969.

Cohen SM, Greenspan EM, Weiner RJ: Triple combination chemotherapy of disseminated melanoma. *Cancer* 29:1489–1493, 1972.

Collins CG, Collins JH, Barclay DL, et al: Cancer involving the vulva. A report on 109 consecutive cases. *Am J Obstet Gynecol* 87:762–769,1963.

Collins CG, Hansen LH, Theirot E: A clinical stain for use in selecting biopsy sites in patients with vulvar disease. *Obstet Gynecol* 28:158–162, 1966.

Collins CG, Roman-Lopez JJ, Lee FYL: Intraepithelial carcinoma of the vulva. *Am J Obstet Gynecol* 108:1187–1191, 1970.

Collins CG, Lee FYL, Roman-Lopez JJ: Invasive carcinoma of the vulva with lymph node metastases. *Am J Obstet Gynecol* 109:446–452, 1971.

Creasman WT, Gallager HS, Rutledge F: Paget's disease of the vulva. *Gynecol Oncol* 3:133–148, 1975.

Curry SL, Wharton JT, Rutledge F: Positive lymph nodes in vulvar squamous carcinoma. *Gynecol Oncol* 9:63–67, 1980.

Daly JW, Million RR: Radical vulvectomy combined with elective node irradiation for $T_x N_0$ squamous carcinoma of the vulva. *Cancer* 34:161–165, 1974.

Das Gupta, D'Urso: Melanoma of the female genitalia. *Surg Gynecol Obstet* 119:1074–1078, 1964.

Davos I, Abell MR: Soft tissue sarcomas of vulva. *Gynecol Oncol* 4:70–86, 1976.

Dean RE, Taylor ES, Weisbrad DM, et al: The treatment of premalignant and malignant lesions of the vulva. *Am J Obstet Gynecol* 119:59–68, 1974.

Deligdisch L, Szulman AE: Multiple and multifocal carcinomas in female genital organs and breast. *Gynecol Oncol* 3:181–190, 1975.

Deppe G, Bruckner HW, Cohen CJ: Adriamycin treatment of advanced vulvar carcinoma. *Obstet Gynecol* 50:135–145, 1977.

Dinner MI, Peters CR, Martinbeau P, et al: Perineal reconstruction following extended radical vulvectomy. *Gynecol Oncol* 8:78–83, 1979.

DiPaola GR, Gomez-Rueda N: Relevance of microinvasion in carcinoma of the vulva. *Obstet Gynecol* 45:647–649, 1975.

DiSaia PJ, Rutledge MD, Smith JP: Sarcoma of the vulva. Report of 12 patients. *Obstet Gynecol* 38:180–184, 1971.

DiSaia PJ, Creasman WT, Rich WM: An alternate approach to early cancer of the vulva. *Am J Obstet Gynecol* 133:825–832, 1979.

Dockerty MD, Pratt J: Extramammary Paget's disease. *Cancer* 5:1161–1169, 1952.

Dodson MG, O'Leary JA, Averette HE: Primary carcinoma Bartholin's gland. *Obstet Gynecol* 35:578–584, 1970.

Donaldson ES, Powell D, Hanson M, et al: Prognostic parameters in invasive vulvar cancer. *Gynecol Oncol* 11:184–190, 1981.

Eichner E, Barclay DL, Collins CG: Discussion of intraepithelial cancer of the vulva. *Am J Obstet Gynecol* 86:95–106, 1963.

Elias EG, Mukund SD, Goel IP: A clinicopathological study of prognostic factors in cutaneous malignant melanoma. *Surg Gynecol Obstet* 114:327–334, 1977.

Encalada J, Bigalli A, Fernandez CA, et al: Clinical study of treatment with bleomycin in malignant tumors. *Acta Folha Med* 67:25–29, 1973.

Fenn M, Morley GW, Abell MR: Paget's disease of the vulva. *Obstet Gynecol* 38:660–670, 1971.

Fetherston WC, Friedrich EG: The origin and significance of vulvar Paget's disease. *Obstet Gynecol* 39:735–744, 1972.

Figge DC, Gaudenz R: Invasive carcinoma of the vulva. *Am J Obstet Gynecol* 119:382–395, 1974.

Forney JP, Morrow CP, DiSaia PJ et al: Seven-drug polychemotherapy in the treatment of advanced and recurrent squamous carcinoma of the female genital tract. *Am J Obstet Gynecol* 123:748–752, 1975.

Foye G, Marsh MR, Minhowitz S: Verrucous carcinoma of the vulva. *Obstet Gynecol* 34:484–487, 1969.

Frankendal B, Larsson LG, Westling P: Carcinoma of the vulva: Results of an individualized treatment schedule. *Acta Radiol Ther Biol* 12:165–174, 1973.

Franklin EW, Rutledge FD: Prognostic factors in epidermoid carcinoma of the vulva. *Obstet Gynecol* 37:892–901, 1971.

Franklin EW, Rutledge FD: Epidemiology of epidermoid carcinoma of the vulva. *Obstet Gynecol* 39:165–172, 1972.

Franklin EW: Clinical staging of carcinoma of the vulva. *Obstet Gynecol* 40:277–286, 1972.

Friedrich EG: Topical testosterone for benign vulvar dystrophy. *Obstet Gynecol* 37:677–686, 1971.

Friedrich EG: Reversible vulvar atypia. A case report. *Obstet Gynecol* 39:173–181, 1972.

Friedrich E, Wilkinson E, Steingraeber P, et al: Paget's disease of the vulva and carcinoma of the breast. *Obstet Gynecol* 46:130–134, 1975.

Friedrich EG: New nomeclature for vulvar disease. Report of The Committee on Terminology. *Obstet Gynecol* 47:122–124, 1976.

Friedrich EG, DiPaola GR: Postoperative staging of vulvar carcinoma: A retrospective study. *Int Gynecol Obstet* 15:270–274, 1977.

Friedrich EG, Wilkinson EJ in Blaustein (ed): *The Vulva in Pathology of the Female Genital Tract.* New York, Springer Verlag, Ancel. 1977, Chap 2.

Friedrich G, Wilkinson EH, Fu YS: Carcinoma in situ of the vulva: A continuing challenge. *Am J Obstet Gynecol* 136:830–843, 1980.

Frischbier HJ, Thomsen K: Treatment of cancer of the vulva with high energy electrons. *Am J Obstet Gynecol* 111:431–435, 1971.

Gallousis S: Verrucous carcinoma. *Obstet Gynecol* 40:502–507, 1972.

Goldsmith H: Melanoma, *In Practice of Surgery*. New York, Harper and Row. 1978, pp 1–26.

Gorgun B, Goplerud DR, Watne AL: Intra-arterial chemotherapy in advanced pelvic tumors. *Arch Surg* 94:251–257, 1967.

Gotlieb J, Mendelson D, Serpick A: An evaluation of large intermittent doses of cyclophosphamide (NSC-26271) in the treatment of metastatic malignant melanoma. *Cancer Chemother Rep* 54:365–368, 1970.

Green TH: Carcinoma of the vulva. A reassessment. *Obstet Gynecol* 52:462–469, 1978.

Gumport SL, Harris MN, Roses DF, The diagnosis and management of common skin cancers. *Cancer* 31:79–90, 1981.

Gunn R, Gallager S: Vulvar Paget's disease: A topographic study. *Cancer* 46:590–594, 1980.

Haffner WHJ, Frick HC: Intermittent intravenous methotrexate in the treatment of advanced epidermoid carcinoma of the cervix and vulvovagina. *Cancer* 26:812–815, 1970.

Hart WR, Norris HJ, Helwig EB: Relation of lichen sclerosus et atrophicus of the vulva to development of carcinoma. *Obstet Gynecol* 45:369–377, 1975.

Hart WH, Millman J: Progression of intraepithelial Paget's disease of the vulva to invasive carcinoma. *Cancer* 40:2333–2337, 1977.

Hay DM, Cole FM: Postgranulomatous epidermoid carcinoma of the vulva. *Am J Obstet Gynecol* 108:479–484, 1970.

Helgason NM, Hass AC, Latourette HB: Radiation therapy in carcinoma of the vulva: A review of 53 patients. *Cancer* 30:997–1000, 1972.

Helwig EB, Graham JH: Anogenital (extramammary) Paget's disease. *Cancer* 16:387–403, 1963.

Hilgers RD, Malkasian GD, Soule EH: Embryonal rhabdomyosarcoma (botryoid type) of the vagina. *Am J Obstet Gynecol* 107:484–502, 1970.

Hunter DJS: Carcinoma of the vulva: A review of 361 patients. *Gynecol Oncol* 3:117–123, 1975.

Ichikawa T: Discovery of clinical effect of bleomycin against squamous cell carcinoma and further development of its research. *Asian Med J* 13:210–221, 1970.

Iverson T, Abeler V, Kolstad P: Squamous cell carcinoma in situ of the vulva. A clinical and histopathological study. *Gynecol Oncol* 11:224–229, 1981.

Jafari K, Cartnick E: Microinvasive squamous cell carcinoma of the vulva. *Gynecol Oncol* 4:158–166, 1976.

Japaze H, Garcia-Bunuel R, Woodruff JD: Primary vulvar neoplasia. *Obstet Gynecol* 49:404–411, 1977.

Jeffcoate TNA, Woodcock AS: Premalignant conditions of the vulva with particular reference to chronic epithelial dystrophies. *Br Med J* 2:127–134, 1961.

Jeffcoate TNA: Chronic vulvar dystrophies. *Am J Obstet Gynecol* 95:61–74, 1966.

Jimerson GK, Merrill JA: Multicentric squamous malignancy involving the cervix and vulva. *Cancer* 26:150–153, 1970.

Josey WE, Nahmias AJ, Naib ZM: Viruses and cancer of the lower genital tract. *Cancer* 38:526–533, 1976.

Kaplan AL, Kaufman RH: Management of advanced carcinoma of the vulva. *Gynecol Oncol* 3:220–232, 1975.

Karlen JR, Piver MS, Barlow JJ: Melanoma of the vulva. *Obstet Gynecol* 45:181–185, 1975.

Katayama KP, Woodruff JD, Jones HW: Chromosomes of condyloma acuminatum, Paget's disease, in situ carcinoma, invasive squamous cell carcinoma and malignant melanoma of the human vulva. *Obstet Gynecol* 39:346–356, 1972.

Kaufman RH, Gardener HL, Brown D, et al: Vulvar dystrophies: An evaluation. *Am J Obstet Gynecol* 120:363–367, 1974.

Koss LG, Ladinsky S, Brockunier A: Paget's disease of the vulva. Report of 10 cases. *Obstet Gynecol* 31:513–525, 1968.

Kovi J, Tillman RL, Lee SM: Malignant transformation of condyloma acuminatum. *Am J Clin Pathol* 61:702–710, 1974.

Krupp PJ, Lee FYL, Bohm JW, et al: Prognostic parameters and clinical staging criteria in epidermoid carcinoma of the vulva. *Obstet Gynecol* 46:84–88, 1975.

Krupp PJ, Lee F, Bohm JW et al: Therapy of advanced epidermoid carcinoma of vulva. Report of 13 patients, with review of recent literature. *Obstet Gynecol* 46:433–438, 1975.

Krupp PJ, Bohm JW, Lee FYL: Current status of the treatment of epidermoid cancer of the vulva. *Cancer* 38:587–595, 1976.

Krupp PJ, Bohm JW: Lymph gland metastases in invasive squamous cell cancer of the vulva. *Am J Obstet Gynecol* 130:943–952, 1978.

Kumar AP, Wrenn EL, Fleming ID, et al: Combined therapy to prevent complete pelvic exenteration for rhabdomyosarcoma of the vagina or uterus. *Cancer* 37:118–122, 1976.

Kunschner A, Kanbour AI, David B: Early vulvar carcinoma. *Am J Obstet Gynecol* 132:599–606, 1978.

Lash AF, Zibel M: Carcinoma of the vulva in a young woman. *Am J Obstet Gynecol* 62:216–219, 1951.

Lee SC, Roth LM, Ehrlich C: Extramammary Paget's disease of the vulva. *Cancer* 39:2540–2549, 1977.

Lister UM, Akinla O: Carcinoma of the vulva in childhood. *J Obstet Gynecol Brit Comm* 79:470–473, 1972.

Lucas WE, Benirschke K, Lebherz TB: Verrucous carcinoma of the female genital tract. *Am J Obstet Gynecol* 119:435–440, 1974.

Luce JK, Thurman WB, Isaacs B, et al: Clinical trials with the antitumor agent 5(3,3 dimethyl-1-triazeno) imidazole 4-carboxamide (NSC-45388). *Cancer Chemother Rep* 54:119–123, 1970.

Lundwall R: Cancer of the vulva. A clinical review. *Acta Radiol Suppl* 208:1–218, 1961.

Magrina JF, Webb MJ, Gaffey TA: Stage I squamous cell cancer of the vulva. *Am J Obstet Gynecol* 134:453–459, 1979.

Mann PR, Cowan MA: Ultrastructural changes in four cases of lichen sclerosus et atrophicus. *Br J Dermatol* 89:223–231, 1973.

Masterson JG, Gross AS: Carcinoma of the Bartholin's gland. Review of the literature and report of a new case in an elderly patient treated by radical operation. *Am J Obstet Gynecol* 69:1323–1332, 1955.

Masterson JG, Nelson HJ: The role of chemotherapy in the treatment of gynecologic malignancy. *Am J Obstet Gynecol* 93:1102–1111, 1965.

McAdams AJ, Kistner BH: Relationship of chronic vulvar disease, leukoplakia and carcinoma in situ to carcinoma of the vulva. *Cancer* 11:740–757, 1958.

McKelvey JL: Carcinoma of the vulva: Classification, treatment and results. *Proc Natl Cancer Conf* 6:361–364, 1970.

Merrill JA, Ross NL: Cancer of the vulva. *Cancer* 14:13–20, 1961.

Miller TR, Pack GT: The familial aspect of malignant melanoma. *Arch Derm* 86:35–43, 1962.

Morley GW: Infiltrative carcinoma of the vulva: Results of surgical treatment. *Am J Obstet Gynecol* 124:874–888, 1976.

Morris JM: A formula for selected lymphadenectomy. Its application to cancer of the vulva. *Obstet Gynecol* 50:152–158, 1977.

Morrow CP, Rutledge FN: Melanoma of the vulva. *Obstet Gynecol* 39:745–752, 1972.

Morrow CP, DiSaia PJ: Malignant melanoma of the female genitalia: A clinical analysis. *Obstet Gynecol Survey* 31:233–271, 1976.

Morton DL, Eilber FR: Immunological factors which influence response to immunotherapy in malignant melanoma. *Surgery* 68:158–164, 1970.

Mosher MG, Deconti RC, Bertino JR: Bleomycin therapy in advanced Hodgkin's disease and epidermoid cancers. *Cancer* 30:56–60, 1972.

Nakao C, Nolan J, DiSaia PJ: "Microinvasive" epidermoid carcinoma of the vulva with an unexpected natural history. *Am J Obstet Gynecol* 120:1122–1123, 1974.

Nathanson L, Hall TC, Vaniter GF, Farber S: Melanoma as a medical problem. *Arch Intern Med* 119:479–492, 1967.

Pack GT, Oropeza R: A comparative study of melanoma and epidermoid carcinomas of the vulva: A review of 44 melanomas and 58 epidermoid carcinomas (1930–1965). *Rev Surg* 24:305–324, 1968.

Parker RT, Duncan I, Rampone J: Operative management of early invasive epidermoid carcinoma of the vulva. *Am J Obstet Gynecol* 123:349–355, 1975.

Parmley TH, Woodruff JD, Julian CG: Invasive vulvar Paget's disease. *Obstet Gynecol* 46:341–346, 1975.

Piver MS, Xynos FP: Pelvic lymphadenectomy in women with carcinoma of the clitoris. *Obstet Gyencol* 49:592–595, 1977.

Plentyl A, Friedman E: *Lymphatic System of the Female Genitalia.* Philadelphia, W.B. Saunders, 1971, pp 27–50.

Rivard G, Ortega J, Hittle R, et al: Intensive chemotherapy as primary treatment of rhabdomyosarcoma of the pelvis. *Cancer* 36:1593–1597, 1975.

Roth L, Lee S, Ehrlich C: Paget's disease of the vulva. *Am J Surg Path* 1:193–206, 1977.

Rutledge FN, Sinclair M: Treatment of intraepithelial carcinoma of the vulva by skin excision and grafts. *Am J Obstet Gynecol* 102:806–818, 1968.

Rutledge FN, Smith J, Franklin EW: Carcinoma of the vulva. *Am J Obstet Gynecol* 106:1117–1130, 1970.

Sackett NB: Carcinoma primary in Bartholin's gland: Case report. *Am J Obstet Gynecol* 75:183–188, 1958.

Schneider J, Gerhartz H: Treatment of squamous epithelial carcinoma with bleomycin. *Verh Dtsch Ges Inn Med* 78:163–166, 1973.

Seski JC, Reinhalter ER, Silva J: Abnormalities of lymphocyte transformations in women with intraepithelial carcinoma of the vulva. *Obstet Gynecol* 52:332–336, 1978.

Shingleton HM, Fowler WC, Palumbo C, et al: Carcinoma of the vulva. Influence of radical operation on survival cure rate. *Obstet Gynecol* 35:1–6, 1970.

Sirisabya N: Clinical trial of bleomycin on female genital cancer: A preliminary report. *J Med Assoc Thai* 57:135–138, 1974.

Smith FR, Pollock RS: Carcinoma of the vulva. Results of treatment and effect of special factors on results. *Surg Gynecol Obstet* 84:78–83, 1947.

Srivannaboon S, Boonyanit S, Vatananusara C, et al: A clinical trial of bleomycin on carcinoma of the vulva: A preliminary report. *J Med Assoc Thai* 56:101–108, 1973.

Taki I, Janovski N: Paget's disease of the vulva: Presentation and histochemical study of 4 cases. *Obstet Gynecol* 108:385–391, 1961.

Taussig FJ: Leukoplakia and cancer of the vulva. *Arch Dermatol Syphilol* 21:431–445, 1930.

Taussig FJ: A study of the lymph glands in cancer of the cervix and cancer of the vulva. *Am J Obstet Gynecol* 36:819–832, 1938.

Taussig FJ: Carcinoma of the vulva. An analysis of 155 cases 1911–1940. *Am J Obstet Gynecol* 40:764–779, 1949.

Taylor P, Stenwig JT, Klausen H: Paget's disease of the vulva. A report of 18 cases. *Gynecol Oncol* 3:46–60, 1975.

Tchang F, Okagaki T, Richart R: Adenocarcinoma of Bartholin's gland associated with Paget's disease of the vulvar area. *Cancer* 31:221–225, 1973.

Thornton WN, Flanagan WC: Pelvic exenteration in the treatment of advanced malignancy of the vulva. *Am J Obstet Gynecol* 117:774–781, 1973.

Tojo S, Matsuura Y, Oku T: Therapeutic effects of bleomycin on vulvar carcinoma. *Advan Obstet Gynecol* 24:236–246, 1972.

Tompkins MG, Conklin FJ, MacLeod S: Vulvar carcinoma. *Am J Obstet Gynecol* 82:16–23, 1961.

Tsukada Y, Lopez R, Pickren JW, et al: Paget's disease of the vulva. A clinicopathologic study of 8 cases. *Obstet Gynecol* 45:73–78, 1975.

Wharton LR, Everett HS: Primary malignant Bartholin's gland tumors. *Obstet Gynecol Survey* 6:1–8, 1951.

Wharton JT, Gallager S, Rutledge FN: Microinvasive carcinoma of the vulva. *Am J Obstet Gynecol* 118:159–164, 1974.

Williams GA, Richardson AC, Hathcock EW: Topical testosterone in dystrophic diseases of the vulva. *Am J Obstet Gynecol* 96:21–30, 1966.

Woodruff JD, Baens JS: Interpretation of atrophic and hypertrophic alterations in the vulvar epithelium. *Am J Obstet Gynecol* 86:713–723, 1963.

Woodruff JD: Pathology of malignant melanoma, part II. *Clin Bull* 7:52–59, 1976.

Woodruff JD, Julian CG, Puray T: The contemporary challenge of carcinoma in situ of the vulva. *Am J Obstet Gynecol* 115:677–686, 1973.

Yackel DB, Symmonds RE, Kempers RD: Melanoma of the vulva. *Obstet Gynecol* 35:625–630, 1970.

Yazigi R, Piver MS, Tsukada Y: Microinvasive carcinoma of the vulva. *Obstet Gynecol* 51:368–370, 1978.

Zelle K: Treatment of vulvar dystrophies with topical testosterone proprionate. *Am J Obstet Gynecol* 109:570–573, 1971.

zur Hausen H: Condylomata acuminata and human genital cancer. *Cancer Res* 36:794, 1976.

12 Trophoblastic Disease

Michael B. Hanson

During the past two decades, there have been significant advances in the diagnosis and therapy of patients with gestational trophoblastic disease. Notable among these advances have been: 1) the development of a clinical classification system based on the extent and location of disease rather than on the pathology of trophoblastic tumors, 2) the development of chemotherapeutic agents which are highly effective against both localized and metastatic trophoblastic disease, and 3) the perfection of a specific radioimmunoassay for human chorionic gonadotropin (hCG), thereby allowing its use as a reliable method to monitor the response of trophoblastic malignancy to treatment. These advances have resulted in a marked increase in the survival of patients with trophoblastic tumors. However, a significant number of patients with trophoblastic disease are still misdiagnosed each year, and such errors in diagnosis often result in morbidity and even mortality. A most fundamental prerequisite to a thorough understanding of trophoblastic disease is the realization that patients with these tumors present with a variety of different symptoms.

In this chapter the common symptoms of patients with trophoblastic

328

disease will be reviewed. Special sections will be devoted to the etiology, evaluation, and therapy of trophoblastic tumors. As in other types of gynecologic cancer, therapy must be strictly individualized according to the anatomic extent and malignant potential of each trophoblastic tumor.

ETIOLOGY

The etiology of gestational trophoblastic disease remains unknown. However, the geographical distribution of patients with trophoblastic disease has been defined and endemic areas identified. The prevalence of gestational trophoblastic disease ranges from 1 in 80 pregnancies in Southeast Asia, Mexico, and India to 1 in 4000 pregnancies in Northern Europe (Table 12-1). In the United States, trophoblastic disease occurs with a frequency of 1 per 2000 live births. In general, it occurs most frequently in populations with low socioeconomic status and a high incidence of malnutrition (Teoh 1971, Marquez-Monter 1968, Acosta-Sison 1949). Commonly available staple foods in endemic areas are rice, corn, and beans. A dietary relationship to hydatidiform mole may not exist as an inherent deficiency of a specific type of food, but rather may reflect the methods by which foods are prepared (Reynolds 1976). One nutritional deficiency associated with trophoblastic abnormalities is that of folic acid (Hibbard 1965). Folic acid is required for cellular metabolism, and its deficiency can prevent normal replication of any rapidly dividing cells including the trophoblast. Prolonged boiling of rice, beans, and corn, as practiced in many areas endemic for hydatidiform mole, destroys up to 95% of dietary folic acid, and may deprive early embryonic and trophoblastic cells of the nutritional elements required for normal development.

Table 12-1
Prevalence of Hydatidiform Mole According to Geographic Location

Author	Country	Prevalence per Number of Live Births
Wei and Ouyang (1963)	Taiwan	1/80
Acosta-Sison (1956)	Philippines	1/170
Marquez-Monter (1963)	Mexico	1/200
Brindeau et al (1952)	France	1/500
Beischer and Fortune (1968)	Australia	1/695
Teoh et al (1971)	Singapore	1/823
McCorriston (1968)	Hawaii	1/1326
Yen and McMahon (1968)	U.S.A.	1/1450
Hertig and Sheldon (1947)	U.S.A.	1/2050
Brewer and Gerbie (1967)	U.S.A.	1/2100

Certain investigators (Pascasio 1970, Pour-Reza 1974) have reported decreased total protein and albumin levels in patients with gestational trophoblastic disease. To date, however, it remains unclear as to whether protein deficiency is a causative factor in gestational trophoblast disease or if the developing trophoblast simply has an increased demand for protein which leads to a hypoproteinemic state in the patient who already has a dietary deficiency of protein.

Other factors have also been associated with an increased incidence of gestational trophoblastic disease. For example, hydatidiform mole has been shown to be more common in teenagers and in women over the age of 40 (Bagshawe 1976, Teoh 1971). Multiparous women have been reported to have a higher incidence of hydatidiform mole than those of low parity. The reasons for these statistical observations remain to be elucidated. Certain ABO blood group matings have been associated with an increased risk for the development of choriocarcinoma. An analysis of ABO matings in 317 patients with gestational trophoblastic disease by Bagshawe (1976) revealed a relative risk of developing choriocarcinoma in A x O and O x A matings of over 2.0. In a study of 347 patients with hydatidiform mole, however, Curry and co-workers (1975) could find no association between the incidence of gestational trophoblastic disease and age, parity, or blood type. Likewise, specific HLA haplotypes do not appear to be significantly associated with an increased risk for developing trophoblastic malignancy (Bagshawe 1976).

Although the precise etiology of trophoblastic disease is unknown, there is more agreement concerning the underlying pathologic events prior to the development of these tumors. Hertig and Edmonds (1940) and Park (1971) have postulated the two most widely held theories concerning pathogenesis of hydatidiform mole. Hertig advocated that the changes seen in molar pregnancy result from fetal circulatory inadequacy, and that most moles, if examined early enough, contain at least a rudimentary fetal sac. Failure of the growth of fetal vessels into the villous stroma from the intervillous spaces causes the villi to become hydropic, but trophoblasts are "nourished maternally" and continue to proliferate. Park's theory of pathogenesis identifies the trophoblast itself as the causative factor in gestational trophoblastic disease. According to this theory (Park 1971), secretion of fluid by the abnormal trophoblast leads to hydropic degeneration of the chorionic villi, obliteration of villous vasculature, and ultimate death of the fetus. The reasons for excessive trophoblastic proliferation, however, are not specified.

Hydatidiform moles have been divided by Vassilakos and colleagues (1977) into "partial" and "complete" moles. Partial moles have hydropic villi interspersed among normal villi, and are associated with a fetus, cord, or amniotic membranes. Trophoblastic cells are atrophic, and hyperplasia or anaplasia is usually focal. Most partial moles have chromosomal abnormalities, with triploidy and trisomy 16 being the most frequent. A large number of patients with this type of mole have been observed, and malignant degeneration is very rare (Vassilakos 1977, Szulman 1978, Berkowitz 1979).

Complete moles are not associated with a fetus, cord, or amniotic membranes, and all have a 46 XX chromosomal pattern (Vassilakos 1977, Kajii 1977, Jacobs 1978). Both syncytiotrophoblasts and cytotrophoblasts show marked hyperplasia and anaplasia. Patients with complete moles have been shown to develop malignant sequelae (Vassilakos 1977), and these lesions are thought to be precursors of choriocarcinoma. There is no transition between partial and complete moles. The characteristics of a mole are genetically determined and are expressed phenotypically before eight weeks of gestation (Szulman 1978). Complete hydatidiform moles are believed to be a result of androgenesis, ie, the development of an ovum under the influence of a spermatozoon nucleus with the original nucleus of the ovum being either absent or inactivated. Theoretically, this may occur in two ways. First, nondivision at the second meiotic division could result in a diploid sperm for fertilization. Alternatively, a haploid sperm could cause fertilization and subsequently duplicate its chromosomes after meiotic division. Analysis using fluorescent Q and R band polymorphism (Kajii 1977, Jacobs 1978, Wake 1978) indicates that all the chromosomes of complete hydatidiform moles come from the paternal parent. Yamashita et al (1979), studying the presence of HLA antigens on the cell surface, reported that these antigens were identical to those of the father but different from those of the mother. Because the HLA antigens studied were homozygous, these investigators concluded that fertilization must have occurred with a haploid sperm followed by duplication as a postmeiotic event. Since the complete mole appears to be derived entirely from paternal genetic components, it would act as a complete allograft. Therefore, the host could theoretically activate an immune response against the foreign antigenic material present on the cell surface of this type of molar tissue.

PATHOLOGY

For practical purposes, gestational trophoblastic disease can be classified pathologically into hydatidiform mole, chorioadenoma destruens, and choriocarcinoma. Although the histologic characteristics for each of these entities are sufficiently distinct, it should be emphasized that both chorioadenoma destruens and choriocarcinoma may demonstrate metastatic behavior.

Hydatidiform Mole

Both normal and neoplastic trophoblastic cells share certain morphologic characteristics including: 1) rapid proliferation, 2) infiltration,

3) vascular invasion, 4) hematogenous dissemination, and 5) spontaneous regression. However, the normal placenta can be easily differentiated histologically from hydatidiform mole. Unlike the villi of the normal placenta, which are of a delicate branching pattern, the villi of hydatidiform mole are distended by fluid and form grape-like vesicles (Figure 12-1). Each vesicle is a cystic villus with no intrinsic vessels and whose stroma is replaced by fluid. Adjacent vesicles are connected by strands of connective tissue. Vesicles vary in size up to approximately one inch in diameter. Microscopically, three criteria are used to differentiate hydatidiform mole from its normal counterpart:

1. Hydropic swelling of the villous stroma.
2. Marked decrease or complete absence of fetal vessels in the villi.
3. Proliferation of the trophoblast.

Trophoblasts infiltrate the uterus at the implantation site in a manner similar to a normal gestation. However, the total quantity of trophoblastic tissue seen in gestational trophoblastic disease exceeds that of normal gestation (Figure 12-2).

Many investigators have subdivided hydatidiform moles into groups according to the histologic characteristics of the trophoblastic tissue and the amount of its proliferation, in an attempt to determine the biological behavior of each tumor (Hertig and Sheldon 1947, Curry 1975, Driscoll 1977). Driscoll (1977), for example, divided hydatidiform moles according to the degree of hyperplastic and differentiation of the trophoblast.

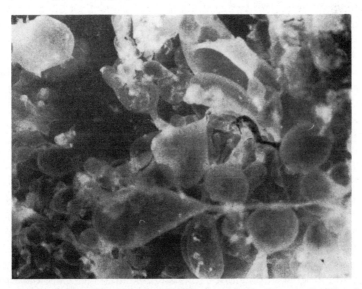

Figure 12-1 Hydatidiform mole. Note the varying sized cystically dilated villi.

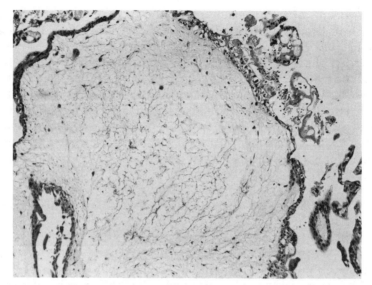

Figure 12-2 Hydatidiform mole. The large avascular hydropic villus is surrounded by trophoblast showing mild proliferation. Hematoxylin and eosin stain (magnification 100 ×).

Grade I tumors were characterized by minimal hyperplasia and well-differentiated trophoblast, while grade III tumors exhibited marked hyperplasia and poorly differentiated trophoblastic cells. These investigators were able to correlate tumor grade with hCG production, potential for malignancy, and prognosis. The degree of hyperplasia and differentiation may also be important in determining the response of complicated trophoblastic disease to chemotherapy. For example, Deligdisch and co-workers (1978) reported that a favorable response to chemotherapy was associated with a plexiform pattern of trophoblastic growth, maturation of the trophoblast, and deposition of fibrin-like material at the interface between the trophoblastic and host tissues. Histologic correlates associated with a poor clinical response were high mitotic activity and vascular invasion by tumor cells.

Chorioadenoma Destruens (Invasive Mole)

The term invasive mole signifies the presence of villi within uterine muscle or its blood vessels (Figure 12-3). It must be emphasized that the presence of villi is the one histopathologic finding which distinguishes chorioadenoma destruens from choriocarcinoma. Diagnosis is usually made on examination of a hysterectomy specimen, since this entity is almost impossible to diagnose from uterine curettage. Chorioadenoma destruens and choriocarcinoma have been shown to have metastatic potential, both locally and to distant sites. Invasion can continue through the full thickness of the myometrium into the peritoneal cavity or broad ligament, resulting in massive hemorrhage. Although biologically more aggressive than a hydatidiform mole, chorioadenoma destruens is not associated with a high incidence of malignant degeneration. Mortality associated with invasive moles relates more to local complications such as hemorrhage or uterine perforation than to progressive metastatic disease (Elston 1972).

Choriocarcinoma

Choriocarcinoma, the most aggressive form of gestational trophoblastic disease, is characterized by myometrial invasion without the presence of villi. Cytotrophoblasts and multinucleated syncytiotrophoblasts must be present to make this diagnosis, and the syncytiotrophoblasts should "cap" the cytotrophoblasts (Figure 12-4). Nodules of choriocarcinoma often reveal central hemorrhage and necrosis. Because choriocarcinoma has no inherent stromal vasculature, malignant trophoblasts are located at the periphery of tumor nodules, and vessels are present only at the tumor-host interface. The lack of native blood vessels and the close association with maternal vessels account for a

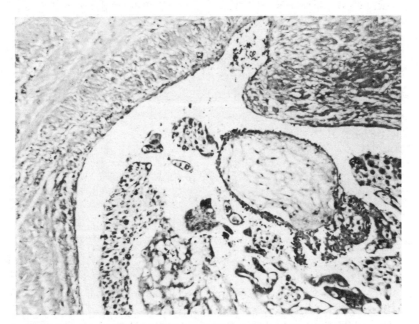

Figure 12-3 Chorioadenoma destruens. Myometrium and myometrial vessels are invaded by villi and proliferating trophoblast. Hematoxylin and eosin stain (magnification 100 ×).

334

high frequency of blood-borne metastases. In contrast, lymph node involvement is infrequent, being reported in 4% to 6% of cases (Novak 1930, Park 1950).

The diagnosis of choriocarcinoma is seldom made by curettage. The patient with this malignancy often presents with metastatic lesions in the absence of demonstrable uterine pathology. Metastases tend to be round, with a central area of hemorrhage and necrosis. The lungs are the most common site of metastatic spread, and pulmonary metastases are found in 80% to 100% of patients dying from their disease (Elston 1977, Ober 1971). Other common metastatic sites are the brain, liver, and vagina. Vaginal metastases occur by the retrograde spread of tumor emboli from the uterus into the paravaginal venous plexus.

Choriocarcinoma is preceded by a hydatidiform mole in approximately one half of the cases, with one-quarter of these tumors each following spontaneous abortions and normal pregnancies. Two percent of choriocarcinomas are preceded by ectopic pregnancies. Choriocarcinoma usually becomes manifest within two years of the preceding pregnancy, but some cases have been reported as long as ten years following the antecedent pregnancy.

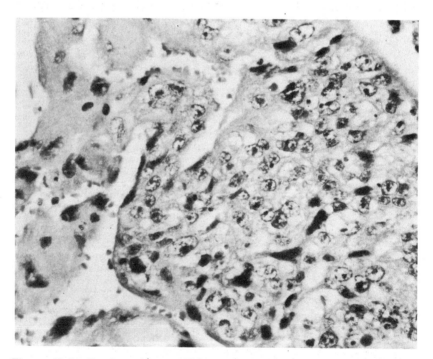

Figure 12-4 Choriocarcinoma. This tumor is characterized by malignant cytotrophoblast and syncytiotrophoblast. The large, multinucleated, synctiotrophoblast cells are seen to the right and exhibit characteristic "capping" of the cytotrophoblast. Hematoxylin and eosin stain (magnification 250 ×).

Theca-Lutein Cysts

Theca-lutein cysts are present in approximately 40% of patients with trophoblastic disease, and are bilateral in the majority of cases (Figure 12-5). Histologically, these cysts are characterized by a prominent lining of luteinized theca cells with regular nuclei and a pale-staining cytoplasm. They apparently originate in atretic follicles in which the cells of the theca-interna have undergone hyperplasia and become luteinized. The luteinization of the theca cells is presumably in response to high levels of hCG produced by the trophoblast (Novak and Koff 1930). Theca-lutein cysts can be produced in experimental animals by the administration of excessive amounts of chorionic gonadotropin (Blaustein 1977). They have also been observed when gonadotropins are used to induce ovulation, and occasionally in erythroblastosis secondary to Rh incompatibility (Girouard 1964). Factors in addition to hCG may be necessary for the development of theca-lutein cysts since they have occasionally been reported in the absence of either trophoblastic disease or increased serum levels of hCG.

Theca-lutein cysts have frequently been mistaken for metastatic spread of trophoblastic disease to the ovaries, and may be unnecessarily removed at time of hysterectomy. With effective treatment of trophoblastic disease, the cysts invariably regress, although this decrease in size may lag behind the fall in serum hCG. Concentrations of hCG have been shown to be elevated in the cyst fluid of theca-lutein cysts, but these levels are usually less than plasma hCG levels (Bagshawe 1969). Ultrasonography is frequently employed to detect theca-lutein cysts, and can be used to follow their regression throughout therapy. Removal of theca-lutein cysts is indicated only in cases of bleeding or torsion.

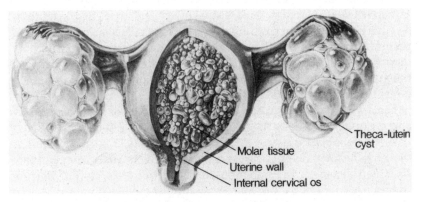

Figure 12-5 Theca-lutein cysts associated with hydatidiform mole. These cysts usually regress following treatment of trophoblastic disease, and surgical excision is not necessary.

Coexistent Pregnancy

An intrauterine pregnancy can coexist with trophoblastic disease in any of its histologic types (Clark et al 1970, Jones and Lauerson 1975). The occurrence of hydatidiform mole with a coexisting fetus is extremely rare, however, varying from 1:9500 to 1:140,000 pregnancies (Bowles 1943, Beischer 1966). In one rather large series of hydatidiform moles from the Royal Womens Hospital in Melbourne, Australia, a coexistent fetus was present in 5.9% of the cases (Beischer and Fortune 1968). Most investigators believe that this event occurs most commonly in a multiple gestation pregnancy in which one ovum dies, and the placenta then undergoes degenerative changes and trophoblastic transformation. There are cases of coexistent pregnancy and trophoblastic disease in which there is only one placenta. In these cases, molar degeneration often involves the entire placenta, resulting secondarily in the death of the fetus. Rarely, viable infants result from coexistent trophoblastic and normal pregnancies (Beischer 1966, Hohe et al 1971). The size and ultimate fate of the fetus depends upon at what point in gestation trophoblastic degeneration of the placenta begins, the rate of its progression, and the amount of placenta involved. Since trophoblastic abnormalities may be caused by defective ova, it is not surprising that an increased incidence of developmental abnormalities has been reported in the surviving fetuses (Beischer 1966). Metastasis of trophoblastic tissue to the fetus has been reported, and these fetuses have occasionally been successfully treated with chemotherapy.

DIAGNOSIS AND EVALUATION

Gestational trophoblastic disease confined to the uterus is usually associated with a well-defined group of clinical signs and symptoms. Vaginal bleeding, often six to eight weeks after a missed menstrual period, occurs in approximately 90% of patients. Bleeding may vary from a scanty, dark brown discharge to profuse, bright red hemorrhage. Passage of molar tissue may accompany any of these bleeding patterns. Uterine size larger than that calculated for the date of gestation is seen in over 50% of patients with molar pregnancy. Also, fetal heart sounds are conspicuously absent. Indicated studies in the initial evaluation of patients suspected of having trophoblastic disease are presented in Table 12-2. In addition to a thorough history and physical examination, CBC, platelet count, urinalysis, blood chemistry determinations, liver function tests, clotting function studies, thyroid evaluation, and serum hCG should be obtained. Also, a chest x-ray and electrocardiogram should be performed when the patient is first evaluated.

When molar tissue has not been passed, a definitive diagnosis of

Table 12-2
Initial Evaluation of Patients with Trophoblastic Disease

1. History and physical examination
2. Cervical cytologic smear
3. Laboratory studies:
   a) CBC, differential, platelet count
   b) serum electrolytes
   c) liver function tests
   d) thyroid function tests (T_3, T_4, T_3-resin uptake)
   e) clotting studies
   f) serum hCG
   g) urinalysis
   h) blood type
4. Chest x-ray, PA and lateral
5. Pelvic ultrasonography

trophoblastic disease can usually be made by ultrasonography. The sonogram of a hydatidiform mole characteristically shows a "snow-storm" pattern consisting of multiple intrauterine echoes (Figure 12-6). The echoes are due to the differential density between trophoblastic villi and the surrounding tissue. This pattern can be differentiated from that of a normal intrauterine pregnancy in which a gestational sac and fetus are present. In those rare cases in which an intrauterine pregnancy coexists with trophoblastic disease, ultrasonography can usually confirm an

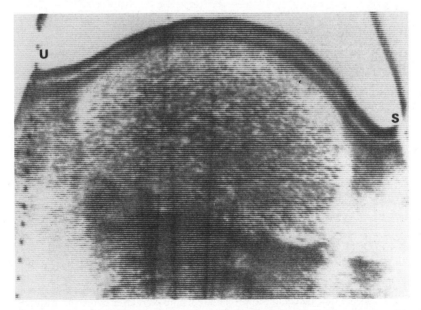

Figure 12-6 Longitudinal sonogram in midline. Note the coarse echo pattern indicative of trophoblastic disease. U = umbilicus, S = symphysis pubis.

338

abnormality because of the increased size of the trophoblast. The value of ultrasonography in identifying the presence of theca-lutein cysts of the ovary has been previously discussed.

Amniography may be used to make the diagnosis of trophoblastic disease if ultrasonography is unavailable. This technique is usually employed in patients with a uterine size of at least 14 weeks, and consists of injecting a radiopaque dye into the uterine cavity. Demonstration of the characteristic "moth-eaten" or "honeycomb" patterns, formed by dye surrounding the translucent grape-like structures of the mole, permits a definitive diagnosis.

Serum concentrations of human chorionic gonadotropin (hCG) can also be helpful in making the diagnosis of trophoblastic disease. It should be emphasized, however, that a single elevated serum hCG value cannot be used as the sole criterion for this diagnosis. Serial serum determinations of hCG, using the specific radioimmunoassay for the beta subunit (Vaitukaitis 1972), should be plotted against the curve for hCG values expected in a normal intrauterine pregnancy (Figure 12-7). A progressive rise in serum hCG after 90 to 100 days of pregnancy (the time at which hCG would plateau in a normal pregnancy) is highly suggestive of trophoblastic disease, provided that multiple gestation has been excluded.

There are also a number of medical complications commonly associated with trophoblastic disease. Preeclampsia characterized by hyperten-

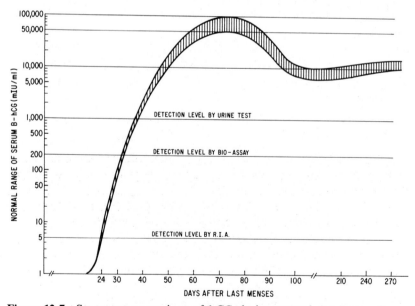

Figure 12-7 Serum concentrations of hCG during normal pregnancy. Serum hCG levels are first detectable approximately nine days after ovulation with peak concentrations occurring at 60 to 80 days' gestation (from Wilson EA, and Jawad MT, unpublished data).

sion, proteinuria, and edema occurs in approximately 20% to 30% of patients with hydatidiform mole (Table 12-3). Symptoms usually appear in the first or second trimester of pregnancy and, unlike preeclampsia associated with a normal pregnancy, occur more frequently in multiparas than in primagravidas. Hypertension usually precedes the onset of edema and proteinuria in patients with trophoblastic disease. Preeclampsia is more commonly observed in hydatidiform moles in which the uterus is greater than the size of a 20-week gestation. This is consistent with other conditions which are known to be associated with a rapid increase in uterine size and preeclampsia, such as polyhydramnios and multiple gestation. Trophoblastic disease should be suspected, therefore, in any patient presenting with the signs and symptoms of preeclampsia during the first 20 weeks of pregnancy. If such a patient has no fetal heart sounds, then ultrasonography should be performed to establish the diagnosis. While preeclampsia is commonly associated with trophoblastic disease, eclampsia is rare. Chesley (1946), in a review of the world literature between 1866 and 1946, reported only 35 cases of eclampsia associated with trophoblastic disease.

Table 12-3
Incidence of Toxemia in Trophoblastic Disease

Author	No. of Patients	Toxemia
Crowell (1955)	15	4 (27%)
Stroup (1956)	38	13 (34%)
Acosta-Sison (1956)	85	31 (36%)
Marquez-Monter (1963)	104	35 (35%)
Chun (1964)	269	135 (50%)
Total	511	218 (42%)

A second medical complication associated with trophoblastic disease is hyperthyroidism. Approximately 70% of patients with trophoblastic disease will have biochemical evidence of hyperthyroidism manifested by elevated serum T_3, T_4, and PBI levels. However, less than 10% of these patients actually display clinical signs of thryotoxicosis such as tachycardia, heat intolerance, fatigue, or nervousness. Although several investigators speculated that a unique thyroid-stimulating hormone (TSH) was synthesized by trophoblastic tissue, recent evidence (Kenimer 1975, Nagataki 1977) suggests that hCG itself may cause hyperthyroidism. The hCG molecule has an alpha chain identical to that of TSH and, therefore, has an inherent capacity to stimulate the thyroid gland.

Hyperemesis, as manifested by increased nausea and vomiting, may also occur in as many as 25% of patients with hydatidiform mole.

Although the exact etiology of hyperemesis is unknown, high levels of hCG have been implicated in its causation. Recently, Kauppila and co-workers (1979) reported that patients experiencing hyperemesis gravidarum had significantly higher serum hCG concentrations than normal pregnant subjects at 7 to 14 weeks' gestation. Hyperemesis was noted to begin concomitantly with the rise in serum hCG levels and occurred most commonly at 10 to 12 weeks' gestation whe.. hCG levels were highest (Figure 12-7). Increased sensitivity of the hypothalamic vomiting center to circulating levels of hCG has also been suggested as an etiologic factor in hyperemesis.

Perhaps the most ominous symptoms are those associated with metastatic trophoblastic disease. Unfortunately, patients with these symptoms are often misdiagnosed, thereby allowing the disease to progress. The most common site of extrapelvic metastases from trophoblastic disease is the lung (Goldstein 1972). Too often, the diagnosis of metastatic trophoblastic disease is not even considered in a patient in the reproductive age group who presents with a pulmonary lesion. In some cases, an unnecessary thoractomy is performed in an effort to establish the correct diagnosis. Complicated trophoblastic disease should be part of the differential diagnosis in a young woman presenting with hemoptysis or a lung lesion, particularly if there is no history of cigarette smoking. A serum hCG should be obtained and, if markedly elevated, a uterine curettage performed to confirm the diagnosis of trophoblastic disease. Recently, Goldenberg and colleagues (1980) have reported the effective photoscan localization of hCG-producing tumors, using radiolabeled anti-hCG antibodies. This method is able to identify metastatic trophoblastic disease without requiring operative intervention.

Patients with metastatic trophoblastic disease may also present with neurologic symptoms. It has been estimated that single or multiple metastases to the brain occur in 14% to 28% of patients with choriocarcinoma (Park and Lees 1950, Bagshawe 1969). Most metastases are to the posterior brain. Presenting symptoms are usually those of intracranial hemorrhage, and include sudden headache, vomiting, impairment of consciousness, or focal neurological signs (Vaughan and Howard 1962, Gurwitt et al 1975). Cerebral involvement, if extensive, may be reflected by the rapid onset of generalized cerebral dysfunction. If a solitary metastasis is involved, evidence of increased intracranial pressure or a specific neurologic deficit may be present. Any woman of childbearing age who presents with signs of acute or subacute intracranial pathology must be suspected of having choriocarcinoma metastatic to the brain. While isolated cases of metastatic cerebral choriocarcinoma without lung involvement have been reported (Sengupta et al 1976), the great majority of patients with cerebral metastases will also have pulmonary involvement (Park and Lees 1950, Weed and Hammond 1980). Choriocarcinoma is thought to spread to the brain via arterial embolization. Arteriovenous shunting may be responsible for those rare cases in which there is central nervous system involvement in the absence of pulmonary disease.

Other less common presenting symptoms of patients with metastatic trophoblastic disease are those of bowel obstruction or intraabdominal bleeding. Trophoblastic disease may involve virtually any organ system and, therefore, can cause a great variety of symptoms. Although trophoblastic disease that follows a hydatidiform mole is usually diagnosed, that which follows a normal pregnancy is often undetected. The diagnosis of trophoblastic disease should be considered in any patient with persistent uterine bleeding following the delivery of an apparently normal intrauterine pregnancy. A serum hCG level should be obtained and a uterine curettage performed, if indicated.

Once evacuation of the uterus has been performed and histologic confirmation of trophoblastic disease obtained, every effort should be made to stage the tumor. Although numerous staging systems have been proposed for trophoblastic disease, we prefer the classification proposed by Hammond and co-workers (1980). According to this system (Figure 12-8), gestational trophoblastic neoplasia is categorized into uncomplicated disease and complicated disease. Complicated trophoblastic disease is further divided into localized or metastatic disease, and metastatic disease into "good" and "poor" prognosis groups. Criteria for inclusion into each of these categories are shown in Table 12-4. Basically, uncomplicated trophoblastic disease consists of hydatidiform mole which is completely removed. Following uterine evacuation, the patient is placed on oral contraceptives and followed with weekly serum hCG determinations. The rate of decline of serum hCG is logarithmic, according to the half-life of the molecule. Approximately 80% of patients with hydatidiform mole will demonstrate nondetectable serum hCG levels by eight weeks after evacuation. A rise or plateau in serum hCG concentrations for at least two consecutive weeks necessitates inclusion of the case into the complicated trophoblastic category.

Patients suspected of having complicated trophoblastic disease

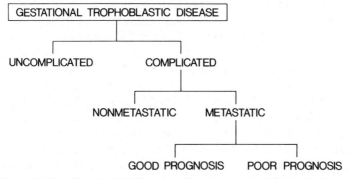

Figure 12-8 Clinical classification of gestational trophoblastic disease.

Table 12-4
Staging System for Gestational Trophoblastic Neoplasia

I Uncomplicated Disease

  A. Hydatidiform mole

  B. Molar degeneration (transitional mole)

II Complicated Disease
(rising or persistently elevated serum hCG values following uterine evacuation)

  A. Nonmetastatic

    1. persistent hydatidiform mole

    2. chorioadenoma destruens (invasive mole)

    3. choriocarcinoma

  B. Metastatic

    1. good prognosis, low risk

      a) initial serum hCG titer < 40,000 mIU/ml or urinary hCG titer < 100,000 IU/24h

      b) duration of symptoms < 4 months

      c) no liver or brain metastases

      d) no previous chemotherapy

    2. poor prognosis, high risk

      a) initial serum hCG titer > 40,000 mIU/ml or urinary hCG titer > 100,000 IU/24h

      b) duration of symptoms > 4 months

      c) liver or brain metastases

      d) previous chemotherapy

      e) disease following term pregnancy

should be admitted to the hospital and have additional staging evaluation to rule out the presence of metastatic disease. The specific studies included in this staging evaluation are illustrated in Table 12-5. These studies are similar to those performed in the initial evaluation of all patients with trophoblastic disease prior to uterine evacuation, but with the addition of specific procedures to rule out the presence of metastases to the lung (Figure 12-9), pelvis, brain, or liver. Any patient with a questionable pulmonary metastasis on chest x-ray should have tomography performed to define more precisely the extent and location of the lesion. Likewise, all patients with complicated trophoblastic disease should have liver and brain scans to localize occult metastases in these organs.

Liver scanning is usually performed using technetium-99 (^{99}Tc)-labeled sulfur colloid (Figure 12-10). The walls of the hepatic sinuses are lined by Kupffer cells whose normal function is phagocytosis. These cells extract about 95% of colloid particles during a single pass through the liver. Therefore, the uptake of colloid tracer as measured by a scintillation camera is a reliable indication of hepatic functional integrity. Computed tomography (CT) scanning or ultrasound is indicated in patients with a localized defect on radionuclide scanning, and can be quite accurate in differentiating metastatic lesions from benign hepatic cysts.

Table 12-5
Staging Evaluation for Patients with Complicated Trophoblastic Disease

1. History and physical examination
2. Cervical cytologic smear
3. Laboratory studies
    a) CBC, differential, platelet count
    b) serum electrolytes
    c) liver function tests
    d) thyroid function tests (T_3, T_4, T_3-resin uptake)
    e) clotting studies
    f) weekly serum hCG
    g) urinalysis
    h) blood type
4. Chest x-ray, PA and lateral, (tomography if indicated)
5. Pelvic ultrasonography
6. Electrocardiogram
7. Intravenous pyelogram
8. Liver-spleen scan (radionuclide or CT)
9. Brain scan (CT or radionuclide)

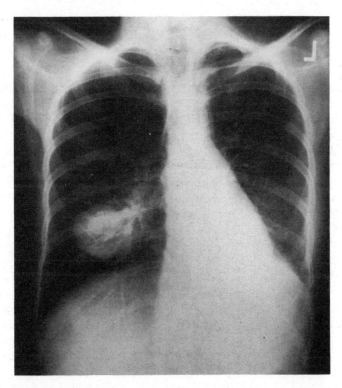

Figure 12-9 Pulmonary metastasis in patient with good prognosis/metastatic trophoblastic disease. Large lobular density in right lower lobe represents metastatic choriocarcinoma.

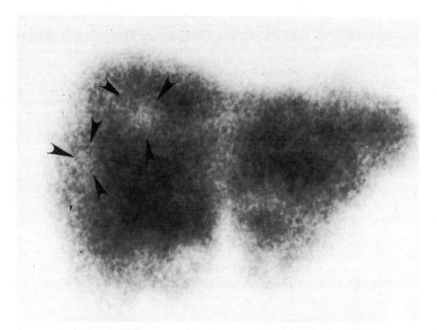

Figure 12-10 Technetium (^{99m}Tc) labeled sulfur colloid scan of liver in a patient with choriocarcinoma metastatic to the liver. Multiple filling defects in liver parenchyma (arrows) are indicative of tumor metastases.

Radionuclide brain scanning has been the most frequently used method to diagnose cerebral involvement by metastatic trophoblastic disease. ^{99}Tc coupled to one of several pharmaceutical agents such as pertechnitate or diethylenetriaminepentacetic acid (DPTA) is administered intravenously in a dose of 10 to 20 mCi. Following injection, these agents are rapidly cleared from the circulation and excreted by glomerular filtration. Normally, the brain vasculature excludes most substances which are not highly lipid-soluble. The capillaries of the brain are lined by endothelial cells which have tight intercellular junctions and a continuous basement membrane which impedes pore filtration (Reese and Karnovsky 1967). With tumor formation, there are a number of factors which allow for effective localization of radionuclides. Tumors in the brain are generally associated with increased vascularity, and the endothelial cells within these new capillaries seem to lack the tight intercellular junctions present in normal vessels (Brightman et al 1970, Long 1970, Shuttleworth 1972). In addition, there is generally increased metabolic activity in tumor cells allowing greater uptake of radiopharmaceuticals and metabolic substrates into the tumor. Technetium is a gamma-emitting agent with a half-life of six hours, which is readily detected by a scintillation camera. Brain scans are generally performed two to three hours after intravenous injection of the labeled tracer. Although radionuclide scanning cannot provide information concerning the morphology of the lesion, the diagnostic accuracy in terms of percentage true positive is 75% to 80% (George and Wagner 1975, Weed and Hammond 1980).

Recently, computerized tomography (CT) scans have been shown to be highly effective in the diagnosis of choriocarcinoma metastatic to the brain. One of the principal advantages of CT scanning is that it accurately delineates the anatomic extent of the tumor metastasis and its relationship to surrounding normal structures (Figure 12-11). Several studies (Mikhael and Mattar 1976, Fordham 1977) have indicated that CT scanning is more accurate than radionuclide scanning in the diagnosis of intracranial tumors. The improved resolution of tomographic scans in the diagnosis of metastatic choriocarcinoma is reflected in a false negative rate of only 4% as compared to a false negative rate of 8% to 15% in technetium scanning (Surwit et al 1980).

An operation is not necessary to confirm the presence of an intracranial metastasis if: 1) there is evidence of metastatic trophoblastic disease on chest x-ray, 2) radionuclide or CT scans are positive, and 3) serum hCG titers are abnormal (Bucy and Stilp 1972). Cerebral angiography may be helpful in those patients who present with intracranial, subarachnoid, or subdural hemorrhage. Bagshawe (1976) concluded that the concentration of hCG in the cerebrospinal fluid (CSF) could be

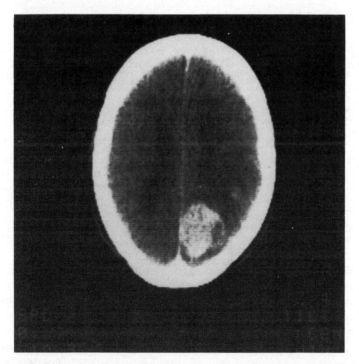

Figure 12-11 Contrast-enhanced CT scan of cerebral metastasis from choriocarcinoma. This densely enhancing lesion involved the parieto-occipital cortex.

helpful in detecting early central nervous system involvement by choriocarcinoma. The CSF/plasma hCG ratio was found to be more diagnostically significant than the absolute concentration of hCG in the CSF. Specifically, a CSF/plasma hCG ratio in excess of 60 was found to be indicative of brain metastases.

It should be emphasized that the previously mentioned staging studies should serve only as a general guide for evaluating the patient with complicated trophoblastic disease. Symptoms indicative of possible metastatic involvement of any specific organ system should be thoroughly evaluated by appropriate tests.

THERAPY

For organization purposes, treatment will be discussed according to the specific stage of trophoblastic disease. Individual sections will be devoted to the therapy of hydatidiform mole, nonmetastatic complicated trophoblastic disease, and metastatic trophoblastic disease, "good" and "poor" prognosis.

Hydatidiform Mole

The major therapy of hydatidiform mole involves evacuation of the uterus. If severe medical complications such as hyperthyroidism, toxemia, or coagulopathy are also present, it may be necessary to stabilize the patient with appropriate medical therapy prior to surgery. It should be pointed out that uterine evacuation itself, with the resultant decrease in serum hCG levels, usually results in prompt improvement of these medical complications. The preferred method of uterine evacuation in most patients is suction curettage. This procedure should be performed under general anesthesia and followed by gentle, sharp curettage of the uterus. Oxytocin should be given immediately after uterine evacuation and continued for 12 to 24 hours to facilitate normal involution. In patients whose uterine size is in excess of that consistent with a 20-week pregnancy, hysterotomy may be used as an alternate method of uterine evacuation, although it is generally not recommended.

The major complication of suction curettage is blood loss. For this reason, ample amounts of appropriately crossmatched blood should be available for immediate transfusion should the need arise. In addition, pulmonary vascular compromise secondary to deportation of trophoblastic tissue has been reported following molar evacuation. This complication requires immediate treatment with digitalis, diuretics, and other cardiopulmonary support measures (Hammond and Currie 1980). If the patient with a hydatidiform mole has completed childbearing, a realistic alternative to uterine evacuation is total abdominal hysterectomy. The ovaries should not be removed unless indicated by additional disease not associated with trophoblastic disease. Theca-lutein cysts, if present, usually undergo rapid regression after removal of the hydatidiform mole.

Following uterine evacuation, the patient should be placed on oral contraceptives for at least six months and, preferably, for one year. These agents are not only the most reliable form of contraception, but also suppress pituitary luteinizing hormone levels. Oral contraceptives may cause a slight delay in the decline of serum hCG following removal of trophoblastic tissue (Stone et al 1976). Serum hCG levels, using the specific beta-subunit radioimmunoassay (Vaitukaitis 1972) should be obtained at weekly intervals until normal. Chest x-rays and pelvic examinations should be performed at monthly intervals until the serum hCG titer returns to normal. Pregnancy tests should not be used to follow hCG levels in patients with trophoblastic disease. Such tests, based on serum determinations of hCG, generally are not sensitive enough to reliably detect hCG concentrations less than 200 mIU/ml. A rise or plateau of hCG levels for two consecutive weeks is indicative of complicated trophoblastic disease, and necessitates further staging evaluation. Approximately 20% of patients with the diagnosis of hydatidiform mole will develop complicated trophoblastic disease.

The use of prophylactic chemotherapy at the time of molar evacuation as a method of reducing the incidence of subsequent complicated trophoblastic disease has been advocated by Goldstein (1972) and Holland (1971). In patients with unevacuated molar pregnancy, a single five-day course of either methotrexate (0.3 mg/kg/day) or actinomycin D (10 to 12 μg/kg/day) was utilized, and evacuation was performed on the third day of treatment. The incidence of complicated trophoblastic disease in patients receiving prophylactic chemotherapy was only 8% as compared to 20% in patients not receiving chemotherapy (Goldstein 1972). Most investigators, however, feel that the added risks of giving prophylactic chemotherapy to all patients with hydatidiform mole outweigh the benefits of reducing malignant sequelae in a relatively small number of them.

Nonmetastatic Complicated Trophoblastic Disease

The diagnosis of nonmetastatic complicated trophoblastic disease is usually made by the observation of persistently elevated or rising serum hCG titers in the absence of signs or symptoms of metastatic disease. However, these patients may have microscopic foci of disease beyond the uterus which simply are not detected by conventional diagnostic techniques. The major treatment modality for these patients is chemotherapy consisting of one of several single-agent regimens (Table 12-6). These include intramuscular methotrexate, 15 to 25 mg daily for five days (Hertz et al 1961), intravenous actinomycin D, 10 to 13 μg/kg/day for five days (Ross et al 1966), or periodic high-dose methotrexate with citrovorum factor rescue (Goldstein et al 1978). These regimens can be repeated every two weeks (nontreatment interval seven to nine days), provided that severe bone marrow, hepatic, or renal toxicity is not present. Treatment is not continued when: 1) the WBC is less than 3000/mm^3, 2) the segmented neutrophil count is less than 1500/mm^3, 3) the platelet count is less than 100,000, or 4) there is evidence of increasing renal or hepatic dysfunction.

Table 12-6
Chemotherapy Protocols Used in Nonmetastatic Trophoblastic Disease and in Good Prognosis/Metastatic Trophoblastic Disease

---

Methotrexate, 15–25 mg (0.4 mg/kg) IM
daily x 5 days

or

Actinomycin D, 10–13 μgm/kg IV
daily x 5 days

or

Methotrexate, 1 mg/kg IM at 4 pm on
days 1, 3, 5, 7
Citrovorum factor 0.1 mg/kg IM at 4 pm
on days 2, 4, 6, 8

Methotrexate with citrovorum factor rescue was initially proposed (Bagshawe and Wilde 1964) as a regimen which could achieve a high degree of antitumor activity with minimal toxicity. In a group of 32 patients with nonmetastatic trophoblastic disease, Goldstein and coworkers (1978) noted a 91% remission rate using this protocol. There was no evidence of bone morrow or hepatic toxicity in any patient regardless of the total dose or number of courses utilized. Serum levels of hCG should be obtained at weekly intervals throughout treatment, and chemotherapy continued until three consecutive negative titers have been obtained. Pelvic examination and chest x-rays should be performed at least every two weeks during treatment, and the patient maintained on oral contraceptives for a period of one year. Once remission (three consecutive negative serum hCG levels) has been achieved, hCG determinations should be obtained monthly for three months, and bimonthly for six months.

The role of hysterectomy in the treatment of nonmetastatic trophoblastic disease has been emphasized by Hammond et al (1980). These authors reported that a sustained remission was achieved by chemotherapy alone in 87% of patients with this disease. In a second group of patients with localized disease who underwent initial elective hysterectomy at the time of institution of systemic chemotherapy, remission was obtained in 100% of cases. Furthermore, the number of courses of chemotherapy necessary to achieve remission was reduced to 2.2 in the hysterectomy group, as compared to 4.0 in patients not undergoing primary removal of the uterus. For this reason, hysterectomy is advocated midway during the first course of chemotherapy in patients with nonmetastatic trophoblastic disease who have completed their childbearing function.

Patients demonstrating a rising serum hCG titer or the development of new metastases while being treated with single-agent chemotherapy, should receive multiagent therapy.

Good Prognosis/Metastatic Trophoblastic Disease

Patients with metastatic trophoblastic disease whose initial serum hCG prior to treatment is less than 40,000 mIU/ml, whose duration of disease is less than four months, and who have no evidence of liver or brain metastases, are placed in the good prognosis group. In general, patients with good prognosis/metastatic disease can be treated with any of the chemotherapy regimens utilized in the therapy of localized complicated trophoblastic disease. The same guidelines for the administration of chemotherapy also apply to these patients. Cyclic chemotherapy is continued until three consecutive negative, weekly serum hCG titers have been obtained, and there is no evidence of metastatic disease. Likewise, the patient should be given oral contraceptives for at least one year after institution of therapy. Since pulmonary metastases are the most common site of extrapelvic disease in these patients, chest x-rays should be performed at least every two weeks throughout therapy. The size of the metastatic lesions as well as the serum hCG titer should be compared serially to assess response to chemotherapy.

Although by definition there is a metastatic component of the disease in each patient within this group, there is evidence to suggest that primary hysterectomy may also be useful as an adjunctive therapeutic method in these cases. Hammond and colleagues (1980) reported that 35 of 40 patients (87%) with good prognosis/metastatic disease achieved remission by chemotherapy alone. The additional five patients required subsequent hysterectomy for cure of disease.

In a second group of patients with this stage of disease, hysterectomy was performed initially during the first course of chemotherapy. Subsequent courses were then given and the progress of disease monitored biochemically by serial serum hCG determinations. Remission occurred in all of these patients.

In the primary hysterectomy group, the average total hospital stay, including that for surgery and chemotherapy, was 56.6 days as compared to 76.6 days in patients receiving chemotherapy alone. Likewise, the initial use of hysterectomy significantly reduced the number of courses of chemotherapy necessary to achieve remission from 5.9 to 3.8. For these reasons, the performance of hysterectomy on the third day of the initial course of chemotherapy is advocated in those patients with good prognosis/metastatic trophoblastic disease who have completed childbearing. Approximately 5% of these patients will develop tumor recurrence after initial remission (Hammond et al 1980). Following remission, serum hCG levels should be obtained monthly for three months, and bimonthly for six months.

One of the apparent explanations for tumor recurrence is that a small number of viable tumor cells may remain despite nondetectable hCG concentrations in the serum. It has been estimated that the average trophoblastic tumor cell produces no more than 5×10^{-4} IU hCG per day. Therefore, persistent tumor cells can theoretically be present without being detected by biochemical monitoring. For this reason, it is recommended that all patients with good prognosis/trophoblastic disease be given at least one course of chemotherapy after serum hCG concentrations have fallen to nondetectable levels.

Poor Prognosis/Metastatic Trophoblastic Disease

Poor prognosis/metastatic trophoblastic disease is defined by: 1) the presence of cerebral or hepatic metastases, 2) duration of symptoms in excess of four months, 3) prior unsuccessful chemotherapy, 4) an initial serum hCG titer prior to treatment in excess of 40,000 mIU/ml, or 5) metastatic disease following a term pregnancy.

Metastatic trophoblastic disease occurring after a term pregnancy is included in this high-risk group for several reasons. The disease is often misdiagnosed after a term pregnancy because of a low index of suspicion and the fact that the patient can present with a great variety of symptoms, including liver failure, hemorrhage, or focal neurologic signs. Consequently, the disease is often widely metastatic by the time the patient is first treated. There is also recent evidence to suggest that choriocarcinoma after a term pregnancy may differ genetically from that occurring following a hydatidiform mole (Patillo et al 1981). Choriocarcinomas occurring after a term pregnancy were found to have both maternal and paternal chromosomes and, therefore, represented only a partial allograft. In contrast, choriocarcinoma following hydatidiform mole was found to have only paternal chromosomes, thereby comprising a complete allograft. The implication of these findings is that the host may not be able to mount an effective immunologic response against a choriocarcinoma following a term pregnancy because it is an incomplete allograft.

It should be emphasized that patients with poor prognosis/ metastatic disease comprise a high-risk group often requiring several modalities of therapy, including multiple agent chemotherapy, surgery, and radiation therapy. Consequently, it is strongly recommended that patients with this type of advanced trophoblastic disease be treated at a major hospital or cancer center by a qualified gynecologic oncologist. In this way, the most advanced facilities are available not only for primary therapy, but also for the treatment of complications which may result from the required use of intensive chemotherapy.

The basic treatment for patients with poor prognosis/metastatic trophoblastic disease is combination multiagent chemotherapy. Attempts to treat these patients with single-agent chemotherapy have generally been unsuccessful. Hertz and colleagues (1961), for example, reported that only 1 of 7 patients (17%) with cerebral metastases achieved remission when treated by methotrexate alone. Likewise, the response rate of patients whose metastatic disease had occurred more than four months prior to treatment was only 31% when they were given single-agent chemotherapy alone.

The specific chemotherapy protocols utilized in poor prognosis metastatic trophoblastic disease are illustrated in Table 12-7. At present,

Table 12-7
Chemotherapy Protocols Used in Poor Prognosis/Metastatic Trophoblastic Disease

Methotrexate, 12–15 mg IM
Actinomycin D, 8–10 μg/kg IV
Chlorambucil, 8–10 mg PO
                daily $\times$ 5 days

                  or

Methotrexate, 12–15 mg IM
Actinomycin D, 8–10 μg/kg IV
Cyclophosphamide, 150–250 mg IV
                daily $\times$ 5 days

                  or

Cisplatin, 20 mg/m^2 IV daily $\times$ 5 days
Bleomycin, 20 U/m^2 IV day 1 and weekly thereafter
Vinblastine, 9 mg/m^2 IV day 1

                  or

Hydroxyurea, 500 mg. P.O. days 1,2
Vincristine, 1 mg/m^2 IV day 3
Methotrexate, 100 mg/m^2 IV day 3 (7:00 am)
            200 mg/m^2 12 hr infusion day 3 (7:00 pm)
Folic Acid, 12 mg/m^2 IM q12hr starting 12h after
            MTX days 5,6,7
Actinomycin D, 10 μg/kg IV days 5,6,7
Cyclophosphamide, 600 mg/m^2 IV day 5
Doxorubicin, 30 mg/m^2 IV day 10

the two chemotherapy regimens of choice are the methotrexate-actino-mycin D-chlorambucil (MAC) combination proposed by Hammond and colleagues (1973) and the CHAMOMA protocol initially reported by Bagshawe (1964) and later modified by Surwit and co-workers (1979). Patients not responding to any of these regimens can be treated with the Cisplatin-vinblastine-bleomycin combination used initially in the treatment of testicular germ cell cancer by Einhorn and Donohue (1977). It should be remembered that each of these regimens is quite toxic. Hammond and co-workers (1980) noted that 5 of 63 patients with poor prognostic/metastatic disease died of chemotherapy-induced toxicity. Therefore, bone marrow, hepatic, and renal toxicity should be monitored closely by appropriate laboratory tests. Treatment courses can be repeated after an interval of ten days without chemotherapy, provided that signs of toxicity are not present. Also, prolonged combination chemotherapy may cause profound electrolyte imbalance and protein depletion. Every effort should be made to utilize antiemetic agents such as phenothiazine or droperidol during chemotherapy. Likewise, total parenteral nutrition may be necessary to provide the essential caloric and nitrogen balance in these patients.

Radiation therapy should be given to the brain or liver if trophoblastic metastases are present in these organs. Brace (1968) first reported the advantages of adding adjunctive, whole brain irradiation to chemotherapy in patients with metastatic cerebral choriocarcinoma. These investigators gave an initial course of 2000 rad, so that a repeat course could be given without damaging normal brain tissue. It is now recommended that 3000 rad whole brain radiation be given at a dose rate of 300 rad per day (Hammond et al 1980). This is the equivalent of giving 4000 rad at a rate of 180 to 200 rad per day, and is both hemostatic and tumoricidal. Radiation therapy should be given simultaneously with the beginning of multiagent chemotherapy. Using this combination, Weed and Hammond (1980) reported a survival rate of 50% in patients with cerebral metastatic choriocarcinoma. Surgical intervention should be limited to those patients who demonstrate progressive neurologic deterioration secondary to intracranial bleeding. Intracranial hemorrhage remains a common cause of death in patients with cerebral choriocarcinoma, and emergency craniotomy may be necessary to stabilize the patient so that chemotherapeutic cure can ultimately be achieved (Gurwitt et al 1975).

Trophoblastic disease metastatic to the liver has the potential not only of replacing normal hepatic parenchyma and causing end-organ failure, but also of producing massive intraabdominal hemorrhage. Both of these conditions can be fatal. It is therefore recommended that patients with hepatic metastases from trophoblastic disease be treated by whole liver irradiation. A total hepatic dose of 2000 rad should be given simultaneously with the onset of chemotherapy at a dose rate of 180 rad per day. Care should be taken not to exceed normal liver tolerance (2500 rad), and liver function studies should be monitored closely throughout therapy. Hepatic radiation, when given in these doses, is not tumoricidal (Brace 1968, Hammond et al 1980). However, when radiation is combined with chemotherapy, it is curative in up to 50% of cases. Rarely, trophoblastic disease metastatic to the liver will cause severe intraabdominal bleeding. In these cases, surgical therapy should be directed toward hemostasis while preserving as much normal liver parenchyma as possible. An alternative method of therapy for hepatic hemorrhage secondary to metastatic disease has been proposed by Grumbine and co-workers (1980). These investigators were able to produce selective hepatic artery occlusion using detachable silicone balloons. Occlusion for ten days was associated with permanent arterial obliteration and was effective in controlling hemorrhage in over 90% of these cases. Parenchymal damage did not occur because hepatic portal blood flow was maintained during arterial occlusion.

The role of primary tumor debulking in poor prognosis/metastatic trophoblastic disease has been emphasized by Hammond and co-workers (1980). Initial elective hysterectomy in these patients reduced both the average number of days of hospitalization and the number of courses of chemotherapy required to produce remission. Tumor reductive surgery was generally most effective when performed at the time of initial chemotherapy. Other primary surgical procedures included thoracotomy, craniotomy, and exploratory laparatomy with tumor excision. There was no increase in postoperative complications or delayed wound healing when surgery was performed during the initial course of chemotherapy.

As in other less malignant types of trophoblastic disease, the patient should be maintained on oral contraceptives throughout therapy, and response to treatment monitored by serial hCG determinations. Again, remission is defined as three consecutive negative serum hCG levels in the absence of detectable metastatic disease. Hammond and co-workers (1980) have reported that over 20% of patients with poor prognosis/ metastatic trophoblastic disease develop recurrent disease after an initial remission. The majority of these recurrences occurred within one year of the original diagnosis of remission. Therefore, it is recommended that at least three courses of multiagent chemotherapy be given after remission has first been achieved in patients with poor prognosis/metastatic disease. In these patients, contraception should be continued for a minimum of one year following remission.

SURVIVAL AND FOLLOW-UP

The remission rate of patients with complicated trophoblastic disease is presented in Table 12-8. In most recent series, the initial remission rate of patients with localized complicated trophoblastic disease and good prognosis/metastatic disease is in excess of 95% and, with the addition of primary adjunctive surgery, virtually all of these cases will be cured (Hammond et al 1980). However, the response rate of patients with poor prognosis/metastatic disease to combination therapy is only 65% to 70%. Furthermore, a significant number of these patients will develop recurrent disease after initially achieving remission.

Table 12-8
Remission Rates in Patients with Complicated Trophoblastic Disease

Classification	Number of Patients	Remission (%)
Nonmetastatic*	293	96.36%
Metastatic		
Good Prognosis**	83	99.99%
Poor Prognosis†	80	68.94%

*Hammond (1967, 1970), Brewer (1971), Goldstein (1972, 1978), Osathanondh (1975), Hatch (1978)
**Hammond (1973), Hatch (1978)
†Hammond (1973), Hatch (1978), Surwit (1979, 1980)

As has been stated previously, all patients with complicated trophoblastic disease should be followed with serial serum hCG titers throughout therapy and for at least one year after remission. The frequency with which hCG determinations are obtained depends upon the individual case. However, levels are generally obtained weekly until remission, then every month for three months, and bimonthly for six months. In addition, some investigators believe that serum hCG determinations should be obtained every six months for life in patients with poor prognosis/ metastatic trophoblastic disease.

Contraception, preferably with oral contraceptive agents, should be maintained for one year following remission. If there is a medical contraindication to oral contraceptives, the patient should be encouraged to use other reliable contraceptive methods. The use of the intrauterine contraceptive device is discouraged because the patient may experience bleeding and other complications which could make evaluation of trophoblastic disease more difficult.

At the present time, there is little evidence to suggest that successfully treated, complicated trophoblastic disease is associated with an increased incidence of infertility or fetal wastage (Pastorifide et al, Hammond 1980). The outcome of pregnancies in women previously treated for complicated trophoblastic disease is shown in Table 12-9. No increase in spontaneous abortions, congenital anomalies, stillbirths, perinatal morbidity, or neonatal morbidity has been noted. Likewise, no particular chemotherapeutic agent has been associated with subsequent fetal wastage or infertility (Van Thiel 1970, Walden 1976). The use of contraception for one year following remission has been credited with keeping reproductive function normal in patients previously treated for trophoblastic disease.

It is quite likely that any mature ovum affected by chemotherapy would be eliminated during this time period. Other oocytes in the resting phase (prophase, meiosis I) are thought to be quite resistant to the effects of chemotherapy. The incidence of other primary malignancies has not been shown to be increased in patients with trophoblastic disease.

Table 12-9
Pregnancy Following Chemotherapy for Trophoblastic Disease

Authors	Number of Pregnancies	Live Term Births	Spontaneous Abortions	Stillbirths
Van Thiel (1970)	88	71 (81%)	15 (17%)	2 (2%)
Pastorfide (1973)	118*	73 (62%)	18 (15.1%)	1 (< 1%)
Walden (1976)	64*	45 (70.3%)	10 (15.6%)	4 (6.3%)
Ross (1977)	96	78 (81%)	15 (16%)	3 (3%)
Hammond et al (1980)	31	28 (90%)	3 (10%)	0 (0%)

*Includes premature births not listed

REFERENCES

Acosta-Sison H. Statistical study of chorioepithelioma in the Philippine General Hospital. *Am J Obstet Gynecol* 58:125–132, 1949.

Acosta-Sison H, Manila PI. The relationship of hydatidiform mole to preeclampsia and eclampsia. *Am J Obstet Gynecol* 71:1279–1282, 1956.

Acosta-Sison H. The chance of malignancy in a repeated hydatidiform mole. *Am J Obstet Gynecol* 78:876–880, 1959.

Ausman JI, Levin VA, Brown WE. Brain tumor chemotherapy: Pharmacological principles derived from a monkey brain-tumor model. *J Neurosurg* 46:155–164, 1977.

Bagshawe KD, Wilde CE. Infusion therapy for pelvic trophoblastic tumor. *Br J Obstet Gynecol* 71:565–570, 1964.

Bagshawe KD. *Choriocarcinoma. The Clinical Biology of the Trophoblast and Its Tumours.* Baltimore: Williams and Wilkins Company, 1969, pp 93–94.

Bagshawe KD. *Choriocarcinoma.* London, William Clowes, 1969, pp 930–994.

Bagshawe KD, Wilson H, Dublon P, et al. Follow-up after hydatidiform mole: Studies using radioimmunoassay for urinary human chorionic gonadotropin (hCG). *J Obstet Gynecol Br Commw* 80:461–468, 1973.

Bagshawe KD, Walden PAM. Monitoring of choriocarcinoma. *Proc Br Inst Radiol* 49:291–292, 1976.

Bagshawe KD. Risk and prognostic factors in trophoblastic neoplasia. *Cancer* 38:1373–1385, 1976.

Bagshawe KD, Harland S. Detection of intracranial tumours with special reference to immunodiagnosis. *Proc Roy Soc Med* 51–53, 1976.

Bagshawe KD. Treatment of trophoblastic tumors: Recent results. *Cancer Res* 62:192–199, 1977.

Beischer NA. Hydatidiform mole with coexistent fetus. *Aust NZ J Obstet Gynaecol* 6:127–141, 1966.

Beischer NA, Fortune DW. Significance of chromatin patterns in cases of hydatidiform mole with associated fetus. *Am J Obstet Gynecol* 100:276–282, 1968.

Berkowitz RS, Goldstein DP, Bernstein M. Natural history of partial hydatidiform moles. *Lancet* 1:717–721, 1970.

Blaustein A. *Pathology of the Female Genital Tract*. New York, Springer-Verlag, 1977.

Bowles HE. Extensive hydatidiform mole formation with living child. *Am J Obstet Gynecol* 46:154–159, 1943.

Brace KC. The role of irradiation in the treatment of metastatic trophoblastic disease. *Radiology* 91:539–540, 1968.

Brewer JI, Smith RT, Pratt GB. Choriocarcinoma. Absolute 5-year survival rates of 122 patients treated by hysterectomy. *Am J Obstet Gynecol* 85:841–843, 1963.

Brewer JI, Gerbie AB. Early Development of choriocarcinoma. In Holland JF, Hreshchyshyn MM (eds): *Choriocarcinoma: Transactions of a Conference of the International Union Against Cancer,* Berlin, Germany, Springer-Verlag, 1967.

Brewer J, Eckman TR, Dolkart RE, et al. Gestational trophoblastic disease. *Am J Obstet Gynecol* 109:335–340, 1971.

Brightman MW, Klatzo I, Olsson Y, et al. The blood-brain barrier to proteins under normal and pathological conditions. *J Neurol Sci* 10:215–239, 1970.

Brindeau A, Hinglais A, Hinglais M. La mole hydatidiform. *Bull Fed Soc Gynecol Obstet De Langue Française.* 4:3–36, 1952.

Bucy PC, Stilp TJ. Metastatic choriocarcinoma of the brain: Its recognition, treatment and cure and other matters. *Schweiz Arch Neurol* 18:201–232, 1975.

Chesley LC, Cosgrove SA, Preece J. Hydatidiform mole, with special reference to recurrence and associated eclampsia. *Am J Obstet Gynecol* 52:311–320, 1946.

Chun D, Broga C, Chow C, et al. Clinical observations on some aspects of hydatidiform moles. *J Obstet Gynaecol Br Commw* 71:180–184, 1964.

Clark PB, Gusdon JP, Burt RL. Hydatidiform mole with coexistent fetus: Discussion and review of diagnostic methods. *Obstet Gynecol* 35:597–600, 1970.

Corder MP, Hively LF, Stone WH, et al. Methotrexate with leucovorin rescue in the treatment of gynecologic malignancies. *Oncology* 32:275–282, 1975.

Crowell JA. Hydatidiform mole and toxemia of pregnancy. *North Carolina Med J* 16:11–17, 1955.

Curry SL, Hammond CB, Tyrey L, et al. Hydatidiform mole: Diagnosis, management and long-term follow-up of 347 patients. *Obstet Gynecol* 45:1–8, 1975.

Das PC. Hydatidiform mole: A statistical and clinical study. *J Obstet Gynaecol Br Commw* 45:265–280, 1938.

Delfs E. Quantitative chorionic gonadotropin: Prognostic value in hydatidiform mole and chorioepithelioma. *Obstet Gynecol* 9:1–24, 1957.

Deligdisch L, Driscoll SG, Goldstein DP. Gestational trophoblastic neoplasms: Morphologic correlations of therapeutic response. *Am J Obstet Gynecol* 130:801–806, 1978.

Driscoll SG. Gestational trophoblastic neoplasms: Morphologic considerations. *Am J Pathol* 8:529–539, 1977.

Einhorn LH, Donohue J. *Cis* diamine-dichloroplatinum, vinblastine, and bleomycin combination chemotherapy in disseminated testicular cancer. *Ann Intern Med* 87:293-298, 1977.

Elston CW, Bagshawe KD. The value of histologic grading in the management of hydatidiform mole. *J Obstet Gynaecol Br Commw* 79:717-724, 1972.

Elston CW. The histopathology of trophoblastic tumors. *J Clin Pathol* [suppl] 10:111-113, 1977.

Fordham EW. The complementary role of computerized axial transmission tomography and radionuclide imaging of the brain. *Semin Nucl Med* 7:137-159, 1977.

Geographic variations in the occurrence of hydatidiform mole and choriocarcinoma. The joint project for study of choriocarcinoma and hydatidiform mole in Asia. *Ann NY Acad Sci* 80:178-196, 1956.

George RO, Wagner HN. Ten years of brain tumor scanning at Johns Hopkins 1962-1972, in DeBlanc HJ Jr, Sorenson JA (eds): *Noninvasive Brain Imaging: Computed Tomography and Radionuclides.* Acton, Mass, Publishing Sciences Group, 1975, p 147.

Girouard DP, Barclay DL, Collins CG. hyperreactio luteinalis. Review of literature and report of 2 cases. *Obstet Gynecol* 23:513-525, 1964.

Goldenberg DM, Kim EE, DeLand FH, et al: Clinical radioimmunodetection of cancer with radioactive antibodies to human chorionic gonadotropin. *Science* 208:1284-1286, 1980.

Goldstein DP, Reid DE. Recent developments in the management of molar pregnancy. *Clin Obstet Gynecol* 10:313-322, 1967.

Goldstein DP. The chemotherapy of gestational trophoblastic disease. Principles of clinical Management. *JAMA* 220:209-213, 1972.

Goldstein DP. Prevention of gestational trophoblastic disease by use of actinomycin D in molar pregnancies. *Obstet Gynecol* 43:475-479, 1974.

Goldstein DP, Saracco P, Osathanondh R, et al. Methotrexate with citrovorum factor rescue for gestational trophoblastic neoplasms. *Obstet Gynecol* 51:93-96, 1978.

Grumbine FC, Rosenshein NB, Brereton HD, et al. Managment of liver metastasis from gestational trophoblastic neoplasia. *Am J Obstet Gynecol* 137:959-961, 1980.

Gurwitt L, Long JM, Clark R. Cerebral metastatic choriocarcinoma. *Obstet Gynecol* 45:583-588, 1975.

Hammond CB, Hertz R, Ross GT, et al. Primary chemotherapy for nonmetastatic gestational trophoblastic neoplasms. *Am J Obstet Gynecol* 98:71-78, 1967.

Hammond CB, Borchert LG, Tyrey L, et al. Treatment of metastatic trophoblastic disease: Good and poor prognosis. *Am J Obstet Gynecol* 115:451-457, 1973.

Hammond CB, Weed JC, Currie JL. The role of operation in the current therapy of gestational trophoblastic disease. *Am J Obstet Gynecol* 136:844-858, 1980.

Hatch KD, Shingleton HM, Austin JM, et al. Southern Regional trophoblastic disease center, 1972-1977. *South Med J* 71:1334-1336, 1978.

Hertig AT, Edmond HW. Genesis of hydatidiform moles. *Arch Pathol* 31:260-291, 1940.

Hertig AT, Sheldon WH. Hydatidiform mole: A pathologicoclinical correlation of 200 cases. *Am J Obstet Gynecol* 53:1-36, 1947.

Hertig AT, Mansell H. Hydatidiform Mole and Choriocarcinoma, in *Tumors of the Female Sex Organs, Atlas of Tumor Pathology.* Armed Forces Institute of Pathology, 1956.

Hertz R, Lewis JL, Lipsett MB. Five years' experience with the chemotherapy of metastatic choriocarcinoma and related trophoblastic tumors in women. *Am J Obstet Gynecol* 82:631–640, 1961.

Hibbard BM, Hibbard ED, Jeffcoate TN. Folic acid and reproduction. *Acta Obstet Gynecol Scand* 44:375–400, 1965.

Hohe PT, Cochrane CR, Gmelich JT, et al. Coexistent trophoblastic tumor and viable pregnancy. *Obstet Gynecol* 38:899–904, 1971.

Holland JF. E pluribus unim: Presidential address. *Cancer Res* 31:1319–1329, 1971.

Jacobs P, Hassold T, Matuyama A, et al. Chromosome constitution of gestational trophoblastic disease. *Lancet* 2:49, 1978.

Jones WB, Lewis JL. Treatment of gestational trophoblastic disease. *Am J Obstet Gynecol* 120:14–20, 1974.

Jones WB, Lauerson NH. Hydatidiform mole with coexistent fetus. *Am J Obstet Gynecol* 122:267–272, 1975.

Kajii T, Ohama K. Androgenic origin of hydatidiform mole. *Nature* 268:633–634, 1977.

Kauppila A, Huhtaniemi I, Ylikorkala O. Raised serum human chorionic gonadotropin concentrations in hyperemesis gravidarum. *Br Med J* 1:1670–1671, 1979.

Kenimer JG, Hershman JM, Higgins HP. The thyrotropin in hydatidiform moles is human chorionic gonadotropin. *J Ce M* 40:482–491, 1975.

Lambert B, Debrux J. Theca-lutein cysts of pregnancy without mole of chorioepithelioma. *Obstet Gynecol* 22:643–647, 1963.

Lewis J, Hertz R. Effects of early embryectomy and hormonal therapy on the fate of the placenta in pregnant rhesus monkeys. *Proc Soc Exp Biol Med* 123:805–809, 1966.

Lewis JL, Ketcham AS, Hertz R. Surgical intervention during chemotherapy of gestational trophoblastic neoplasms. *Cancer* 19:1517–1522, 1966.

Lewis JL. Current status of treatment of gestational trophoblastic disease. *Cancer* 38:620–626, 1976.

Li MC, Hertz R, Spencer DB. Effect of methotrexate therapy upon choriocarcinoma and chorioadenoma. *Proc Soc Exp Biol Med* 93:361–366, 1956.

Long DM. Capillary ultrastructure and the blood-brain barrier in human malignant brain tumors. *J Neurosurg* 32:127–144, 1970.

Marquez-Monter H, Alfaro de la Vega G, Robles M, et al. Epidemiology and pathology of hydatidiform mole in the general hospital of Mexico: A study of 104 cases. *Am J Obstet Gynecol* 85:856–864, 1963.

McComb P, Yuen BH, Boyes D, et al. Recurrence of metastatic trophoblastic disease after negative plasma human chorionic gonadotropin β-subunit assay. *Gynecol Oncol* 9:114–116, 1980.

McCorriston CC. Racial incidence of hydatidiform mole. *Am J Obstet Gynecol* 101:377–382, 1968.

Mikhael MA, Mattar AG. Sensitivity of radionuclide brain imaging and computerized transaxial tomography in detecting tumors of the posterior fossa. *J Nucl Med* 18:26–28, 1977.

Miller JM, Surwit EA, Hammond CB. Choriocarcinoma following term pregnancy. *Obstet Gynecol* 53:207–212, 1979.

Nagataki S, Mizuno M, Sakamoto S, et al. Thyroid function in molar pregnancy. *J Ce M* 44:254–263, 1977.

Natoli WJ, Rashad MM. Hawaiian moles. *Am J Roentgenol Rad Ther Nucl Med* 114:142–144, 1972.

Novak E, Koff AK. Ovarian and pituitary changes associated with hydatidiform and chorioepithelioma. *Am J Obstet Gynecol* 20:481–499, 1930.

Novak E, Koff AK. Chorioepithelioma with special reference to disappearance of the primary uterine tumor. *Am J Obstet Gynecol* 20:153–164, 1930.

Ober WB, Edgcomb JH, Price EB. The pathology of choriocarcinoma. *Ann NY Acad Sci* 142:299–321, 1971.

Okudaira Y, Strauss L. Ultrastructure of molar trophoblast. Observations on hydatidiform mole and chorioadenoma destruens. *Obstet Gynecol* 30:172–187, 1967.

Osathanondh R, Goldstein DP, Pastorfide GB. Actinomycin D as the primary agent for gestational trophoblastic disease. *Cancer* 36:863–866, 1975.

Pallias JE, Pellet W. Brain Metastases, in Vinken PJ, Bruyn GW (eds). *Handbook of Clinical Neurology, Vol. 18*. New York, American Elsevier, 1975, pp. 201–232.

Park WW, Lees JC. Choriocarcinoma: A general review with an analysis of 516 cases. *Arch Pathol* 49:73–104, 1950.

Park WW, Lees JC. Choriocarcinoma: A general review with an analysis of 516 cases. *Arch Pathol* 49:205–241, 1950.

Park WW. *Choriocarcinoma: A Study of Its Pathology*. Philadelphia, Davis, 1971.

Pascasio FM, Suarez R, Manuel-Limson GA, et al. Serum protein changes in hydatidiform mole. *Am J Obstet Gynecol* 107:972–973, 1970.

Pastorfide GB, Goldstein DP. Pregnancy after hydatidiform mole. *Obstet Gynecol* 42:67–70, 1973.

Pour-Reza M, Agheli N, Vaghefi SB. Serum creatinine, urea and protein level changes in hydatidiform mole. *JAMA* 230:580–581, 1974.

Pratt RA, DiChiro G, Weed JC. Cerebral necrosis following irradiation and chemotherapy for metastatic choriocarcinoma. *Surg Neurol* 7:117–120, 1977.

Pritchard JA. Blood volume changes in pregnancy and the puerperium. IV. Anemia associated with hydatidiform mole. *Am J Obstet Gynecol* 91:621–629, 1965.

Ratnam SS, Teoh ES, Dawood MY. Methotrexate for prophylaxis of choriocarcinoma. *Am J Obstet Gynecol* 111:1021–1027, 1971.

Reese TS, Karnovsky MJ. Fine structural location of a blood-brain barrier to exogenous peroxidase. *J Cell Biol* 34:207–217, 1967.

Reynolds SRM. Hydatidiform mole: A vascular congenital anomaly. *Obstet Gynecol* 47:244–250, 1976.

Ross GT, Stolbach LL, Hertz R. Actinomycin D in the treatment of methotrexate-resistant trophoblastic disease in women. *Cancer Res* 22:1015–1017, 1962.

Ross GT, Goldstein DP, Hertz R, et al. Sequential use of methotrexate and actinomycin D in the treatment of metastatic choriocarcinoma and related trophoblastic diseases in women. *Am J Obstet Gynecol* 93:223–229, 1965.

Ross GT, Hammond CB. Chemotherapy of metastatic and nonmetastatic gestational trophoblastic neoplasms. *Tex Rep Biol Med* 24:326–338, 1966.

Schlaerth JB, Morrow CP, DePetrillo AD. Sustained remission of choriocarcinoma with *cis*-platinum, vinblastine and bleomycin after failure of conventional combination drug therapy. *Am J Obstet Gynecol* 136:983–985, 1980.

Schreiber JR, Rebar RW, Chen HC, et al. Limitation of the specific serum radioimmunoassay for human chorionic gonadotropin in the management of trophoblastic neoplasms. *Am J Obstet Gynecol* 125:705–707, 1976.

Sengupta BS, Chatterjee D, Persuad V. Primary neurological manifestation of choriocarcinoma. *Int Surg* 61:88–94, 1976.

Shuttleworth EC. Barrier Phenomena in Brain Tumors. *Prog Exp Tumor Res* 17:279–290, 1972.

Sicuranza BJ, Tisdall LH. Hydatidiform mole and eclampsia with co-existent living fetus in the second trimester of pregnancy. *Am J Obset Gynecol* 126:513–514, 1976.

Stone M, Dent J, Kardana A, et al. Relationship of oral contraception to development of trophoblastic tumour after evacuation of hydatidiform mole. *Br J Obstet Gynaecol* 83:913–916, 1976.

Stroup PE. Study of thirty-eight cases of hydatidiform mole at the Pennsylvania Hospital. *Am J Obstet Gynecol* 72:294–303, 1956.

Surwit EA, Suciu TN, Schmidt HJ, et al. A new combination chemotherapy for resistant trophoblastic disease. *Gynecol Oncol* 8:110–118, 1979.

Surwit EA, Hammond CB. Treatment of metastatic trophoblastic disease with poor prognosis. *Obstet Gynecol* 55:565–570, 1980.

Szulman AE, Serti V. The syndromes of hydatidiform mole. I. Cytogenetic and morphologic correlations. *Am J Obstet Gynecol* 131:665–671, 1978.

Taliadouros GS, Canfield RE, Nisula BC. Thyroid-stimulating activity of chorionic gonadotropin and luteinizing hormone. *J Ce M* 47:855–860, 1978.

Teoh ES, Dawood MY, Ratnam SS. Epidemiology of hydatidiform mole in Singapore. *Am J Obstet Gynecol* 110:415–420, 1971.

Vaitukaitis JL, Braunstein GD, Ross GT. A radioimmunoassay which specifically measures human chorionic gonadotropin in the presence of human luteinizing hormone. *Am J Obstet Gynecol* 113:751–758, 1972.

Van Thiel DH, Ross GT, Lipsett MB. Pregnancies after chemotherapy of trophoblastic neoplasms. *Science* 169:1326–1327, 1970.

Van Thiel DH, Grodin JM, Ross GT, et al. Partial placenta accreta in pregnancies following chemotherapy for gestational trophoblastic neoplasms. *Am J Obstet Gynecol* 112:54–58, 1972.

Vassilakos P, Riotton G, Kajii T. Hydatidiform mole: Two entities. *Am J Obstet Gynecol* 127:167–170, 1977.

Vaughan HG, Howard RG. Intracranial hemorrhage due to metastatic chorionepithelioma. *Neurology* 12:771–777, 1962.

Wake N, Takagi N, Sasaki M. Androgenesis as a cause of hydatidiform mole. *JNCI* 60:51–53, 1978.

Walden PAM, Bagshawe KD. Reproductive performance of women successfully treated for gestational trophoblastic tumors. *Am J Obstet Gynecol* 125:1108–1114, 1976.

Weed JC, Hammond CB. Cerebral metastatic choriocarcinoma: Intensive therapy and prognosis. *Obstet Gynecol* 55:89–94, 1980.

Wei P, Ouyang PC. Trophoblastic disease in Taiwan: A review of 157 cases in a 10-year period. *Am J Obstet Gynecol* 85:844–849, 1968.

Yamashita K, Wake N, Araki T, et al. Human lymphocyte antigen expression in hydatidiform mole. Androgenesis following fertilization by a haploid sperm. *Am J Obstet Gynecol* 135:597–600, 1979.

Yen S, MacMahon B. Epidemiologic features of trophoblastic disease. *Am J Obstet Gynecol* 101:126–132, 1968.

13 Sarcoma of the Female Genital Tract

Hugh R. K. Barber

Sarcoma of the uterus is a malignant tumor rising from the connective tissue or muscles of that organ. This is a rare disease, in contrast to the common benign tumor of connective tissue and muscle, the fibromyoma or fibroid. Sarcomas account for approximately 3% to 5% of all malignant tumors of the uterine corpus. They are among the most lethal tumors encountered in gynecology. It is difficult, however, to quote precise statistics because what many clinics consider low-grade sarcomas, others would merely call cellular benign myomas. This obviously affects not only the incidence but also the survival rate, because most individuals with cellular benign myomas do well.

The patient is usually over age 50, and presents with the complaint of recent, heavy vaginal bleeding that is often accompanied by pain. A suggestive, but not conclusive, sign is a rapid increase in the size of a fibroid.

In general, sarcomas are usually not diagnosed until the uterus has been removed at the time of hysterectomy. There is no specific clinical feature that is identified with sarcoma of the uterus except heavy bleeding, pain, rapid increase in the size of the fibroid, and a high degree of suspicion on the part of the responsible physician.

Sarcomas are more common in nulliparous women. They differ from epithelial tumors in that they have an increased propensity to metastasize via the blood stream. Thus, hepatic, pulmonary, and cerebral metastases are more common.

The pelvic examination usually reveals a large pelvic mass. On inspection with a speculum, there may be a friable polyp palpable through the os. The tumor may originate from the vagina in younger women and from the cervix in the child, but these are rare conditions.

Until recently, the only available treatment for uterine sarcoma has been surgical excision, which is effective only in neoplasms confined to the uterus. Advances in chemotherapy and radiation therapy have made these modalities worthy of therapeutic trial, either singly or in combination. Currently, there is a trend to follow surgery with chemotherapy because of the propensity of these tumors to metastasize widely, usually through the blood.

STAGING

There is no official clinical staging system for sarcomas of the uterus. Cavanaugh (1979) has reported that the following is the most commonly applied, whatever the histopathologic type. It correlates well with prognosis.

Stage I   Sarcoma confined to the uterus.

Stage II   Sarcoma involving the corpus and cervix.

Stage III   Sarcoma extending outside the uterus, but confined to the pelvis.

Stage IV   Sarcoma extending beyond the true pelvis.

In this classification, Stage I includes those patients whose tumors are confined to the uterine corpus, whether the uterus is enlarged or not. This is a practical method of clinical staging, despite the fact that enlargement for sarcoma would obviously carry a much worse prognosis than enlargement from associated leiomyomas. The staging is surgical and retrospective. The prognosis in sarcoma of the uterus is not only related to the clinical stage of disease, but also to the histopathology present in the tumor.

Classifications

There are two classifications of uterine sarcoma, one compiled by Ober, as listed in Table 13-1, and another (Table 13-2), which is a modification of this extensive classification, and has been reported by Kempson and Bari (1970). Ober's classification, reported in 1959, groups tumors according to whether they are pure homologous, pure heterologous, or mixed homologous and mixed heterologous. It serves to clarify and establish a common classification, permitting institutions to compare their results.

Table 13-1
Ober's Classification of Uterine Sarcomas

I. Leiomyosarcoma
  A. Arising in a leiomyoma
  B. Arising diffusely in the uterine wall

II. Mesenchymal sarcoma
  A. Pure homologous
    1. Endometrial stromal sarcoma
    2. Stromal endometriosis (endolymphatic stromal myosis)*
    3. Sarcoma botryoides (without heterologous elements)
  B. Pure heterologous
    1. Rhabdomyosarcoma
    2. Chondrosarcoma
    3. Osteosarcoma
    4. Liposarcoma (not reported)
  C. Mixed homologous
    1. Carcinosarcoma
      a. Adenocarcinoma plus stromal sarcoma
      b. Adenoacanthoma plus stromal sarcoma
      c. Squamous carcinoma plus stromal sarcoma
      d. Sarcoma botryoides plus neoplastic epithelium and without heterologous elements
  D. Mixed heterologous
    1. Carcinosarcoma (as above, with one or more heterologous elements)
    2. Mixed mesenchymal sarcoma
      a. Stromal sarcoma plus one or more heterologous elements
      b. Two or more heterologous elements without mesenchymal "myxomatous" stromal sarcoma
    3. Sarcoma botryoides (with heterologous elements)†

III. Blood vessel sarcomas**
  A. Hemangiosarcoma (hemangioendothelioma)
  B. Hemangiopericytoma*

IV. Lymphomas
  A. Reticulum cell sarcoma
  B. Lymphosarcoma
  C. Leukemic infiltration

V. Unclassified sarcoma

VI. Metastatic sarcoma (not reported)

*These tumors are not uniformly malignant.
†Cartilage and striated muscle are the most frequent heterologous elements. Bone is occasionally seen. Heterologous lipoblastic elements are difficult to evaluate.
**Lymphangiosarcoma has also been reported.
(Ober WB: *Ann NY Acad Sci* 75:568, 1959.)

Table 13-2
Modified Classification of Uterine Sarcomas

I. Pure sarcomas
   A. Pure homologous
      1. Leiomyosarcoma
      2. Stromal sarcoma
      3. Endolymphatic stromal myosis*
      4. Angiosarcoma
      5. Fibrosarcoma
   B. Pure heterologous
      1. Rhabdomyosarcoma (including sarcoma botryoides)
      2. Chondrosarcoma
      3. Osteosarcoma
      4. Liposarcoma
II. Mixed sarcomas
   A. Mixed homologous
   B. Mixed heterologous
   C. Mixed heterologous sarcomas with or without homologous elements
III. Malignant mixed Müllerian tumors (mixed mesodermal tumors)
   A. Malignant mixed Müllerian tumor, homologous type
      1. Carcinoma plus leiomyosarcoma
      2. Stromal sarcoma or fibrosarcoma
      3. Mixtures of these sarcomas
   B. Malignant mixed Müllerian tumor, heterologous type
      1. Carcinoma plus heterologous sarcoma with or without homologous sarcoma
IV. Sarcoma, unclassified
V. Malignant lymphoma

---

*This tumor was benign in this series, but has been classified as sarcoma because of reported recurrences and metastases.
(Kempson RL, Bari W: *Human Pathol* 1:331, 1970.)

HISTOGENESIS

Leiomyoma and leiosarcoma may be accurately separated in most instances. In most cases, histogenesis is straightforward once the neoplasm has been classified correctly. For example, leiomyosarcoma, the most frequently encountered form, is derived from adult smooth muscle. Tumors of blood vessel origin are derived from preexisting adult blood vessels, which are ubiquitous in the uterus, as in any other viscus. The few instances of lymphosarcoma or reticulum cell sarcoma that arise in the uterus either de novo or as part of multicentric tumorgenesis, are derived from lymphoid or reticuloendothelial cells, which are likewise ubiquitous. The only group of uterine sarcomas that pose a histogenetic problem is the group of so-called mixed, mixed mesenchymal, or mixed mesodermal tumors. This group is of particular importance because, historically, there has been much debate concerning its nature, particularly with respect to the explanations for the diversity of cellular elements it may contain, and with respect to the problem of the relationship of malformation to tumor.

Many of the theories of the histogenetic aspects of uterine sarcomas have been discarded as either not probable or not provable. Cohnheim's theory of displaced rest is not given much credence today. Wilms's theory, which is really a version of the rest theory, implied an invisible rest, ie, a group of cells indistinguishable from normally matured cells, but lacking the capacity for a coordinated response to normal stimuli for growth and differentiation. Wilms explained the presence of cartilage and bone in mixed tumors on the basis of inclusion of structures from the sclerotome in the caudal portion of the growing Wolffian duct. Sweet applied Wilms's ideas to Müllerian duct derivatives as well. It is difficult to know whether Sweet and Wilms thought their theories were a further differentiation of Schwalbes's concept of a dysontogenetic field, or as something opposed to it. Robert Meyer (1919) advanced theories of displacement still further by postulating "illegal" cell connections between the Wolffian and Müllerian systems as the origin of mixed tumors. Some reinforcement of Meyer's theory can be found in the observation of Gruenwald (1941) who demonstrated that the growing caudal end of the Müllerian duct is in contact with and surrounded by the same basement membrane as the growing end of the Wolffian duct. Ober states that Meyer's illicit cell connections may not prove to be as "illegal" as the embryologic knowledge of his day permitted him to think.

Theories based on rest are no longer in vogue. However, they do surface from time to time, especially when somebody reports that, in the middle of a poorly differentiated neoplasm with many atypical, bizarre cells, there is a structure composed of three plates of well-differentiated cartilage, surrounded by a membrane suggestive of perichondrium. The question is then raised, Is this truly a rest that had been there before the tumor developed, and, if so, does it have anything to do with the development of the tumor?

Contemporary with the theories of cell rests have been ideas that weighed it more in terms of the dynamics of cell growth. Pfannenstiel believed that the varied components of these tumors arose on the basis of metaplasia. His report antedates Wilms's publications. Schwalbes's idea of dysontogenetic fields is an effort to reconcile these divergent emphases on the mechanism of tumor formation. Albrecht considered tumor formation to be a repetition of organ-forming processes, representing organoid formation in excess on the basis of an embryonic or a postembryonic error in development, never a primary error or malformation of a cell. He recognized the importance of postnatal pathological processes in tumor formation.

Nickelson (1918) expanded on Albrecht's theories. In addition to the theories of anomalous blending, he also described anomalies of bulk, position, and differentiation. Nickelson ascribed the rich variety of cellular elements to a process of dedifferentiation and rejuvenescence, a process that assumes particular significance in the light of subsequent discoveries about the lack of a sharp division between stromal and epithelial cell forms.

Willis (1948) has expressed himself with characteristic emphasis, stating that many workers have followed Wilms in supposing the uterine mixed tumors to arise from developmentally misplaced tissues. Currently, the opinion is that this idea should be discarded, since it is discredited by the researchers of experimental embryology, and it is as unnecessary as it is improbable. It is difficult to accept the fact that undifferentiated rests of heterotopic tissues may remain in the endometrium for the entire span of a woman's reproductive life. This would mean that the rest had survived multiple pregnancies, and eventually produced a mixed tumor at the age of 50, 60, or 70. This theory is not scientifically sound. This is particularly true insofar as the postmenopausal woman is concerned. An argument can be advanced as to whether or not this should apply to histogenetically similar tumors, such as juvenile sarcoma botryoides.

Theories of histogenesis are constantly being challenged and outdated. However, it is important to keep in mind that the endometrial stroma and its congeners distributed throughout the genital tract, although mature, are the least highly specialized adult derivatives of the mesenchyma of the urogenital ridge. The distribution of the tissue beneath the peritoneal surfaces of the uterus and other pelvic structures (forming subcoelomic mesenchyme) is the basis for the occurrence of histologically and histogenetically similar tumors arising outside the uterus and its accessory passages.

Ober (1959) has reported on Gruenwald's demonstration that, in the human embryo, the mesenchyme around the Müllerian duct is derived from the coelom, even as duct epithelium itself. As the duct develops, there are continuing contributions from the surrounding mesenchyme to the ductal epithelium and vice versa. It might be said that they have the capacity for morphologic intermutability or liability. A question is raised relative to this theory. To some extent, this property must be lost as cell maturation and specialization progress, for pathologists do not see epithelium regenerating from stroma, or vice versa, in endometrium examined after curettage or during the puerperium. Even if the glands and stroma were not related ontogenetically, one can conceive of tumorgenic stimuli that are either selective and specific, or the converse. Tissues have a limited number of responses to stimuli, and neoplastic growth is only one of these.

It is interesting to note that mixed tumors are not reported in the Fallopian tube, the unfused portion of the Müllerian apparatus, whereas a surprising number arise either in the anterior or posterior midline of the uterus or at the junction of the upper third and lower two thirds of the vagina. Whether there is increased cellular lability at lines of fusion, or whether there is an anomaly of blending at these sites, remains an unanswered question.

Ober has stated that the taxonomic study of tumors is largely within the province of surgical pathology. Insofar as uterine sarcomas are concerned, Ober stressed the importance of anatomically studying well-oriented sections, of studying multiple sections, of realizing the value of special stains and demonstrating specific features of the cells and ground substance, and of noting the distribution and composition of metastases in the postmortem studies which furnish the necessary information regarding distant metastases, the natural history of the disease, and the mechanism of death.

Ober has divided uterine sarcomas into six major classes. Of these, leiomyosarcoma is the most frequently encountered, but, histologically, it is the least varied. The family of mesenchymal sarcomas is the next most frequent and is histologically the most complex. Tumors of blood vessel origin are extremely rare, but they present a few interesting relationships. Lymphomas are included for the sake of completeness. Ober also has reported that there is no case of metastatic sarcoma (unless one includes leukemic infiltration). Unclassified sarcomas are always a problem, not only in their identification but also in management and projection of a prognosis.

PATHOLOGY

Leiomyosarcoma, statistically the most frequently encountered uterine sarcoma, comprises from 50% to 75% of various large series. It may arise in a preexisting leiomyoma or, less frequently, may arise diffusely in a wall of a nonleiomatous uterus. In some instances, it may be difficult to determine from the gross appearance whether it arose in a leiomyoma or not.

Smooth muscle tumors that have invaded contiguous organs or blood vessels are malignant. If invasion is not present, the mitotic rate is evaluated. Tumors with less than five mitoses per ten-high-power field are benign. Those with higher mitotic counts are malignant. The prognosis for a leiomyosarcoma with greater than ten mitoses per ten-high-power field is poor, and metastases are frequent. The behavior of smooth muscle tumors with mitotic counts between four and nine per ten-high-power field is less certain, but some tumors with this level of mitotic activity will metastasize.

Patients with malignant mixed Müllerian tumors of the homologous type that are small and noninvasive or have invaded the myometrium only superficially, may be cured by hysterectomy. If the tumors are large and highly invasive, the outlook is almost hopeless, despite any therapy. Heterologous, malignant, mixed Müllerian tumors with chondrosarcoma as the heterologous element and without significant invasion, may also be cured. The presence of osteoid, bone, or rhabdomyoblast, indicates a highly malignant neoplasm with an almost certain fatal outcome. Reports indicate that all such tumors are large at the time of initial diagnosis. Recent work with combination chemotherapy has shown some improvement, especially in those patients whose gross tumor has been removed.

Infiltrating stromal tumors with mitotic counts of about 20 per ten-high-power field all metastasize. Those with five or less per ten-high-power field have not metastasized or have recurred after therapy. These criteria provide a sharp dividing point between endolymphatic stromal myosis and endometrial stromal sarcoma. The behavior of tumors with mitotic counts of 6 to 20 per ten-high-power field is unknown, but they may have a better prognosis than stromal tumors with higher counts.

Accurate diagnosis and classification of any group of tumors is essential before effective therapy can be determined. Establishing accurate diagnostic criteria for uterine sarcomas has been particularly difficult because of the large number of different histologic patterns that occur, and because of the difficulty of separating benign from malignant mesenchymal neoplasms.

If tumors with similar origins or behaviors are classified separately, or if tumors of divergent origin and behavior are classified together, the results of therapy will not be valid. Pure sarcomas contain only a single recognizable sarcomatous element, whereas mixed tumors contain two or more different malignant elements. The malignant cells in homologous tumors are morphologically recognizable as being derived from the mesenchymal tissue normally present in the uterus.

HOMOLOGOUS SARCOMAS

The pure homologous tumors have been reviewed by Ober and Jason (1953), and by Symmonds and Dockerty (1955). While some growths are exophytic with limited invasive activity, others may be extremely invasive and give rise to both pelvic and distant metastases. In general, the degree of malignancy of endometrial stromal sarcoma is less accurately predicted from close examination of its cellular features than from careful gross and microscopic evidence of invasiveness. An unusual member of this series is the so-called stromatous endometriosis (or endolymphatic stromal myosis), a proliferative lesion of endometrial stroma which has a limited capacity for autonomous growth. Whether or not the endolymphatic pattern should be construed as evidence of reduced malignancy is an important question that remains to be solved. Dockerty and his colleagues classify stromatous endometriosis as a sarcoma-like lesion and, until more cases are followed to a determinate end point, one cannot say more. In some cases of stromatous endometriosis, one can see an epithelium-like pattern differentiating from the matrix of "juvescent" stromal cells, and, on occasion, peculiar vascular patterns may be observed. This coincides with Gruenwald's observations of the lability of the stroma-epithelium relationship. A pure homologous sarcoma is composed of a single-cell type, resembling the mesenchymal tissue found in the normal uterus (smooth muscle in a pure leiomyosarcoma).

HETEROLOGOUS SARCOMAS

Heterologous tumors contain cells differentiated into mesenchymal structures not normally present in the uterus, such as bone, striated muscle, or cartilage. A pure heterologous tumor contains a single type of heterologous sarcoma. Pure heterologous tumors differ chiefly in a quantitative way from the mixed mesenchymal sarcomas. Rhabdomyosarcoma is the most frequent member of this group. In the past, most of these cases proved to be fatal within a year, but, with triple and quadruple chemotherapy, the salvage rate is improving. Chondrosarcoma is less common than the rhabdomyosarcoma. The extent to which the heterologous elements found in such tumors reflect local environmental factors that promote cell specialization along a given pathway remains debatable. Osteosarcoma is likewise very rare. Liposarcoma is so rare that no unequivocal case has yet been reported as being primary in the uterus. It occurs rarely as a component in mixed tumors, but, in general, it is difficult to be certain whether fat in a rapidly growing neoplasm is due to cellular degeneration or whether the cells are truly lipoblastic.

MIXED SARCOMAS

The mixed sarcomas contain tumor cells that are differentiated into at least two different types of homologous or heterologous sarcomas without evidence of epithelial elements. An example of this would be a sarcoma containing mixtures of leiomyosarcomas, or stromal sarcoma and rhabdomyosarcoma. The mixed sarcomas comprise about 60% of the group of mesenchymal tumors. Mixed tumors include carcinosarcoma, mixed mesenchymal sarcoma, and sarcoma botryoides. The first two types occur chiefly in the uterine corpus in postmenopausal women; sarcoma botryoides occurs chiefly in infants and children, usually in the vulvovaginal region, less often in the cervix of younger women, and rarely with its distinctive gross appearance in the corpus uteri. Most commonly, sarcoma botryoides contains some heterologous element, and is best considered the juvenile version of a mixed mesenchymal sarcoma.

The malignant, mixed Müllerian tumors contain carcinomas and sarcomas mixed together. The carcinoma may be adenocarcinoma, squamous carcinoma, undifferentiated carcinoma, or any mixture of these. The sarcoma may be pure or mixed, homologous or heterologous. There is never evidence of ectodermal or endodermal tissue in teratomas. This group of tumors is often designated as mixed mesodermal tumors; the best histogenetic term is malignant, mixed Müllerian tumors.

The pure sarcomas, whether homologous or heterologous, should be designated by their familiar names, such as leiomyosarcoma, stromal sarcoma, or rhabdomyosarcoma. The mixed sarcomas without carcinoma are designated as mixed sarcoma, homologous or mixed sarcoma, or heterologous sarcoma. Neoplasms with carcinoma and sarcoma are designated as malignant, mixed Müllerian tumors, homologous type; or malignant, mixed Müllerian tumors, heterologous type; depending upon the differentiation of the sarcomatous tissue.

Some sarcomas are composed primarily of undifferentiated cells, and many sections must be examined to find diagnostic areas. Histochemical stains are often needed to prove differentiation of malignant tissue. In spite of thorough sectioning and staining, some sarcomas of the uterus are composed entirely of tumor tissue so poorly differentiated that they defy classification. These tumors should be listed as sarcomas, unclassified. The majority of uterine sarcomas will be leiomyosarcomas; malignant, mixed Müllerian tumors; or stromal sarcomas. Other types are rarely encountered.

Terms such as carcinosarcoma and sarcoma botryoides should be discarded. Sarcoma botryoides is a clinical term for grape-like tumors, and should not be used morphologically. Most cases of botryoides sarcoma in children are embryonal rhabdomyosarcomas, and those in adults are usually malignant, mixed Müllerian tumors.

LEIOMYOSARCOMA

Malignant degeneration of the myoma is exceedingly rare, probably occurring in 0.2% or less of patients. But the great frequency of uterine myomas still makes this the most common type of uterine sarcoma. Leiomyosarcoma is statistically the most frequently encountered uterine sarcoma and comprises from 50% to 75% of various large series. In some instances, it may be difficult to ascertain from the gross appearance whether the tumor arose in a leiomyoma or not. Corscaden and Singh (1958) have distinguished between lethal and innocuous cases. They point out that, when the sarcoma is defined as cellular atypical lesions confined to a leiomyoma without evidence of invasion of the surrounding myometrium, the tumor is harmless. Usually, such cases are discovered by the pathologist on histologic examination of one or more myomata in a uterus removed without clinical or even gross pathologic suspicion of malignancy. This is a form of pathologist's cancer.

The opposite picture is presented by leiomyosarcomas that are grossly and diffusely invasive. These sarcomas tend to appear clinically as large, multinodular masses, often with a history of recent rapid growth. At exploration, they are often adherent to adjacent structures or have infiltrated widely, and casual gross inspection leaves little doubt as to their malignant nature. In Corscaden's series, all of the patients died of their disease in short order.

The postmenopausal growth of a previously known myoma or rapid growth of a static tumor may suggest the possibility of malignant change. The diagnosis of leiomyosarcoma is rarely made preoperatively, because the symptoms and physical findings are attributed to myoma. Actually, the diagnosis is made so infrequently at the time of surgery because there is usually nothing distinctive about sarcomatous degeneration. A firm diagnosis is made only on histologic examination. The triad of bleeding, pain, and rapid growth within the uterus should alert the clinician to the possibility of sarcoma of the uterus.

Clinical Features

The most frequent sign of leiomyosarcoma is profuse vaginal bleeding. The patient often presents with a very low hemoglobin, is pale, and fatigues very easily. Pelvic pain, if present, is the result of rapid enlargement of the tumor. In many respects the clinical findings are indistinguishable from those produced by benign uterine tumors. A rapid increase in uterine size may be the only clue that a sarcoma is present.

If the tumor is submucosal, the preoperative diagnosis may be made by curettage or endometrial biopsy. Most often, the tumor is intramural or subserosal, and diagnosis by curettage is impossible. Occasionally, a leiomyosarcoma may form a fleshy mass which protrudes through the cervix and can be biopsied.

Pathogenesis

There has been speculation as to whether the sarcoma arises from the mature muscle cells of the uterine wall or myoma, or whether it evolves from nests of undifferentiated cells in the myometrium. Ober (1959) states categorically that leiomyosarcoma is the most frequently encountered form of uterine sarcoma. The consistent elements of the uterus — muscle, connective tissue, epithelium, and blood vessels — are of mesodermal origin, and undoubtedly all neoplasms develop from undifferentiated cells. It may be expected that a pure sarcoma or a mixed tumor could arise from the basic element, the type depending upon the lability of the originating cell. A multitude of diverse patterns are noted in these unusual, mixed uterine malignancies.

Pathology

Gross   Leiomyosarcomas may be grossly indistinguishable from leiomyomas. Although, on occasion, the leiomyosarcoma may be somewhat softer, yellowish, and have a cystic inconsistency, on cutting into it, it is often found to be rather pulpaceous, necrotic, and cystic. The leiomyosarcoma is occasionally recognized grossly, but is most frequently an unexpected finding at microscopic examination. Ideally, every myomatous uterus should be opened in the operating room.

Marked softening and grayish-blue discoloration of myoma, especially if associated with a history of rapid or postmenopausal growth, should suggest malignant change. Cutting across a suspicious myoma and finding a mushy, necrotic, raw-pork appearance with hemorrhage, should arouse suspicions of a sarcoma; the surgeon may then wish to extend the scope of his operation. Frequently, the changes in the myoma are hyaline, cystic, or hemorrhagic, but occasionally malignant alteration is responsible.

Microscopic   The microscopic appearance of leiomyosarcoma is similar to that of sarcomas in general, the constituent cell being spindle, round, or giant cell in type. Some of the cells appear to blend with mature muscle cells. The cellular morphology makes division of the sarcomas into separate subgroups difficult, because frequently a tumor is composed of more than one cell type.

Instead of the uniform, consistent, innocuous pattern seen with benign myoma, one finds extreme pleomorphism and marked hyperchromatosis in a sarcoma; giant cells are frequent as a result of coalesced, degenerative nuclei. Mitotic activity is common and of considerable prognostic importance.

Aaro (1966) has reported that the number of mitoses is a reliable basis for the separation of leiomyomas from leiomyosarcomas. Others have depended upon pleomorphism, invasion, and the presence of giant cells, as reliable criteria. At the other extreme, Corscaden and Stout (1929) maintain that recurrences or metastases, or both, are the only valid evidence of malignancy.

The number of mitoses is the single most accurate criterion for the diagnosis of leiomyosarcoma. When there are ten or more mitoses per ten-high-power field, the vast majority of uterine smooth muscle tumors will behave aggressively, regardless of cellular atypism, presence of giant cells, or confinement of tumor to the uterus at the time of surgery. Tumors with mitotic counts about ten per ten-high-power field are classified as leiomyosarcomas. Reports indicate that tumors with five to nine metastases per ten-high-power field usually behave aggressively and metastasize. Uterine smooth muscle tumors with fewer than five mitoses per ten-high-power field are almost always benign.

The rare tumor which has fewer than five mitoses per ten-high-power field and is aggressive, will fall into the category of the so-called benign, metastasizing leiomyoma and intervenous leiomyomitoses. In these patients, mctastascs usually appear at long intervals after the initial surgery and can often be controlled by surgical excision. There is no way to separate these rare, histologically benign, but biologically malignant, tumors from leiomyomas, unless the tumor has invaded contiguous structures at the time of initial surgery.

The presence or absence of giant cells does not correlate with survival. A large number of giant cells may be found in tumors with few mitoses and a benign course. The degree of cellular atypism appears to be of limited value in determining the malignancy of smooth muscle tumors. Some leiomyosarcomas demonstrate minimal or no cellular pleomorphism, whereas smooth muscle cells and leiomyomas may be markedly atypical. In general, tumors with high mitotic counts most often contain a great number of markedly atypical cells.

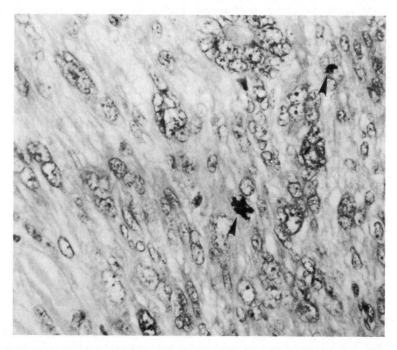

Figure 13-1 Uterine leiomyosarcoma: The tumor cells are spindle shaped with moderate nuclear atypia. The diagnosis of malignancy is established by the mitotic activity of the tumor (arrows).

The following conclusion can be drawn about uterine smooth muscle tumors: true invasion of contiguous organs or blood vessels is indicative of malignancy, regardless of mitotic counts or the presence of atypical tumor cells. Invasive leiomyosarcomas must be carefully separated from parasitic leiomyomas, which may also grow onto other organs. If invasion is not demonstrated, the mitotic count is evaluated. Tumors with zero to four mitoses per ten-high-power field are benign, regardless of the degree of cellular atypism. The uterine smooth muscle tumor with five to nine mitoses per ten-high-power field and stromal cell pleomorphism is regarded as malignant. Tumors with more than nine mitoses per ten-high-power field must be regarded as being malignant, regardless of whether atypism is present. They should be diagnosed as leiomyosarcoma. By the use of these criteria, the future behavior of almost all uterine smooth muscle tumors can be accurately predicted.

Treatment

Modern clinicians agree that the primary mode of therapy is total hysterectomy and bilateral salpingo-oophorectomy. The use of roentgen therapy alone has been abandoned, except in late cases where it is palliative. Pelvic irradiation as an adjuvant to surgery in leiomyosarcoma does not appear to increase the survival rate.

Chemotherapy is of increasing importance following primary surgery for uterine sarcomas. There is a variety of combinations of agents that are employed for the treatment of sarcomas. One regimen that is under study is the combination of cyclophosphamide, doxorubicin, and cis-platinum. Another combination that has been widely employed is vincristine, actinomycin, and cyclophosphamide. Vincristine, doxorubicin, and dimethyltriazenoimidazole carboximide (DTIC), has been reported to provide a high rate of complete or partial remission.

Survival

The overall survival rate for uterine sarcomas is approximately 20% to 30%. In leiomyosarcomas, there is a clearly increasing mortality with an increasing number of mitoses. It is evident that not all leiomyosarcomas grow and infiltrate at the same rate. Very rarely, one encounters a case in which leiomyomata have been removed for 10, 15, or 20 years before a large pelvic recurrence develops. On closer examination and further sectioning of the original tissue, one may find areas of cellular atypism that, in retrospect, can be reclassified as sarcomatous.

ENDOMETRIAL STROMAL SARCOMA

As its name implies, this sarcoma apparently arises from the endometrial stromal cell. Endometrial stromal sarcoma and its variant, endolymphatic stromal myosis, comprise the pure homologous type of endometrial sarcoma.

These tumors are usually classified into two groups on the basis of morphology and behavior. Endolymphatic stromal myosis is an infiltrating stromal lesion with an indolent course, and has been reported occasionally to recur and metastasize, usually after long periods of time. Endometrial stromal sarcoma infiltrates the myometrium more widely, and has a more aggressive course, frequent metastases, and higher mortality. Both these tumors have many features in common, including the presence of tumor cells within lymphatic spaces, and there is doubt that they represent separate entities. The number of mitoses per ten-high-power field is an accurate method of diagnosing these two neoplasms.

It must be remembered that there is a benign endometrial stromal tumor, the so-called stromal nodule, which does not infiltrate lymphatic spaces or the myometrium, and which has a low mitotic count.

Clinical Features

Endometrial stromal sarcoma occurs from adolescence to old age. Most patients are perimenopausal, but about one-third are postmenopausal. Irregular bleeding is the most common symptom. Abdominal or pelvic pain is present in a very small number of patients. The pelvic examination usually reveals a diffusely, moderately, or nodular enlarged uterus which, in advanced cases, may be fixed to other pelvic structures or the pelvic wall. Because many of these tumors protrude into the endometrial cavity, curettage or endometrial biopsy is often diagnostic. It has been reported that approximately 60% of the patients have an enlarged uterus, and that in about 20% a mass is visible in the cervical canal on vaginal speculum examination. Endometrial stromal sarcoma represents about 0.2% or less of uterine sarcomas.

Pathology

This endometrial tumor is often polypoid, and one or more polyps may actually protrude out of the cervix. The tumor may form a soft mass with extensive hemorrhage and necrosis. The mass may be well or poorly circumscribed, and may involve the myometrium alone, or both the endometrium and the myometrium, with protrusion into the endometrial cavity.

The endolymphatic stromal myosis variant may produce only a focal or diffuse thickening of the myometrium, or there may be grossly visible cords of tumor within the myometrium and the parametrial vessels.

Histologically, both groups of infiltrating stromal tumors are composed of monotonous sheets of cells of basophilic nuclei and indistinct cytoplasm. Some tumors contain predominantly round masses of tumor cells, with no infiltration at the points of contact with the myometrium. Foreign strands of reticulum surrounding individual tumor cells, or small clumps of tumor cells, can be seen with silver stains. In each case, the tumor is demonstrated within the lymphatics or lymphatic-like spaces. No heterologous elements are observed in the tumor. Lymphatic permeation can be seen, and may simulate the more benign lesion called endolymphatic stromal myosis.

In the better differentiated tumors, the cells may show some similarity to normal endometrial stroma, but as dedifferentiation progresses this might become less apparent. Hyperchromatism, pleomorphism, mitotic activity, giant cells, and very abnormal cells are apparent. On occasion, both stromal and glandular elements are stimulated to malignant degeneration by what appears to be both an endometrial sarcoma and an adenocarcinoma.

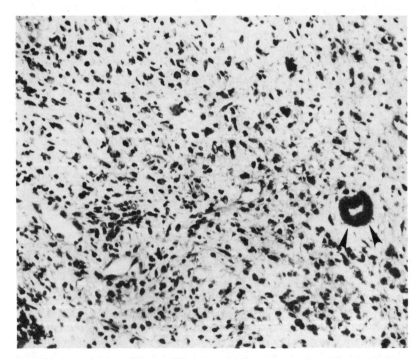

Figure 13-2 Endometrial stromal sarcoma: The tumor consists of a proliferation of small cells with hyperchromatic nuclei which surround a normal endometrial gland (arrows).

The stromal tumors are divided into two groups on the basis of mitotic counts in the most active areas of the tumor. All stromal sarcomas contain more than 20 mitoses per ten-high-power field; endolymphatic stromal myosis shows five or fewer. Reports in the literature do not reveal any tumors with counts of 6 to 12 mitoses per ten-high-power field.

Histologically, endometrial stromal sarcoma and, occasionally, endolymphatic stromal mycosis, may be confused with malignant lymphoma or undifferentiated small carcinoma of the cervix. Separation of the latter from stromal sarcoma may be a difficult problem because stromal sarcoma can invade the cervix. It has been reported that the reticulum stain is the best available method to distinguish carcinoma from stromal sarcoma.

Treatment

Total abdominal hysterectomy and bilateral salpingo-oophorectomy are recommended for the treatment of endometrial stromal sarcoma. Some consider preoperative radiotherapy, when possible, to be indicated. Because these sarcomas can frequently be diagnosed by endometrial sampling, a program for preoperative radiation can be instituted immediately.

External radiation therapy has been replaced by a combination of hormone therapy such as progestational treatment (medroxyprogesterone acetate, 400 mg intramuscularly per week, and/or megestrol acetate, 40 mg orally three times a day), and triple chemotherapy. The latter should include an alkalating agent as well as doxorubicin. The addition of actinomycin D and vincristine has provided some improvement in survival rates.

Recurrent or metastatic endometrial sarcomas should be managed with progestational therapy and combination chemotherapy, as outlined for adjunct therapy following primary radiation surgery. Because these tumors are occasionally radiosensitive, radiation therapy may be included as part of the regimen, if there is a lesion present in the pelvis.

MIXED MESODERMAL TUMORS

Mixed mesodermal tumors are uterine sarcomas mixed with various types of carcinoma. They are composed of mesodermal elements arising from the endometrial stromal cells, and epithelial elements arising from the cells of the endometrial glands. Ober (1959) has separated mesenchymal sarcoma into homologous and heterologous tumors of the uterus. Homologous mixed mesodermal tumors are tumors with nonspecific sarcomatous and carcinomatous elements; they are often referred to as carcinosarcomas. Heterologous mixed mesodermal tumors are those tumors having a combination of carcinomatous and heterologous sarcomatous elements such as striated muscle, cartilage, osteoid, bone, or fat.

The wide variety of histologic patterns encountered in malignant, mixed Müllerian tumors has created problems in accurate diagnosis and classification. One such problem is whether the presence or absence of a specifically differentiated tumor element is an important indication of future behavior. The answer will determine the extent to which these tumors should be subclassified. Data are also needed concerning the response of specific homologous or heterologous elements to therapy.

Basic Principles

Formerly, mixed mesodermal tumors were thought to have originated from embryonic cell rests. However, most investigators now believe that these tumors originate from undifferentiated stromal cells which have the capacity to differentiate into both epithelium and stroma.

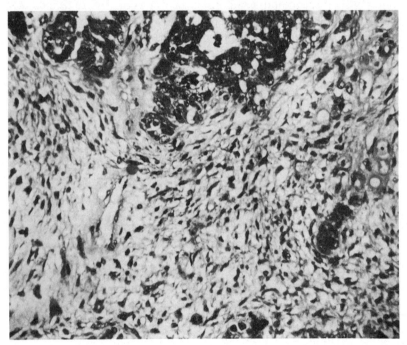

Figure 13-3 Mixed mesodermal tumor of uterus: Multiple different histologic patterns can be seen in these neoplasms. This example shows malignant glandular epithelium in the upper portion of the photomicrograph with malignant stromal cells resembling malignant smooth muscle cells seen in the midportion of the picture. This is an example of a malignant mixed mesodermal tumor of homologous type.

The pathogenesis of this tumor is not definitely known. However, a current explanation favors the theory of the growth of this tumor from pluripotential subepithelial cells.

The incidence of the tumor is increased in postmenopausal women. Many of these patients have a history of radiotherapy of the genital organs for benign gynecologic disease. A causal relationship between occurrence of carcinosarcoma and estrogen treatment of the endometrium is not mentioned in the literature.

These tumors have been subdivided into two groups: homologous and heterologous. Tumors are not placed in the heterologous group unless there is definite histologic evidence of differentiation into tissue not normally present in the uterus, such as bone, cartilage, or skeletal muscle. The type of carcinoma present is usually an adenocarcinoma. Although the term applied to these tumors is less than satisfactory, it does group together a complex of related neoplasms with similar clinical behaviors, and avoids the objectionable and imprecise term, carcinosarcoma.

The average age for the appearance of these tumors is identical to that of adenocarcinoma of the endometrium, the middle of the sixth decade. Nevertheless, it must be recognized that sarcoma botryoides of the cervix and upper vagina is a variant of the mixed tumor that usually occurs during the first decade of life. Almost all patients are postmenopausal. Sternberg (1954) has reported that these tumors occur more frequently in blacks, whereas Chuang (1970) reported the incidence in blacks to be only 2%.

Histogenesis

Meyer has explained the morphology of the mixed mesodermal tumor on the basis of three possibilities: 1) collision tumors result from two independently developing tumors that invade one another; 2) combination tumors result from two different blastomatous elements derived from one stem cell (comparable to a Wilms's tumor); and 3) composition tumors result when both the parenchyma and stroma become blastomatous. It has been suggested by Hertig (1960) that collision tumors and composition tumors are essentially similar histologically, except in the anatomic site at which the epithelial and stromal elements of the tumor arise. The combination tumor arising from a single stem cell (considered by modern investigators to be the endometrial stromal cell), is analogous to the true carcinosarcoma of the endometrial stromal origin.

Clinical Features

Mixed mesodermal sarcomas are extremely malignant and spread early to regional lymph nodes and adjacent stroma. Although the spread pattern is similar to adenocarcinoma of the endometrium, it is more aggressive. Vascular invasion is common, and lung, liver, and bone metastases occur. The most common complaints are abnormal bleeding, vaginal discharge, pelvic pressure and pain, symptoms referable to the urinary tract or intestine, and abdominal enlargement. Some patients give a history of having passed large fragments of necrotic tissue, and patients with extensive disease may complain of weakness, lassitude, and anorexia. Only a few patients are asymptomatic.

Pelvic examination may reveal enlargement of the uterus or prolapse of polypoid masses from the vagina. The irregularity produced by the tumor may be mistaken for leiomyoma. Parametrial extension may cause thickening or nodularity. Metastases to the external genitalia are rare.

Cases in the literature suggest t' at prior uterine radiation therapy (to control dysfunctional bleeding) may have an etiologic role in the development of this tumor.

Diagnosis is usually established by curettage or endometrial biopsy in a postmenopausal, bleeding patient with an enlarged uterus. The uterine cavity usually contains a necrotic, polypoid, friable tumor, which may protrude beyond the external os.

Pathology

Gross   Endometrial sarcoma and mixed tumor, present as a grayish-pink, polypoid, excrescence, often extruding from the cervical os or vaginal introitus. There may be areas of hemorrhage and necrosis. The tumors invariably involve the endometrium, and often extend into the myometrium for visible distances. Inversion of the uterus may develop as a complication, although it is not frequently recognized until the time of surgery. The malignant nature of these polypoid lesions is generally not recognized until excision or biopsy of the polyp is carried out.

Microscopic   In an excellent review of mesenchymal tumors, Ober and Tovell (1959) emphasize that the common denominator of all tumors is the endometrial stroma. Elements which are homologous (indigenous to the uterus) or heterologous (foreign to the uterus), such as cartilage and striated muscle, may be found. In homologous tumors, a carcinosarcoma evolves; in the heterologous, a mixed mesodermal tumor results. It must be restated that these two lesions are clinically and histologically similar, being variants on a theme.

It has been reported that there are varying degrees of malignancy in neoplasms of endometrial stroma, with all intermediate gradations between stromal endometriosis and frank endometrial sarcoma. Reports indicate that low-grade, pure tumors are much more common in younger women, and are relatively innocuous. The heterologous and mixed sarcomas afflict an older age group, and the prognosis is much worse.

Mixed mesodermal sarcomas are variants of endometrial sarcomas; in addition to sarcoma, they exhibit the other heterologous elements noted previously. Bone, cartilage, striated muscle, and other mesodermal elements may be found, but it is no longer believed that the demonstration of rhabdomyoblasts (striated muscle cells) is necessary for diagnosis. Nevertheless, rare malignancies of these elements, the rhabdomyosarcoma, osteosarcoma, chondrosarcoma, and liposarcoma are variants of the mixed tumors. Tumors of the so called mixed type have been divided into composition, combination, and collision types as previously described.

Electromicroscopic studies have revealed cells similar to adenocarcinomatous cells, sarcomatous cells with increased number of microvesicles, and intermediate cells. Growth of carcinosarcoma in tissue culture has revealed sarcomatous and carcinomatous cell types, but no evidence of intermediate or transitional cells.

COURSE OF THE DISEASE

The classification of the various groups of tumors into specific pathologic types is difficult, because many authors believe they are variants of the same disease. Histologically, this is undoubtedly true. Nevertheless, there are grades of malignancies similar to those noted with other tumors, and, although the clinical course depends largely on the extent of the disease at the time of therapy, the degree of anaplasia must play a role.

The low-grade endometrial sarcoma that is confined largely to the cavity, offers a much better prognosis than the bizarre mixed mesodermal tumor that has extended into the adjacent tumors. In general, the overall survival rate is poor, and early recurrences are the rule; a very high percentage of these patients die within two years of the initial treatment. It should be noted that, regardless of the initial patterns, the metastatic lesions resemble adenocarcinoma in 75% to 80% of the cases. In one reported series, the survival rate of patients with homologous tumors was 27%, and those with heterologous tumors was 15%, an insignificant difference because of the small numbers of patients that have been reported.

If heterologous elements are present, and if these are rhabdomyoblasts or osteoblasts, the prognosis is extremely grave. In one reported series, all patients whose tumors contained rhabdomyosarcoma or osteosarcoma have died. On the other hand, the only survivors in another series were patients whose tumors contained chondrosarcoma as the heterologous element. A determination of the extent of myometrial invasion is equally as important to the prognosis as is subdivision of these tumors on the basis of differentiation of the tumor cell.

Patients with homologous tumors who have survived in a reported series are those whose tumors have invaded no further than one half the distance to the myometrium at the time of hysterectomy. Tumors extending beyond this point result in death. Superficial or no myometrial invasion does not necessarily mean that the patient will survive, because some deaths and metastases occur in the absence of invasion.

For patients with heterologous tumors, the extent of the tumor at the time of therapy is also important. The only survivors reported in a series of heterologous tumors had small superficial tumors with chondrosarcoma as the only heterologous element. All reported tumors that contained rhabdomyosarcoma or osteosarcoma had extended outside the uterus, and were larger than 4 cm at the time of diagnosis.

Treatment

Generally, therapy consists of total hysterectomy, bilateral salpingo-oophorectomy, and, in selected patients, irradiation. These tumors have not responded well to external x-ray therapy. However, striking local regression of stromal sarcoma has been reported after radiation therapy, but metastases often appear outside the pelvis, even though the primary tumor has decreased in size.

Currently, encouraging results have been reported with combination chemotherapy, including an alkylating agent, actinomycin D, vincristine, and doxorubicin. The role of cis-platinum remains to be evaluated. If these patients are to be treated with chemotherapy, at least a three-drug or four-drug regimen is indicated. In some sarcomas, the use of progestational agents has had a beneficial effect on the stroma of the tumor.

HEMANGIOPERICYTOMA

Hemangiopericytoma is a rare but widely distributed connective tissue tumor, composed of nonneoplastic capillary endothelium, surrounded by collars of neoplastic capillary pericytes. It is closely related to the glomus tumor. The first report of this tumor in the uterus was by Greene and Gerbie (1954), who presented five well-illustrated, well-documented cases. In general, these seem to be discrete, well demarcated, spherical tumors, grossly similar to leiomyomas, although possibly with a less whorled texture. They are more cellular than the average myoma.

Pathology

Gross   These tumors are not grossly pathognomonic and may be mistaken for leiomyomas, but they are usually less discrete, softer, and yellow. They vary in size from 1.5 cm to 8 cm, and are nonencapsulated.

Microscopic　The tumors exhibit a proliferation of medium-sized, ovoid, perivascular cells, presumably derived from the pericytes of Zimmermann. Sections show numerous nonneoplastic capillaries, often collapsed and surrounded by reticulum sheaths. The reticulum sheath separates the endothelium from the surrounding collars of neoplastic pericytes. These tumor cells, each surrounded by reticulum fibers, are epithelioid or spindle-shaped, with uniform, round, or oval nuclei. Mitoses are rarely seen. The variable amount of collagen, not indigenous to the tumor, is compressed by the collar-like masses of pericytes. Reticulum stains to demonstrate the single layer of endothelial cells on an argyrophilic membrane are useful in distinguishing this type of tumor from proliferations of endothelial origin. The perivascular pattern is quite distinctive. Because hemangiopericytomas are characterized histologically by concentric arrangement of pericytes around capillaries, differential stains are often necessary to distinguish them from stromatosis or vascular myomas. Although generally benign, this lesion should be regarded as a low grade (20% to 25%) malignancy.

Treatment and Prognosis

In general, hemangiopericytomas are unpredictable in terms of local recurrence and metastasis. None of the cases described so far in the uterus has displayed invasive or recurrent potentialities. A circumscribed tumor within the myometrium is more likely to be benign than, for example, a tumor of similar histologic appearance that is locally infiltrative in soft tissue. As a rule, these tumors are usually found incidentally, and the prognosis is good. Surgery is the treatment of choice; radiation therapy has not been particularly effective. Chemotherapy remains to be evaluated in this small group of tumors. If it is used, it should be used as a multi-drug regimen.

BENIGN METASTASIZING LEIOMYOMA

This tumor has often been called an intravascular fibromyoma, metastasizing fibromyoma, a metastatic myoma, or a recurring fibromyoma. This is a very rare condition in which a leiomyoma, apparently histologically benign, extends locally by way of blood vessels or lymphatics, or metastasizes to more distant organs. Usually, when such a case is described, doubt is expressed as to whether the tissues examined microscopically were representative of the entire tumor, or whether an area of sarcoma might have been overlooked. This is a fascinating type of intravenous myomatous lesion that has been intermittently reported for the past 70 years. The intravenous leiomyomatosis presents a rather typical gross appearance; cords of tumor extending through the myometrium and into the broad ligaments. Thromboembolic complications have rarely been associated with this tumor.

Treatment

Total hysterectomy and bilateral salpingo-oophorectomy is the treatment usually chosen. The question of radiation therapy is raised, but is usually not employed because of the intravascular infiltration of this tumor. Chemotherapy would seem to be the treatment of choice as an adjuvant type of therapy, but its role remains to be evaluated.

LYMPHOMA

This is an extremely rare tumor and is usually associated with generalized lymphoma, but it may occur alone. The lymphoma has a tendency to spread by the hematogenous route, and, therefore, involvement of the liver and lungs is common. Malignant lymphoma in the female genital tract poses the unanswerable question of primary site vs multicentric origin. In cases of leukemia, the female genital organs are found at autopsy to be involved by leukemic infiltrates in proportion to the assiduity with which search is made for such manifestations. Very rarely, a lymphoma may appear to be primary in the uterus, as in one of the uterine leiomyosarcomas or in reticulum cell sarcoma. There are very few cases in the literature, and, in most of them, the uterine lymphoma was part of a generalized disease which was present concurrently or manifested itself soon thereafter.

A chest film is mandatory in any suspected case of lymphoma of the pelvis. The survival rate is usually low, and, in an overall series, is about 25%.

Symptoms

There are no characteristic symptoms. Bleeding may occur and, if curettage is carried out, the diagnosis is usually made. Occasionally, vaginal bleeding may be a presenting symptom of an underlying leukemia of lymphomatosis.

Treatment

Total hysterectomy, bilateral salpingo-oophorectomy, and postoperative irradiation to the pelvis are recommended.

Because this tumor is inclined to have a hematogenous spread, chemotherapy is indicated, since it is known that a lymphoma responds well to it. At present, there are no data to support the use of chemotherapy for uterine lymphomas, except to equate the possibility of response with the good response from chemotherapy of lymphoma present elsewhere in the body.

METASTATIC SARCOMA AND UNCLASSIFIED SARCOMA

Ober has reported that he has never seen or heard of sarcoma metastatic to the uterus, unless one includes leukemic infiltrates or multicentric lymphoma. He also stated that the group of unclassified sarcomas is placed in the classification both as a warning and as a safety valve.

BIBLIOGRAPHY

Aaro LA, Symmonds RE, Dockerty MB: Sarcoma of the uterus: A clinical and pathological study of 177 cases. *Am J Obstet Gynecol* 94:101, 1966.

Azizi F, Bitran J, Javehari G, et al: Remission of uterine leiomyosarcomas treated with vincristine, adriamycin, and dimethyl-triazeno-imidazole carboximide. *Am J Obstet Gynecol* 133(4):379, 1979.

Barber HRK (ed): Sarcoma of the uterus, in *Manual of Gynecologic Oncology*. Philadelphia, J.B. Lippincott Co, 1980, Chap 24.

Belgrad R, Elbadai N, Rubin P: Uterine sarcoma. *Radiology* 114:181, 1975.

Cavanagh D, Praphat H, Ruffolo EH: *Sarcoma of the Uterus*. New York, Appleton-Century-Crofts, 1979.

Chuang JT, VanVelden DJJ, Graham JD: Carcinosarcoma and mixed mesodermal of the uterine corpus: A review of 49 cases. *Obstet Gynecol* 35:769, 1970.

Corscaden JA, Stout AP: Sarcoma of the uterus. *Am J Roentgenol* 21:155, 1929.

Corscaden JA, Singh BP: Leiomyosarcoma of the uterus. *Am J Obstet Gynecol* 75:149, 1958.

DiSaia PJ, Castro JR, Rutledge FN: Mixed mesodermal sarcoma of the uterus. *Am J Roentgenol Radium Ther Nucl Med* 117:632, 1973.

Gilbert HA, Kagan AR, Lagasse L, et al: The value of radiation therapy in uterine sarcoma. *Obstet Gynecol* 45:84, 1975.

Greene RR, Gerbie AB: Hemangiopericytoma of the uterus. *Obstet Gynecol* 3:150, 1954.

Gruenwald P: The relation of the growing Müllerian duct to the Wolffian duct and its importance for the genesis of malformation. *Anat Record* 81:1, 1941.

Hart WR, Yoonessi M: Endometrial stromatosis of the uterus. *Obstet Gynecol* 49:393, 1977.

Hayes D: Mixed Müllerian tumor of the corpus uteri. *J Obstet Gynecol Brit Commonw* 81:160, 1974.

Hertig AT, Gore H: Tumors of the female sex organs, Part 2, in *Tumors of the Vulva, Vagina and Uterus*. Washington, Armed Forces Institute of Pathology, 1960.

Johnson CE, Soule EH: Malignant lymphoma as a gynecologic problem. *Obstet Gynecol* 9:149, 1957.

386

Kempson RL, Bari W: Uterine sarcomas: Classification, diagnosis and prognosis. *Human Pathol* 1:331, 1970.

Mazur MT, Askin FB: Endolymphatic stromal myosis. Unique presentation and ultrastructural study. *Cancer* 42:2661, 1978.

Meyer R: Beitrag zur verständigunz uber die namengebunz in der geschwlstlehre. *Zentr Allgen Path* 30:291, 1919.

McGowan L (ed): *Sarcoma of the Uterus: Gynecologic Oncology*. New York, Appleton-Century-Crofts, 1978.

Mortel R, Koss L, Lewis JL Jr, et al: Mesodermal mixed tumors of the uterine corpus. *Obstet Gynecol* 43:248, 1974.

Mosel A: Endometrial carcinosarcoma in a young woman with Turner's syndrome. *Geburts Frauenheilkd* 39(3):217, 1979.

Nicholson GW: Multiple mesodermal mixed tumors of the uterus, associated with pleuricentric carcinomata. *Guy's Hosp Rept* 69:173, 1918.

Ober WB: Uterine sarcoma: Histogenesis and taxonomy. *Ann NY Acad Sci* 75:568, 1959.

Ober WB, Jason S: Sarcoma of the endometrial stroma. *AMA Arch Pathol* 56:301, 1953.

Ober WB, Tovell HMM: Mesenchymal sarcomas of the uterus. *Am J Obstet Gynecol* 77:246, 1959.

Silverberg SG: Leiomyosarcoma of the uterus. A clinico-pathologic study. *Obstet Gynecol* 38:613, 1971.

Silverberg SG: Reproducibility of the mitosis count in the histological diagnosis of smooth muscle tumors of the uterus. *Human Pathol* 7:451, 1976.

Silverberg SG: Malignant mixed mesodermal tumor of the uterus: An ultrastructural study. *Am J Obstet Gynecol* 110:702, 1971.

Smith JP, Rutledge F, Delclos L, et al: Combined irradiation and chemotherapy for sarcoma of the pelvis in females. *Am J Roentgenol Radium Ther Nucl Med* 123:571, 1975.

Smith JP: Chemotherapy in gynecologic cancer. *Clin Obstet Gynecol* 18:109, 1975.

Sternberg WH, Clark WH, Smith RC: Malignant mixed Müllerian tumors (mixed mesodermal of the uterus). A study of 21 cases. *Cancer* 7:704, 1954.

Symmonds RE, Dockerty MB: Sarcoma and sarcoma-like proliferation of the endometrial stroma. I. A clinico-pathologic study of 19 mixed mesodermal tumors. *Surg Gynecol Obstet* 100:232, 1955.

Taylor HB, Norris HJ: Mesenchymal tumors of the uterus. IV. Diagnosis and prognosis of leiomyosarcomas. *Arch Pathol* 82:40, 1966.

Taylor CW: Müllerian mixed tumor. *Acta Pathol Microbiol Scand* 80 (suppl 23):48, 1972.

Williamson EO, Christopherson WM: Malignant mixed Müllerian tumors of the uterus. *Cancer* 29:585, 1972.

Willis RA: *Pathology of Tumors*. London, Butterworth, 1948, p 754.

14 Childhood Gynecologic Tumors

Hugh R. K. Barber

Cancer, rather surprisingly, is now one of the most important causes of death in childhood. This is due to the decrease in infant mortality from infectious diseases in the past quarter of a century. Although cancer is primarily an adult disease, it kills more children between the ages of 3 and 14 than any other disease. Incidence and mortality have declined slightly over the years, but, in 1981 cancer is expected to afflict some 6200 children and kill about 2300 of them. Common childhood cancers include leukemia (accounting for one half of the deaths), and cancer of the brain and central nervous system, soft tissue, kidney, and bone. For all forms of cancer occurring in children under age 15, the five-year survival rate adjusted for normal life expectancy is 39%. For the most frequent forms, the rate ranges from zero for some leukemias to 84% for eye tumors. In some medical centers, the five-year survival rate for acute lymphocytic leukemia — the most common childhood type — is 50% to 75%. In the age group 1 to 15, tumors are exceeded in lethality only by accidents.

It should be noted that a primary care physician is unlikely to see more than a couple of cases in a working lifetime. Diagnosis is usually difficult, since the early signs tend to be vague — pallor, unsteadiness, loss of appetite, headache — all of which are common to many other disorders. In most cases, the mode of origin of the growth differs from that in adults, being a developmental malformation (which may even be present at birth), rather than a result of chronic irritation. Hence, epithelial, ie, surface tissues, which are the usual sufferers from chronic trauma, are not generally the sites of origin.

Immunological factors are also probably important. The antibody recognition and defense systems are immature in the young child, and this may account for the frequency of acute lymphoblastic leukemia. Whether virus infection plays any part in induction is still uncertain and unproved, though the idea is very tempting, especially since comparable leukemias can certainly be induced by viruses in laboratory animals. Just as normal growth in children is more pronounced than in adults, some malignant growths tend to develop rapidly and metastasize early. They are correspondingly radiosensitive, but this unfortunately does not mean radiocurability.

The term childhood or adolescent gynecological tumors is used to indicate any new growth (benign or malignant) occurring between birth and age 14. (Some consider adolescence to extend to age 16). This implies the growth of newly formed cells derived from normal body cells or preceding developmental cells. Benign neoplasm indicates a tumor that does not in itself destroy the host, while a malignant neoplasm, if left untreated, destroys the host.

The American Cancer Society is currently establishing advisory committees on childhood cancer throughout the country at the Division level. These committees will determine the most urgent needs of children with cancer, as well as those of their families, and the best ways of meeting these needs. A National American Cancer Society Advisory Committee on Childhood Cancer will assist in the development of the Division committees, and serve as a forum for communication between cancer specialists and others involved in the care of children with malignancies.

About 3% of malignancy in childhood and adolescence is related to the gynecologic system. Even the busy gynecologist, unless he specializes in pediatric gynecology, sees relatively few tumors of the genital tract in children during any one year. Since the average pediatrician also has marked limitations in exposure to pediatric gynecologic oncology, he should refer any case in which the diagnosis is in doubt and the therapy beyond his capabilities, to a qualified specialist or clinic.

It must be emphasized that in some cases time is the essence between localized and widespread disease. Procrastination and hoping that time will take care of the disease is fraught with great dangers for the patient; and, from the physician's standpoint, this exposes him or her not only to the disappointment, frustration, and emotional turmoil of having missed an important diagnosis, but also to the threat of a large malpractice award for many years in the future. It is important to remember that if in doubt, obtain a consultation!

Statistics show that cancer originating in the reproductive system in childhood and adolescent age groups is characterized by rapid growth, early spread, and frequently a fatal outcome. There are basic differences between pelvic cancer in the adult and in pediatric and adolescent groups. These are:

1. There is limited space available for tumor expansion.
2. The effect of therapy, especially radical surgery or irradiation (with respect to further development of the individual), is different.
3. There is a high degree of malignancy in cancer of the young.
4. The most commonly seen neoplasms are special types of ovarian and uterovaginal sarcoma.
5. The immunologic surveillance mechanism is very inefficient in childhood.

EMBRYOLOGY

In order to understand completely gynecological neoplasms in children, a brief review of the embryology of the female genital tract is relevant. The urogenital organs include two separate systems with wholly different functions, but they are so closely related embryologically and anatomically that it is impossible to study one and, at the same time, ignore the other. While mesoderm is the major component in the development of the urogenital system, the entoderm and ectoderm also make important contributions.

The urogenital fold or mesonephric ridge is a large and important body occupying the posterior or dorsal portion of the primitive peritoneal cavity. This structure lies on each side of the midline, and runs the entire length of the fetus. From this urogenital fold arise the ovaries, kidneys, Fallopian tubes, uterus, and part of the vagina. Even in the later stages of fetal development, the distance between the structures is measured in millimeters. The urogenital fold serves to explain the interrelationship between these structures, as well as the possibility for congenital rests between organ systems.

Development of the Ovary

The germ cells which will eventually inhabit the gonads originate from the primitive hindgut. They appear around the 25th day. By 30 days, the gut, complete with mesentery, has been formed. The germ cells now migrate from the gut to the root of the mesentery. At the same time, the celomic epithelium proliferates and forms thickenings, the genital ridges, together with the underlying mesenchyma on either side of the mesenteric root near the developing kidney.

At this stage the primitive gonad (genital ridge) consists of mesoderm (celomic epithelium plus mesenchyme) covered by celomic epithelium. The germ cells now migrate from the root of the mesentery to the genital ridge. The celomic epithelium growing into the genital ridge forms so-called sex cords, which enclose each germ cell. Up to this time, around the seventh week, the gonad is of indifferent type, male being indistinguishable from female. The germ cells and most of the sex-cord cells remain in the superficial part, the future cortex of the ovary. The cords lose contact with the surface epithelium and form small groups of cells, each with its germ cell, a primitive follicle. Some of the sex cords grow into the medulla. These tend to regress and form rudimentary tubules, the rete.

As the ovary grows, it projects increasingly into the peritoneal (celomic) cavity, thus forming a mesentery. At the same time, the ovary descends extraperitoneally into the abdominal cavity. Two ligaments develop, and these may help to control its descent, guiding it to its final position and preventing its complete descent through the inguinal ring, in contrast to the testis. The first structure is the suspensory ligament, attached to the anterior (cephalic) pole of the ovary and connecting it with its site of origin, the genital ridge. Another ligament or gubernaculum develops at the posterior caudal end of the ovary. At first attached to the genital ridge, it later becomes attached to the developing uterus and follows the latter.

Development of Uterus and Fallopian Tubes

When the embryo reaches the size of 10 mm at 35 to 36 days, a longitudinal groove appears on the dorsal aspect of the celomic cavity lateral to the Wolffian (mesonephric) ridge. This groove or fold becomes sealed off to form a tube, the paramesonephric or Müllerian duct. The tube is open at its upper end, communicating with the future peritoneal cavity. The lower end forms a solid tip (Müllerian tubercle).

The Müllerian ducts from either side grow in a caudal direction, extraperitoneally. They also bend medially and anteriorly, and ultimately fuse in front of the hindgut. The mesonephric duct becomes involved in the walls of the paramesonephric ducts. At first, there is a septum separating the lumina of the two ducts. Later, the septum disappears, and a single cavity is formed, the uterus. The upper parts of both ducts retain their identity and form the Fallopian tubes. While this is happening, the ovary is also affected. Its gubernaculum is ultimately attached to the Müllerian duct at the cornua of the developing uterus. Its effect is to pull the ovary medially, so that its long axis becomes horizontal.

The lower end of the fused Müllerian ducts beyond the uterine lumen remains solid, proliferates, and forms a solid cord. This cord will develop a canal to form the vagina, which opens into the urogenital sinus. At the point of entry into the urogenital sinus, part of the Müllerian tubercle persists and forms the hymen.

Development of External Genitalia

At an early stage, the hindgut and the various urogenital ducts open into a common cloaca. A septum (urorectal) grows down between the allantois and the hindgut during the fifth week.

Eventually this septum fuses with the cloacal membrane, thus dividing the cloaca into two compartments—the rectum dorsally and the urogenital sinus ventrally. At the same time, the developing uterus grows down and makes contact with the urogenital sinus. At the end of the seventh week, the urogenital membrane breaks down so that the urogenital sinus opens onto the surface. The developing uterus and vagina push downward and cause an elongation and narrowing of the upper part of the urogenital sinus. This will form the urethra.

Meanwhile, on the surface of the embryo, around the urogenital sinus, five swellings appear. At the cephalic end, a medial line swelling grows, the genital tubercle, which will become the clitoris. Posterior to the genital tubercle and on either side of the urogenital membrane a fold is formed—the urethral fold. Lateral to each of these, a further swelling appears—the genital or labial swelling. These swellings approach each other at their posterior ends, fuse, and form the posterior commissure. The remaining swellings become the labia minora.

Certain small but clinically important glands are formed in and around the urogenital sinus. In the embryo, epithelial buds arise from the urethra and also from the epithelium of the urogenital sinus. In the male, these two sets of buds grow together and give rise to the glands of the prostate. They remain separate in the female, the urethral buds forming the urethral glands and the urogenital buds giving rise to the paraurethral glands of Skene. Later, the ducts open into the vestibule on either side of the urethra. Two other small glands arise by budding from the epithelium of the posterior part of the vestibule, one on either side of the vaginal opening. These are the greater vestibular or Bartholin's glands. Similar, smaller glands also arise in the anterior portion of the vestibule.

Development of the Kidneys

The three embryonal kidneys arise from the mesonephric area in succession: the pronephros, the mesonephros (Wolffian body), and the metanephros, the permanent kidney. The metanephros has a double origin. The ureter, pelvis, calyces, and collecting tubules arise as an outgrowth of the Wolffian duct, whereas the secreting parts of the tubules are formed directly from the posterior end of the intermediate cell mass.

Development of the Adrenal (Suprarenal Gland)

Although the adrenal gland is not a part of the urogenital system, its proximity, overlapping function, and propensity for producing aberrant rests in the reproductive system proper, make it appropriate to include a brief outline of its development.

The adrenal gland is formed by a combination of mesodermal elements which develop into the cortex, and an ectodermal portion which forms the medulla. Mesothelial cells located between the root of the mesentery and the developing gonad begin to proliferate during the fifth week of development, and penetrate the underlying mesenchyme. Here they differentiate into the formation of the fetal or primitive cortex. Shortly thereafter, a second wave of cells from the mesothelium penetrates the mesenchyma and forms the definitive cortex of the gland. During the time that the cortex is developing, cells originating in the sympathetic system (ectoderm) invade its medial aspect and become arranged in cords and clusters, forming the medulla.

TUMORS OF THE VULVA

Genital neoplasms occur very rarely in human females less than 16 years of age; they are seldom encountered, even in large pediatric clinics and hospitals. Despite their rarity, almost every type of genital tumor, and certainly all of the common ones occurring in adults, have been discovered in girls less than 16 years of age. Although genital tumors in such girls is rare, each type of growth has been reported, and the fact remains that the immature genitalia have the potentiality for developing all varieties of neoplasms.

Approximately one half of the tumors discovered in children under age 16 are potentially malignant. Many histologically benign tumors in this age group are as lethal as cancers, because of the rapidity of their development or because their size or location interferes with or destroys vital physiologic functions. More neoplasms in childhood are composed of morphologically immature, dysontogenetic tissues than are new growths in adults. In this regard, it may be pointed out that 90% of all malignant neoplasms in all age groups are carcinomas. In children, however, the ratio between sarcomas and carcinomas is reversed: 90% of all malignant neoplasms in childhood are sarcomas.

It has been suggested that many malignancies found in infants actually start before birth. Both benign and malignant tumors have been discovered in fetal organs. The preponderance of dysontogeneic tumors in infancy and childhood implies that most childhood neoplasms have their origin in an embryonic nidus. In infancy, most teratomas are composed of immature tissues which give evidence of arising from embryonic elements and which develop potentialities for differentiating in directions other than those taken by the normal tissues surrounding them.

Whenever a girl up to age 16 presents with any swelling or ulceration, the diagnosis of a malignant change must be entertained, and adequate measures taken either to rule this diagnosis in or out.

As in the adult, early diagnosis and prompt, effective treatment of genital tumors improves the prognosis in children. All too often, the fact that neoplasms of the genital organs in children are so rare may lead to a delay in the diagnosis. New growths in childhood usually are more advanced when first diagnosed because of the reluctance on the part of parents and physicians to accept the fact that this is abnormal and will not disappear.

CLASSIFICATION

Benign

1. Cyst of the canal of Nuck
2. Epithelial occlusion cyst
3. Paraurethral cyst
4. Cyst of Bartholin's glands
5. Hidradenoma
6. Fibroma
7. Lipoma
8. Hemangioma
9. Labial papilloma
10. Hymenal tags
11. Lymphangioma
12. Condylomata
13. Fibroepithelial tabs
14. Granular cell myeloblastoma
15. Granulomatous lesions
16. Lesions of the integument
17. Herpesvirus complicating condylomata

Malignant

1. In situ carcinoma
2. Invasive carcinoma
3. Sarcoma

Benign Tumors

Relatively few benign tumors of the vulva occur during childhood. The sebaceous and sweat glands from which some benign vulval neoplasms develop do not become active until after menarche. Bartholin's cysts or tumors are very rare in childhood.

Any variation in the vulva that is considered abnormal by parents results in a visit to the physician. Benign and malignant tumors are rare in children. However, an overall knowledge of the significant pathology, as well as the variations that can exist in this area, is important. It serves for an informed and intelligent decision (both diagnostic and therapeutic) about pathologic conditions arising in the vulva.

White lesions are uncommon, but may occur. They represent a thinning of the integument in the area, and biopsy readily establishes the diagnosis. Unless distressing symptoms occur, therapy is not necessary. It is reported that many cases recover spontaneously in the postmenarchal years. Despite the young age of these patients, any persistant ulceration or tumor formation should be biopsied.

Granulomatous lesions are of two varieties, pyogenic granulomata and the nonspecific chronic granulomatous lesions. Biopsy readily makes a specific diagnosis and excludes more serious problems. The former responds to cauterization and either local or systemic antibiotics. The nonspecific type usually responds to estrogen ointments.

Tumors of the vulva may originate in the labia, vulval glands, vestibule, or clitoris. They may remain localized or extend locally or to distant lymph nodes or organs. Benign tumors of the vulva run the whole gamut seen in the adult.

The most common benign lesion of the vulva is the *hemangioma*. The cavernous variety is more difficult to treat. However, the port-wine and strawberry hemangiomas can be controlled by cryotherapy with carbon dioxide ice or newer forms of cryosurgical apparatus. Recently, spectacular results have been reported with the CO_2 laser beam as a method of treating large hemangiomas and lymphangiomas.

Epithelial inclusion cysts may develop from bits of vulvar or vaginal epithelium buried beneath the mucosa at the time of a laceration or other trauma. They are seldom more than a few centimeters in diameter, lie against the covering mucosa, and contain thick, caseous material. They have a smooth, inner surface lined by squamous epithelium. An epithelial inclusion cyst is treated by simple excision.

Lymphangiomas may be single or multiple. The majority are manifested as a localized swelling. Basically, the histology is not unlike an hemangioma, except that the tumor sinuses are filled with lymph instead of blood. Good results have been reported in treating these with the CO_2 laser beam.

Hidradenomas are derived from apocrine sweat glands, and are found in the labia. They are usually small, subcutaneous, cystic tumors that protrude and have a characteristic umbilication. Occasionally, they may be pedunculated. They are benign and respond to simple excision if their size becomes a problem.

Fibromas (papillomata) are seen as solid, fibrous masses, usually on a pedicle. Small, asymptomatic tumors require no therapy. If they become enlarged, excision is indicated. The same basic principles apply to fibroepithelial polyps. Labial papillomas are similar to squamous papillomas found elsewhere in the body, but must be differentiated from sarcoma in the vulva. Lipomas are also fairly common. Again, no therapy is indicated for these small, rounded, soft, fatty tumors. With increasing size, simple excision is indicated.

Leiomyomata are relatively rare, but have been reported. The finding of a harder, circumscribed, subcutaneous tumor might suggest the diagnosis, but also raises the possibility of sarcoma. Removal by local excision is not indicated unless there is rapid growth or a change in the appearance of this small nodule. Usually, the exact diagnosis is not made until the time of excision and laboratory examination.

Myoblastoma (granular cell myoblastoma) of the vulva is uncommon, usually a benign tumor that may develop in the skin, subcutaneous tissue, and voluntary muscles. A few malignant myoblastomas which metastasize have been reported; local recurrence because of incomplete excision is not unusual. A number of tumors of this type have been found in the vulvar tissue of adults but they are quite rare in children. The tumors are usually less than 2 cm in diameter and present as globular, distinctly outlined, grayish-yellow nodules that cause the child no distress. They may be mistaken for a sebaceous cyst in an older girl. Histologically, the microscopic picture may suggest striated muscle at first glance, but there are no crossed striations in this tumor. The origin of granular cell myoblastoma is uncertain. While some suggest that they originate from muscle, the present concensus is that they arise from neurologic tissue, probably from the nerve sheath. Treatment consists of local excision. The margin of the growth may be indefinite. It may recur unless the line of excision is well beyond its visible edge.

Cysts of the canal of Nuck (hydrocele of the vulva) originate as a cystic dilatation of the closed end of the hernia sac with atrophy of the proximal portion, as indicated by a fibrous tissue band leading proximally into the inguinal canal. They are usually found in the labia majora. A hydrocele of the vulva is not a true tumor. A swelling due to a vulvar hydrocele is more common in the right than in the left labium. It is located more anteriorly than a cyst of the major vestibular (Bartholin's) gland duct. It may extend upward to the inguinal ligament. When exposed surgically, it is found to be a pendant-shaped sac, largest at its dorsal end and terminating anteriorly in a long thin strand. The latter turns laterally and courses towards the inguinal region. The terminal end of the round ligament lies along one side of the cyst, which is covered by a thin layer of muscle formed by the outer part of the vestibular bulb. The sac has a smooth lining resembling peritoneum and is filled with clear fluid. Unless their size dictates intervention, they can be disregarded. The differential diagnosis includes a labial hernia. A hernia contains an ovary, bowel, omentum, or other viscera, and is usually reducible. A hydrocele contains only fluid.

Paraurethral cysts (inclusion cysts) usually occur when the paraurethral glands become infected, and there is closure of the proximal ends leading into the urethra. They are occasionally seen in adolescents. Unless they become symptomatic, they have no clinical importance. With infection, simple excision and drainage controls this condition. If diverticuli occur, they should be excised.

The diagnosis of a paraurethral duct cyst is made on the basis of its location in relation to the urethra, and on the histologic appearance of its lining if it is excised. Most paraurethral cysts are found in the urethrovaginal wall dorsal to the outer third of the urethra. There is seldom any difficulty in differentiating them from the mesonephric (Gartner's) ducts that are almost always located along the lateral sides of the vagina, or from the paramesonephric cysts that are more often near the cervix.

The treatment should be conservative, if possible. However, if a large paraurethral cyst blocks the vagina or compresses the urethra sufficiently to block it partially or completely, it must be excised or marsupialized. The dissection is difficult because of the limited size of the area and the hazard of injury to the urethra. If the cyst is causing no trouble, it should not be removed until after the menarche. It is excised at that time so that, with coitus or delivery, it will not rupture into the urethra.

Condyloma acuminatum has been uncommon in the past. However, with the new sexual revolution, it is being seen with increasing frequency. When complicated with herpesvirus 2, it gives a very ominous clinical appearance. The multiple, wart-like excrescences sometimes respond to local hygiene and sulfa cream, but generally their removal by electrodesiccation and curettement is indicated. Follow-up attention to hygiene is necessary if a recurrence of the condyloma is to be prevented. Some physicians use podophyllin in oil locally, but unless the lesion is very small, the results usually are unsatisfactory.

Condyloma acuminatum is a common, venereally transmitted lesion of the cervix due to a human papilloma virus. It can be diagnosed on Pap smears during mass screening programs, localized colposcopically, and confirmed by tissue biopsies. Patients with this lesion must be followed carefully, since they seem to be at an increased risk for cancer of the cervix, due to the possible oncogenic role of the condyloma virus.

When condyloma acuminatum is detected cytologically, the patient is referred for colposcopy, since the lesions are not usually visible with the speculum. Four types of condylomatous lesions can be identified with the colposcope: the typical florid condyloma acuminatum, the early condyloma, the flat condyloma, and the "condylomatous vaginitis."

The specific presentation of condyloma acuminatum on Pap smears, at colposcopy, and on cervical biopsies has only recently been recognized. These lesions were often previously misdiagnosed as dysplasia. Therefore, differential morphologic diagnosis between condyloma acuminatum and dysplasia is of great importance, particularly because the former is a self-limited disease which regresses spontaneously within 6 to 18 months. Condyloma acuminatum is found in younger age groups than dysplasia, and is seen quite frequently in the sexually active, young teenager.

Hymenal tags are a relatively common minor developmental anomaly. Lesions appearing at the hymenal ring are usually judged to be hymenal tags. This may cause a delay in making a diagnosis and, therefore, a delay in treatment if the condition is more serious. Since they may be confused with a neoplasm of the vulva, it is preferable to excise them and have the tissue diagnosed histologically.

Malignant Tumors

Carcinoma of the vulva in children is extremely rare, but a few cases of carcinoma in situ and even invasive cancer have been reported in the literature. These lesions have an extremely malignant clinical course, and widespread local and distant metastases must be ruled out before radical therapy is undertaken. Adequate surgery consists of a radical vulvectomy, including superficial nodes and, if indicated, deep node dissection.

Embryonic tumors of the perineum are extremely rare. However, a malignant teratoma of the perineum is occasionally reported in the literature. Teratomas in this area are more likely to be seen overlying the dorsal aspect of the sacrum and coccyx, or as retroperitoneal teratomas located between the rectum and the sacrococcygeal spine.

CLASSIFICATION OF TUMORS OF THE VAGINA AND HYMEN

Benign

1. Hematocolpos
2. Congenital cyst
3. Mesonephric (Gartner's) duct cyst
4. Epithelial inclusion or retention cyst
5. Polyps

6. Angioma
7. Lipoma
8. Fibroma
9. Lymphangioma
10. Paramesonephric (Müllerian) duct cyst
11. Vaginal polyps
12. Vaginal condyloma acuminatum

Malignant

1. Squamous carcinoma
2. Adenocarcinoma
3. Clear-cell carcinoma
4. Rhabdomyosarcoma (sarcoma botryoides)

Benign Tumors

Benign tumors of the vagina in children usually are unilocular cysts of remnants of the mesonephric ducts or, rarely, accumulations of fluid in a portion of an unfused paramesonephric duct. *Congenital cysts* of the hymen are occasionally seen, measuring 2 to 8 mm in diameter. They usually occur on the external surface, but may occur on the inner surface. Squamous cell papillomas and granulation polyps of the vagina are rare in children. Congenital cysts are usually epithelial inclusion cysts or retention cysts, and may disappear or drain spontaneously. If necessary, they can be easily removed.

One of the more common conditions seen in pediatric gynecology is congenital obstruction of the lower vaginal tract by an *imperforate hymen.* A bulging membrane is seen, and, in the newborn or neonatal period, the fluid behind the hymen is nonsanguineous. Simple incision and drainage usually solves the problem (hydrometrocolpos). The fluid retention may involve not only the vagina but the uterus as well, presenting as an abdominal tumor.

Cystic enlargements of remnants of a mesonephric duct, although infrequently seen in infants, children, and adolescents, are, nevertheless, the commonest type of benign vaginal swelling encountered in infancy and childhood. They are retention cysts, but not true neoplasms. It will be recalled that in the embryonic life, a mesonephric duct extends along the lateral side of each unfused paramesonephric (Müllerian) duct and, also, that shortly after fusion of the paramesonephric ducts, the lowest portions of the mesonephric ducts regress. However, some portions do not regress, and form clear-cell cysts along the lateral part of the vagina. The mesonephric duct cyst usually needs no treatment and, if it is to be treated, it should be marsupialized.

Cystic remnants of unfused paramesonephric ducts (Müllerian) are rarely encountered in patients of any age. They seem to cause most trouble at menarche, when the cavity of the unfused remnants becomes filled with menstrual blood. It will be recalled that the paramesonephric ducts of the embryo are paired and lie against each other in the lower portion of the urogenital cord. The medial walls of the two ducts break down during embryonic growth and the united ducts become the ureterovaginal canal. Later, the epithelium of the urogenital sinus grows upward and replaces the original paramesonephric epithelium lining the canal. Occasionally, a remnant of one of the ducts that did not undergo fusion and that was not replaced by urogenital sinus epithelium, persists alongside the vagina, and becomes cystic.

Treatment is usually conservative management and observation. However, a paramesonephric duct cyst that becomes filled with menstrual blood may extend from the lower vagina upward into the pelvis above the level of the cervix. These are most difficult dissections, and all that should be attempted is to marsupialize them so that there is no reaccumulation of fluid.

The main solid tumors of the hymen and vagina are *polyps* and *angiomata*. Again, therapy depends on the size, symptomatology, and the patient's anxiety.

Granulation polyps and *squamous cell papillomas* of the vagina are extremely rare during childhood. Any polypoid tumor of the vagina in a child or adolescent, regardless of its apparently innocent gross and histologic appearance, is more likely to be sarcomatous than benign. The lesion should be biopsied so that there will be no delay in diagnosis and treatment.

Condyloma acuminatum of the vagina is less common than those of the vulva. When they do occur, they tend to be more friable, and they grow more rapidly than those on the external genitalia. It is important to evaluate pediatric and adolescent patients who have vaginal condyloma to rule out any sort of systemic disease. These patients are very often immunosuppressed, and they should be evaluated for any lymphomatous or leukemic process. The treatment should consist of cryotherapy, or hot cauterization and electrocoagulation, depending upon the extent of the lesion and its location. Some of these patients, indeed most, will have to be admitted to the hospital for proper evaluation and treatment.

Adenosis of the vagina has been identified with increasing frequency since 1970. However, it was first reported in 1877 and, in 1927, Plaut and Dreyfus proposed the term adenosis. This has since been the term used for the benign form of the disease. As early as 1940, Plaut also proposed that adenosis might be a premalignant disease and a forerunner of adenocarcinoma. However, this progression has not been confirmed after many hundreds of cases have been followed. In 1968, Sandberg reported an incidence of 41% of benign occult adenosis at autopsy in surgically sectioned, postpubertal vaginas, but was unable to identify this process in any prepubertal vaginas.

Vaginal adenosis (the abnormal presence of glands in the vagina) is commonly found in adolescent females whose mothers were given diethylstilbestrol early in pregnancy. These glands are found in the superficial portions of the subepithelial layer of the vagina, and can be differentiated histologically from mesonephric duct remnants; they appear endocervical, but a tubal or endometrial type of epithelium may also be observed. The epithelial appearance of these glands suggest a Müllerian (paramesonephric) rather than a mesonephric origin. The histologic, visual, and colposcopic features have now been identified and will be discussed later.

The pathogenesis of vaginal adenosis is unknown, but animal experiments have given some indication of how it occurs. The vagina originates from the Müllerian tissue, proximally and dorsally, from the urogenital sinus. As the urogenital sinus tissue grows upward, the columnar epithelium is normally replaced to the level of the squamocolumnar junction. However, it is found that in the transformation zone, there is a considerable amount of columnar epithelium interspersed with stratified squamous epithelium. In the anterior part of the vagina, the vaginal fornices, and the uterine cervix, there are large regions with heterotopic columnar epithelium, with beginning development of gland-like downgrowths into the stroma.

The developmental mechanism of this heterotopic columnar epithelium, as well as its future potencies, has now been documented clinically. It has been shown that the mitotic rate is inhibited in the vaginal and cervical regions in those girls whose mothers took diethylstilbestrol, and that the epithelium does not undergo a transformation. Studies point to the mitotic activity as an important prerequisite for the epithelial transformation and differentiation. Changes in the epithelium follow, and the rate of mitotic inhibition is irreversible.

The histology of the vaginal adenosis consists of the presence of glandular epithelium replacing the squamous lining of the vagina, or forming glands beneath it. It is characterized by mucus-filled cells resembling endocervical epithelium and/or mucus-free columnar cells (ciliated or nonciliated) resembling tubal or endometrial epithelium. On visual examination, vaginal adenosis appears either as a red granular mucosa, small cyst, or a papillary lesion, often multicentric in appearance. On colposcopic examination, the tissue is characteristic of that seen from the endocervix, and is a columnar epithelium. It is identified as ectopy on the cervix and, on the vagina, it is called adenosis.

Having identified the adenosis histologically from representative fields, no additional treatment is needed, and the patient can be followed with close observation.

Malignant Tumors

Carcinoma of the vagina is extremely rare in childhood but, again, a few cases have been reported. While some of these arise in squamous epithelium, most of the reported cases in children are adenocarcinoma which develop from Müllerian or Wolffian remnants. Both of these lesions are highly malignant, and extensive metastases are frequently present at the time of the initial diagnosis.

Herbst (1970) reported seven girls, 15 to 22 years of age, with adenocarcinoma of the vagina (clear-cell or endometrial type) between 1966 and 1969.

Despite the fact that at least two million women took diethylstilbestrol, there are fewer than 400 cases of clear-cell adenocarcinoma listed in the Registry for research on hormonal transplacental carcinogenesis. Approximately two thirds of the investigated cases are associated with intrauterine exposure to diethylstilbestrol or a related nonsteroidal estrogen. The youngest DES-exposed patient in the Registry was seven years old and the oldest was 27 at the time of diagnosis. The age incidence begins to rise sharply at 14, with a peak at 19, followed by a drop to the age of 22. Less than 10% of cases have occurred prior to age 14, and the shape of the curve beyond age 22 is uncertain. All girls born after 1940 should be considered suspect for their mother's having ingested diethylstilbestrol. In these patients, pelvic examination should start at puberty or at any age if there are any symptoms such as discharge of any type and, particularly, if there is any bloody discharge. The important criteria for a good prognosis depends upon: 1) the degree of mitotic activity, 2) the presence of involved regional lymph nodes, and 3) the stage of the disease. The treatment chosen most often for these patients is radical hysterectomy, partial or total vaginectomy, and pelvic lymph node dissection. Vaginal reconstruction can be performed immediately or delayed for a period of time. Radiation therapy has been shown to give equally good results, but the side effects on these young children is greater than those following surgery.

Endodermal sinus tumors have been observed in pediatric and adolescent patients. It is not possible to distinguish histologically the endodermal sinus tumor of the vagina from that of the ovary. The question of histogenesis remains controversial, as the tumor's histologic appearance suggests a germ-cell origin. It has been proposed that there is a lack of embryonic organizers during a critical period of germ-cell migration and that the germ cells are misdirected into the region of the upper vagina.

The tumor is rarely encountered. Most cases are in infants less than two years of age. The age peak is consistent with the age peak of other germ-cell tumors originating in infancy, ie, sacrococcygeal teratomas and embryonal carcinomas of the infantile testis. A differential diagnosis should be made between sarcoma botryoides or rhabdomyosarcoma. The optimal form of treatment is unknown. Currently, a combination of surgery and multiple chemotherapeutic agents has given some promise for cure.

The botryoid form of embryonal rhabdomyosarcoma (sarcoma botryoides) is the most common malignant tumor of the vagina during the first decade of life. It is a pure heterologous sarcoma, and classically occurs in children. While occasionally seen within a few days after birth, most cases develop before the age of five. The lesion usually originates in the subepithelial layers of the vagina, and expands within the limits of that organ. When seen in the vagina, it usually starts as a small, broad-based, polypoid mass, and, as it grows, takes on the typical appearance of a lobulated mass of vesicular or hemorrhagic polyps which soon fill the vagina and project through the vaginal introitus. Widespread metastases are the rule rather than the exception, and the only cases treated successfully are those diagnosed early. The most common metastatic sites are the lung and the regional nodes. Bloody discharge, vaginal bleeding, and/or a mass is the most common sign. Since the earliest sign may be only a few spots of blood, it is important to investigate this thoroughly without delay. Pain is usually not present until the lesion is far enough advanced to produce bladder or bowel symptoms.

Vaginal examination is often very difficult. Following sedation of the patient, if it is not possible to visualize the vagina by the use of a pediatric speculum or small urethroscope, the patient should be admitted to the hospital and then examined under general anesthesia. This is generally necessary if the bulk of the tumor is excessive and does not permit easy visualization of its site of origin. Under these circumstances, on the basis of our experience, the following technique is suggested.

If one attempts to remove the tumor a bit at a time to visualize the base and decrease the mass, excessive bleeding soon becomes a problem. If cauterization is attempted, the pelvic structures and planes soon become very edematous. Therefore, the mass is grasped by a series of climbing sponge sticks to control the tumor until the base can be palpated, and the stalk is turned slowly, compressing the blood supply. The neoplasm can then be removed almost bloodlessly. The vagina is washed with saline, followed by ether and, again, saline. After drying the area, it can be inspected in detail.

Until recently, total pelvic exenteration with a complete pelvic node dissection, total vaginectomy, and simple vulvectomy were considered the ideal treatment. However, with the spectacular response of these tumors to certain combinations of chemotherapeutic agents, the current method of management is surgery combined with chemotherapy.

A fourth tumor which may originate in the subepithelial connective tissue layer of the vagina is the *mesonephroma*. This tumor develops from persistent remnants of the mesonephric duct following its degeneration dur-

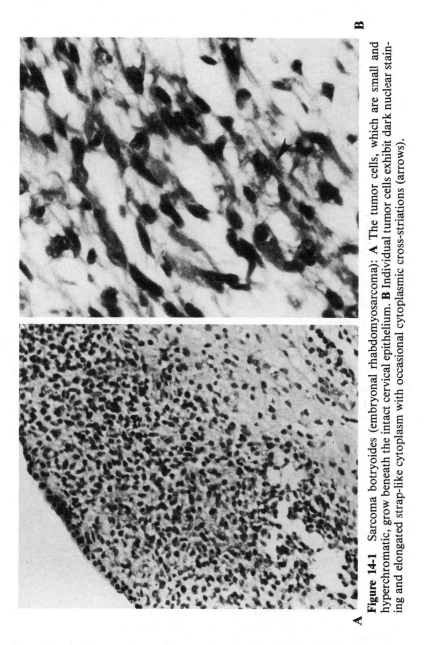

Figure 14-1 Sarcoma botryoides (embryonal rhabdomyosarcoma): **A** The tumor cells, which are small and hyperchromatic, grow beneath the intact cervical epithelium. **B** Individual tumor cells exhibit dark nuclear staining and elongated strap-like cytoplasm with occasional cytoplasmic cross-striations (arrows).

ing embryonic and fetal life. There is confusion regarding the relationship of mesonephroma to embryonal and adolescent tumors, as discussed above. Certain evidence indicates that a mesonephroma is histologically different. The relationship between a true mesonephroma and the other tumors is limited to its origin in the subepithelial connective tissue layer of the vagina. Most arise in the cervix or at levels above the cervix, ie, in the broad ligament. There is very little evidence for mesonephric duct remnants in the vagina; therefore, the chance of finding a true mesonephroma of the vagina appears slim. The treatment for the mesonephroma is essentially the same as it is for the Müllerian duct type of clear-cell adenocarcinoma.

TUMORS OF THE CERVIX

Benign tumors of the cervix and the body of the uterus are rare in children. Most uterine neoplasms that occur during youth are malignant. Few adenocarcinomas have been reported but, as in other organs, most malignant new growths of the uterus are sarcomatous during the premenarcheal period. Malignant tumors of the cervix and vagina so often fill the vaginal canal in children that it is impossible to tell where the growth originated. Rhabdomyosarcoma is generally considered a cervical neoplasm but, as a rule, tumors of this type in youngsters start in the vagina.

CLASSIFICATION

Benign

1. Polyps
2. Squamous papilloma
3. Mesonephric cyst
4. Hemangioma
5. Leiomyoma
6. Hypertrophy and hyperplasia of cervical glands
7. Condylomata
8. Leukoplakia
9. Endometriosis

Premalignant

1. Dysplasia
2. Carcinoma in situ

Malignant

1. Squamous carcinoma
2. Adenocarcinoma

a) Mesonephric origin
b) Müllerian origin
3. Sarcoma botryoides or rhabdomyosarcoma

Children almost never develop benign tumors of the cervix. However, they do develop malignant lesions in the cervix. The most commonly seen benign lesions are polyps, squamous papilloma, mesonephric duct cysts, hemangioma, leiomyoma, hypertrophy and hyperplasia of the cervical glands, condylomata, leukoplakia, and endometriosis. Although undue concern usually occurs when these lesions are discovered, biopsy and removal when indicated promptly resolves the anxiety and identifies the pathologic state.

Dysplasia and carcinoma in situ is now being reported at earlier age groups. However, Nealon and Christopherson (1979) report that, in spite of the revolutionary changes in the mores and practices of adolescent sexuality, there has not been a significant increase in the rates of cervical cancer precursors in a study of 29,600 young women under age 21. The study represents women from families of lower socioeconomic status. Over a 21-year period, no cases of cancer in situ or invasive cancer occurred. The dysplasia rate was low (0.9 per 1000), and, when prerevolutionary and revolutionary periods were compared, there was no significant difference in the rates. However, these investigators did caution that an attempt should be made to monitor these young women of the sexual revolution, since the effects of their past and current participation might not be discernible for years to come. Epidemiologically, it is evident that dysplasia and carcinoma in situ of the cervix are taking on the characteristics of a venereal disease, and a great deal of caution should be exercised in following these patients.

Although rare, both squamous cell carcinoma and adenocarcinoma of the cervix have been reported. Huffman has reported 32 cases through 1966. Pollack and Taylor (1947) reviewed the literature on cervical cancer in the first two decades of life, and found only 30 cases with the survival of four children for five years. All were of mesonephric origin and adenocarcinoma.

Cancer of the cervix in children is rarely diagnosed early, and the disease progresses so rapidly that metastasis has usually occurred by the time the initial diagnosis is made. Any malodorous or bloody vaginal discharge in a child should be investigated promptly. Since all children born after 1940 are suspect for having been exposed to diethylstilbestrol in utero, it is most important that investigation be started immediately. While the majority of discharges will probably be due to retention of a foreign body, cancer will sometimes be present. In those instances where tissue is passed, this may be the first indication of trouble, and the disease is often far advanced. Even under these circumstances, however, the patient is still entitled to a thorough diagnostic workup and evaluation for therapy.

Rhabdomyosarcoma and clear-cell Müllerian duct adenocarcinoma have been discussed under malignant neoplasms of the vagina. The workup and treatment are essentially the same for the cervix as for the vagina.

Treatment of cancer of the cervix in this age group ideally is radical hysterectomy and pelvic node dissection. If the tumor has infiltrated other structures, pelvic exenteration must be considered as offering the best chance of survival. There is some reluctance on the part of clinicians to give radiation therapy to children because of the effects on bone epiphyses, as well as the other organs in the pelvis. Multiple-drug chemotherapy has given promise for prolonging survival among these children.

TUMORS OF THE UTERINE FUNDUS

Several types of benign uterine tumors have been found in children but they are very uncommon. There have been practically no reports of uterine myomas in children since the world's literature was reviewed in 1930.

CLASSIFICATION

Benign

    1. Fibroids
    2. Endometriosis
    3. Polyps

Premalignant

    1. Endometrial dysplasia
    2. Endometrial carcinoma in situ

Malignant

    1. Adenocarcinoma
    2. Sarcoma
    3. Metastatic lesions

Uterine tumors are extremely rare, but the majority of those reported are malignant. The main benign tumors are fibroids, endometriosis, and polyps. Fibroids have been reported in a girl aged 11. There are also rare reports of tumors arising from the epithelial or mesodermal elements of the uterine wall, but they are so rare that they are medical curiosities.

Premalignant Although the invasive type of endometrial cancer encountered in the adult is practically unknown in the teenage patient, dysplasias and carcinoma in situ have been reported. This usually occurs in, but not necessarily caused by, an estrogen environment. The patient has some or all of the following findings: hirsutism, obesity, anovulation, amenorrhea followed by hypermenorrhea, and infertility. If the bleeding is excessive, the patient should have a curettage and careful study of the endometrium. Prophylactically, the patient should be cycled by use of a progestational agent or an antiestrogen agent such as clomiphene. Hormone assay studies reveal an occasional patient who may be controlled by cortisone therapy.

Malignant tumors of the uterine body may be primary or secondary. Primary adenocarcinoma of the uterus has been reported in a two-year-old child. Primary sarcoma of the uterus in children is also seen, but, fortunately, only rarely. Silverberg and Makowski (1975) have reported 21 cases of endometrial cancer in young women taking oral contraceptive agents. The majority of these patients were receiving sequential agents, not the combined type of pill. Patients receiving diethylstilbestrol as replacement therapy for Turner's syndrome have developed cancer of the uterine corpus. These have been adenosquamous types of cancer.

Therapy for cancer of the uterus is total extirpation of the uterus, adnexa, and upper vagina, preceded or followed by external cobalt therapy, depending upon the depth of penetration of the lesion into the myometrium. However, in the under-age-25 group, with evidence of superficial invasive cancer of the endometrium, a careful therapeutic trial, under close observation, with progestins or clomiphene is justified. Kistner (1971) has reported success in this group, and quotes Arthur Hertig's statement that pregnancy would be the best treatment for these patients.

A point to emphasize is that young people with cancer confined to the endometrium may be the victims of continuous, uninterrupted, anovulatory cycles and will be cured by sloughing or curetting the endometrium, and then cycling the patient with a progestational agent.

FALLOPIAN TUBES

A search of the literature has failed to find any report of a primary malignancy of these organs in a child. Of course, secondary invasion is seen. The most common lesion around the adnexal area (excluding the area itself) is a paraovarian cyst arising from the paraoophoron. These cysts may attain a large size and, on occasion, demand surgical extirpation.

OVARIAN CANCER

The difficulty of diagnosing ovarian cancer in a child is surpassed only by confusion over its treatment. Although ovarian tumors comprise not more than 1% of all new growths in children who are less than 16 years of age, they are, nevertheless, the most frequent genital cancer during childhood and adolescence. In spite of their rarity, they are included in the differential diagnosis of many abdominal disorders. Because they are infrequent, the diagnosis may be missed. When they *are* overlooked, they tend to create special problems. Fortunately, only one in ten is malignant.

Approximately 30% of all ovarian tumors in children and adolescents are cystic teratomas or dermoids. The remainder include all sorts of benign and malignant ovarian neoplasms. The most common malignant neoplasm found in childhood probably is the dysgerminoma. Some of the more unusual tumors are represented in the literature by only one or two case reports but, when they are included, it can be said that every type of ovarian neoplasm seen in adult women has been encountered in girls less than 16 years of age.

Ovarian neoplasms may occur at any age in childhood or adolescence, but tend to be more frequent between the ages of 10 and 14 years. This finding suggests that release of a control mechanism or pituitary stimulation of a latent factor may trigger tumor development.

Ovarian cancer poses certain problems in children that are not as significant in adults. These are: 1) increased cachexia and ascites, 2) relatively greater pressure symptoms and dyspnea with larger tumors, 3) more rapid evolution, 4) limited space for tumor expansion, 5) a higher degree of virulence, 6) less effective immunologic defense, and 7) the effects of therapy on the child's future development.

Classification

1. Tumors of epithelial and stromal origin
    A) Serous
    B) Mucinous
    C) Endometrioid
    D) Clear-cell (mesonephric)
2. Germ-cell tumors
    A) Dysgerminoma
    B) Tumors in teratoma group
        (1) Extraembryonal forms
            a) Endodermal sinus tumor (mesoblastoma vitellium, yolk sac carcinoma, extraembryonic membrane tumor)
        (2) Embyonal teratoma, solid and cystic

        (3) Adult teratoma
           a) Solid
           b) Cystic (dermoid cyst)
              1. Benign
              2. With malignant change
        (4) Struma ovarii
        (5) Carcinoid
      C) Mixed forms of the above
  3. Gonadoblastoma
      A) With germinoma
      B) Without germinoma
  4. Sex cord-Mesenchyme tumors (mesenchymoma; gonadal stromal tumors)
      A) Female cell types
        (1) Granulosa cell tumor
        (2) Thecoma-fibroma type
      B) Male cell types
        (1) Sertoli-Leydig-cell tumor (arrhenoblastoma; androblastoma)
        (2) Sertoli-cell tumor (androblastoma tubulare)
        (3) Hilus-(Leydig)-cell tumor
      C) Mixed cell types (gynandroblastoma)
      D) Indeterminate cell types
  5. Tumors not specific for ovary
      A) Lymphoma
      B) Burkitt's lymphoma
  6. Miscellaneous
      A) Sarcoma
      B) Fibroma
  7. Metastatic tumors
      A) Krukenberg
      B) Choriocarcinoma

Signs and Symptoms

Ovarian new growths in children may produce minimal symptoms in their early state of development. The degree of symptomatology and the physical findings are in direct relation to the rapidity of growth, position, degree of malignancy, potentially produced hormones, and possible accidents associated with these neoplasms (torsion, rupture, hemorrhage, infection, etc). Since ovarian tumors are frequently abdominal and have their embryologic origin from the level of T-12, it is not surprising that abdominal pain and abdominal tumors are commonly seen. Pain may be related to the relatively small pelvic and abdominal cavities, which cause a new growth to stretch the peritoneum and produce pressure on adjacent organs. Rectal examination often reveals the pelvis to be free of tumor. However, a negative rectal examination does not rule out an ovarian neoplasm because, frequently, the ovarian tumor will present only as an abdominal mass during childhood. The hormone-producing tumors, although rare, and then only rarely functioning, produce a clinical picture related to the type of hormone being secreted.

Physical Findings

A general physical examination, including pelvic and rectal examinations, is essential. Rectal examination often indicates that the pelvis is free of tumor, but a negative finding does not rule out an ovarian neoplasm since it frequently presents as an abdominal mass in the early stages. In most children it is impossible to palpate normal ovaries; therefore, if an ovary can be palpated, it is abnormal. The size determines whether it can be felt abdominally or by rectal-abdominal palpation.

Diagnostic Procedures

Baseline blood counts, urinalysis, and blood chemistries must be obtained. A flat plate of the abdomen may help determine whether a dermoid cyst is present or not. If time permits, intravenous pyelograms and x-ray studies of the bone age may be useful in patients suspected of having a hormone-producing tumor. A hormone assay profile may also be valuable in diagnosis; the alpha-fetoprotein titer has been found to be elevated in extraembryonal endodermal sinus tumors, as well as in certain embryonal carcinomas. Although rare, the hormone-producing tumors present a clinical picture related to the hormone they produce. However, only about 25% of the hormone-associated tumors are functioning, and they produce hormones that give rise to a definite type of clinical picture. Pneumoperitoneum has been used to outline small tumors but, recently, ultrasonic methods and a CAT scan have been introduced, superceding the pneumoperitoneum as a diagnostic test. The role of laparoscopy in abdominal and pelvic problems remains to be determined for this age group.

Differential Diagnosis

The clinical picture and physical findings usually point to the diagnosis. Differential diagnosis includes appendiceal abscesses, intussusception, obstruction, salpingitis, hematometra, pyelonephritis, Wilms's tumor, neuroblastoma, and retroperitoneal sarcoma.

STAGE GROUPING FOR PRIMARY CARCINOMA
OF THE OVARY IN COMMON EPITHELIAL OVARIAN CANCER

Stage I	Growth limited to the ovaries.
Stage Ia	Growth limited to *one* ovary; no ascites.
	(i) No tumor on the external surface; capsule intact.
	(ii) Tumor present on the external surface and/or capsule ruptured.
Stage Ib	Growth limited to *both* ovaries; no ascites.
	(i) No tumor on the external surface; capsule intact.
	(ii) Tumor present on the external surface and/or capsule(s) ruptured.
Stage Ic	Tumor either Stage Ia or Stage Ib, but with ascites* or positive peritoneal washings.
Stage II	Growth involving one or both ovaries with pelvic extension.
Stage IIa	Extension and/or metastases to the uterus and/or tubes.
Stage IIb	Extension to other pelvic tissues.
Stabe IIc	Tumor either Stage IIa or IIb, but with ascites* or positive peritoneal washings.
Stage III	Growth involving one or both ovaries with intraperitoneal metastases outside the pelvis and/or positive retroperitoneal nodes; tumor limited to the true pelvis, with histologically proven malignant extension to small bowel or omentum.
Stage IV	Growth involving one or both ovaries with distant metastases. If pleural effusion is present, there must be positive cytology to allot a case to Stage IV; parenchymal liver metastases classified in Stage IV.
Special category	Unexplored cases which are thought to be ovarian carcinoma.

---

*Ascites is peritoneal effusion which, in the opinion of the surgeon, is pathologic and/or clearly exceeds normal amounts.

It has been shown that there is no correlation between the clinical and histologic malignancy in many of the ovarian tumors. This is true for various types of neoplasm, but especially for epithelial tumors, granulosa-cell tumors, and virilizing tumors. It has been recommended that cases of germ-cell tumors, hormone-producing neoplasms, and metastatic carcinomas should be excluded from therapeutic statistics on ovarian epithelial tumors. However, this does focus attention for careful evaluation of the extent of all ovarian cancers.

There are seven primary points that should be emphasized concerning ovarian tumors in childhood.

1. The ovary is the most common site of new growths in childhood, involving the gynecologic organs.

2. The ovary in a child is essentially an abdominal organ, and tumors are abdominal rather than pelvic.

3. Ovarian tumors in childhood are especially susceptible to torsion due to a longer ovarian suspensory ligament.

4. About one in ten ovarian neoplasms are malignant and, therefore, as a general rule, the odds are good that the tumor is benign. Panic is not justified, but judicious concern is indicated.

5. The evolution of ovarian tumors in children is more rapid because of the contracted spatial relationships.

6. Large tumors produce relatively greater pressure symptoms and dyspnea.

7. There is increased cachexia and ascites.

Proposed Grouping for Malignant Ovarian Tumors in Childhood

Group	Extent of Disease
I	Disease limited to one ovary. Negative peritoneal washing.
II	Disease limited to one ovary and ipsilateral paraaortic nodes. Bilateral primary ovarian tumors without pelvic extension, with or without paraaortic node involvement. Negative peritoneal washing.
III	Disease spread to pelvis, mesenteric and paraaortic nodes, abdominal wall, peritoneum, diaphragm, liver, and other organs in the peritoneal cavity.
IV	Distant metastases (lung, bone, brain, peripheral nodes).

This grouping has been proposed by Wollnar and co-workers (1976). They considered the new approach more useful in planning therapy; it is also applicable to the extent and locations of disease found at the time of disease recurrence, which is the time when most of these patients are first seen at comprehensive cancer centers.

TUMORS OF EPITHELIAL AND STROMAL ORIGIN

Although epithelial tumors comprise 90% of ovarian tumors, they are rarely seen in children, particularly before puberty. Among the common epithelial tumors, about 8% occur under the age of 35 and, of this number, very few occur in pediatric and adolescent groups. In these age groups, the tumor of the common epithelial variety most often seen is a mucinous or serous cystadenocarcinoma. If an encapsulated, unilateral, mucinous cystadenocarcinoma is found in a child in the absence of positive cells in the pelvis, particularly if it is of low grade malignancy, unilateral salpingo-oophorectomy with bisection and biopsy of the opposite ovary is sufficient treatment. If there is any evidence of spread beyond the ovary, a total hysterectomy, bilateral salpingo-oophorectomy, appendectomy, and omentectomy (if an omentum has been developed), should be performed. The roles of phosphorus-32 and prophylactic chemotherapy remain to be evaluated.

Germ-Cell Tumors

Germ-cell tumors are almost always found in children and adolescents, rather than in adults. A knowledge of their natural history guides the surgeon in treatment. Dysgerminomas are the most common malignant germ-cell tumors encountered in the pediatric and adolescent age group. They are usually highly radiosensitive and have a bilateral rate of only 5% to 10%.

Although controversial, therapy for an encapsulated, unilateral dysgerminoma in the young girl consists of unilateral salpingo-oophorectomy. This is based on the assumption that there are no tumors in the opposite ovary, no positive paraaortic nodes, and no positive cells in the pelvis, although some investigators dispute the value of cytology in these tumors. These patients should be followed every two months for the first two years, with chest x-rays every six months. If there is any evidence of spread at the time of the original surgery, total hysterectomy and bilateral salpingo-oophorectomy is advised. Whether postoperative x-ray therapy is administered can best be determined individually. Since these tumors are known to recur late, the question has been raised whether, after these patients have had their family, it is not in their best interest to consider hysterectomy and removal of the remaining ovary. The role of the second-look operation must be considered in patients who have had a dysgerminoma, particularly in pediatric and adolescent patients. If, at the time of the original operation, the mass is greater than 15 cm in diameter, and the pathologist's report indicates a triad of anaplasia, medullary structures, and numerous mitoses, then an exploration is indicated 8 to 12 months later.

Embryonal teratomas as well as the extraembryonal tumors, endodermal sinus and choriocarcinoma, and polyvesicular vitalline tumors, are highly malignant. When unilateral and encapsulated, treatment by unilateral salpingo-oophorectomy is as effective as total hysterectomy and bilateral salpingo-oophorectomy. Surgery at any time and radiation have little to offer since these tumors are relatively radioresistant. The role of multiple-drug chemotherapy has given some surprisingly good results, and should be made part of the regimen in the treatment of these patients.

More than 50% of ovarian tumors in children and adolescents are of the germ-cell variety. Benign cystic teratomas make up the majority of these tumors. They can be excised simply, with preservation of the ovary in most cases. In the occasional cancer arising in a cystic teratoma, unilateral salpingo-oophorectomy is indicated if there is no evidence of spread.

Gonadoblastoma

Gonadoblastomas are composed of both germ cells and gonadal stromal cells in approximately equal proportions. Most of these patients are intersexual, have primary amenorrhea, and are unable to reproduce. Therefore, there is no need for conservation in managing these patients. Approximately 90% of the cases are chromatin-negative. The most frequently encountered karyotypes are 46 XY, 45 XO, and/or 46 XY. Hyaline bodies that simulate Call-Exner bodies are typically present, and foci of calcification are common. The calcifications may be demonstrated by x-ray of the pelvis and abdomen. The malignant potential is determined by the type of germ cell present. Approximately one half of the gonadoblastomas are associated with dysgerminoma, and are therefore relatively benign. Occasionally, endodermal sinus tumors, choriocarcinomas, and embryonal carcinomas may represent the germ-cell type present in the gonadoblastoma. The malignancy rate in such cases is increased. Since these tumors are found in the intersex patient, bilateral salpingo-oophorectomy is indicated.

Gonadal Stromal Tumors (Sex-Cord Mesenchymal Tumors) Female Type

Gonadal stromal tumors make up the category of tumors which include those tumors of the female type, such as the granulosa, granulosa-thecoma, or male-cell types such as the Sertoli-Leydig cell (arrhenoblastoma), Sertoli, and hilus-(Leydig)-cell tumors. These are not as common as the germ-cell tumors, nor are they as malignant.

Granulosa-Cell Tumors

Although approximately 100 granulosa-cell tumors in children have been reported in the literature, only three have proved to be malignant. The histologic and clinical findings of the granulosa-cell tumor give no indication of the clinical course that the patient will have. Hertig (1961) has called the granulosa-cell tumor the most glamorous of all neoplasms. They are infrequent in childhood and account for few cases of precocious puberty. Only approximately 25% of these tumors are functional. The startling secondary sexual changes that they produce in children are dramatic. From 5% to 10% of the tumors occur before the patient reaches the age of puberty. When they are functional, they produce a feminine habitus, maturation of the genitalia, and enlargement of the breasts. Pubic hair is scant. Vaginal bleeding may occur. However, precocious puberty is usually constitutional, and only about 2% result from an ovarian tumor. More often, the diagnosis is made after an abdominal and pelvic mass is discovered. On exploration, the tumor is rounded or lobulated, with a smooth surface. On cutting, the tumor is found to have a thin capsule, and the bulk of the tumor may be solid or present with numerous cystic spaces which may be filled with clotted blood. These cysts may rupture, causing an acute abdomen from the hemoperitoneum. The tumors are bilateral in only about 5% of the cases.

Treatment of the unilateral, encapsulated tumor is unilateral oophorectomy with wedge resection of the opposite ovary. In the presence of spread beyond the ovary to pelvic structures, hysterectomy and bilateral salpingo-oophorectomy should be carried out. The use of postoperative x-ray therapy should be individualized. The tumor in general has a good prognosis. The malignancy rate in adults is about 25% but is less in children, ranging from about 3% to 6%. Recurrences are usually local, and distant metastases are rare. Recurrences may occur at any time, but they develop very slowly, and often take many years to develop.

The histologic appearance of a tumor of this group is no index of its final behavior. These tumors are sensitive to x-rays, which should be employed if widespread metastases or recurrent cancer are present. It is important to follow these children for life. Vaginal cytology in the premenopausal child will reveal increasing estrogen stimulation if recurrence is developing. Since these patients are characterized by a late recurrence, few recurring under five years, it is suggested that, after childbearing is completed, the uterus and opposite ovary be removed.

Sertoli-Leydig-Cell Tumor

This term has been selected instead of the more familiar term, arrhenoblastoma, since many of these are nonfunctioning or have estrogenic effects rather than masculinizing tendencies. In those tumors with a predominance of functioning Sertoli cells, the effect may be that of a feminizing tumor. However, if the Leydig cells are predominant and functional, the patient first is defeminized (atrophy of the breast, loss of female contour, amenorrhea), followed by masculinization (hirsutism, hypertrophy of the clitoris, and voice changes).

The tumor usually affects women of the childbearing age and is very rare in childhood. It is bilateral in ony 5% of the cases. When these tumors show malignant behavior (ranging from 3% to 20%), it is usually manifested by intraabdominal spread rather than by distant metastases.

The plan of management outlined for the granulosa-cell tumor can be applied to this tumor. Signs and symptoms regress after excision. However, the patient may be left with increased hirsutism and voice changes. Since these tumors have a history of late recurrence, the question is raised (but cannot be answered at this time) relative to reexploration after the patient has had her children, followed by hysterectomy and removal of the opposite ovary.

Gynandroblastoma (Mixed Type)

Gynandroblastoma should contain typical aggregates of granulosa cells with Call-Exner bodies in either hollow tubules or Leydig-cell-containing crystalloids of Reinke. There are no reports of this tumor in childhood, but there is no reason to believe that they would differ in behavior either from the granulosa-cell or Sertoli-Leydig-cell tumor.

TUMORS NOT SPECIFIC FOR THE OVARY

The ovary may be involved as part of disseminated Hodgkin's disease. These tumors are usually seen among the adult population. However, ovarian involvement has been reported among children suffering from Burkitt's tumor. It is interesting that the first human virus to be suspected of causing a human cancer was isolated as a result of epidemiologic observations made in populations of tropical Africa, particularly in patients with Burkitt's tumor. The particular distribution of the tumor from a geographic and ecological standpoint, as well as its age distribution, typical of an infectious disease, has led to the suspicion that Burkitt's tumor may be caused by an infectious agent. A concerted effort resulted in the isolation of a virus (EB virus) from Burkitt's tumor cells. Cyclophosphamide is very effective as treatment, and often these tumors melt away. However, a large tumor causing symptoms should be excised.

MISCELLANEOUS

Sarcoma

Ovarian sarcomas occur more frequently in children than in adults. They are relatively rare. Usually primary, they may be the result of secondary malignant changes in a fibroma or teratoma. The tumor is highly malignant, and patients rarely survive five years. If encapsulated and unilateral, there is no advantage to radical over conservative surgery. However, with evidence of spread, total hysterectomy and bilateral salpingo-oophorectomy are indicated. Combination and multiple-drug chemotherapy have given optimism for some success in treating these highly malignant and rare tumors.

Metastatic Cancer

Metastases to the ovaries do occur in children; there are reports of Krukenberg tumors with the primary lesion in the upper gastrointestinal tract. As much of the primary tumor as possible, as well as any metastases, should be removed surgically. Krukenberg tumors are characterized histologically by large, swollen, signet-ring-like cells which lie in clumps within areas of mucoid degeneration. They are scattered throughout an edematous stroma-like matrix. Only tumors meeting these criteria should be included. Krukenberg tumors are bilateral, and are grossly kidney-shaped.

Metastases to the ovaries may be secondary to cancer anywhere in the abdomen, breast, or thyroid. Ovarian metastasis should be removed if possible.

INTRAABDOMINAL MASSES IN CHILDREN — A SYSTEMATIC ROENTGENOGRAPHIC APPROACH

An intraabdominal mass in an infant or young child can be malignant, and should be carefully and immediately evaluated. However, through a concern for thoroughness, numerous studies may be ordered, some of which are both physically and emotionally traumatic to the child and her family. These more complicated procedures are frequently unnecessary and often yield information that could have been obtained by the selective use of less dramatic techniques. By following a stepwise procedure, each new step being related to findings obtained in earlier studies, most of the complicated and evasive procedures can be avoided.

Abdominal masses in pediatric and adolescent patients commonly involve the kidneys and bladder; adrenal lesions are less common. Other tumors such as lymphoma, teratoma, lymphangioma, rhabdomyosarcoma, or lipoma are rarely found in the retroperitoneal space in children. Sacrococcygeal teratomas are infrequently encountered.

When an abdominal mass is palpated, roentgenograms can usually pinpoint its location, especially if several views including supine, prone, oblique, and upright are taken.

If abdominal x-rays fail to define the structures adequately, other invasive techniques are indicated for diagnostic purposes. An intravenous pyelogram (IVP) outlines intrarenal areas and demonstrates the effect of the mass on the urinary tract system. Radioisotope scans of the kidney demonstrate the blood flow to the renal mass that was not visualized in expiratory pyelography. Imaging with an isotope such as technetium-99m glucohepatonate can differentiate renal tumors from pseudotumors. This modality is also useful in detecting incomplete rotation of the kidney. Only rarely, when the disease process complicates interpretation of these studies, are further invasive methods, such as angiography, necessary. Complete evaluation and a minimum number of procedures are the goals of a systematic approach to diagnosing intraabdominal masses in children. It should be remembered that cancers are rare, and that most tumors in children are benign.

Ultrasonography records sound reflections at tissue interfaces. Normal physiologic function is not necessary to obtain these recordings. The density of the tissue and its elasticity, as well as the orientation of the ultrasound beam to tissue, must be evaluated. With B-mode ultrasonography, cystic structures appear as echo-free areas (anechoic) and solid structures as dots (echoic). Low-grain study of the ultrasonogram indicates the size of a mass; high-grain study indicates that it is solid. Real-time ultrasound can detect motion within a mass. The CAT scan remains to be evaluated in the diagnosis of masses in the abdomen of a child.

All tissues in the body are liable to undergo malignant change and all cells have an inherent potential for the development of cancer. The origin may be unicentric or multicentric. All of the known carcinogenic factors, ie, viruses, chemicals, ionizing radiation, genetic factors, which are associated with cancer in the adult, are also found in the child. The theory of misplaced blastomeres may take on added significance in this age group.

The most common abdominal mass in children is renal in origin. An expiratory pyelogram with early-phase, total body opacification provides findings within three broad categories that distinguish various types of renal abnormalities. These include: 1) caliceal distortion from hydronephrosis, cystic kidney disease, abscess, benign and malignant renal tumors, as well as infiltrative disease such as lymphomas and leukemia, 2) nonvisualization caused by total obstruction of the urinary tract, renal vein thrombosis, or replacement of the kidney by infiltrating tumor, and 3) duplication of part of the urinary system.

Enlargement of the adrenal gland is far less common than enlargement of the kidney. Overall, the most likely cause of an enlarged adrenal gland in a newborn infant is hemorrhage, often associated with jaundice. Adrenal insufficiency is occasionally evident, but only when hemorrhage is bilateral. Neuroblastoma, which comprises approximately 10% of all childhood cancers, is another cause of adrenal enlargement. Adenoma, carcinoma, and pheochromocytoma of the adrenal gland may also be present.

An enlarged bladder is the most common cause of a pelvic mass and may be found in patients with three types of clinical findings, those with normal spines, abnormal spines, and displacement of the bladder.

RADIATION THERAPY FOR GYNECOLOGIC TUMORS IN CHILDHOOD AND ADOLESCENCE

Radiation therapy is used both for definitive and palliative treatment. There is great reluctance to give radiation therapy to an infant, a young child, or an adolescent child. Not only are there immediate problems, such as skin reactions, bone marrow depression, and gastrointestinal symptoms, but also the delayed problems of inhibition of growth, radiation nephritis, bone changes, and gonadal damage, with the possibility of later production of a compromised offspring.

Therefore, prophylactic postoperative radiation to the pelvis is not indicated in this age group and should be discouraged. However, if radiation therapy is definitely indicated as definitive or palliative treatment, there should be no hesitancy in using it.

In those patients who receive radiation therapy as definitive treatment, a postradiation state will exist. The patients must be followed at regular intervals for the rest of their lives, since the complications may take 30 to 40 years to develop.

In summary, it can be stated that when surgery can provide adequate treatment, it should be the treatment of choice, without additional prophylactic radiation therapy. However, when radiation therapy is indicated, it should be given as definitive or prophylactic treatment, accepting and anticipating the possibility of postradiation syndrome.

ANTITUMOR CHEMOTHERAPY OF GYNECOLOGIC TUMORS IN CHILDHOOD AND ADOLESCENCE

Exclusive of choriocarcinoma, anticancer chemotherapy is not used as definitive treatment of solid tumors of the genital tract in children, but is administered either prophylactically or as a palliative.

The indications for chemotherapy include those patients in whom all gross disease has been removed, but the natural history of the disease is such that it is associated with a high recurrence rate, ie, rhabdomyosarcoma and the embryonal ovarian cancers. Chemotherapy should be used in inoperable cases in order to shrink the volume of mass prior to radiation, in combination with radiation therapy, or to decrease the mass in anticipation of changing a clinically inoperable to an operable situation.

420

The indications for chemotherapy and the type given to children with various kinds of tumor should be carefully evaluated before therapy is instituted. Children and adolescents share the same problems that occur in adults. In no greater degree does the term "little people" apply than in evaluating new growths in the pediatric patients.

The small size of the child markedly limits the available room for growth of the tumor, resulting in grotesque deformity produced by only moderately sized tumors. Tumors parallel the rapid growth of children and usually possess a high degree of malignancy, resulting in rapid clinical deterioration.

The margin of safety for the anticancer drugs is slightly less than that in the adult. Radical surgery and/or radiation therapy may have far-reaching effects on future development. In dealing with problems in this age group, the same principles of judging operability, indications, and contraindications must be followed as in treatment of the adult.

This approach offers the patient the maximum opportunity for treatment without an inordinately high morbidity and mortality rate. However, if any chance for survival is to be given to the patient, comprehensive treatment must be carried out within a reasonable length of time.

The ancient philosophy of medicine of not inflicting harm must be respected, and this broad principle, applicable to all disciplines of medicine, continues to serve as a guide for clinical judgment in treating childhood and adolescent gynecologic tumors.

BIBLIOGRAPHY

Arje SL: *The Challenge of Childhood Cancer.* New York, American Cancer Society, 1972.

Barber HRK, Graber EA: Gynecological tumors in childhood and adolescence. *Obstet Gynecol Surv* 28:357, 1973.

Barber HRK: Ovarian cancer, part II. *Ca-A Cancer Journal for Clinicians.* 30:2, 1980.

Barber HRK: Foreword. *Clin Obstet Gynecol* 12:929, 1969.

Barber HRK: *Ovarian Carcinoma: Etiology, Diagnosis and Treatment.* New York, Masson Publishing USA, Inc, 1978.

Barber HRK: A guide to ovarian tumors in children. *Consultant* 15:88, 1975.

Barber HRK, Graber EA: Managing ovarian tumors of childhood and adolescence. *Contemp Ob/Gyn* 3:123, 1974.

Barber HRK, Kwon T: Current status of the treatment of gynecologic cancer: By site. *Cancer* 38:610, 1978.

Barber HRK, Graber EA, Kwon T: *Ovarian Cancer.* New York, American Cancer Society, 1975.

Barber HRK: *Ovarian Cancer in Children—Guide for a Difficult Decision.* New York, American Cancer Society, 1975.

Barclay DL, Macey HB, Reed RJ: Lichen sclerosus et atrophicus in the vulvae of children. *Obstet Gynecol* 27:637, 1966.

Cancer Facts and Figures 1980. New York, American Cancer Society, 1979.

Cham WC, Exelby P, Clark D, et al: Patterns of extension as a guide to radiation therapy in the management of ovarian neoplasms in children. *Cancer* 37:1443, 1976.

Cohen JF, Klein MD, Laver MBD: Cysts of vagina in the newborn infant. *Surg Gynecol Obstet* 94:322, 1957.

Craig JM: Tumors of the lower genitourinary tract. *Pediatr Clin North Am* 6:491, 1959.

Cutler BS, Forbes AP, Ingersoll FM, et al: Endometrial carcinoma after stilbestrol therapy in gonadal dysgenesis. *N Engl J Med* 287:628, 1972.

de Alvarez R: Adolescent gynecology. *Clin Obstet Gynecol* 9:709, 1966.

Dodds GS: *The Essentials of Human Embryology,* Third Edition. New York, John Wiley & Sons, Inc, 1946.

Fechner RE, Kaufman RH: Endometrial adenocarcinoma in Stein-Leventhal syndrome. *Cancer* 34:444, 1974.

Graber EA, Barber HRK, O'Rourke J: Simple surgical treatment of condyloma acuminatum of vulva. *Obstet Gynecol* 27:247, 1967.

Grossman H: *Evaluating Common Intraabdominal Masses in Children — A Systematic Roentgenographic Approach.* New York, American Cancer Society, 1976.

Haines RW, Mohinddin A: *Handbook of Human Embryology,* ed 3. Baltimore, The Williams & Wilkins Co, 1965.

Herbst AL, Scully RE: Adenocarcinoma of the vagina in adolescence. *Cancer* 25:745, 1970.

Hertig AT, Gore H: *Tumors of Female Sex Organs III. Tumors of the Ovary and Fallopian Tube.* Washington, DC, Armed Forces Institute of Pathology, 1961.

Hilgers RD, Malkasian GD Jr, Soule EH: Embryonic rhabdomyosarcoma of vagina. *Am J Obstet Gynecol* 107:484, 1970.

Huffman JW: Management of malignant genital tumors in female children. *Clin Obstet Gynecol* 14:1088, 1971.

Huffman JW: *Gynecology of Childhood and Adolescence.* Philadelphia, WB Saunders, 1968.

Jeffcoate TNA: Chronic vulvar dystrophies. *Am J Obstet Gynecol* 95:61, 1966.

Joannides G: Hidradenoma papilleferum. *Am J Obstet Gynecol* 94:849, 1966.

Kistner RW: The effects of progestational agents on hyperplasia and carcinoma in situ of the endometrium, in Barber HRK, Graber EA (eds): *Gynecological Oncology.* New York, Excerpta Medica, 1970, pp 141–155.

Langman J: *Medical Embryology — Human Development — Normal and Abnormal.* Baltimore, The Williams & Wilkins Co, 1963.

Nealon NA, Christopherson WM. Cervix cancer precursors in young offspring of low-income families. *Obstet Gynecol* 54:135, 1979.

Ober WB, Edgecomb JH: Sarcoma botryoides in the female urogenital tract. *Cancer* 7:75, 1954.

Peterson E: Endometrial carcinoma in young women. *Obstet Gynecol* 31:702, 1968.

Plaut A, Dreyfus ML: Adenosis of the vagina and its relation to primary adenocarcinoma. *Surg Gynecol Obstet* 21:756, 1940.

Pollack RS, Taylor HC: Carcinoma of the cervix in the first two decades of life. *Am J Obstet Gynecol* 53:135, 1947.

Sandberg EC: The incidence and distribution of occult vaginal adenosis. *Am J Obstet Gynecol* 101, 322, 1968.

Silverberg SG, Makowski EL: Endometrial carcinoma in young women taking oral contraceptive agents. *Obstet Gynecol* 46:503, 1975.

Wollner N, Exelby PR, Woodruff JM, et al: Malignant ovarian tumors in childhood. *Cancer* 37:1953, 1976.

15 Gynecologic Tumors in Pregnancy

Hugh R. K. Barber

Gynecologic cancer complicating pregnancy was surrounded by controversy just one decade ago. The controversy usually concerned the question of whether an abortion was therapeutic in women with a cancer or whether it constituted unnecessary interference. This posed a difficult decision for the clinician faced with this problem. With the liberalized abortion law, the woman takes it upon herself to have an elective abortion whenever a diagnosis of cancer is made. It is rare that an abortion committee has to deal with the decision of whether to abort or not. There are some patients who elect to continue the pregnancy and seek help from a clinician experienced in managing a patient with cancer complicating pregnancy.

A degree of uncertainty exists with respect to the treatment of cancer associated with pregnancy. Furthermore, collective experience in the management of gynecologic cancer in pregnancy is limited. Therefore, it is important to collate the data from the literature and make an informed decision that will answer the question for the patient and her family.

The most malignant cancer sites in the major age groups for women are: under age 15, leukemia, brain and central nervous system, kidney, bone, and connective tissue; ages 15 to 34, leukemia, breast, brain and central nervous system, uterus, and Hodgkin's disease; ages 35 to 54, breast, lung, colon and rectum, uterus, and ovary.

When malignant disease is associated with pregnancy, the majority of pregnancies are complicated by breast cancer, lymphoma, malignant melanoma, gynecologic cancer, and bone cancer. Pregnancy represents a major physiologic process for the maintenance of the race, and cancer is a major pathologic process accounting for numerous deaths—the struggle leading to biologic immortality or destruction. In summary, there is a combination of a controlled growth—pregnancy, and an uncontrolled growth—cancer, in the same host, providing a setting for a project that is stimulating, and which will undoubtedly be rewarding and answer some important questions relative to both the pregnancy and the cancer.

The opinions expressed in the literature of the effects of pregnancy on the malignant process range from those who feel that pregnancy increases resistance to cancer, to the other extreme that pregnancy has a stimulating effect. The lack of agreement makes it difficult, if not impossible, for the average physician to plan treatment of such patients. Unfortunately, these decisions are based all too often on emotion rather than on recorded, objective scientific data, of which there is little available.

Cancer complicating pregnancy is best divided into pelvic and extrapelvic malignancy. Pelvic cancer complicating pregnancy is most often treated by surgery. The rationale for this is based upon the following arguments:

1. It would appear that the preferred treatment for cancer is to excise it widely when this can be done without inordinate mortality and morbidity.

2. Surgery provides an all-embracing approach in the shortest period of time.

3. When cancer and pregnancy co-exist, the principle of eradication of the cancerous organ still obtains.

In the past 25 years there has been an improvement in the treatment for cancer in general. It follows that more women will become pregnant during treatment of cancer, or during subsequent follow-up. The impact of greater emphasis on cancer detection remains to be evaluated, but early reports indicate that cancer in pregnancy is increasing, due in no small measure to diligent screening programs.

It is important to establish a firm histologic diagnosis. Having established the diagnosis, the philosophy must be to treat the cancer and ignore the pregnancy. However, in certain instances, therapy may result in the interruption of pregnancy. Since there is no direct attack on the fetus, and since this approach is medically sound, it is accepted but not necessarily condoned by the clergy.

The pregnant state is divided into the standard three trimesters plus a fourth postpartum period which extends for four months. There are now well-established guidelines for treatment in each trimester, and principles should be adapted to patients on an individual basis.

There is an increasing body of evidence in the current literature which favors primary surgery as the preferred method of treatment for gynecologic cancers complicating pregnancy. Radiation therapy has its optimal effect in well-oxygenated tissue that is undergoing rapid growth. As soon as the pregnancy is damaged by radiation, involution follows, creating an anoxic type of tissue. This is a poor setting to achieve a good radiation effect.

Cancer in pregnancy is increasing because of the greater emphasis on cancer detection. It is also increasing because women are delaying the time of their first pregnancy until they are in their mid or late thirties. Many of these individuals are career women and have the knowledge that they can be protected through amniocentesis against delivering an anomalous baby. They elect to wait until they are older to start their families. When cancer complicates pregnancy, three questions constantly arise, ie, does the pregnancy affect prognosis, what effect will the cancer have on the fetus, and what will treatment do to the fetus? These questions will be answered as the different cancers are discussed.

GENITAL CANCER COMPLICATING PREGNANCY

The cancers that are included in this group are those of the lower genital tract and of the upper genital tract. Cancers of the lower genital tract include those of the vulva, vagina, and cervix. Cancers of the upper genital tract include those of the endometrium, ovary, and breast. The rectum is also included in the discussion of cancers of the pelvis, although it is not truly a genital tract cancer.

Cancer of the Vulva

Cancer of the vulva accounts for only 1% of all cancers, and 3% or 4% of all gynecologic cancers. There are only 500 deaths from cancer of the vulva in the United States each year. It is usually encountered late in life; approximately 85% of the cases occur after the menopause, particularly in the seventh decade. Cancer of the vulva is rare in women before the age of 45, and extremely rare in pregnancy. When it does occur in pregnancy, the patients are surprisingly young.

Shannon collected five cases from the literature in 1941 and added one case. The average age of these six patients was 21.5 years. The average age in the Memorial-James Ewing Hospital series was 27.3 years. The infrequent occurrence of cancer of the vulva complicating pregnancy also may be appreciated by a survey of Way's large personal series of cases in which there were only four instances.

The major histologic type is squamous cell carcinoma, constituting about 82%. The average age for women with this cancer is 65 years for whites, and 55 years for blacks.

With the current sexual revolution and the initiation of intercourse at earlier ages than previously reported, the incidence of abnormal cytology and histology of the vulva may increase. This can be anticipated if the same association that has been observed for abnormal cytology in herpesvirus 2 in the cervix is reported. Preliminary observations have indicated a similar association. The chronic irritation brought about by the wearing of nylon stockings and pantyhose, creating an environment for the growth of bacteria and viruses, may increase the number of cancers of the vulva that will be seen in the future.

Barclay (1974), in a review of the literature, found only 31 women with vulvar cancers associated with pregnancy. Of these cases, only 12 were actually diagnosed and treated during pregnancy, with another two being treated following termination of pregnancy. Lutz et al, in 1977, reported five vulvar cancers associated with pregnancy, of which three were diagnosed and treated during pregnancy, and two within six months postpartum. The authors reported on three cases of cancer of the vulva associated with pregnancy. Two were diagnosed prior to pregnancy, and one in the fifth month of pregnancy.

The author's plan of management for patients who are pregnant and have a diagnosis of cancer of the vulva is as follows:

1. First trimester: Radical vulvectomy and bilateral superificial node dissection. A deep node dissection is carried out only if the highest node is positive (so-called Cloquet's node) or if several nodes are present.

2. Second trimester: The same treatment as for the first trimester. However, it may be technically impossible to do an adequate node dissection. If so, a radical vulvectomy should be done and the node dissection delayed until after delivery.

3. Third trimester: If the lesion is small and will not interfere with vaginal delivery, this method of delivery should be permitted. Radical vulvectomy and node dissection should be carried out in the immediate postpartum period within two to four weeks.

4. Postpartum: Radical vulvectomy and bilateral superficial and deep node dissection.

5. Subsequent pregnancy: Cesarean section should be reserved for obstetrical indications in those patients where scarring might present a hazard.

Cancer in situ of the vulva can be followed safely during pregnancy or, if very localized, can be treated at that time. With the aid of colposcopically directed biopsies to rule out invasive cancer, definitive therapy might well be delayed until the postpartum period.

Cancer of the Vagina

Cancer of the vagina is extremely rare, comprising less than 1% of all genital malignancies. To date, there have been approximately 300 deaths from cancer of the vagina reported in the United States. The anticipated impact from cancer of the vagina and cervix in those individuals whose mothers took diethylstilbestrol has not materialized. Currently, the ratio of cancer of the cervix to vaginal cancer is approximately 50:1. It is often difficult to tell whether the tumor arises primarily in the vaginal epithelium or extends to it from the primary locus in the cervix. When both are involved, the cervix is considered the primary site.

Cancer of the vagina has been found mainly in women over the age of 50. The average age was 61 years for white women and 58 years for blacks.

Recently, adenosis and adenocarcinoma (Müllerian clear-cell carcinoma) have been reported in young women whose mothers took diethylstilbestrol (DES) during pregnancy. This unusual relationship may alter the normal age distribution reported for cancer of the vagina. Currently, the author knows of only one case of adenocarcinoma of the Müllerian duct complicating pregnancy. This was treated at term by cesarean section followed by a radical hysterectomy, bilateral pelvic node dissection, and vaginectomy.

Collins and Barclay (1973) reported ten vaginal carcinomas associated with pregnancy collected from the literature. Lutz et al (1977) reported one such case. Among those reported with follow-up, the prognosis was not good.

The collected experience in managing vaginal cancer complicating pregnancy makes it difficult to suggest a plan for therapy. However, it should be treated in general as though the patient were not pregnant. It is recommended that if the fetus is viable, delivery by a high vertical cesarean section should be performed and therapy started as if the patient were not pregnant. If the infant is not viable or near viable age, external therapy should be started, followed by radium or cesium application, which must take into consideration the location of the lesion. In the rare instance where the patient does not abort spontaneously following the external therapy, the uterus should be emptied before the radium application is made. If the lesion is early (Stage I) and located in the upper part of the vagina, it can be managed by radical hysterectomy, vaginectomy, and pelvic node dissection.

Herbst et al (1971) recorded seven girls, 15 to 22 years of age, with adenocarcinoma of the vagina (clear-cell, Müllerian type) between 1966 and 1969. The association between diethylstilbestrol and this type of clear-cell adenocarcinoma has been repeatedly documented. The first results of an HEW-funded study made public recently have confirmed that the synthetic estrogen diethylstilbestrol, while a cancer threat to daughters of women who took the drug during pregnancy to prevent miscarriages, may pose less risk than earlier anticipated. DES was once widely prescribed for the prevention of miscarriages. An estimated four to six million persons—women who took the drug during pregnancy and their children—are believed to have been exposed to it, chiefly between 1945 and 1955, but some as late as the 1970s. To date, there have been less than 400 cases of adenocarcinoma reported in this group.

It is recommended that when adenocarcinoma is diagnosed in these patients, the management should be the same as in the nonpregnant state, ie, radical hysterectomy, vaginectomy, and pelvic node dissection. If the diagnosis is made at friability, a cesarean section should be carried out, followed immediately by the treatment outlined above.

Cancer of the Cervix

Diligent screening programs are detecting cancer of the cervix in all stages from 0 to IV. Since the natural history for the development of invasive cancer ranges from 5 to 20 years, a certain number of women in this group will become pregnant in the presence of fungating advanced cervical cancer. Approximately one pregnancy in 3000 is complicated by cervical cancer. The disease is not different from that diagnosed in the nonpregnant state.

Reports collected from the literature suggest that the incidence of positive nodes is greater during the pregnant state. Comparison of comparable stages of the disease in the pregnant and nonpregnant patient does not show any difference. Prognosis depends on the extent of disease. Accurate tissue diagnosis is important. In the presence of an obvious lesion, biopsy is indicated, whether the Pap smear is negative or not. Local punch biopsy must be performed, and, if positive for invasion, no further biopsies are necessary. If the biopsy is positive for an in situ lesion, and it can be carefully outlined and followed by colposcopy, this is the method that should be chosen. If the lesion is extensive, multiple punch biopsies are indicated. Cone biopsy is hazardous in pregnant patients. Fortunately, the squamocolumnar junction and the transformation zone are easily seen by colposcopic examination, and directed biopsies can be obtained if indicated. The frequent and safe utilization of colposcopy during pregnancy for examination of the patient at risk or under suspicion is one of its most valuable uses. If the diagnosis of an in situ lesion is accurately made, the patient can be safely followed during her pregnancy and delivered from below, with cesarean section reserved for any obstetrical indication.

The diagnosis is often delayed in pregnancy. The youth of these patients and their accompanying pregnancy undoubtedly play a role in the reluctance of the responsible physician to examine the cervix at the first sign of abnormal bleeding. It is important to investigate excessive discharge and vaginal bleeding during pregnancy. Speculum examination is indicated in all pregnant women, particularly those with symptoms. More frequent cytologic studies should be carried out. Schmitz and his co-workers' experience along these lines, in which 25 cases of cancer in the cervix were detected among smears taken on 10,369 pregnant patients, bears this out. Stage for stage, there is no difference in the prognosis and survival between the pregnant and the nonpregnant patient.

Although surgery is the preferred method of treatment in the author's experience, radiation therapy is generally accepted as the method of choice. Both methods are presented in outline form:

Surgical treatment

1. First trimester and early part of the second trimester: Radical hysterectomy and pelvic node dissection with the fetus in utero.

2. Late second trimester: Await viability of the fetus, and then do a classical cesarean section, followed immediately by a radical hysterectomy and pelvic node dissection.

3. Third trimester: Classical cesarean section followed immediately by a radical hysterectomy and pelvic node dissection.

4. Postpartum: Radical hysterectomy and bilateral pelvic node dissection.

Radiation therapy

1. Nonviable fetus, first and second trimesters: External radiation with at least 3000 rad to the uterus. Spontaneous evacuation is preferred to intervention. Tandems and colpostats are then used. Following this, booster doses are given over the nodal area to increase the dosage to at least 5000 rad.

2. Viable fetus, third trimester: Classical cesarean section, followed immediately by external therapy. On completion of this, use radium or cesium insertion.

3. Postpartum: Radiate as in the nonpregnant patient. Because of the danger of infection, the radium is usually divided into several applications.

Currently, most radiation therapists are starting treatment with external therapy, followed by intrauterine and intravaginal application of radium or cesium.

Cancer of the Rectum

Cancer of the rectum complicating pregnancy is not strictly a gynecologic or a genital cancer, but actually is a pelvic cancer. Therefore, it is included in the discussion.

There have been more than 200 cases reported in the literature. The extremely low incidence is reflected in the figures reported by McLean, in which he states that there is one cancer of the rectum for every 50,000 cases of pregnancy. Although cancer of the rectum and/or colon is a rare complication of pregnancy, it should be included in the differential diagnosis for a patient with colonic symptoms. The presence of rectal bleeding, abdominal pain, changing bowel habits, weight loss, palpable abdominal mass, and/or persistent nausea and vomiting in late pregnancy, should alert the obstetrician to the possibility of a bowel lesion. The consideration of a colonic cancer is particularly important in a patient with factors known to predispose to malignant changes.

Unless the symptoms improve, a thorough investigation should be carried out. Harm to the fetus from barium studies must be weighed against the fetal outcome of not diagnosing a cancer of the bowel in its early stage. The role of colonoscopy as a diagnostic procedure in these cases has not been established. Once the diagnosis has been made, it is important to proceed with treatment. A suggested plan of management is presented:

1. First and second trimesters: An abdominal-perineal resection or an anterior resection is carried out, depending upon the position of the lesion and its extent.

2. Late second and third trimesters: If possible, management should be delayed until the fetus is viable. However, complications related to the cancer may require prompt treatment. These include hemorrhage, obstruction, and perforation. Cesarean section is usually required to facilitate the technical aspects of the operation if the pregnancy is beyond the first or second trimester. An abdominal-perineal or an anterior resection is the treatment usually chosen. If there is any evidence of local spread, total hysterectomy and bilateral salpingo-oophorectomy may also be required. In the presence of large bowel carcinoma, there is increasing evidence indicating that bilateral oophorectomy should be carried out in order to remove the ovary as a major site for metastasis.

Cancer of the Upper Genital Tract

Adenocarcinoma of the endometrium with intrauterine pregnancy is extremely rare. Karlen et al (1972) reviewed the literature since 1900, summarized five acceptable cases, and added a sixth. A unique case of corpus cancer associated with a tubal pregnancy was reported by Tracy in 1932, but the pathologic findings were not illustrated. Sandstrom and coworkers reported one case and found six others reported in the literature. Four of the seven tumors were adenoacanthomas. Follow-up on four of the six previously reported patients indicated that three are in good health more than five years after diagnosis. Barber and Brunschwig (1962) reported one case that was discovered after curettage for spontaneous abortion.

It is interesting to note the high frequency of occurrence of squamous differentiation in tumors discovered in pregnancy. Glücksman (1959) noted a similar high frequency of squamous differentiation in tumors of the cervix in pregnancy. This may be related to the hormonal milieu present during the gravid state.

Patients reported in the literature were all Caucasian and ranged in age from 21 to 43 years. The majority complained of dysmenorrhea, irregular menses, or hypermenorrhea of recent onset and short duration. The prior menstrual and medical histories were generally unremarkable with the exception of one patient who had genital tuberculosis. Except for obesity, constitutional factors associated with endometrial carcinoma, such as hypertension and diabetes mellitus, have not been reported.

Cancer of the Ovary

Cancer of the ovary accounted for approximately 5% of all cancers among women. It accounted for 20% of the genital cancers among whites, and 12% among blacks.

Analysis of ovarian cancers by histologic type shows notable racial variations. Although papillary serous cystadenocarcinomas made up about one fourth of all ovarian cancers in both races, a higher percentage of these tumors were classified as localized among black women than among white women. Papillary carcinomas occurred more frequently among white than black women, and were often diagnosed in a localized stage among whites (27% vs 19%). There was a much higher percentage of papillary cystadenocarcinoma of the ovary among black women (15%) than among white women (2%); 31% were localized among whites and only 16% among blacks.

When diagnosed with localized disease, white women with mucinous cystadenocarcinomas and granulosa-cell carcinomas had relatively good survival rates. The most lethal tumors were the unclassified carcinomas and adenocarcinomas; only 10% and 18%, respectively, of the patients with these tumor types lived for five years. However, about three fourths of these patients were diagnosed after the disease had metastasized to distant sites.

Deaths from ovarian cancer have increased slowly over the last 40 years, and the rate is now 2.5 times that of 1930. In 1981, it is anticipated that there will be 18,000 new cases and about 11,400 deaths from cancer of the ovary. It is now the leading cause of death from gynecologic cancer. Early diagnosis is the key to successful treatment. This is a matter of chance rather than a scientific method. When ovarian cancer is diagnosed in its early stages, it is considered a surgical disease; the standard treatment is total hysterectomy, bilateral salpingo-oophorectomy, and omentectomy.

Ovarian cancer occurs in about 1 in 18,000 pregnancies. In the nonpregnant state, about 20% of ovarian tumors are found to be malignant, but in the pregnant state the rate drops to 5%. There is no explanation for this at the present time.

Chung and Birnbaum (1972) found that fewer than 40 cases of ovarian cancer complicating pregnancy had been recorded between 1963 and 1972. There were an additional ten cases during, and four after pregnancy. Beischer (1971) recorded 164 gonadal tumors diagnosed during pregnancy or in the puerperium at the Royal Women's Hospital in Melbourne during the years 1947 to 1969. More than 50% were either adult cystic teratomas or mucinous cystadenomas, and only four (2.4%) were malignant. They commented on the difficulty of establishing a definite diagnosis during pregnancy, and concluded that the size of the tumor was not a reliable criterion of malignancy. Novak and his co-workers reported 100 examples of ovarian neoplasm associated with gestation. The absolute five-year survival rate in these 100 cases was 76%. Such excellent salvage is a reflection of the favorable pathologic type of tumors encountered in these patients.

It is generally accepted that ovarian cancer has become the most lethal primary genital cancer and results in more deaths than malignancy arising in both the cervix and the corpus combined. Uterine neoplasms often produce abnormal bleeding and may, in a majority of cases, be detected by study of vaginal cytologic preparations. Most ovarian tumors are silent, and symptoms develop only when there has been spread of the neoplasm or the mass becomes palpable. Thus, a majority of such lesions prove to be inoperable at the time of initial surgery.

The problems are compounded when ovarian tumors coexist with pregnancy, since the gravid uterus may prevent adequate palpation of a coexistent adnexal mass, especially if it is cystic and small. In such cases it may seem to be a portion of the enlarged, softened corpus. Consequently, as in the nonpregnant state, most ovarian neoplasms during pregnancy are not detected until they are well advanced. The signs and symptoms are not basically different from those occurring in the nonpregnant woman. The presenting symptom may be a complication of the tumor, such as torsion, rupture, hemorrhage, or infection.

The pelvic findings are important in the decision whether to operate immediately or to observe the patient for a period of time. A unilateral, encapsulated, freely movable mass of uniform consistency and less than 10 cm in size, can be kept under observation until the second trimester. If it decreases in size, presumably it represented a corpus luteum cyst. However, progressive growth requires exploration without further delay. On the other hand, a hard, knobby, fixed mass of variegated consistency (a tumor that has hard areas, soft areas, rubbery areas, and cystic areas is suspect), or signs of fluid are indications for surgical intervention despite the stage of the pregnancy.

The management of cancer of the ovary complicating pregnancy can be summarized as follows:

1. Treat as in the nonpregnant state.
2. General workup and exploratory laparotomy.
3. Aspiration of the pelvis and abdomen when the peritoneum is opened.
4. If the tumor is low-grade, unilateral, and encapsulated perform unilateral salpingo-oophorectomy and biopsy of the opposite ovary. If negative, consider the treatment to be adequate and allow the pregnancy to go to term.
5. If the lesion has extended beyond the ovary, aspirate for cytology, perform an exploratory laparotomy with careful staging, bilateral salpingo-oophorectomy, appendectomy, and omentectomy. Chemotherapy should be given as indicated.

Routine inspection of the tubes and ovaries is mandatory at the time of cesarean section.

Novak (1975) has reported the absolute survival rate in 100 cases as 76%. This excellent salvage rate is a reflection of the favorable pathologic type of tumors encountered in these women. The series included 45 common epithelial tumors, 14 gonadal stromal tumors, 33 germ-cell tumors, 2 sarcomas, 2 metastatic Krükenberg type of tumor, and 4 metastatic tumors, including 2 which were unclassifiable.

Every effort should be made to avoid surgery in the first trimester of pregnancy to minimize the possibility of abortion. At this time, most cystic masses are corpora luteum of pregnancy. The latter are often larger during the second month of pregnancy as a result of the striking thecal luteinization associated with the high levels of chorionic gonadotropin. On the other hand, prolonged procrastination is unwarranted since, on occasion, an ovarian enlargement has been followed, only to discover an advanced lesion when definite surgery was performed at term. There is no question that the pregnancy deserves special consideration; however, the ground rules for the management of ovarian tumors should not be neglected.

Results from numerous investigations suggest the possibility that the immune reaction is suppressed during pregnancy. This has been reported by Anderson et al (1974) who treated pregnant women with recurrent herpesvirus type 2 with BCG and obtained dramatic responses, suggesting a diminished cell-mediated immunity during pregnancy. There have been other supporting data. The role that such reactions may play in the course of an ovarian tumor during pregnancy remains to be documented, but introduces a challenge in the prognosis.

In most reported series, approximately one third of the cases are Stages III or IV at operation. One must be prepared for this volume of tumor before the initial operation. The most aggressive cancers in terms of early spread are the solid adenocarcinomas and serous cystadenocarcinomas. Survival in patients with ovarian cancer in pregnancy is no different than in the nonpregnant group. The type of tumor and its anatomical spread determines the five-year cure rate.

Breast Cancer

Over 106,000 new cases of breast cancer are diagnosed in the United States each year. One of every six cases occurs in a woman less than 45 years of age. It is not surprising that in this fertile population pregnancy sometimes coincides with malignancy or follows its treatment.

Among women in the United States who are 25 to 74 years of age, the breast is the leading site of cancer mortality; in women 39 to 44 years of age, it is the leading cause of death. Breast cancer mortality and incidence rates increase with age, but the rates of increase are greater during the reproductive years. The age-specific incidence and mortality rates for breast cancer, beyond 40 years of age, are consistently higher in women who never marry, experience their pregnancy at a later age, and have fewer children. The relative risk in married women who are first pregnant under 20 years of age, is about one third less than in women who are first pregnant when they are 35 or older. However, the most discriminating risk factor, with respect to marital and reproductive history, is the age of the women at first birth. Recent studies have indicated no protective effects of lactation on the development of breast malignancy.

The association of breast cancer with pregnancy is a special situation that has plagued physicians with both ethical and therapeutic uncertainties. The physician is confronted with the responsibility for two lives, with the unlikely prospect that both can be served equally well. He is also faced with the potentially lethal, hormonal-sensitive tumor in a host undergoing complex, progressive, and progressively adverse, endocrine and hormonal changes.

The obstetrician-gynecologist feels secure in managing the pregnant woman with pelvic cancer. However, he is less secure in his management and control if the patient has an extrapelvic malignancy. If castration or termination of the pregnancy is indicated, the obstetrician-gynecologist is the technician, and all too often the patient is then managed by a medical oncologist. When a surgeon undertakes a radical approach to breast cancer, the obstetrician-gynecologist becomes a bystander. The hematologist-oncologist is consulted to treat and follow the patient. This is not ideal for the patient's management and is not in the best interest of the patient. The obstetrician-gynecologist is best qualified to serve as the primary care physician and should control and coordinate the care of the pregnant patient with a neoplasm. As specialists are consulted, their role should be as a *consultant* and not as the physician in charge of the care of the patient. The obstetrician-gynecologist must continue as the responsible physician, all orders and treatment controlled by him.

Management of breast cancer associated with pregnancy may be a severe test for any clinician. Widely different views are held by surgeons, gynecologists, and radiotherapists about its treatment and prognosis. In addition, nonclinical, religious, psychological, and socioeconomic considerations undoubtedly influence the choice of management. Breast cancer in pregnancy is a difficult clinical problem which requires skill and good judgment.

In the United States, 3% of newly diagnosed breast cancers are accompanied by pregnancy, the concurrence favoring women in the fourth decade of life. This is relevant at present because women are having their first babies later in life than formerly. They are now delivering their first child in their 30s, and often in their late 30s. This increases the chance of an associated cancer complicating pregnancy.

Holleb and Farrow (1962) grouped patients into the following groups: simultaneous pregnancy, postpartum pregnancy, and subsequent pregnancy. The overall five-year survival rates for these major groups were 33%, 29%, and 52%, respectively. When there were positive nodes: 21%, 15%, and 30%, were reported. It should be noted that the frequency of positive nodes (70% on the cases) is somewhat higher than in the usual nonpregnant group.

The outlook for such patients is less favorable than that of the nonpregnant, nonlactating woman, probably because the stage of disease is more advanced at the time of discovery. The most significant factor in the poorer prognosis is physician delay in diagnosis and therapy. If age and stage of disease are taken into account, pregnancy itself seems to have a negligible influence on prognosis. Radical mastectomy can be expected to be almost as curative for pregnant patients with operable cancer as for others, and presents little chance for fetal loss. Reports from the literature indicate that therapeutic abortion does not improve the chance for cure, although in effect it is prophylactic castration. Studies on the use of estrogen receptors and triple-agent chemotherapy remain to be evaluated insofar as they relate to cancer of the breast complicating pregnancy.

The important questions in regard to pregnant or lactating women with proven cancer of the breast are:

1. How should the pregnant patient with breast cancer be treated?
2. Is waiting for the termination of pregnancy indicated or even desirable before mastectomy is performed?
3. Does accepted treatment by today's standards alter the life expectancy of women?

4. If the woman is pregnant at the time of diagnosis or subsequent to mastectomy, is termination of pregnancy indicated?
5. Should the surgeon plan to castrate surgically the woman with treated breast cancer for therapeutic reasons, or primarily to prevent future pregnancies?

Some of these questions have already been answered. The consensus of opinion from the literature is that patients presenting with early breast cancer in the first trimester should be treated in the same manner as nonpregnant patients. There is no harm in allowing the pregnancy to continue. Termination, if elected, is based on social, economic, and psychologic factors. However, in several centers, patients with operable tumors and positive nodes, are receiving adjuvant chemotherapy. If this regimen is followed there may be an argument for aborting the fetus, provided the disease is treated in the first trimester, because of the teratogenic risk of the drug to the fetus.

There does not seem to be any special risk in treating patients with breast cancer in the second half of pregnancy rather than waiting for the postpartum period. A modest delay in therapy to allow for delivery probably has no deleterious effects.

Patients with Stages III and IV cancer have such a poor prognosis that a uniform plan of therapy is difficult to outline. After a frank discussion with the patient and her husband, the decision may be to accept treatment, knowing that there is a risk of teratogenesis. Other patients may elect termination of the pregnancy followed by aggressive therapy. There may be a place for prophylactic castration in the treatment of disseminated disease, but its role is yet to be clearly defined.

The association of pregnancy with breast cancer does not constitute a significantly increased risk. Subsequent pregnancies are not associated with decreased survival, whether or not regional lymph nodes were involved at the time of the original operation. Treatment during the first trimester need not be delayed, but treatment during the second and third trimesters is associated with poor survival, although it is not dissimilar to that obtained within three months of delivery. Therefore, delay, if expedient, is permissible, but treatment should be completed in the shortest possible time. Therapeutic abortion does not add to survival, and ovarian ablation does not recommend it.

Breast cancer in association with both pregnancy and lactation is rare, but presents a therapeutic problem of considerable magnitude. The outlook for such patients is less favorable than that of the nonpregnant, nonlactating woman, probably because the stage of disease is more advanced when it is discovered. The most significant factor in the poorer prognosis is often physician delay in diagnosis and therapy.

When mastectomy is carried out early in pregnancy, the operation can be as effective as in nonpregnant women of the same age group. It is to be emphasized that, when pregnancy and breast cancer are found concurrently, prompt therapy for the cancer should be undertaken.

Interruption of pregnancy in nondisseminated breast cancer is of little value. If pregnancy is near term when the diagnosis of breast cancer is made, the desire of the husband and wife for a child should be considered. A modest delay in therapy to allow for delivery should have no deleterious effect.

Castration should be withheld and used only for the patient with metastatic disease. There may be a place for prophylactic castration in the treatment of disseminated disease, but its role has yet to be clearly defined.

Subsequent pregnancy may be permitted. An interval of at least two years should elapse between treatment and the start of a new pregnancy. Nature will eliminate patients with aggressive tumors. It is a method of selecting patients with a better prognosis. Patients who had positive nodes at the time of treatment for their breast cancer have a high rate of treatment failure and decreased rate of survival, both in the pregnant and nonpregnant state.

Prompt evaluation of a breast mass during pregnancy is indicated. The pessimistic outlook reported in the past is not justified. Better diagnosis and therapy can give respectable survival rates.

FETAL AND PLACENTAL TRANSMISSION OF MALIGNANCY

Metastasis to the fetus and/or placenta has stimulated a great deal of interest and considerable controversy. When cancer complicates pregnancy, it is common for the afflicted woman and/or her family to ask whether the cancer will spread to the baby. In addition, they ask if it will have an indirect or delayed effect on the child. Fortunately, this is extremely rare. There are probably fewer than 40 reported cases of metastatic disease having been identified within the placenta. The most common lesions are metastatic melanoma, breast cancer, and tumors of the leukemia-lymphoma groups.

Many theories and interpretations have been advanced to explain the paucity of documented cases of placental and fetal metastasis: 1) Most placentas probably are not carefully examined by both gross and histologic evaluation; 2) The possibility of active resistance by the trophoblast has been proposed, 3) The fetal environment may be unfavorable for the rare cancer cell that crosses the barrier established by the placenta, 4) Reynolds and Pack (1955) and Scharnagel (1951) have proposed that the tumor cells have the potential to invade the chorionic villi and penetrate the intravillous capillaries, thus becoming blood-borne via the umbilical vein to the liver of the fetus, and 5) In our present state of knowledge, it is wise to accept the fact that unknown factors control metastasis to the placenta or fetus.

If the sinuses around the villi are large and circulation is sluggish, the presence of tumor cells in these sinuses does not truly represent metastasis to the placenta. The designation should be reserved for the intravillous destruction and invasion of tumor cells. Using these criteria, few of the cases reported actually qualify for the diagnosis of metastasis to the placenta.

Metastasis from the mother to the fetus is indeed rare. There have been about two dozen cases reported in the literature. Criteria include maternal and placental invasion, and the occurrence of the same cancer in the baby within one year of birth. Beyond one year, viral transmission, genetic transmission, or altered immunity are considered factors in the development of cancer. The case most often referred to was reported by Sir Eardley Holland (1949), where maternal, placental, and fetal disease were all documented.

RADIOTHERAPY AND ANTINEOPLASTIC THERAPY

Surgery and radiation are effective forms of treatment for localized cancer. Chemotherapy can be used for disseminated as well as localized tumors. Exclusive of breast cancer and rare instances of ovarian cancer, surgery and/or radiation therapy, by its direct or indirect attack on the fetus, eliminates the fetus as a consideration in the overall management of the neoplastic process. The use of radiation therapy and surgery has been covered earlier in the chapter. It is rare that antineoplastic therapy would be used in cases of genital cancer. However, in breast and ovary cancer, it might be considered rarely as a modality of treatment. In these instances, a single drug should be used; alkylating agents are the ones usually chosen. Antifolic acid drugs are contraindicated in the first trimester of pregnancy because of their teratogenic effect and their propensity to produce an abortion.

BIBLIOGRAPHY

Introduction

Barber HRK, Brunschwig A: Gynecologic cancer complicating pregnancy. *Am J Obstet Gynecol* 85:156, 1962.

Betson JR, Golden ML: Cancer and pregnancy. *Am J Obstet Gynecol* 81:718, 1961.

Boronow RC: Extrapelvic malignancy and pregnancy. *Obstet Gynecol Sur* 19:1, 1964.

Cancer—A Manual for Practitioners, ed 5. Boston, American Cancer Society, Massachusetts Division, 1978.

Golomb HM, Ultmann JE: An approach to general oncology: Principles and procedures. *J Reprod Med* 17:191, 1976.

Phelan JT: Cancer and pregnancy. *NY State J Med* 68:3011, 1968.

Vulva

Barclay DL: Surgery of the vulva, perineum and vagina in pregnancy, in Barber HRK, Graber EA (eds): *Surgical Disease in Pregnancy.* Philadelphia, W.B. Saunders Co, 1974, pp 310–335.

Collins CG, Barclay DL: Cancer of the vulva and cancer of the vagina in pregnancy. *Clin Obstet Gynecol* 6:927, 1973.

Collins JH: Pregnancy and delivery following extensive vulvectomy. *Am J Obstet Gynccol* 80:187, 1960.

Shannon WF, Marting E: Primary epidermoid carcinoma of vulva complicating pregnancy. *Am J Obstet Gynecol* 41:117, 1941.

Vagina

Collins CG, Barclay DL: Cancer of the vulva and cancer of the vagina in pregnancy. *Clin Obstet Gynecol* 6:927, 1973.

Herbst AL, Ulfelder H, Poskanzer DC: Carcinoma of the vagina. *N Engl J Med* 284:878, 1971.

Lutz MH: Genital malignancy in pregnancy. *Am J Obstet Gynecol* 129:536, 1977.

Cervix

Glucksman A: Symposium on histomorphology of cervical carcinoma during pregnancy. *Acta Cytologica* 3:54, 1959.

Green TH Jr: Carcinoma of the cervix in pregnancy, in Barber HRK, Graber EA (eds): *Surgical Disease in Pregnancy.* Philadelphia, W.B. Saunders Co, 1974, pp 354–371.

McDuff HC, Carney WI, Waterman GW: Cancer of the cervix and pregnancy. *Obstet Gynecol* 8:196, 1956.

Sablinska R: Invasive carcinoma of the cervix associated with pregnancy. Correlation between patient age, advancement of cancer and gestation, and results of treatment. *Gynecol Oncol* 5:363, 1977.

Endometrium

Karlen JR, Sternberg LB, Abbott JN: Carcinoma of the endometrium coexisting with pregnancy. *Obstet Gynecol* 40:334, 1972.

Sandstrom RE: Adenocarcinoma of the endometrium in pregnancy. *Obstet Gynecol* 53(suppl):73S, 1979.

Schumann EA: Observations upon the coexistence of carcinoma fundus uteri and pregnancy. *Trans Am Gynecol Soc* 52:245, 1927.

Tracy SE: Carcinoma of the uterus complicated by tubal gestation. *Am J Obstet Gynecol* 23:223, 1932.

Wall JA, Lucci JA: Adenocarcinoma of the corpus uteri and pelvic tuberculosis complicating pregnancy. *Obstet Gynecol* 2:629, 1953.

Westman A: A case of simultaneous pregnancy and cancer of the corpus uteri. *Acta Obstet Gynecol Scand* 14:191, 1934.

Ovary

Beischer HA: Growth and malignancy of ovarian tumors in pregnancy. *Aust NZ J Obstet Gynaecol* 11:208, 1971.

Betson JR Jr, Golden ML: Primary carcinoma of the ovary coexisting with pregnancy: Report of three cases. *Obstet Gynecol* 12:589, 1958.

Chung A, Birnbaum SJ: Ovarian cancer associated with pregnancy. *Obstet Gynecol* 41:211, 1972.

Novak ER: Ovarian tumors in pregnancy. An ovarian tumor registry review. *Obstet Gynecol* 46:401, 1975.

White HC: Ovarian tumors in pregnancy. *Am J Obstet Gynecol* 116:544, 1973.

Colon

Barber HRK, Brunschwig A: Carcinoma of the bowel. *Am J Obstet Gynecol* 100:926, 1968.

Levin B: Aspects of gastrointestinal tumors during reproductive years. *J Reprod Med* 17:233, 1976.

McLean DW, Arminski TC, Bradley GT: Management of primary carcinoma diagnosed during pregnancy. *Am J Surg* 90:816, 1955.

Breast

Donegan WL: Breast cancer and pregnancy. *Obstet Gynecol* 50:244, 1977.

Holleb AI, Farrow JH: The relation of carcinoma of the breast and pregnancy in 283 patients. *Surg Gynecol Obstet* 115:65, 1962.

Hubay CA, Barry FM, Marr CC: Pregnancy and breast cancer. *Surg Clin North Am* 58:819, 1978.

Ribeiro GG, Palmer MK: Breast carcinoma associated with pregnancy: A clinician's dilemma. *Br Med J* 2:1524–1527, 1977.

Trevis N, Holleb AI: A report of 549 cases of breast cancer in women 35 years of age or younger. *Surg Gynecol Obstet* 107:271, 1958.

Miscellaneous

Anderson FD, Usliyima RN, Larson CL: Recurrent herpes genitalis: Treatment with BCG. *Obstet Gynecol* 43:797, 1974.

Coombes GB: Phaeochromocytoma presenting in pregnancy. *Proc Roy Soc Med* 69:8, 1976.

Finkbeiner JA: Antineoplastic chemotherapy in pregnancy, in Barber HRK, Graber EA (eds): *Surgical Disease in Pregnancy.* Philadelphia, W.B. Saunders Co, 1974, pp 711–718.

Holland E. A case of transplacental metastasis of malignant melanoma from mother to fetus. *J Obstet Gynecol Br Empire* 56:529, 1949.

Jafari K, Lash AF, Webster A: Pregnancy and sarcoma. *Acta Obstet Gynecol Scand* 57:265–271, 1978.

Jaffe HL, Reddi PR: Radiation therapy in pregnancy, in Barber HRK, Graber EA (eds): *Surgical Disease in Pregnancy.* Philadelphia, W.B. Saunders Co, 1974, pp 727–736.

Nicholson HD: Cytotoxic drugs in pregnancy. *J Obstet Gynecol Br Commonw* 75:307–312, 1968.

Pack GT, Scharnagel IM: The prognosis for malignant melanoma in the pregnant woman. *Cancer* 4:324, 1951.

Pang C: Transplacental metastases of the Brown Pearce rabbit tumor. *Bull Tulane Med Fac* 17:31, 1957.

Pizzarello DJ, Witcofski RL: *Medical Radiation Biology*. Philadelphia, Lea & Febiger, 1972, p 59.

Plummer G: Anomalies occurring in children exposed in utero to the atom bomb on Hiroshima. *Pediatrics* 10:687–693, 1952.

Pratt CB, Rivera G, Shanks E: Osteosarcoma during pregnancy. *Obstet Gynecol* 50(suppl 1):24S, 1977.

Reynolds AG: Placental metastases from malignant melanoma. Report of a case. *Obstet Gynecol* 6:205, 1955.

Smythe AR II, Underwood PB Jr, Kreutner A Jr: Metastatic placental tumors: Report of three cases. *Am J Obstet Gynecol* 125:1149, 1976.

Sokol JE, Lessman EM: Effects of cancer chemotherapeutic agents on the human fetus. *JAMA* 172:1765–1769, 1960.

Stewart A, Kneale GW: Radiation dose effects in relation to obstetric x-rays and childhood cancers. *Lancet* 1:1185–1188, 1970.

Sweet DL Jr, Kinzie J: Consequences of radiotherapy and antineoplastic therapy for the fetus. *J Reprod Med* 17:241, 1976.

16 Cancer of the Breast

Hugh R. K. Barber

More than 48 million American women have passed their 35th birthday. In the next year, women in this age bracket will develop about 110,000 new breast cancers, and approximately 36,800 of these women will die of the disease. It is therefore understandable that this diagnosis is devastating to any woman who is told that she has a cancer of the breast. All too often, it is synonymous with death. Newer advances in diagnosis, therapy, and follow-up offer hope for longer survival, more cures, and a better quality of life for patients with breast cancer.

Breast cancer is the most prevalent cancer in women in the United States today. It constitutes approximately 28% of all cancers in women. Breast cancer has remained constant in incidence, prevalence, and mortality during a period in which death in middle-aged women from other causes has decreased. During the last 15 years breast cancer has emerged in the United States as the most common malignant tumor of women and is the commonest cause of death among white women between ages 40 and 65.

As an unsightly malignant growth on an easily visible external organ, the crab-like progress of breast cancer is dramatic to anyone who has seen a case. Of the major cancers we tend to modify by management, it is also the one that appears to be the most amenable to diagnostic and therapeutic efforts. Despite this, cancer of the breast remains a study in therapeutic controversy. Although it is the most frequent cancer in women, there have not been enough reports of a definitive nature in the literature to settle the many arguments related to proper therapy. Currently, we still can expect approximately 50% of the women with breast cancer to die of this disease within five to ten years of the diagnosis and treatment.

Although radical mastectomy has been the mainstay of treatment of operable, early cases, some surgeons feel this form of treatment is too radical, while others feel it is not radical enough. Many modifications have been proposed, and even simple excision of the mass with radiation has the support of an increasing number of surgeons. Some statisticians argue that no method of treatment has affected survival rates.

The use of adjunctive chemotherapy in combination with surgery for operable cases is under investigation. Another major advance is the ability to predict response to hormone treatment. The identification of the estrogen receptor mechanism has provided a method for identifying those cancers that are hormone-dependent. The recent identification of progesterone receptors in breast cancer cells has added to the ability to predict the response that a tumor will have to hormones or their withdrawal.

During the past ten years a better informed public and medical profession have brought a great deal of the attention to problems relative to the breast. In the last few years, the occurrence of the disease in socially and/or politically prominent figures has focused even more attention on the breast.

For all of these reasons, breast cancer is among the most important problems in the United States, one which tests the ability both of the biologic scientist and the practicing physician. Clinical evaluation of the breast is difficult at best, and failure to make a diagnosis is tragic to the patient, embarrassing to the physician, and often fraught with the problems of medicolegal retaliation. It should be emphasized that even when the diagnosis is properly made, suitably established under the microscope, and proper and adequate treatment is given by the best available method, the outcome will all too frequently be failure. Physicians and patients are always delighted when there is a long-term survival. However, although there is a certain pride in this achievement, there must be an equal amount of humility because the reason for success is still as mysterious as the cause of failure.

The pathologic categories of breast cancer include a large number of cystologic types of epithelial neoplasms (infiltrating duct, lobulary carcinoma, colloid carcinoma, medullary carcinoma, comedo carcinoma, and papillary carcinoma), as well as malignant neoplasms of mesenchyme origin (sarcomas). However, the predominant cell type is infiltrating duct carcinoma.

BASIC PRINCIPLES

Statistics suggest a rise in the number of breast carcinomas in regard to: 1) incidence — 72 per 100,000 females (new cases diagnosed in a given year); 2) prevalence — 100 per 100,000 females (number with the disease in a given year); and 3) mortality — 27 per 100,000 females (number dying with the disease in a given year). One out of every 13 women, or about 7%, will develop cancer of the breast. There are approximately 110,000 new cases reported in the United States each year, and more than 36,000 deaths. Approximately every 15 minutes a woman dies of cancer of the breast. Among women in the United States who are 25 to 74 years of age, breast cancer is the leading cause of cancer mortality. It is the leading cause of deaths in women between 40 and 44 years of age. The incidence of breast cancer increases with age. A woman of 70 has six times the chance of harboring a breast cancer as has a woman at age 40. The death rate from breast cancer has been steady over the past 40 years in spite of advances in surgical, radiotherapeutic, and chemotherapeutic techniques.

More than 90% of breast cancer is detected initially by the patient herself. Among those not carrying out routine self-examination, the discovery is accidental and often too late.

Several curious facts are now substantiated. Cancer of the breast is more common on the left side, in outer quadrants, in women without children, and in those who have not suckled. It is bilateral and successive in 4% or more of cases, more prevalent in those with a family history of breast cancer, and more common in those with endometrial and ovarian cancer. The male-to-female ratio is 1:100. The risk of breast cancer increases with the increase in age at which a woman bears her first full-term child. Women who are first parous before age 18 have a risk of developing breast cancer that is approximately only 0.3 times the risk of those whose first delivery of a full-term child is at the age of 35 or older. MacMahon's data surprisingly suggest that initial full-term pregnancy occurring after the age of 30 carries a risk of breast carcinoma greater than that of women who have never been pregnant at all. Women with a low urinary excretion ratio of estriol to the sum of estradiol plus estrone have a higher risk of cancer.

ETIOLOGY

Despite extensive epidemiologic studies and knowledge of patterns of population distribution, no common causative agent is evident. Etiologic factors currently being investigated include hormonal mechanisms, viral agents, and immunologic processes. Recent studies indicate the possibility that postmenopausal estrogen therapy may contribute to the development of breast cancer, but this has not been substantiated.

Thus, the etiologic background of breast cancer may be thought of as having a triangular configuration. One side of the triangle includes genetic factors or ethnic background and family history. The second side is the endocrine factor, including the presence of ovaries, the adverse effects of late pregnancy, nulligravidity, and the increased incidence of the disease in the menopause. The third side of this etiologic triangle include the carcinogenic factors such as external ionizing radiation. There is also increasing evidence that a virus is involved.

Bilaterality is a common feature of breast cancer. Approximately 1% of women presenting with breast cancer have frank clinical disease on both sides; approximately 15% of those who survive the treatment of an initial breast cancer for three or more years will develop cancer in the opposite breast. Urban has confirmed that, by prompt contralateral biopsy, contralateral occult cancers are seen in about 25% of patients with breast cancer recently proved on one side.

DIAGNOSIS

A thorough history and clinical examination is required whenever there is a suggestion of breast disease. Yet, more than 90% of breast cancers are discovered by the patient herself. A well-informed public who is taught self-examination of the breast will identify lumps at an earlier period than previously and will seek help earlier.

The typical presentation is a lump in the breast which, in the early stages, is isolated, freely movable, and painless. Later, the more dramatic findings that are identified with breast cancer will appear. About 50% of patients will present with their cancer in the upper outer quadrant, 20% centrally, 10% in the lower outer quadrant, and 20% in the medial half. If the patient reports that the lump has been present for at least one month, axillary nodes are positive in 50% of the cases. If the lump has been present for six months or more, axillary nodes are positive in about 70% of the cases.

In addition to careful examination of the breast, mammography, xerography, and thermography are available as modalities for making a diagnosis. The final decision as to whether it is a cancer or not depends upon excisional biopsy. Recommendations have been advanced for doing contralateral biopsies in any woman found to have a cancer of the breast, because there is a pickup rate of between 10% and 15% of simultaneous bilateral breast cancer. Aspiration biopsy of breast or nodal masses is advocated by certain centers in the United States.

Differential Diagnosis and Characteristic Symptom Complexes

Fibrocystic diseases

1. Commonly bilateral and multiple.

2. Characterized by dull heavy pain, a sense of fullness, and tenderness.

3. Symptoms and size of the mass commonly increase at the time of the menses.

4. Tenderness is common.

5. Axillary nodes should be absent, or at least not palpable.

The lumps are cystic to palpation, tender, well delineated, mobile, and transilluminate clearly. Aspiration reveals a typical turbid, nonhemorrhagic, yellow-greenish or brownish fluid.

Fibroadenoma

1. Very mobile, solid, firm, rubbery, regular, well delineated, and nontender.

2. Multiple and bilateral in 14% to 25% of patients. They occur in women between 15 and 39 years of age, with a median age of 20.

Cystosarcoma phyllodes

1. A rare variant of fibroadenoma.

2. May cause massive enlargement of the breast, particularly in pregnancy.

3. The skin is seldom involved, and the axilla is usually clear.

4. Venous engorgement and skin inflammation may be present.

Intraductal papilloma

1. Present with a serous, serosanguineous, sanguineous, or watery type of nipple discharge.

2. The discharge is usually from a single duct, and is commonly unilateral.

3. No lump can be felt in most patients. The median age is 40 years.

Duct ectasia

1. Duct ectasia (commonly known as mastitis) also is commonly manifested with nipple discharge.

2. The discharge is usually multicolored and sticky, bilateral, and from multiple ducts.

3. The patient often experiences burning, itching, or a dull, drawing type of pain around the nipple and the areola.

4. When more advanced, they can resemble locally advanced breast cancer.

Galactocele

1. Typically occurs following lactation.

2. Usually found beneath the areola.

3. Occasionally tender.

Cysts of the glands of Montgomery

1. Essentially a sebaceous cyst involving paraareolar glands and presenting under the areola.

2. Usually very small.

3. May be fixed to the skin, but not to the chest wall.

4. Benign process.

Fat necrosis

1. Usually results from trauma.

2. Characteristic skin dimpling and a firm, distinct mass.

3. May be very difficult to differentiate from cancer.

4. Lesion is occasionally tender.

Mondor's disease

1. Caused by superficial thrombosis of veins overlying the breast; may produce skin dimpling.

2. Typically, tenderness is present in early phases.

3. Lesion is self-limited and disappears with time.

Cancer

1. Usually presents as a solitary, unilateral, solid, hard, irregular, poorly delineated, nonmovable, painless, and nontender lump.

2. Usually in the upper outer quadrant of the breast.

3. As it advances, the signs become more pronounced.

4. Certain cancers of the breast, however, do not conform to this clinical picture. For example, Paget's disease presents with eczema of the nipple.

5. Medullary, colloid, papillary cancers can be present with a well-delineated mass that is not hard and gives the impression of mobility.

6. Sarcoma also presents with a well-delineated mass and closely resembles a fibroadenoma.

Patients at high risk to develop breast cancer include:

1. Women

2. Those over 40 years of age

3. Family history of breast cancer

4. Nulliparous women or those with first parity after age 34.

5. Previous history of cancer in one breast

6. Those with a precancerous mastopathy type of fibrocystic disease

7. Those with adverse hormonal milieu

8. Those with lowered immunologic competence

9. Patients with excessive exposure of the breast to ionizing radiation

10. Those exposed to carcinogens

11. Those with endometrial or ovarian cancer

12. Those with high dietary intake of fat

13. Patients with chronic psychologic stress, and those living in the western hemisphere or cold climates

14. Those belonging to the upper socioeconomic group of the white race

15. Those infected with a breast tumor virus (more indefinite).

Biopsy is mandatory in patients with:

1. True, three-dimensional, dominant lumps, even if diagnostic aids are negative

2. Excluding cysts which can be aspirated safely under controlled conditions

3. Suspicious lesions found by diagnostic aids, even if there are no clinical findings

4. Serous, serosanguineous, bloody, or watery nipple discharge, even if there are no palpable masses, and negative cytology and breast x-ray studies

5. Adverse signs such as eczema of the nipple, unexplained retractions or elevations, suspicious axillary enlargement, redness of the skin of the breast, underlying induration without signs of infection, and unexplained skin dimpling or a persistent dominant area of unexplained thickening of the breast (Table 16-1).

Mammography: Benefits vs Risk

X-ray studies of the breast are advisable: for all patients over 50 years of age on a yearly basis; for symptomatic breasts that are difficult to diagnose clinically; if there is an abnormal thermogram; for factors related to increased risk of breast cancer; preoperatively when a breast lump is present, except when a patient is under 25 years of age; after cyst aspiration; in cases of multinodular breast, large pendulous breast, and areas of thickening without a true mass; in breasts with thin scar formation due to previous biopsies or trauma; and for patients who are in a high-risk group for breast cancer.

Indications for mammography

1. Women over age 50 years
2. Previous mastectomy
3. Sister, mother or both, with premenopausal breast cancer
4. Nulliparity
5. First child born after age 30
6. Menstruation at age 11 or under
7. History of previous benign tumors
8. Presence of lumps, discharge, severe pain, or cystic breast
9. At any age, if the patient is concerned and a mammography has been recommended by her physician
10. Presence of large breasts. Mammography is particularly important, regardless of age, because it is much more difficult to find the lump by palpation in these patients.

Table 16-1
Comparison of Special Histologic Types of Infiltrating Breast Carcinoma

Parameter	Histologic Type					
	Infiltrating Duct Carcinomas	Infiltrating Lobular Carcinomas	Medullary Infiltrating	Colloid Infiltrating	Comedo Carcinoma Infiltrating	Papillary Infiltrating
Node involvement (%)	60	60	44	32	32	17
Crude survival, 5 years (%)	54	50	63	73	73	83
Actuarial survival, 5 years (%)	59	57	69	76	84	89
Percent, total	78.1	8.7	4.3	2.6	4.6	1.2

11. If the patient is aged 35 to 50, has no signs or symptoms, and no increased risk factors, she should have a complete examination including history, palpation, thermography, and the option of mammography.

Risk of breast cancer *vs* risk of mammography More and more women look to the gynecologist as their primary physician for detection of breast disease. More and more gynecologists examine the breasts as part of the routine gynecologic examination. Interest is increasing in developing expertise in palpation and teaching breast self-examination, as well as in the study of ancillary diagnostic procedures such as thermography and mammography. Screening is simply a procedure to detect undiagnosed disease in an apparently well individual. With the increased use of mammography as a screening device, controversy has arisen about the risks involved. The average American woman faces a 7% chance of developing breast cancer in her lifetime. The benefit vs risk must be evaluated against this background.

With up-to-date equipment, one rad is the approximate dose absorbed by each breast during one mammogram. Since the average woman already faces a 7% chance of getting breast cancer, one mammogram would theoretically raise her risk to 7.07% (7% plus 7% multiplied by 1% [.07 + .07 × .01 = .0707, or 7.07%]). Fifteen mammograms (one every year for 15 years) would theoretically raise the average woman's risk from 7% to 8%. With the most modern equipment, measurements indicate a reduction in radiation levels of 0.2 to 0.3 rad to the skin. Such skin radiation, with low kilovoltage from molybdenum anode tubes and compression techniques, delivers doses to the midbreast of 0.2 to 0.3 rad for a right-angle pair of films.

There are numerous benefits of mammography. Most cancer experts believe that early detection offers the best cure rate. In American Cancer Society and National Center Institute screening centers, 45% of palpable breast cancers have been confirmed by mammography. For earliest breast cancers — called minimal tumors — which cannot be felt and are only detectable through mammography, five-year cure rates of up to 95% have been reported, compared with only 45% after the disease has spread to nearby lymph nodes.

Thermography is not an indicator of cancer as such; however, it does alert the clinician to the possibility of disease. Clinical examination and/or mammography is needed for more definitive diagnosis and localization. Approximately 20% to 25% of abnormal thermograms are found in patients with no abnormal findings from other methods. These need to be watched more closely, and may represent a high-risk group. Some observers have found occasional cancers becoming apparent clinically one to three years after positive thermograms.

What results can be expected from screening? Strax (1976) has reported that some idea of the type of benefits to be derived from screening can be obtained by examining the results obtained at the Guttman Institute in New York. Of 126,472 examinations done in 1971 to 1976, 61,994 were initial studies, and 64,478 were subsequent examinations. Of 4501 recommendations for biopsy or aspirations, 2815 were done, and 641 cancers were found.

Schematic Anatomical Staging Outline
(Clinical Observations)

The term clinical staging refers to a method of staging that applies only to clinical examination prior to histologic assessment of regional lymph node areas.

Clinical diagnostic staging systems have been devised by the American Joint Committee for Cancer Staging and End Results Reporting; the TNM classification. For the gynecologist, this is a fairly elaborate type of staging. The following is proposed as a simplified method.

Stage I — Breast mass localized, all nodes negative.

Stage II — Breast mass localized, axilla positive.

Stage III — Breast mass locally extensive; axilla, supraclavicular, and internal mammory nodes positive.

Stage IV — Distant metastases.

In addition to the above classifications, there is the postsurgical-treatment, pathologic staging system of the American Joint Committee for Cancer Staging and End Results Reporting; the TNM classification. These elaborate stagings have value when a detailed study of cancer of the breast is being conducted. However, the simpler classification meets the needs for the practicing gynecologist.

TYPE OF SURGERY

The operation is tailored to the type of lesion and extent of disease. If a patient has localized breast cancer without grave signs suggesting or establishing curability by regional means of therapy, many treatment alternatives are available and a choice must be made. There are data suggesting there is no particular advantage of any given approach, but there are few reliable data for establishing truly optimal treatment.

Treatment alternatives vary from lumpectomy to extended radical mastectomy or supraradical mastectomy. Data at this time appear to have reliably answered some of the questions raised by consideration of these treatment alternatives. There is general agreement that: 1) no benefit from surgical removal of the internal mammary lymph nodes (as a routine operative approach) has been demonstrated, 2) no benefit has been demonstrated in the administration of postoperative radiation therapy or prophylactic castration after radical mastectomy, and 3) radiation therapy can control breast cancer effectively, but its relative effectiveness, in comparison to that of surgical methods, has not been completely clarified.

Lumpectomy has two disadvantages. One is that cancer of the breast is often diffuse, and there may be more cancer present than appreciated. Between one third and one half of breast tumors are found outside the original site. The other disadvantage is that nodes are not removed and examined; thus there is no way of knowing if the nodes are involved.

With a reasonably early lesion, a modified radical mastectomy, leaving the pectoralis major muscle intact, is being selected with increasing frequency. This avoids the major defect in the axilla and affords a rather good cosmetic result. The nodes are taken out and are available for pathologic examination.

The nature and description of the various methods of treatment of breast cancer which apply to the tumor itself are reviewed as follows:

1. Extended radical mastectomy or supraradical mastectomy— surgical removal of the internal mammary chain of lymph nodes, the entire involved breast, the underlying chest muscles, and the lymph nodes in the axilla.

2. Halsted radical mastectomy—surgical, en bloc removal of the entire involved breast, the underlying chest muscles, and the lymph nodes in the axilla.

3. Modified radical mastectomy—surgical removal of the entire involved breast and the lymph nodes in the axilla. The underlying chest muscles are removed in part or left in place after removal of the axillary nodes.

4. Simple mastectomy (more recently called total mastectomy)— surgical removal of the entire involved breast. The underlying chest muscles and the lymph nodes in the axilla are not removed.

5. Limited procedures have a variety of names including lumpectomy, local excision, partial mastectomy, and tylectomy (comparable to lumpectomy). In each instance, the tumor is surgically removed with a varying amount of surrounding tissue.

Note: All of the above procedures completely remove the involved breast.

There are unanswered and partially answered questions about available treatment strategies, but in spite of this the clinician must decide on the primary therapy for his patient with breast cancer. In this regard, it seems fair to make the following statements about therapy for breast cancer patients with clinically localized disease:

1. Partial mastectomy, with or without radiation therapy, should not be employed on a general basis until clinical trials have established that this is equal or superior to methods employing removal of the entire breast.

2. Mastectomy with or without axillary dissection is indicated if no clinically involved axillary nodes are present.

3. Mastectomy with axillary node dissection (radical mastectomy or modified radical mastectomy), or mastectomy combined with adequate postoperative x-ray therapy, should be performed if axillary lymph nodes are clinically palpable.

4. Adjunctive systemic chemotherapy should be employed in addition to mastectomy in patients who have histologically demonstrated axillary lymph node mestastases.

Adjunctive systemic chemotherapy is administered postoperatively to patients with pathologic evidence of axillary lymph node metastases. If the initial reported clinical results can be substantiated, this is more likely to improve the overall results than any of the modifications of regional treatment that have been discussed.

A reasonable alternative to the above plan is elimination of axillary dissection in patients with a clinically negative axilla, but logic would mandate adjunctive chemotherapy for all patients, since there is no way to determine which patients have lymphatic metastases. It should also be stressed that the extent of regional treatment of breast cancer must be modified on occasion by age and concurrent medical problems.

ESTROGEN RECEPTOR (ER) ASSAY

The tissue-estrogen receptor assay (TERA) in mammary tumor tissue provides the physician with the most important single indicator yet devised for assessing the likelihood that the breast patient would benefit from endocrine therapy. The cytoplasmic estrogen receptor protein is labile and requires explicit guidelines in regard to specimen handling and processing. A properly chilled segment of the surgical specimen must be delivered to avert a false-negative assay result. There is evidence that the estrogen-binding protein being measured is, in fact, a receptor. The parameters provided in evidence are the affinity constant for hormone binding as determined from Scatchard plots and sedimentation velocity exhibited by the protein-hormone complex during ultracentrification on a sucrose gradient. The endocrine status of the patient must be considered in interpreting TERA results.

Mechanism

Estrogen-receptor assays make it possible to predict, with a greater degree of confidence than was previously possible, the response of a given tumor to endocrine treatment. Estrogens, whether administered pharmacologically or secreted by an endocrine-active tissue, or carried bound to a protein, transport protein.

The nature of hormone receptors shows that 20% to 40% of carcinomas of the breast exhibit objective regression when subjected to some form of antiestrogen or estrogen-ablative therapy. Such tumors are assumed to be hormone-dependent. Experimental and clinical studies have demonstrated that hormone-dependent tumors have a strong affinity for estrogen.

The discovery of estrogen-binding receptors in mammary carcinomas has lead to the development of sensitive quantitative assays. These assays can be performed on tumor tissue excised by biopsy. The results of these assays have been evaluated as a possible prognostic index of clinical response to antiestrogen or estrogen-ablative therapy. Tumors that have a strong affinity for estrogen are more likely to regress when estrogen levels are significantly decreased.

Estrogens are carried bound to plasma-transport protein. The ability of the tissue to bind hormones is secondary to specific hormone receptors located within or on the surface of cells. These receptors apparently interact with a given hormone by combining with it, thereby initiating the biochemical events characteristic of the function of that particular hormone.

It is believed that estrogens may be able to enter the cytoplasm of all cells, whether they are target tissues or not. The steroid hormone enters the cell, presumably by passive diffusion, and combines with specific receptor proteins that are termed receptors (estrogen receptors [ER]). This reaction is labelled *uptake*. Following this initial binding step, the steroid receptor complex undergoes a temperature-dependent activation. This *activation* allows the steroid receptor complex to enter the nucleus of the cell and bind to the chromatin, the genetic information of the cell. This is labelled *translocation*. Once inside the nucleus, the steroid hormone receptor complex associates with the nuclear chromatin; this is labelled *retention*. Once bound to the chromatin by a little-understood process, the interaction in the steroid receptor complex with the genetic information of the cells leads to an elaboration of new species of messenger RNA. These messenger RNA molecules can be *translated* on polysomes into new proteins. It is these new proteins that lead to the induced effects of the steroid hormone.

From current knowledge of hormone receptor interactions, it is obvious that a cell will not respond to a specific steroid unless the cell contains specific receptors. In the absence of specific receptors, the cell will not respond to the hormone. This is true of neoplastic as well as normal cells.

Antiestrogens have been introduced as a therapeutic modality in the treatment of breast cancer. The mechanism of action simply indicates that antiestrogens, in part, competitively prevent the binding of estrogen to the receptor protein. However, the action is slightly more complicated than described by this simplistic statement.

Antiestrogens, when administered pharmacologically, are also transported in the plasma and readily enter all cells, whether they be target tissue or not. Once again, as with estrogens, these molecules can bind to the estrogen receptor. However, their action is greater than simply prevention of binding of radioactive estrogens to the receptor. Recent experiments have shown that antiestrogen can bind to the receptor and activate, and that the antiestrogens bound to the estrogen receptor can then translocate to the nucleus and also bind to chromatin sites. At this time, there is no absolute clear-cut documentation of what is happening. In terms of two criteria, nuclear occupancy time and salt extractability, these complexes are very different in their biologic behavior from that of the normal estrogen receptor complex. Additional activity of these anti-estrogen compounds involves this nuclear interaction.

In summary, antiestrogens can exert their effect by two mechanisms. They can compete with biologically active estrogens for the receptor protein and thus prevent their binding, or the antiestrogen compounds can bind to the receptors themselves. These antiestrogen, vertical-line estrogen receptor complexes can translocate the nucleus, where they can alter the transcriptive processes of the cell in a manner that leads to tumor regression.

The assay for hormone receptors usually calls for a minimum of 500 mg of tumor tissue. The tumor must be frozen within 15 minutes after removal from the breast by biopsy. It is better to perform the assay on a biopsy specimen rather than a mastectomy specimen. The pathologist should trim off normal tissue from the biopsy specimen and make certain that the specimen is truly neoplastic.

The estrogen receptor mechanism is very useful in clinical practice. The following are generally accepted guidelines for therapy from the estrogen receptor assay:

1. If a tumor is positive for estrogen receptors, there is a 50% to 60% chance that the tumor will respond favorably to antiestrogen or estrogen ablative therapy.

2. If a tumor is negative for estrogen receptors, there is less than a 10% chance that the tumor will respond to similar therapy.

3. Postmenopausal women tend to have a higher rate of positive estrogen receptor results (60%) than premenopausal women (45%). Invasive lobular carcinomas have a high incidence of positive results (90%), whereas tumors with a high lymphocytic content, notably medullary carcinoma, have a low incidence of positive results (25%).

Other morphologic features, such as histologic grade and involvement of axillary nodes, show no correlation with the presence or absence of estrogen receptors.

It is to be re-emphasized that there is almost constant correlation between lack of response to hormone manipulation and lack of receptor. Fewer than 10% of patients with tumors lack estrogen receptors that respond to hormonal therapy, whether ablative or additive. One might question why even 10% respond if they lack receptor, but, as has been pointed out, there is no clear-cut definition what constitutes positive or negative. One possibility is that the receptor may be present in a sample in such small quantities that it is below the limit of detectability of the assay, but the tumor cells themselves may contain sufficient receptor. It is particularly important to recall that the assays are performed on heterogeneous tissue. A metastatic skin nodule in a patient with breast cancer, for example, might contain 10% to 15% breast cancer cells, or even less. The pathologist has no trouble identifying these cells in a biopsy, and the cells might have receptors and be quite capable of responding to hormonal therapy, showing a clear-cut clinical response. However, the number of cells in the sample assay may be simply too small to yield a positive assay.

If the patient's tumor is positive for estrogen receptors, an assay for progesterone receptor should also be done. Clinical studies have shown that the response to endocrine manipulation is higher in tumors that are both estrogen- and progesterone-receptor positive (70%) than tumors that are only estrogen-receptor positive (55%).

TREATMENT OF ADVANCED BREAST CANCER

Before anticancer drugs were available, the treatment of advanced breast cancer was confined to manipulation of the hormonal balance of the patient. In menstruating women, oophorectomy was a primary treatment, with a goal of reducing circulating estrogens. Approximately 30% to 40% responded to such ablative treatment. In the postmenopausal woman, bilateral adrenalectomy was performed to eliminate the adrenal source of estrogen precursors, or, alternately, hypophysectomy was done to achieve remission by mechanisms that are poorly understood even today.

Physicians were disappointed that surgical ablative procedures yielded objective remissions of only 20% to 40% in unselected patients. In addition, the procedure was never predictable and had to be carried out to find out whether there was any hope for a remission. During that time many physicians preferred to administer high doses of estrogen, progesterone, androgens, and glucocorticoids to postmenopausal patients, which would yield similar rates of tumor regression but with less morbidity than the surgical procedure.

With the advent of combination chemotherapy, alternatives to endocrine manipulations became available. Although cytotoxic drugs were often associated with bothersome and sometimes even life-threatening side effects, tumor-response rates in metastatic cancer were considerably better than endocrine therapy in unselected patients. This observation brought about a change in the management of these patients. Combination chemotherapy has now become the primary treatment for metastatic breast cancer, leaving endocrine therapy for those patients where cytotoxic therapy has failed.

Recently, the management of these patients has been changing. Continued improvement is anticipated. The discovery that the use of estrogen receptors in a breast tumor specimen can be used to predict the response to endocrine therapy may make the choice between chemotherapy and endocrine therapy much less empirical and now enables the physician to make this decision on a rational basis.

In patients whose tumors lack estrogen receptor (ER), the response to endocrine-ablative or hormonal therapy has been negligible. Logically, ER-negative patients should not receive endocrine therapy; chemotherapy should be selected as the first-line treatment.

In patients with ER-positive tumors, the response rate to endocrine therapy is respectable. It is about 60% in most series, and compares favorably with response to chemotherapy in unselected cases. It is obvious that patients with ER-positive tumors should receive endocrine therapy, preferably as the initial treatment for metastatic disease. Those ER-positive patients who fail to respond to endocrine therapy, or whose disease progresses after a favorable response, should then receive chemotherapy.

Estrogen receptor assay findings obtained from primary breast tumor specimens can be employed to predict which patient will have an early recurrence following mastectomy. Historically, the only reliable guide for the physician to determine whether the disease might recur was the presence of metastatic cancer to the axillary nodes. Irrespective of a patient's age, tumor size, or lymph node status, the absence of estrogen receptor in the primary tumor specimen is predictive of a higher early recurrence rate, compared to patients with estrogen receptor-positive tumors.

Many experimental clinical trials are now in progress in an attempt to determine whether systemic chemotherapy or endocrine therapy given to axillary node-positive patients following mastectomy, may delay or prevent recurrence. Estrogen receptor data have the potential to identify a high-risk patient. They may also provide a rational basis to decide what type of adjuvant therapy is indicated.

Tumor receptors to progesterone have also been demonstrated. Preliminary reports indicate that the presence of progesterone receptors, in addition to estrogen receptors, may add further specificity in predicting the response to endocrine ablation. Clinical studies have shown that the response to endocrine manipulation is higher in tumors that are both estrogen and progesterone receptor-positive (70%) than in tumors that are only estrogen receptor-positive (55%).

Other receptors to hormones such as corticoid steroids, growth hormone, androgen, and insulin are being sought. It is hoped that one or more of these may offer a still more sensitive indicator of clinical response to endocrine therapy for metastatic breast cancer.

ADJUNCT THERAPY FOR WOMEN WITH POTENTIALLY CURABLE BREAST CANCER

Systemic or local treatment in addition to the primary surgical treatment is defined as adjunct therapy. In the majority of cases, breast cancer presents clinically as a lump in the breast. Only 10% of all patients have demonstrable distant metastases at the time of their initial presentation, 45% have disease limited to the breast, and 43% have regional disease. Survival at five years is related to the extent of disease at the time of diagnosis.

Breast cancer causes death by spreading throughout the body rather than by local growth. Fatal dissemination can occur even when local growth is minimal at the time of diagnosis. Only 75% of patients with histologically negative lymph nodes are without recurrence for ten years. More disappointing are the results in patients with axillary lymph node involvement. Only 25% of all such patients and about 10% with four or more positive nodes are disease free at ten years. Mortality due to breast cancer continues for more than 20 years following mastectomy.

The most compelling argument for the use of systemic therapy in the management of early breast cancer is that the disease in most patients is probably disseminated at the time of clinical presentation. Cancer arises when one or more normal cells are transformed into a malignant neoplastic cell clone. Approximately 30 doublings of tumor cell clones are required to produce a tumor of minimal size for clinical diagnosis. Experimental studies have shown that even small tumors shed cancer cells into the circulation. One animal model has demonstrated that 1 cc of tumor sheds 10,000 cells in 24 hours. Although many of these cells do not remain viable, others do survive, and cause micrometastases that are initially undetectable but eventually result in clinically overt cancer. Local and regional lymph nodes are not effective mechanical barriers to sustain tumor cell dissemination in breast cancer patients.

CHEMOTHERAPY

Chemotherapy, in theory, is a primary systemic attack, and should be more effective than the local approach. Earlier studies in patients receiving thiotepa suggested that there was a delay in recurrence. This is observed only in premenopausal patients. There is much controversy about the effectiveness of adjuvant chemotherapy and, for a while, this approach was abandoned. It has now been resurrected.

A more recent study using L-phenylalanine mustard as adjunctive therapy for an extended period (for more than a year after mastectomy) again demonstrated a beneficial effect (delay of recurrence) in premenopausal women with high-risk breast cancer. Postmenopausal patients receiving postoperative L-phenylalanine treatment showed no significant increase in the recurrence-free period as compared to the controlled group which did not receive adjuvant chemotherapy.

A trial of drug combinations such as cyclophosphamide, methotrexate, and fluorouracil (CMF) as adjuvant therapy following mastectomy in women with high-risk breast cancer has yielded results similar to those seen in the study using L-phenylalanine mustard.

Both clinical and laboratory studies have shown that cytotoxic alkylating agents and antimetabolites induce marked suppression of ovarian function and cessation of menstruation. It is possible that the beneficial effect of adjuvant chemotherapy in premenopausal women is due partly to the suppression of ovarian activity by these drugs.

Currently, cytotoxic chemotherapeutic agents are used as adjuvant therapy in high-risk breast cancer patients only when their tumors are found to be negative for estrogen receptors. In those patients whose tumors contain estrogen receptors, endocrine ablation therapy is chosen as adjuvant therapy in the high-risk patient.

The Rationale of Adjuvant Chemotherapy

The principles for the systemic treatment of micrometastases with drugs are now well established. First, cancer chemotherapeutic agents kill by the first order of cell kinetics. This means that a given dose of a drug kills a constant fraction, not a constant number, of susceptible cells that are in cycle at that time. It follows from this principle that the duration of treatment is as important as the selection of effective drugs. Second, the susceptibility of tumors to anticancer drugs is related to growth kinetics. Small tumor cell populations have a high proportion of cells and active cellular anabolism leading to cell division (high-growth fraction). As the tumor mass increases, the growth fraction decreases. Many anticancer drugs are effective only against proliferating cells. Therefore, micrometastases that have a high-growth fraction should be much more susceptible to the killing effects of drugs than are clinically apparent tumors. Moreover, experimental data are available to demonstrate this principle in a variety of animal tumor systems.

At present, premenopausal patients show a much better response to chemotherapy than do postmenopausal patients. There is no real explanation for this important difference. It seems most likely that the effectiveness of chemotherapy in premenopausal women is due in part to an influence on the endocrine factors. In support of this hypothesis is the fact that the drug treatment produced amenorrhea in 78% of premenopausal patients in the CMF (cyclophosphamide, methotrexate, and fluorouracil) trial. Another recent study demonstrated that 81% of premenopausal patients developed amenorrhea or oligomenorrhea within six months of treatment with adjuvant chemotherapy. In that study, serial plasma hormone determinations indicated that menstruation was suppressed by direct effect of chemotherapy on the ovaries.

RADIATION THERAPY

The use of radiation therapy as an adjuvant to surgery has been debated from the beginning of clinical x-ray therapy. A higher survival rate has been reported for patients with a large primary tumor and extensive axillary involvement when they receive postoperative radiation therapy, not only to the regional nodes but also to the chest wall. Radiation therapy is usually given postoperatively to patients with inner-quadrant, infiltrating cancer regardless of axillary nodal status, and also to those with outer-quadrant lesions with multiple, positive axillary nodes.

Other indications for considering postoperative x-ray therapy are large primary tumors (more than 5 cm in size), cancer cell permeation of intramammary lymphatic vessels, skin involvement or ulceration, chest wall invasion, or massive axillary involvement.

As tests such as the estrogen receptors become better understood and more readily available in predicting accurately biologic behavior of an individual's breast cancer, a rational approach to therapy can be established. At that time, the role of chemotherapy, immunotherapy, castration, and radiation therapy can be presented accurately.

Radiotherapy *vs* Mastectomy

Bloomer (1976) has reported encouraging preliminary results with radiotherapy as primary care for women with Stage I, II, and III disease. He has shown that an adequate dose of radiation is essential for success. The breast usually retains a good cosmetic appearance. The addition of chemotherapy may in the future further improve survival.

The treatment consisted of external beam irradiation using a 4-MEV linear accelerator, supplemented in many cases with interstitial implantation of iridium-192 ribbons or radium needles. Two opposed, tangential portals included the breast, chest wall, adjacent pleura, and ipsilateral internal mammary lymph node chains. Wedge filters were used as compensators to achieve homogeneity of dose within the tangential breast portal. A third portal encompassed the axillary and supraclavicular nodes.

Bloomer reported that, with the use of supervoltage irradiation, there is only minimal breast retraction and no significant skin discoloration. Despite radiographic changes of fibrosis in the skin, subcutaneous tissue, and supporting stroma, definitive radiation therapy often produces a breast that is cosmetically acceptable in appearance. This is especially true with Stage I and II tumors.

This investigator also reported that no local failures developed in 64 patients with Stage I or II disease. Of the 86 patients with locally advanced and unresectable Stage III tumors, 70% had local control. These results have been obtained after a minimum follow-up period of one year in 100 patients followed for at least two and a half years. This was a preliminary study, but it is encouraging that, in the experience of many centers, most local recurrences occur within the first two years of treatment. Based on this, Bloomer believed that local control is likely to be excellent in patients with operable breast cancer.

Calle and Pilleron (1979) have reported that exclusive radiation is a difficult procedure, and is more complex than lumpectomy followed by irradiation. First of all, the irradiation technique requires a great deal of supervision. Tumor doses must be adequate for local control, but must not jeopardize the chances of performing salvage surgery if radiotherapy fails to control the tumor. Because of the high doses delivered to the breast and nodes, radiation sequelae are more severe, and cosmetic results are not as good as those obtained by lumpectomy followed by irradiation. Second, surgery after irradiation is more difficult to perform than primary surgery and, at ten years, 50% of the patients required such secondary surgery. In contrast, only 16% of the cases treated by lumpectomy required secondary surgery. Of the two regimens, lumpectomy followed by irradiation appears to be an excellent therapeutic modality and has a definite place in the treatment of breast carcinoma. On the other hand, exclusive irradiation is more complex than the combination of surgery and irradiation, and the author does not encourage its general use. It requires a meticulous technique, and cosmetic results are not as satisfactory. When utilizing radiation therapy, it is advisable not to promise the patient conservation of her breasts, but rather to propose an attempt to do this.

Palliation

X-ray therapy has been employed as a palliative measure in the treatment of local recurrence in soft tissue metastases, and for osseous and visceral metastases. The majority of patients with widespread metastatic breast cancer often have painful and disabling bone lesions. Although disseminated osseous metastases must be treated by systemic therapy, irradiation to localized symptomatic areas offers the greatest chance for relief. Subjective improvement, as evidenced by a decrease in pain, is achieved in the majority of patients.

Radiation should also be given to relatively asymptomatic, weight-bearing bone lesions which appear likely to cause a pathologic fracture. At times, prophylactic nailing of a long bone should be carried out prior to irradiation.

Oophorectomy has been employed for palliation in the patient with advanced breast cancer. If an estrogen receptor assay has been done and is positive, the chance for palliation is great. However, if an estrogen receptor assay has not been done, L-dopa given by mouth may help in making the decision. L-dopa is an estrogen-blocking agent at the pituitary level. If the bone pain disappears promptly after a fairly small dose of L-dopa, it can be assumed that it was due to estrogen suppression. These patients usually respond to oophorectomy.

A certain number of elderly, postmenopausal women have better results from adrenalectomy than do younger women. One predictive test is to give high doses of cortisone over a short period of time and, if the bone pain eases, they can be considered candidates for adrenalectomy.

Hypophysectomy suppresses prolactin and growth hormone. For practical purposes, adrenalectomy and hypophysectomy seem to provide the same effects insofar as tumor stimulation is concerned. If one is not effective, the other will offer little if anything.

IMMUNOTHERAPY

Immunotherapy for human cancer is not new. The concept that the immune response plays a principal role in the defense against neoplastic cells was formulated by Paul Ehrlich in 1908. In 1959, Thomas elaborated upon this theory and developed the concept of immunologic surveillance, which was later expanded by Burnet (1970). In general, this theory states that an immune response destroys cancer cells during early tumor formation. Thomas and Burnet stated that malignant cells may differ antigenetically from normal cells, and behave as a graft. There are many experiments both in animals and man that tend to support the concept of immune surveillance.

Despite the encouraging trends and remission rates from combinations of chemotherapeutic drugs, the duration of these responses has been short, with a median of five to ten months. The overall median survival period with combination chemotherapy programs has increased to approximately 10 to 12 months.

Currently, programs of chemoimmunotherapy have been initiated for disseminated breast cancer. These combine BCG with various regimens of multiple drug combinations. A study by Gutterman (1976) has indicated that the prognosis for patients with disseminated breast cancer has been significantly improved by the addition of immunotherapy with living BCG organisms to combination chemotherapy. The duration of remission and the overall survival of patients on chemoimmunotherapy are superior to this investigator's results with chemotherapy alone, as well as compared with the results of combination chemotherapy or single-agent chemotherapy programs as reported in the literature.

THE GYNECOLOGIST AND BREAST DISEASE

The designation of the obstetrician-gynecologist as the primary physician for women may seem to impose new responsibilities on these physicians, but, in reality, it merely reaffirms what most have long regarded as standard practice. The gynecologist has always insisted that examination of the breast is an integral part of his evaluation of every patient, and that a basic knowledge of breast disease is certainly as essential as an understanding of obstetrical and gynecological problems.

Because of the large number of women who come under their observation, gynecologists are in a uniquely favorable position to contribute to the early diagnosis of breast cancer. They are concerned with the routine monitoring and screening of all of their patients, with the appropriate monitoring of those who are at particular risk for the development of breast cancer. They are responsible for the proper disposition of those patients in whom abnormalities are found.

The American College of Obstetricians and Gynecologists has adopted as one of its major goals for the next decade a 50% reduction in breast cancer mortality. Although this is an ambitious goal, it should be an achievable one, based upon the earliest possible detection of breast cancer.

As an initial step toward this goal, the College has formulated a statement of policy regarding the obstetrician-gynecologist's role in early breast cancer diagnosis. These principles apply to the asymptomatic mastectomy patient as well as to the patient who has never had the disease. The principles are:

1. Breast examinations are an integral part of the routine gynecologic examination of all patients.

2. Patients should receive instructions in the technique of life-long, periodic, breast self-examination.

3. Proper ambulatory surgical facilities suitable for performing breast biopsies should be developed.

4. The final diagnosis of pathology rests on a careful histologic examination of a biopsy specimen. Biopsy is necessary for all true, solid, three-dimensional masses.

5. Research, both basic and clinical, in etiology, diagnosis, and treatment of breast lesions is to be encouraged. Innovative screening programs for high-risk patients might be included in this effort.

6. Residency training programs in obstetrics and gynecology should include specific instruction in early detection techniques for breast cancer.

Although the radiologist is responsible for the x-ray interpretation, the pathologist for the biopsy readings, and the surgeon for definitive treatment, the primary physician is usually called upon to coordinate these efforts. Furthermore, he is best able to provide the emotional support so essential to his patient. Local breast disease does not in itself cause death. This optimism and hope must be conveyed to the patient.

No woman should be allowed to enter treatment with unfounded fears. Radical surgery is not always necessary for breast lumps. And when it is, it need not be psychologically traumatic.

The gynecologist should include a breast examination as part of every office visit made by a female patient. Although there are many ways to examine a breast, a standard breast examination has been published by the American Cancer Society. This is listed in step-like fashion as follows:

1. Have the patient sit on the examining table facing you. Adequate lighting is essential. Palpate for enlarged upper, middle, and lower cervical lymph nodes gently and methodically. Pay special attention to the area immediately above the clavicle, a frequent site of metastases from primary breast cancer.

2. Inspect the breast, by first examining the patient with her arms at the side. Inspect the contours of the breast, from the axillary fold to the midline, for bulges, skin dimpling, or areas of surface flattening.

3. Next, ask the patient to raise her arms high over her head, chest forward, to expose the extreme lateral portions and undersurfaces of the breast. This technique emphasizes any surface flattening or skin dimpling. Look for redness, ulceration, edema (orange-peel appearance), surface erosion, or dilated veins. Also, note unilateral elevation of the nipple line or a change in the direction of the axis. The nipple is often pulled toward an adjacent malignant tumor. A *pointing* nipple may be a preliminary clue to the specific location of a breast cancer.

4. Palpate the breast with the patient seated. (Remember that it is not advisable to perform a breast examination when the patient is immediately premenstrual, since tenderness and engorgement may preclude adequate evaluation.)

With the patient still seated, have her put her hands behind her head. Gently palpate the breast with four fingers of your slightly extended hand. Using a rotary or transversely linear motion, examine the breast quadrant by quadrant or in decreasing concentric circles ending at the nipple.

5. Compress the nipple. Place it between your index finger and thumb; gently apply pressure to elicit discharge, and evaluate elasticity and possible fixation at the base of the nipple.

Note the general characteristics of the breast. Is it smooth, granular, or nodular? If you encounter a mass, record its size and consistency; determine whether it is fixed to the skin or pectoralis fascia. Gently press the skin together on either side of the mass to elicit skin flattening or dimpling. Skin dimpling may also become apparent by elevating the breast with your hand, or by asking the patient to press her hands against her hip, thereby contracting the pectoral muscles.

6. Examine the axilla. Facing the patient, support her arm with yours. Then, abduct her arm and place your hand flat against the chest wall and high in the axilla. Press hand inferiorly. A careful examination is essential since nodes in the axilla or behind the pectoralis muscle may be easily missed. Note the number, consistency, movability, and size of the axillary lymph nodes.

7. Palpate the breast with the patient supine. Instruct her to lie supine with her right hand under her head, and her elbow flat on the examining table. Put a small pillow beneath the right shoulder to distribute the breast tissue more evenly over the chest wall. Examine the breast using the technique described earlier. Now, reverse the process and examine the left breast.

Teach Breast Self-Examination (BSE)

Following the physical examination, explain to the patient the importance and technique of breast self-examination. Advise her to examine herself once a month, at a time in her menstrual cycle when the breasts are neither engorged nor tender. If the patient is postmenopausal, the birthdate can be selected as the appropriate date of the month for the breast self-examination.

First, instruct the patient to examine herself while bathing, since a mass is more easily felt when both the hand and breast are wet. Next, have her sit before a mirror and inspect her breasts with her arms at her sides, and then with her arms raised. Advise her to look for a change in contour, dimpling, or nipple abnormality.

Now, tell the patient to lie supine with a small pillow under her shoulder on the side to be examined. Instruct her to palpate the entire right breast with the flat of the fingers of the left hand. Then guide her through palpation of the entire left breast in the same manner, but using the right hand.

Point out areas of clinically unimportant thickening, ie, the inframammary ridge, so that such findings do not worry the patient. Also, carefully describe the suspicious signs of breast cancer.

If the patient discovers a mass or other findings, advise her not to become alarmed, but *do* emphasize the need to see a physician *immediately*. It is for this reason that the patient should examine herself in the morning, rather than night. If she does find a mass, she can have it examined the same day, instead of lying awake all night worrying about whether or not she has any disease in her breast.

BIBLIOGRAPHY

Beatson GT: On the treatment of inoperable cases of carcinoma of the mamma: Suggestions for a new method of treatment, with illustrative cases. *Lancet* 2:104, 1896.

Bloomer WD: Radiotherapy vs mastectomy. *The Female Patient* 1:35–38, 1976.

Bonadonna G, Brusamolino E, Valagussa P, et al: Combination chemotherapy as an adjuvant treatment in operable breast cancer. *N Engl J Med* 294:405, 1976.

Burnet FM: The concept of immunological surveillance. *Prog Exp Tumor Res* 13:1, 1970.

Burnet FM: *Cellular Immunology.* Cambridge, Melbourne University Press, 1969.

Calle R, Pilleron JP: Radiation therapy, with and without lumpectomy of operable breast cancer: Ten-year results. *Dis Breast* 5:2, 1979.

Cosimi AB, Brunstetter FH, Kemmerer WT, et al: Cellular immune competence of breast cancer patients receiving radiotherapy. *Arch Surg* 107:531, 1973.

Ehrlich P: On immunity with special reference to cell life. *Proc Roy Soc London (Biol)* 66:424, 1906.

Fisher B: Postoperative radiotherapy in the treatment of breast cancer: Results of NSABP clinical trial. *Ann Surg* 172:711, 1970.

Fisher B, Carbone O, Economou SG, et al: L-phenylalanine mustard (L-Pam) in the management of primary breast cancer. *N Engl J Med* 292:117, 1975.

Gutterman JU, Mazligit GM, Burgess MA, et al: Immunotherapy of breast cancer, malignant melanoma and acute leukemia with BCG: Prolongation of disease-free interval and survival. *Cancer Immunol Immunother* 1:99, 1976.

Holleb AI: The technique of breast examination. *Cancer* 16:7, 1966.

Holleb AI: The technique of breast examination, in *Breast Cancer: Early and Late.* Chicago, Year Book Medical Publishers Inc, 1970, pp 71–75.

Holleb AI: Restoring confidence in mammography. *Cancer* 26:376, 1976.

Horowitz KB, McGuire WL: Specific progesterone receptors in human breast cancer. *Steroids* 25:497, 1975.

Israel L, Edelstein R: Nonspecific immunostimulation with C. parvum in human cancer, in *Immunologic Aspects of Neoplasia, 26th Annual Symposium.* Baltimore, Williams & Wilkins, 1975, p 485.

Jensen EV, De Sombre ER: Estrogen-receptor interaction. *Science* 182:126, 1973.

Klein E, Holtermann OA: Immunotherapeutic approaches to the management of neoplasms. *Natl Cancer Inst Monogr* 35:379, 1972.

Leis HP Jr: Risk factors in breast cancer. *AORN J* 22:723, 1975.

Leis HP Jr: *Diagnosis and Treatment of Breast Lesions.* New York, Medical Examinations Co, 1970.

Leis HP Jr, Pilnick S, and Black MM: Diagnosis of breast cancer. *Hosp Med* 10:33, 1974.

MacMahon D, Cole P, Brown J: Etiology of human breast cancer. A review. *J Nat Cancer Inst* 50:21, 1973.

MacMahon D, Fineleib M: Breast cancer in relation to nursing and menopausal history. *J Nat Cancer Inst* 24:733, 1960.

MacMahon D, Lin TM, Lowe CR: Lactation and cancer of the breast. A summary of an international study. *Bull WHO* 42:185, 1970.

468

McGuire WL, Carbone PP, Vollmer EP (eds): *Estrogen Receptors in Human Breast Cancer*. New York, Raven Press, 1975.

Nathanson L: Immunology and immunotherapy of human breast cancer. *Cancer Immun Immunotherapy* 2:209, 1977.

Oettgen HF, Old LJ, Farrow JH, et al: Effects of dialyzable transfer factor in patients with breast cancer. *Proc Natl Acad Sci* 71:2319, 1974.

Rojas AF, Feierstein JN, Michiewicz E, et al: Levaminsole in advanced human breast cancer. *Lancet* 1:211, 1976.

Russell KP: The gynecologist and the asymptomatic patient. *Doctor* 4:48, 1976.

Schottenfeld D: Epidemiology of breast cancer. *Clin Bull* 5:135, 1976.

Schwartz GF: Evaluation of the patient with a breast tumor. *Surg Clin North Am* 53:717, 1973.

Smithline F, Sherman L, Kolodny D: Prolactin and breast carcinoma. *N Engl J Med* 292:784, 1975.

Strax P: Results of mass screening for breast cancer in 50,000 examinations. *Cancer* 37:30, 1976.

Stutman O, Heberman RB: Immunological control of breast cancer: Discussion. *Cancer Res* 36:781, 1976.

Urban JA: Management of operable breast cancer. *Cancer* 42:2066, 1978.

17 Surgical Procedures in Gynecologic Malignancies

Hugh R. K. Barber

Today surgery offers patients with many types of cancer more chances for cure than any other known treatment. For this reason, surgery is the most widely used form of cancer therapy. Surgical procedures have inherent limitations in the total cure of the cancer patient, but their importance in the management of early cancer now and in the foreseeable future makes it imperative that all areas of possible improvement be exploited.

The magnitude of the problem of genital cancer in the United States is reflected in the following annual figures. There are a total of 76,400 genital cancers. These include: cervix 16,000, endometrium 38,000, ovary 18,000, and other and unspecified genital cancers 4400. To this must be added the 45,000 new cases of carcinoma in situ of the uterine cervix reported each year. Since the breast is included as part of the upper genital tract, this adds another 110,000 cases to the list, bringing the total to 231,400 cases. Surgery is the treatment that is most often used in all of these genital cancers.

To cure a cancer by surgery, treatment must take place before the cancer has spread and becomes established beyond the tissues that can be removed. During the past century, increasingly expensive operations for cancer were devised and evaluated, and such procedures are now carried out wherever good cancer care is practiced. Despite the increasing extent of the procedures, the risk of surgical operations for cancer has been and still is being progressively reduced. This has permitted application of surgical procedures to more and more persons whose cardiovascular status, kidney function, or general metabolism is seriously impaired. Such concomitant handicaps are, of course, frequent in the older age groups. This lowering of the operative risk is absolutely crucial to the application of preventive surgery, the removal of suspicious tumors or ulcerations, and the removal of certain pathologic areas which predispose to cancer.

Recent attempts to develop even more extensive surgical procedures have not resulted in increased rates of cure, and there now appears to be relatively little prospect of major advances from more extensive removal of tissues.

PREVENTIVE SURGERY

Surgery is becoming increasingly more valuable as a prophylactic procedure in cancer therapy. For instance, at one university hospital, 13% of the operations done on the surgical service were prophylactic in nature in 1935, 23% in 1945, and about 30% in 1955 and 1965. This vital role of prevention is not reflected in survival figures, since cancer has actually been prevented. Avoiding the future development of cancer by the timely removal of precancerous growths may eventually be surgery's greatest contribution to the control of cancer.

RECONSTRUCTIVE SURGERY AND REHABILITATION

A major frontier in the surgical therapy of cancer is reconstruction. Plastic and reconstructive surgeons are incresingly finding ways to restore either function or appearance, or both, after extensive surgical procedures. The knowledge that such reconstruction is possible often determines whether or not a patient will accept an otherwise incapacitating procedure. Perfection of reconstructive surgical techniques performed immediately after cancer removal has markedly shortened the convalescent time of patients who have experienced major surgical losses. By the use of new skin graft techniques and the new anatomical understanding of the source for tissue flaps, it has been possible to reconstruct vaginas at the time of the definitive surgery. Such speedy reconstruction markedly aids in rehabilitation, allows earlier, additional treatment for the cancer when necessary, and shortens hospital stay.

PALLIATIVE SURGERY

In addition to his role in saving lives by eradicating cancer, the surgeon is also frequently called upon to improve the remaining months or years of a patient whose cancer cannot be eradicated. Much judgment must be exercised, however, because the objective is to prolong an enjoyable and productive life — not to prolong agony.

For those patients in whom the growth of cancer leads to pain, the neurosurgeon can often bring great relief by dividing the nerve pathways which carry the painful sensations. In the lower two thirds of the body, this can usually be done with minimal impairment of other functions. Numerous other surgical procedures, which are classified under the general designation of palliative surgery, are of great help to individual patients. They often contribute significantly to longevity and, if they can bring comfort and usefulness back to the patient, they are worth the considerable effort which is often involved.

Surgical procedures used in the treatment of gynecologic malignancy include: cervical amputation, cone biopsy, total hysterectomy and bilateral salpingo-oophorectomy, Wertheim hysterectomy, radical hysterectomy, salpingo-oophorectomy and pelvic lymph node dissection, excision of the cervical stump with pelvic lymph node dissection, radical resection of the cervical stump, radical vaginal hysterectomy (Schauta operation), anterior pelvic exenteration, posterior pelvic exenteration, total pelvic exenteration, Schauta operation with extraperitoneal node dissection, and radiation therapy combined with bilateral pelvic node dissection, as well as radical vulvectomy with superficial and deep node dissection. Radical hysterectomy and pelvic node dissection with total vaginectomy, and radical vaginectomy with pelvic lymph node dissection are sometimes indicated. There are a variety of palliative and reconstructive surgical procedures carried out in the presence of gynecologic malignancy. These include repair of ureteral fistulas, closure of intestinal fistulas, repair of rectovaginal fistulas, urinary diversions, and colostomies. A variety of surgical procedures are used to construct a vagina.

When Meigs reintroduced radical surgery for cancer of the cervix in 1939, an additional useful modality became available. In order to institute a surgical program for gynecologic malignancies, it is necessary to employ a wide range of operations from a radical hysterectomy to pelvic exenteration. From a review of the results of surgery, it is now evident that selection of patients for the different forms of surgical procedures is not only justified but indicated. The indications for radical surgery in lieu of radiation therapy for cancer of the cervix include the following conditions: 1) Stage I and IIa, and selected patients with Stage IV cancer of the cervix with fistula formation, 2) young and/or pregnant individuals, 3) atrophic conical, inelastic vagina, 4) radioresistant cervical cancer, 5) pelvic infections (salpingitis) or simultaneous ovarian or uterine pathology, 6) recurrent cervical cancer after prior irradiation, 7) prior radiation for other reasons, and 8) obesity.

SURGICAL PROCEDURES

It is appropriate to review the five reasons (presented in Meigs' original paper in 1944) for surgery. It was his opinion that they proved satisfactory and therefore are repeated here verbatim:

1. If the cervix has been removed, there is no chance for a recurrence in it.
2. If the cervix has been removed, no new cervical cancer can develop in it.
3. Certain cancers of the cervix are radiation resistant, a fact proved at Pondville Hospital where multiple biopsies are performed at the time the x-ray and radium treatment is being carried out.
4. There will be less damage to the bowel if surgery is undertaken.
5. From the work of both Bonney (1941) and Taussig (1943), it is obvious that patients with lymph node metastases can be cured in some instances, and I believe that it is not possible to cure cancer in lymph nodes deep in the pelvis with radiation.

Exenteration Procedures

Pelvic exenteration was born out of frustrations resulting from the inadequacy of therapy available for patients undergoing the ravages of recurrent gynecologic cancer. The operation evolved gradually as a modality of therapy, and in selected patients it is offered as a second chance for life.

Brunschwig is credited with doing the first en-bloc, one-stage pelvic exenteration. He reported that between 1935 and 1937 a few desultory attempts were made to excise the bladder, prostate, and colon for advanced cancer of the colon by a three-stage operation (first, colostomy; second, cutaneous uterostomies and nephrostomies; and third, excision of pelvic organs); but the results were disappointing and the technique was not pursued further. Brunschwig returned to this operation in December 1946, and carried out an en-masse, one-stage excision of bladder, vagina, uterus, lower ureters, and rectocolon, with thorough node excision. He subsequently did two more operations in early 1947. Later, at the Memorial Hospital, New York, the one-stage procedure was performed as frequently as patients presented with the proper indications, and the first clinical report was published in 1948. A less radical procedure, the anterior pelvic exenteration, was devised and reported in 1950.

Techniques   The technique of pelvic exenteration has been described in great detail by several authors. Essentially, there are three types: anterior, posterior, and total pelvic exenteration. Total pelvic exenteration is a synthesis of three major procedures: 1) radical hysterectomy with bilateral pelvic node dissection and excision, and bilateral salpingo oophorectomy, 2) total cystectomy, and 3) combined abdominal-perineal resection of the rectum. Anterior pelvic exenteration is employed to encompass disease that is located in the region of the bladder; it is a fusion of radical cystectomy, radical hysterectomy, bilateral pelvic node dissection, bilateral salpingo-oophorectomy, and partial vaginectomy. In those instances in which the malignant disease arises in the posterior part of the fornix and involves the rectovaginal septum and rectum, posterior pelvic exenteration is indicated to excise the disease en bloc. In posterior exenteration, which is merely an extended form of abdominal-perineal resection, a radical excision in the lower bowel and rectum is carried out along with radical hysterectomy, bilateral pelvic node excision, bilateral salpingo-oophorectomy, and vaginectomy.

Total pelvic exenteration, which encompasses excision of the bladder, rectum, uterus, tubes, ovaries, and pelvic nodes en mass is described below. Most anterior and posterior pelvic exenterations are less formidable procedures, and will not be discussed separately.

Listed below are the steps in total pelvic exenteration.

1. The abdomen and pelvis are explored carefully.

2. The self-retaining retractor is set in place and the intestines are carefully packed out of the pelvis. Adequate exposure is the keystone of success.

3. The posterior peritoneum is picked up lateral to the infundibulopelvic ligament at the pelvic brim, and is incised superficially, allowing the areolar tissue to fall away.

4. The peritoneum is incised to the round ligament.

5. The round ligament is clamped, cut, and ligated. The incision in the perineum is carried to the inguinal area.

6. The ureter is dissected medially with finger dissection, care being taken to keep the ureter attached to the peritoneum.

7. The common and external iliac vessels are freed from the pelvic wall by incising the tissue between the vessels and pelvic wall. The tissue is separated by finger dissection from the pelvic wall down to the pelvic floor, thus exposing the lateral edge of the sacroiliac nerve plexus (sciatic nerve).

8. The tissue between the rectosigmoid and hypogastric artery is incised and then, by blunt dissection with the index finger, is separated to the pelvic floor.

9. By identifying the distal portion of the obliterated vessels along the lateral edge of the bladder, another relatively avascular plane is located, and the dissection is carried down to the pelvic floor. This facilitates identification and isolation of the obturator vessels and nerves.

10. The common and external iliac vessels are dissected by starting at the origin of the common iliac artery and continuing along the external artery to the inguinal ligament.

11. At the distal end of the external iliac vein, the pelvic tissue is dissected from the vein and removed from the obturator and levator ani muscles by finger dissection. This, in combination with the previous dissection, mobilizes the entire area.

12. The distal dissection is carried along the proximal part of the vein to the level of the hypogastric vessels. As the dissection is carried higher, care must be employed to prevent damage to the hypogastric vein where it joins the common iliac vein. The obturator nerve is identified and protected from injury while the obturator vessels are clamped, cut, and ligated at the obturator foramen.

13. The hypogastric artery is ligated either at its origin from the common iliac artery or wherever it can be mobilized easily, while the vein is ligated distally and then excised proximally.

14. The vessels over the sacroiliac plexus are ligated individually. The entire side now has been mobilized, and a similar procedure is carried out on the contralateral side.

15. The colon is mobilized at the pelvic brim, clamped and transected, after the inferior mesentery artery and vein have been ligated.

16. The rectocolon is freed from the posterior pelvis down to the coccyx; injury to the middle sacral veins must be avoided.

17. The ureters are divided at a level below the pelvic brim.

18. The bladder is mobilized readily from the posterior part of the pubis and is retracted backward.

19. The mass of pelvic viscera is now freed from its attachment to the pelvic floor, and the dissection is carried to the perineum, including the vulva.

20. A pack is placed in the pelvis.

21. Urinary diversion is carried out, usually a segment of ileum or sigmoid being used.

22. A colostomy stoma is placed on the left side at a different level from that of the ileal stoma (for urinary diversion); this usually is brought out to the skin surface in the right lower quadrant.

23. The perineal phase may or may not be done, as the surgeon sees fit.

24. The abdomen is closed in layers with interrupted retention sutures.

Radical Hysterectomy

Radical hysterectomy and pelvic lymphadenectomy is carried out in Stages Ib and IIa cases if the patient has no medical contraindications. In microinvasion, in which the lymphatics and/or blood vessels have been invaded, the tumor covers a wide area, or the basement membrane has been penetrated in several areas. This is probably best treated by radical hysterectomy and pelvic node dissection.

The workup prior to surgery is outlined elsewhere in this book. The surgical procedure is carried out as follows:

The steps in radical hysterectomy and pelvic node dissection are the same as those listed for the pelvic exenteration down to step 14. From there on, the procedure is modified.

15. The cul-de-sac is identified, the peritoneum over the ureters incised, and the dissection is carried down to the cul-de-sac.

16. The bladder flap is developed, and the bladder is dissected down from the operative field.

17. The ureter is freed from its tunnel, using a Mixter clamp. The veins of the vesical uterine ligament are clamped, cut, and ligated. The path of the ureter can now be followed down to its point of entry into the bladder wall.

18. The bladder is now freed from the lower end of the cervix and the upper part of the vagina.

19. The rectum is freed from the vagina. Special attention must be directed to freeing the rectum from the uterosacral ligaments. A sponge on a sponge stick can often roll the rectum off the uterosacral ligaments after the plane has been opened by sharp dissection.

20. The uterosacral ligaments are now clamped close to the sacrum, cut, and suture-ligated.

21. The cardinal ligaments are clamped as close to the pelvic wall as possible. The ureter has now been completely freed and can be easily lifted away from the dissection.

22. The specimen is held only by the vagina. Right-angle clamps, usually Kocher clamps, are placed across the vagina. The upper third of the vagina is included with the specimen.

23. The vagina is left open and hemostasis is obtained, using a continued lock stitch around the vagina.

24. The pelvis is carefully irrigated with saline. A two-inch pack is placed in each pelvic gutter and brought out of the vagina beneath the ureter.

25. The pelvis is now carefully peritonealized.

Radical Vaginal Hysterectomy (Schauta Operation)

An extended vaginal hysterectomy is occasionally performed in highly selected cases. It is known as a Schauta operation, but because of its technical difficulties and the impossibility of gland dissection by the vaginal route, it is little practiced in the United States today. Those few surgeons who have experience with it, have reported good results, although no better than abdominal surgery or radiotherapy.

The vaginal approach is excellent for patients with cancer of the cervical stump, but this can also be accomplished by the vaginal method with satisfactory removal of nodes. If node dissection is to be done at all, Navratil (1966) definitely advises that it be done first. Mitra (1953) has combined the Schauta operation with an extraperitoneal lymphadenectomy. For obese patients or patients who are poor risks, the vaginal operation has much to offer. The operation should be confined to very early Stage I or II cases. It would seem, however, that every surgeon should have a working knowledge of this operation since, on occasion, it may be advantageous to be able to perform it.

The steps in the operation will not be outlined in detail but merely summarized:

1. The operation is begun with an extended vaginal episiotomy, known as a Schuchardt incision.

2. This incision enlarges the vaginal orifice and allows access to the space between the vagina and the levator ani, and the parametrial tissues it contains.

3. The object is to remove ovaries, tubes, uterus, and vagina through the vulvar opening.

4. The vagina is circumcised, ie, a circular incision is made right around the vaginal wall.

5. The upper part of the vagina is closed by sutures (closing off the cancerous cervix). By traction downwards, the areas of the ureteral canal, vesicoureteral junction, and posteriorly, the uterosacral ligaments, become available for dissection. This is a difficult surgical exercise and may be accompanied by troublesome hemorrhage.

6. When the vagina with its contained cervix has been mobilized from the bowel, bladder, and ureter, the vesicouterine pouch is opened and the uterine fundus pulled down to expose the adnexal ligaments for division. This allows removal of the whole genital tract other than the lower third of the vagina, and the operation area can now be closed.

The remainder of the surgical procedures for definitive treatment are variations of these three types of operations.

Repair of Urinary Fistula

A pathologic connection between the urinary tract and an adjacent structure through which urine escapes is called a urinary fistula (L. a pipe, a tube). A fistula between the bladder base and the vagina is the condition most often seen.

In the treatment of patients with cancer, the most common urinary fistulas are ureterovesical (following radical hysterectomy), and vesicovaginal (following radiation therapy).

Two problems must be overcome in the repair of urinary tract fistulas: 1) access to the fistula, and 2) avoidance of wound tension.

There are many methods for closing vaginal vault fistulas. A few of these will be reviewed.

A vesicovaginal fistula may occur after hysterectomy or, less commonly, after radiation therapy. More and more attention is being given to closing the fistulas by a transvesical approach. However, it might be most easily accomplished, if sexual function is not important, by closure of the vaginal vault. This technique is called a Latzko operation. To permit access to the fistula, an extended episiotomy is made. Retractors and traction sutures are required to aid in the optimal approach to the fistula. The main points are:

1. The fistula is usually very close to the vaginal vault suture line and may also be close to the ureteral orifices.
2. The vaginal vault tissue is removed in quadrants.
3. The fistula is closed with the second row of sutures opposing the raw bladder to rectal wall.
4. The vaginal wall is closed transversely with nonabsorbable sutures.

This technique is applicable only to vault fistulas. If it were applied to a fistula farther down the vagina, the vesicorectal suture line would be under tension. Any colpocleisis will shorten the vagina to some extent.

Occasionally, following radiation therapy or radical surgery, a great deal of trauma may result, which requires some type of interposition operation.

Martins' Operation The interposition of the bulbospongiosus muscle (Martins' operation) involves the pedicle of this muscle and the attached fatty tissue which is interposed as described below:

1. An incision is made lateral to the large labia.
2. A pedicle of musculofatty tissue is prepared; hemorrhage must be prevented.

3. The pedicle is pulled medially under the small labia and sutured over the closed fistula and bladder neck.
4. The incisions are closed and a drain is placed lateral to the labial wound.

Interposition of the gracilis muscle   The next operation is the interposition of the gracilis muscle. This is an adductor and rotator of the thigh, originating from the pubic ramus and inserted into the tibia. Its main blood supply with its nerve enters at the junction of the upper- and middle-third, 12 cm from its origin. This allows the surgeon to detach the distal end and fold the belly of the muscle up into the vagina. If the main blood supply is aberrant and enters distally, the muscle cannot be used in this way. The steps are as follows:

1. The skin is incised from the medial femoral epicondyle to the pubic ramus, and the gracilis muscle is exposed. Its blood supply is carefully investigated. If this is normal, the tendon is divided and the muscle mobilized.
2. The fistula must first be closed. A large episiotomy (Schuchardt incision) is necessary to allow access to the fistula.
3. A fairly large area of sclerotic vaginal wall is removed and the fistula closed with two layers of catgut sutures.
4. A tunnel is dissected under the fascia lata so that the gracilis may be pulled through into the vagina in front of the pubic ramus.
5. The muscle is sutured across the fistulous area and the vaginal wall closed over it.

Interposition of the rectus muscle   Interposition of the rectus muscle is sometimes done. If there has been no abdominal radiation, this muscle has advantages over the gracilis. The blood supply is multiple, and the point of entry of the arteries is not critical. In addition, it is more accessible. The one disadvantage is the likelihood of ventral hernia. The steps are as follows:

1. The fistula is mobilized and repaired.
2. Using an abdominal and vaginal approach, a tunnel is dissected from the space of Retzius to the vagina.
3. The rectus sheath is opened and the lower half of one muscle is mobilized and pulled into the vagina.
4. The muscle is sutured across the fistula and the vagina closed.

Interposition of omental fat   Interposition of omental fat (method of Bastiaanse) must sometimes be employed. This technique was developed to deal with large fistulas following combined radium and surgical treatment of cervical cancer. The principle is to introduce into the vagina tissues not damaged by radiation: the bladder fundus, the wall of the sigmoid, and the omentum. A transverse colostomy is made approximately three weeks before the operation so that the vaginal area may be cleared of feces. The steps are as follows:

1. By vaginal dissection, the peritoneal cavity is entered between the bladder and rectal mucosa.
2. By abdominal dissection, the bladder fundus and rectosigmoid are mobilized and an omental pedicle is fashioned.
3. The fistula is closed and the omental fat sutured between them.
4. This type of surgery calls for a very careful dissection in a difficult field of operation. It is best undertaken only by a few surgeons with expertise in this field.

Transvesical repair   Transvesical repair is being employed more commonly now. It is granted that nearly all fistulas can be closed by the vaginal route, but this shortens the vagina, and occasionally it is necessary to open the bladder to gain access to the fistula. Repair by this route is more difficult and should be undertaken only by those with expertise in the field. The steps are as follows:

1. The space of Retzius (suprapubic space) is opened and the bladder incised by a transverse incision.
2. Polyethylene catheters or infant feeding tubes are inserted into the ureters. The vagina should be packed beforehand to push the bladder base upward.
3. The bladder wall is mobilized from the vagina.
4. The vagina is closed with catgut. The bladder wall then is closed with catgut and reinforcing sutures are placed in position.

Rectovaginal Fistula

Rectovaginal fistulas are openings between the rectum and the vagina at any point from the vaginal vault to the outlet. The fistula may vary from one that is of pinpoint size to one that occupies the entire width or length of the vagina.

These fistulas result from a number of causes. No single factor is responsible for many fistulas; however, the total incidence of rectovaginal fistulas is sufficiently high to demand considerable attention from the operating gynecologist. Fistulas may originate from treatment with radiation therapy or radical surgery.

The diagnosis of this condition usually is obvious and simple. The escape of gas and feces is uncontrollable, and there is usually considerable fecal incontinence. A small vesicovaginal fistula may be totally asymptomatic. When the fistula is symptomatic, investigation of both the rectum and vagina is important since the cause(s) must be controlled or quiescent before successful closure may be made.

The condition may be obvious when the labia are spread. A speculum can be rotated to show a high fistula. The vagina may be filled with stool, or the fistula identified by feces coming into the vagina. If the bowel is empty, the dark rectal mucosa may be seen as the fistulous tract, in contrast to the pink mucosa of the vagina. The opening may be small and the tract difficult to outline. The location of the fistula is essential for cure. A small probe placed in the fistula from the vaginal side may be palpated on rectal examination. If difficulties are encountered in following the fistula at operation, injection of indigo carmine into the fistula may aid in identifying it.

The bowel should be well prepared prior to surgery, since healing is helped by reducing the stool content in the colon. Mechanical cleansing with castor oil and enemas is the keystone of the preoperative preparation. Sulfonamides for the bowel and/or neomycin completes the bowel preparation. A few hours before operation, the patient should be given 250 ml of 1% solution of neomycin instilled into the bowel. Currently, povidone-iodine is being used with excellent control of bacteria including *Bacteroides.*

The small rectovaginal fistula can be closed using an approach similar to the Latzko procedure which is performed to close vesicovaginal fistula.

Repair of a large rectovaginal fistula involves more surgery than is required for a small fistula. The preoperative preparation should be carried out as outlined earlier. An incision is made through the sphincter ani muscle, the fistula, and the rectovaginal wall below and above the fistula. This creates an artificial third-degree laceration. One half of the tract of the fistula is cut away with scissors from the left side of the incision, and then the other half from the right side is removed. All scar tissue and a small piece of normal tissue must be excised. The vaginal mucous membrane is dissected back far enough to permit mobilization of the bowel for closure of the fistula. Since the opening in the bowel is too large to be closed by a purse-string suture, it is closed by a series of mattress sutures. The bites in the tissue are taken parallel with the edges of the fistula, but do not enter the lumen of the bowel. The use of #0 chromic catgut is most suitable for these sutures.

The closure can also be made with a continuous suture, the edges being inverted into the lumen of the bowel. After the first layer of sutures has been tied, it is reinforced by a second layer placed in the same way, but taking somewhat coarser bites. Each row should begin and end well beyond the previous line of sutures.

After the mucous membrane has been closed gently and snugly, but not tight enough to strangulate the tissues, the sphincter ani muscle should be approximated. This can be accomplished with a #0 chromic suture that is placed in a curved manner along the external ani sphincter. It is first placed on the patient's left side (the operator's right side), and, after some of the sutures are secured, the suture is brought back in the same manner. It is then placed to secure tissue at the 12 o'clock axis.

At this point the same procedure is carried out on the patient's right side (operator's left) as was done on the left side. This manuever secures the retracted ends of the sphincter. When the suture has been tied, the sphincter is tightened and stabilized. Sutures of the transverse perineal muscles stabilize the base of the urogenital diaphragm. Interrupted sutures placed as a second row improve the chances of cure.

The vaginal wall is approximated by running block-stitch sutures or interrupted sutures from just above the apex of the tear in the vagina down to the remnants of the hymenal ring. Next, fibers of the levator ani are drawn together by three or four widely placed, deep interrupted sutures. From the hymenal ring to the sphincter and down to the anal verge, sutures approximate the superficial muscles, the fascia, and the subcutaneous tissues. It is difficult to identify the individual fibers of the superficial and deep transverse perineal muscles, but it is simple to approximate this tissue. This step brings the investing layers of the urogenital diaphragm into correct apposition. The skin edges are approximated by interrupted sutures by #00 chromic surgical catgut.

Repair of Postradiation Rectovaginal Fistula and Stricture

Postradiation rectovaginal fistulas are notoriously difficult to repair, as are the strictures that are usually associated with them. Previous attempts have involved resection and low anastomosis by various techniques. Patients considered not suitable for resection have been treated by permanent fecal diversion. Bricker recently reported a new technique of repair. It relies on the proximal part of the colon as a vascular pedicle graft, used as a patch to close the rectal defect and provide circumference for relief of any associated stricture.

All of these patients require a preliminary colostomy. In selecting the type of colostomy, due consideration should be given to a possible subsequent repair with the Bricker technique. Thus, a left-sided end-colostomy, leaving a long distal segment with a mucous fistula, makes it possible to proceed at the appropriate time with the fold-over repair. Repair is carried out by mobilizing the fistula. This may have to be accomplished through a combined abdominal and perineal approach. Having transected the normal bowel above the fistula, the normal bowel is opened on the antimesenteric border down to and including the fistula. The area around the fistula is freshened. The proximal end of the colon is folded over and anastomosed onto the fistula. After this is well healed, the terminal colostomy can be mobilized, brought down, and sutured to the fold-over flap after an opening has been made into this piece of fold-over bowel. The anastomosis can be carried out as any end-to-end or end-to-side anastomosis.

Ureterovaginal Fistula

Ureterovaginal fistulas are seen in 3% to 10% of patients who have had radical surgery for cancer of the cervix. Since the blood supply is compromised in this type of surgery, it is best not to try to reanastomose a ureter that has been cut or damaged. It may be wise to leave a ureteral splint in place with the hope that it will heal over. These procedures are acceptable following hysterectomy for benign conditions, but not when radical surgery has been carried out.

When a ureteral fistula occurs after radical hysterectomy, an attempted repair should be delayed from three to six months until all of the reaction has subsided. When it is decided to repair the fistula, the procedure of choice is a submucosal, transversical tunnel reimplantation of the ureter to avoid subsequent reflux. This is preferable to an end-to-end anastomosis of the ureter because it avoids the risk of stenosis. A splint and catheter is left in place for two weeks. Retroperitoneal drainage is advised to promote healing and avoid tissue breakdown and infection by the transient extravasation of urine from the suture line. Tension on the anastomosis can be prevented by mobilizing the bladder, advancing it, and suturing the bladder wall to the psoas muscle. It is very rare that total urinary diversion is required for a ureteral fistula following surgery for cancer of the cervix.

Urinary Diversion Operations

There are a variety of ureterocolic anastomoses; the most commonly employed is the Bricker method. However, more and more procedures have been devised for the complete separation of urinary and fecal tract. The most popular urinary diversion operations are the ileal conduit and the colon conduit.

In the ileal conduit (Bricker) operation, the ureters are anastomosed to an isolated loop of ileum which is implanted in the skin as an ileostomy. The ileal conduit helps to avoid pyelonephritis and chloride absorption which follow bowel implantation, as well as the many complications of permanent cutaneous ureterostomy including stenosis, pyelonephritis, abscess formation, and difficulties in collecting urine.

The ileal conduit is fashioned with a wide stoma (both skin and ureteric), and acts merely as a pipe carrying a free flow of urine, so that there is no stenosis in those spaces, no absorption, no acidemia, no reflux, and no ascending infection. The collecting apparatus consists of a rubber or plastic bag that is held by a water-tight adhesive and supported by a belt. The urine passes into a bag which can be drained without being removed. The most commonly employed type of ileal conduit is that described by Bricker (1950).

Reconstructive Surgery

One of the most common operations for reconstructive purposes following treatment of genital cancer is the construction of a vagina. Many methods have been used, including a segment of large and small bowel to serve as the vagina. Two of the most popular in the field of gynecologic oncology are the McIndoe operation or a modification thereof. In the McIndoe procedure, a split-thickness skin graft of proper size to cover the vaginal form is cut from the superior medial aspect of the patient's thigh. Occasionally, the patient will request that the graft be taken from a buttock.

The vaginal area is now carefully prepared by dissecting between the urethra and bladder anteriorly, and the rectum posteriorly. The dissection is carried up to the peritoneum. It is important to make sure that all bleeding is secured, and that the bed for the graft is completely dry. Some operators prefer to prepare the vagina, pack it open, and change the packing each day for several days until the area is dry and granulation tissue is started. They then return the patient to the operating room, prepare the graft, and insert it. When the technique is carefully carried out, the take of the skin graft is usually well over 90%.

In 1964 Williams devised a brilliantly simple technique which has none of the disadvantages of the other types of operation for reconstruction of the vagina. He keeps the patient in the hospital for only about ten days, creates a functioning vagina from skin richly endowed with nerve endings designed to respond to sexual stimulation, and does not require the assistance of a plastic surgeon. It can be adapted to the needs of the patient who has had a pelvic exenteration and in whom a dissection of the perineal area might lead to fistula formation of the small bowel.

In the Williams operation, the labia majora are separated to display the vulvar area. A crescentic incision is made on the inner aspect of the labia, 5 cm from the midline, and the medial edges are sutured from behind forward to create an adequate, elongated space capable of accom-

484

modating a large obturator or glass dilator. The surrounding tissue and skin edges are finally sutured in layers.

In this operation there is the formation of a cul-de-sac by suturing the labia majora in two layers. This means that the anterior wall of the new vagina is the vulva. It protects the sensitive small labia. It is a simple operation which seems to provide satisfying coitus for both partners.

BIBLIOGRAPHY

Barber HRK: Exenteration procedures in pelvic malignancy, in *Davis' Gynecology and Obstetrics*. Hagerstown, Md, Harper & Row, 1977, vol 3, chap 63.

Barber HRK: Fistulas of the genitourinary tract and complete tear of the perineum, in Goldsmith H (ed): *Practice of Surgery*. Hagerstown, Md, Harper & Row, 1978, chap 24, p 1.

Barber HRK: Pelvic exenteration, in Caplan RM, Sweeney WJ III (eds): *Advances in Obstetrics and Gynecology*. Baltimore, Md, Williams & Wilkins Co, 1978, p 655.

Barber HRK: Relative prognostic significance of preoperative and operative findings in pelvic exenteration. *Surg Clin North Am* 49:431, 1969.

Barber HRK: Treatment of advanced cancer of the cervix by pelvic exenteration. *Bull NY Acad Med* 49(10):870, 1973.

Barber HRK, Brunschwig A: Treatment and results of recurrent cancer of corpus uteri in patients receiving anterior and total pelvic exenteration: 1947–1963. *Cancer* 22:949, 1968.

Barber HRK, Brunschwig A: Pelvic exenteration for advanced and recurrent ovarian cancer. *Surgery* 58:935, 1965.

Barber HRK, Robert S, Brunschwig A: Prognostic significance of the preoperative non-visualizing kidney in patients receiving pelvic exenteration. *Cancer* 16:1674, 1963.

Barber HRK, Brunschwig A: Definitive treatment of radiation necrosis. *Obstet Gynecol* 35:344, 1970.

Barber HRK, Brunschwig A: Results of the surgical treatment of recurrent cancer of the cervix, in Lewis GG Jr, Wentz WB, Jaffe RM (eds): *New Concepts in Gynecological Oncology*. Philadelphia, F.A. Davis Co, 1966, p 145.

Barber HRK, Brunschwig A: Excision of major blood vessels at the periphery of the pelvis in major surgery. *Surgery* 62:426, 1967.

Barber HRK: Results of surgical treatment of cancer of the cervix at the Memorial-James Ewing Hospitals, New York, in Marcus S, Marcus C (eds): *Advances in Obstetrics and Gynecology*. Baltimore, Williams & Wilkins Co, 1967, vol 1, p 622.

Barber HRK, Brunschwig A, Mangioni C: Advanced cancer of the vulva and vagina, treated by anterior and total pelvic exenteration 1947–1962, at the Memorial-James Ewing Hospitals. *Cancer* 22:949, 1968.

Barber HRK, Brunschwig A: Treatment of recurrent corpus cancer by anterior and total pelvic exenteration at the Memorial-James Ewing Hospitals, 1947 through 1962. *Ann Obstet Gynecol* 4:219, 1968.

Bonney V: The results of 500 cases of Wertheim's operation for carcinoma of the cervix. *J Obstet Gynecol Br Empire* 48:421, 1941.

Boronow RC: Management of radiation-induced vaginal fistulas. *Am J Obstet Gynecol* 110:1, 1971.

Bricker EM: Bladder substitution after pelvic exenteration. *Surg Clin North Am* 30:1511, 1950.

Bricker EM, Butcher HR, McAfee A: Results of pelvic exenteration. *Arch Surg* 73:661, 1956.

Brunschwig A: Complete excision of pelvic viscera for advanced carcinoma. *Cancer* 1:177, 1948.

Clark BG, Leadbetter WF: Ureterosigmoidoscopy: Collective review of results in 2897 reported cases. *J Urol* 73:999, 1955.

Clark DH, Holland JB: Repair of vesicovaginal fistula: Simultaneous transvaginal-transvesical approach. *South Med J* 68:1410, 1975.

Coffey RC: Physiological implantation of the severed ureter or common bile duct into the intestine. *JAMA* 56:397, 1911.

Coffey RC: Transplantation of ureters. *Ann Surg* 91:908, 1930.

Coffey RC: Transplantation of ureters into the large intestine. *Surg Gynecol Obstet* 47:593, 1928.

Cordonnier JJ, Lage WT: An evaluation of ureterosigmoid anastomosis by mucosa to mucosa method after two and a half years experience. *J Urol* 66:565, 1951.

Counseller VS: The treatment of vesicovaginal and other pelvic fistulas, in Meigs JV, Sturgis SH (eds): *Progress in Gynecology.* New York, Grune & Stratton, 1950, vol 2, p 702.

Garry MM, Gowan ADT, Hodge CH, et al (eds): *Gynecology Illustrated. Urinary Diversion Operations.* Baltimore, Williams & Wilkins Co, 1972.

Hyman RM: Coagulation therapy for small vesicovaginal fistulas. *Clin Obstet Gynecol* 8:465, 1965.

Latzko W: Bhandlung Hochsitzender blasen und mast darmscheindenffstein nach uteusextipation mit hohen schedienverschluss. *Zbl Gynak* 38:006, 1914.

Mattingly RF: Indications, contraindications and methods of total pelvic exenteration. *Oncology* 21:241, 1967.

Mattingly RF, Borkowf J: Lower urinary tract injuries in pregnancy, in Barber HRK, Graber EA (eds): *Surgical Diseases in Pregnancy.* Philadelphia, W.B. Saunders, 1974.

McIndoe A. Treatment of congenital absence and obliterative conditions of the vagina. *Br J Plast Surg* 2:254, 1950.

Meigs JB: Radical hysterectomy with bilateral lymph node dissections. A report of 100 patients operated on five or more years ago. *Am J Obstet Gynecol* 62:854, 1951.

Mitra S. A new approach to the extended radical vaginal hysterectomy for cancer of the cervix. *Cancer* 6:765, 1953.

Navratil E, Kastner H: Unsere erfahrungen mit 997 amreichschen operationen ber der behandlung des invasiven cervixkarcinoms. *Wien Med Wachenschr* 116:1012, 1966.

Nelson JH: *Atlas of Radical Pelvic Surgery.* New York, Appleton-Century-Crofts, 1969, p 1.

Symmonds RE, Pratt JH, Welch JS: Extended Wertheim operation for primary, recurrent or suspected recurrent carcinoma of cervix. *Obstet Gynecol* 24:15, 1964.

Strean GJ: Transvesical approach to vesicovaginal fistula. *Clin Obstet Gynecol* 8:483, 1965.

St. George J: Face-down position for repair of vesicovaginal fistula. *Obstet Gynecol* 34:495, 1969.

Smout CFV, Jacoby F: *Gynecological and Obstetrical Anatomy,* ed 2. London, Arnold, 1948.

486

Taussig GFJ: Iliac lymphadenectomy for Group II cancer of the cervix. Technique and five-year results in 175 cases. *Am J Obstet Gynecol* 45:733, 1943.

Ulfelder H: Extended radical surgery for recurrent and advanced cervical cancer. *Clin Obstet Gynecol* 10:940, 1967.

Weed JC, Geary WL: Vaginal urinary fistulas and rectovaginal fistulas, in Sciarra JJ (ed): *Gynecology and Obstetrics.* Hagerstown, Md, Harper & Row, 1977.

Williams EA. Congenital absence of vagina: A simple operation for its relief. *J Obstet Gynecol Br Commonw* 71:511, 1964.

18 The Critically Ill Gynecologic Cancer Patient

Hugh R. K. Barber

Exclusive of the patient with malignancy, the gynecologist generally treats patients who are in good health. However, when gynecologic patients become ill, they often become dangerously so because the seriousness of the problem is not realized. This may result from the optimism of all gynecologists who have seen serious problems correct themselves when a course of judicious neglect is followed. The purpose of this chapter is to present material that will serve to identify the patient who is getting into trouble, the prophylaxis, and a plan of therapy for the patient who is critically ill.

The main problems encountered in the gynecologic cancer patient are hemorrhage, ileus, mechanical intestinal obstruction, peritonitis, sepsis and septic shock, disseminated intravascular coagulopathy, and the cardiovascular and respiratory problems that add to these complications. Shock lung has taken on an increasing importance in the management of the gynecologic patient who is critically ill. This condition is sometimes referred to by the catch-all term of adult respiratory distress syndrome (ARDS). The diagnosis of shock lung should be restricted to that episode of respiratory failure associated with shock trauma in the postoperative state. Other cases of acute respiratory failure can usually be ascribed to such problems as aspiration, fat emboli, and specific drugs, including oxygen.

The care of the critically ill patient has become a subspecialty within each discipline of medicine. Many centers have established a critical care unit that serves all of the various disciplines of medicine. The salvage rate has been greatly improved with the establishment of these units. However, it is important to identify the potentially ill patient and institute a prophylactic regimen or, if the emergency has arisen, to have a systematic approach for its identification and immediate care. The patient should be delivered to the critical care unit in the least compromised state possible. It is necessary for each physician to be well trained in the evaluation and management of such clinical problems as respiratory failure, shock and its multitude of sequelae, metabolic disturbances, and renal dysfunction. In addition, the physician should also be well versed in the use of such diagnostic and therapeutic modalities as Swan-Ganz catheterization, constant heparin infusion, and total parenteral nutrition.

FLUIDS AND ELECTROLYTES

The goal of fluid and electrolyte therapy in the critically ill patient is threefold: 1) maintenance of circulating blood volume sufficient to perfuse vital organs, 2) provision of nutrients essential for the maintenance of the internal cellular milieu, and 3) allowance for the transport excretion of waste.

A systematic approach for the replacement of fluids and electrolytes should include: 1) daily baseline requirements, 2) extrarenal losses, and 3) deficits or excesses.

The problem of fluid and electrolyte replacement resolves itself into three parts: a) What are the normal daily baseline requirements?; b) What are the extrarenal losses?; and c) What are the deficits or excesses that are present in the beginning of treatment?

The daily baseline requirements represent the fluid and electrolyte needs for the day of an average patient who is being maintained on parenteral therapy, who has no abnormal losses, and who has not had an excess or deficit present at the start of therapy. The daily baseline requirements include water requirements and electrolyte requirements. The requirements for fluids are based on the observation that the total body water of the adult is usually considered to be 60% of the lean body weight. This is subdivided into intracellular (about 40% of the total body weight) and extracellular (about 20% of the body weight) compartments. The latter may be further broken down into interstitial fluid (about 16% of total weight) and circulating plasma water (4% of total weight). Although the normal adult is capable of excreting wastes in the urine volume of 600 ml per day, producing a concentrated urine, this does not take into account the fact that the critically ill patient may not have optimally efficient kidneys, and will probably be in a catabolic state, requiring excretion of a heavier solute load. In order to insure a urine output of 1200 to 1500 ml per day, the following baseline requirements must be met, ie, insensible loss of 1000 ml and a urinary output of 1500 ml. Therefore, the total requirement of water is 2500 ml. This is replaced as 5% glucose in water. The fluid requirements are calculated on findings that the average adult requires 35 ml of water per kilogram of body weight, and the obese, elderly female requires only 25 ml per kilogram of body weight.

The next daily baseline requirement is that of electrolytes. The maximal need for sodium chloride is 77 mEq of sodium and 77 mEq of chloride. It can be supplied by administering 500 ml of 0.9% sodium chloride. Approximately 30 to 40 mEq of potassium chloride (2 to 3 g of potassium chloride) supplies the daily baseline requirement. A urinary output of at least 1000 ml in 24 hours must be present before potassium can be added safely.

Calories, vitamins, and amino acids must be included in the daily baseline requirement. It is difficult to supply added calories with intravenous fluids. In short term replacement therapy it is not necessary. By giving 100 g of glucose (2000 ml of 5% glucose in water) per day, the nitrogen loss of protein is cut by 50%. One hundred grams of glucose can supply about 400 calories per day. Since the body can only utilize about 0.5 to 0.7 g of glucose per kilogram of body weight per hour, an infusion of 5% glucose in water should be run (no faster than 600 ml per hour) if dehydration is to be prevented.

The average postoperative obstetrical and gynecological patient does not need intravenous vitamin supplements. Vitamins B and C are water soluble and, when given by the intravenous route, are excreted in the urine in high concentrations.

There are practically no indications for the use of amino acids in the average postoperative gynecologic patient. In the immediate postopertive period the enzymes are not working at maximum efficiency and, as a result, the amino acid preparations are excreted at a rapid rate. The reactions associated with protein hydrolysates make their use undesirable, unless they are absolutely needed. Protein supplements are needed, however, for the chronically depleted and malnourished patient.

The extrarenal losses are those losses that are going on under observation; are replaced in kind, in amount, and at a rate equal to that at which they are lost; and are divided into external and internal losses. The external losses include vomitus, fluids from tube suction, surface losses from wounds such as groin dissection wounds, burns, exenterations, and abdominal perineal resections, as well as excessive sweating. Blood from hemorrhage must be replaced at the rate it is lost. The internal losses include losses secondary to ileus, peritonitis, raw pelvic surfaces as seen after a radical hysterectomy, pelvic exenteration, or an abdominal perineal resection.

The excesses and deficits must be included in the regimen for fluid and electrolyte replacement, particularly in the critically ill patient. A fluid excess may result from an expanded extracellular space such as seen in cirrhotics, cardiacs, and nephrotics. The deficit produces dehydration. If the loss is rapid and is less than 48 hours in duration and is diagnosed as an acute obstruction or ileus, it involves mainly the extracellular space. However, if the deficit has developed slowly over a period greater than 48 hours, it involves the intracellular as well as extracellular space.

It is obvious that optimal fluid and electrolyte replacement must include the daily baseline requirement, extrarenal losses, as well as any excesses and deficits.

Aggressive surgery, chemotherapy, and/or radiation therapy for the treatment of pelvic malignancy has given rise to many complications. Among these are bowel fistulas and nutritional deficiencies, which carried a high mortality before the use of hyperalimentation had been researched and instituted. Parenteral hyperalimentation was originally used therapeutically, but more and more it is being used prophylactically to prepare for the anticipated treatment, or for patients who have had a weight loss of 10% or more, or who have trouble with ingestion of food, or who show an inability to absorb from the gastrointestinal tract.

Hyperalimentation is the unique form of intravenous therapy which, parenterally, provides all of the daily nutritional requirements. Although hyperalimentation is discussed elsewhere, it is appropriate to include a brief discussion in this chapter. Parenteral hyperalimentation, or total parenteral nutrition (TPN), is the technique of administering enough calories, amino acids, and other nutrients to provide growth, weight gain and normal healing.

This technique has had a tremendous impact on the critically ill patient who faces slow starvation because of the inability to partake of oral alimentation. If adequate nutrition is available, the body will turn to itself for a source of energy enough to remain alive. A rapid deterioration of lean tissue, muscle, and fat ensues. In the fasting state, the body breaks down approximately 75 g of protein per day (12 g of nitrogen). Liver glycogen stores are depleted within 24 hours. The catabolism of protein to glucogenic amino acids and, finally, to glucose is responsible for the maintenance of serum glucose and starvation. The body turns to stores of lean tissue and muscle for a source of glucose, rather than to fat stores. Therefore, a protein deficiency rapidly develops. As a result, secondary deficiencies develop in tissue synthesis, blood proteins, leukocytes, enzymes, hormones, and antibodies with consequent delay in healing and susceptibility to infection.

The significance of supplying adequate nutrition to the seriously ill patient is quite evident. Severe injury, sepsis secondary to surgery, or other trauma may cause an increased breakdown of body protein and/or nitrogen of up to 50%. Thus, when hyperalimentation is considered, the daily metabolic requirements should also be calculated as 50% greater than normal. Hyperalimentation should be used with extreme caution in patients with 1) impaired renal function, 2) hepatic insufficiency, or 3) diabetes. The purpose of this brief summary is to emphasize the importance of hyperalimentation in managing the debilitated cancer patient.

The surgical technique for the different procedures carried out in the treatment of gynecologic malignancy will not be reviewed. However, two points will be discussed briefly—the removal of a great volume of ascitic fluid, and the start of oozing or bleeding during the operation. The removal of two or more liters of ascitic fluid may lead to an unstable vasomotor system, which may result in shock. Therefore, enough plasma and fluids and electrolytes should be given to correct the imbalance. In those patients in whom it is anticipated that a great amount of ascitic fluid may be removed, Ringer's lactate should be started prior to surgery, and plasma should be available in case it is needed.

The second point concerns the diagnosis and therapy of hemorrhagic disorders that occur during surgery. An acute, unexpected bleeding episode in the absence of injury to any large vessel is a disturbing problem. It may catch the surgeon unprepared and without a definite plan for diagnosis and/or management. In such an emergency, there is usually little time to run a battery of tests—time consuming hematologic tests. The discussion that follows is based on the assumption that bleeding is not from a vessel, but is related to a hemorrhagic disorder.

The plan of action suggested for the management of these patients is based upon three features: 1) clinical judgment, 2) rapid blood tests, and 3) selective therapy.

Clinical judgment is based on a careful workup before operation. Preexisting disorders, congenital or acquired, would presumably be exposed by a thorough history, careful physical examination, and necessary preoperative tests. When preexisting hematologic defects have been ruled out, the causes of unexpected bleeding may be narrowed down to: 1) bleeding from a surgical source, 2) fibrinolysin, 3) defibrination, 4) thrombocytopenia from massive blood bank transfusions, 5) anticoagulants and their antagonists, and 6) mixed clotting problems.

Clotting of blood is complex but, with currently available tests, it is possible to zero in on any deficiency in clotting factors. With knowledge of the deficiencies that alter the prothrombin time, partial thromboplastin time, or thromboplastin generation time, it is possible to make a fairly accurate judgment on what is causing the uncontrolled oozing.

The 12 clotting factors are designated by Roman numerals or generic names. The arrangement of the numbers I to XIII represents the order in which each factor was discovered, and not the time sequence when the factor plays its particular role in coagulation (Factor VI is obsolete).

It is easier to follow the action of these factors when one divides clotting into the three stages:

Stage 1: the generation of thromboplastin. Here, thromboplastin (the word means *clot form*) is generated by both an extrinsic and an intrinsic system. The extrinsic system is simple enough and involves Factors III, IV, and VII. A much more complex intrinsic system involves Factors XII, XI, IX, and VIII, phospholipids from blood platelets, and calcium (Factor IV). The extrinsic and intrinsic systems act together in a final common pathway to create thromboplastin. This final common pathway requires Factors X, V, and IV, and platelet phospholipid.

Stage 2: The conversion of the inactive proenzyme, prothrombin, to active enzyme. This is accomplished by the action of thromboplastin in conjunction with Factors IV, V, VII and X.

Stage 3: The conversion of soluble fibrinogen into insoluble fibrin, which is the polymer formation of the blood clot. Both fibrin, monomer and peptides AB are formed from fibrinogen, but Stage 3 of coagulation is more complicated than this. Factor XIII must be activated to Factor XIII A, a transamidase, by the action of thrombin and calcium. In the meantime, Factor I has been transformed into a fibrin monomer and now proceeds to a fibrin polymer. Through the action of Factor XIII A and calcium, the insoluble fibrin polymer is converted to a crosslinked physiologic fibrin polymer, which is known as the blood clot. Hemostasis involves an interdependence of the blood platelets, the coagulation mechanism, and the blood vessels. The least understood and the least studied factor in hemostasis is that involving the blood vessels.

Blood is a remarkable tissue; it circulates as a fluid, yet remains within the confines of a fragile vascular system. Blood does this by continuously clotting and unclotting. Unclotting, or fibrinolysis, results in the production of fibrin degradation products (FDP). The unclotting or fibrinolytic system has, until recently, been less well studied than the clotting mechanism. Activation of the fibrinolytic system results in degradation of fibrin and fibrinogen. FDP can be quantified in serum and urine. The most common cause of activation of fibrinolysis is activation of coagulation. The secondary activation of fibrinolysis, which normally follows coagulation, has an important homeostatic function: to prevent total thrombosis of the vascular system. Inadequate activation of fibrinolysis, therefore, can lead to further thrombosis, whereas excessive activation can lead to severe hemorrhage.

In summary, clotting consists of platelet aggregation, the formation of the fibrin clot, clot retraction and, in pathologic states, fibrinolysin. It can be assumed that blood loss sufficient to require almost constant transfusion to maintain the blood pressure is attributable to a surgical cause until proved otherwise.

Rapid blood tests should be available within 10 to 15 minutes. Test tubes containing 3.8% sodium citrate solution should be ready in the operating room at all times. Clotting tests, separately or collectively, evaluate the integrity of each of the three stages of blood coagulation. The tests of most value are: 1) prothrombin time, 2) partial thromboplastin time, and 3) thromboplastin generation time.

Selective treatment depends upon identification of all factors which contribute to the bleeding state. As the emergency therapy available is rather limited, it is perhaps best to approach the diagnosis by selective treatment. In using this approach, one assumes that hemophilia or other severe, life-long bleeding disorders would probably have been diagnosed preoperatively.

There are indeed very few therapeutic modalities clinically available at this time: 1) fresh frozen plasma will replace any plasma coagulation factor deficiency, as will antihemophilic plasma; 2) platelet concentrates (or a poor second choice of fresh whole blood) will replace platelets deficient in number or function; 3) epsilon aminocaproic acid, used to arrest fibrinolysins, probably acts by competitive inhibition of plasminogen activators.

The triad of thrombocytopenia, hypofibrinoginemia, and lysis of blood clot within two hours points to the probability of disseminated intravascular coagulation (DIC). Heparin may rapidly restore the platelet count and fibrinogen level, and thus attenuate the bleeding. After heparin has been given, the consumed clotting factor, such as platelets and fibrinogen, may have to be replaced in the form of plasma, platelet concentrates, or fresh blood.

While DIC is being treated, therapy for the precipitating cause (hypovolemic shock) should be carried out. In fact, DIC of short duration can be treated without heparin therapy by removing the precipitating cause. Only in profound and long standing shock and DIC is heparin therapy necessary. Heparin therapy should be considered an adjuvant to treatment, but not a panacea for the patient in hypovolemic shock who needs massive transfusion of blood. In this situation, blood should be given in the amount and at the rate it is being lost.

ILEUS

Ileus is one of the most frequent complications in the postoperative period following surgery for pelvic malignancy. It is often confused with mechanical small bowel obstruction. It is important to make the differential diagnosis between these two. The fluid and electrolyte replacement is the same for both, but the definitive approach to the underlying problem is different.

Ileus is most often preceded by diminution in urine volume. This may be evident for one or two days before the clinical picture of ileus is recognized. Fluids and electrolyte collect in the intestines. The abdomen becomes distended and pushes up the diaphragm with some compromise of the respiratory excursions. This often gives rise to an atelectasis and predisposes to respiratory acidosis.

Paralytic ileus must be differentiated from a mechanical obstruction. Four cardinal symptoms of mechanical intestinal obstruction are: 1) colicky abdominal pain which is intermittent, comes on suddenly, reaches a peak and subsides. Auscultation at the time of pain reveals loud, metallic, high-pitched, peristaltic rushes. This is the most important difference between obstruction and ileus; 2) frequent copious vomiting; 3) distention; and 4) obstipation. After approximately 12 hours, nature compensates and the abdomen is often silent. The patient has entered into a more advanced stage of mechanical obstruction.

The signs and symptoms and findings that are most helpful in judging whether the patient is improving or deteriorating are: 1) pulse rate, 2) respiratory rate, 3) temperature, 4) white count, 5) urinary output, and 6) a followup flat plate of the abdomen.

PERITONITIS

Peritonitis is an inflammation of the peritoneum, a condition marked by exudation of serum and fibrin, cells and pus into the peritoneal cavity. An accurate diagnosis is very important. An awareness of the processes responsible for the clinical findings in peritonitis is vital for rapid diagnosis and institution of proper therapy. Certainly, if the physician can make an accurate estimation of the disease causing peritonitis, treatment may be better directed.

The causes of peritonitis are numerous, and a detailed discussion of each is beyond the scope of this presentation. In general, however, inflammation of the peritoneum is divided into two groups: primary or de novo peritonitis, and secondary or contamination peritonitis. Primary or de novo peritonitis includes primary idiopathic peritonitis and tuberculous peritonitis. Primary idiopathic peritonitis is uncommon and accounts for only 1% of all cases of peritonitis. It is usually due to a hematogenous infection. Tuberculous peritonitis is a disease of declining incidence and now only occurs rarely. Secondary or contamination peritonitis is by far the more common of the two forms of peritonitis. Appendicitis leading to perforation was formerly the most common cause, but has now been supplanted by perforated gastric or peptic ulcer. Other common causes include pancreatitis, gangrenous small bowel from strangulation, obstruction or mesenteric vascular occlusion, perforated colonic diverticulum or carcinoma, ruptured gallbladder, or perforation of any portion of the intestinal tract by an ingested foreign body. Gonococcal salpingitis is a common cause of pelvic peritonitis.

The diagnosis of a full-blown picture of peritonitis is easy, but early diagnosis of this condition may be elusive. The clinical manifestations depend upon the particular etiology of the peritoneal irritation, but certain general clinical findings are present in advancing peritonitis from any cause. The following signs and symptoms may be helpful in diagnosis. Abdominal pain is steady and unrelenting and is aggravated by any movement. Patients often complain of increased pain with any sudden movement during transportation to or within the hospital. Location of pain and rapidity of onset are dependent on etiology. The abdominal pain of peritonitis is almost always accompanied by anorexia, nausea and, frequently, by vomiting.

Physical findings include fever, anxious facial expression, tachycardia, pallor, sweating, rapid and shallow respirations. Abdominal distension is commonly seen, and abdominal muscular rigidity, either local or general, is almost always evident. Rebound abdominal tenderness may be present and is elicited by sudden withdrawal of the examining hand from the abdomen. Percussion is helpful in determining whether a peritoneal irritation is present, as well as in localizing the area of greatest intensity of the pain. Referred abdominal pain is also a common finding and is fairly reliable. Pelvic and rectal examinations are essential to the diagnosis of pelvic peritonitis.

Diagnostic studies include routine blood work, serum amylase determination, abdominal and chest x-rays, and sometimes a peritoneal tap or lavage. Leukocytosis is almost always a constant finding, with polymorphonuclear prominence in the differential count. Blood chemistry determinations are usually normal except for those that reflect dehydration. Urinalysis may show hematuria, pyuria, and increased concentrations of amylase.

The differential diagnosis includes the following: diabetes, pneumonia, pleurisy, acute myocardial infarction, tabes dorsalis, herpes zoster, as well as retroperitoneal diseases.

The mode of therapy for the individual patient with peritonitis is obviously dependent on the etiology, and may vary greatly. The following principles are appropriate for all patients with peritonitis: 1) nasogastric tube for gastrointestinal decompression, 2) intravenous fluids for rehydration, 3) venous pressure monitoring, 4) whole blood or volume expanders for replacement of massive protein losses, 5) urinary catheterization for urinary output measurements, 6) removal of the source of peritoneal contamination or prevention of continued contamination, 7) removal of purulent material, blood, or any intraperitoneal foreign bodies, 8) drainage of any purulent collection to prevent abscess formation, and 9) an antibiotic when appropriate. The management of fluid, electrolyte, and plasma imbalance will not be discussed here in detail. However, the peritonitis patient resembles a 15% to 30% body burn, and the basic principles suggested by Evans for fluid and plasma protein replacement in burn cases can be adapted to the patient with peritonitis.

Evans administered 1 ml of colloid (plasma) and 1 ml of crystalloid (isotonic saline) per kilogram per percent of body burn or, more specifically in these cases, as per percent peritonitis. This is considered the deficit and, in addition to this, there must be added the daily baseline requirement and the extrarenal losses.

POSTOPERATIVE WOUND INFECTION

A collection of blood or serum above or below the fascia may become secondarily infected. This results from bacterial contamination from a variety of sources, and in a large percentage of the cases the result of a break in technique. Infections developing above the fascia and in the subcutaneous fat appear within a few days after surgery, often preceded by low-grade temperature and, later, with evidences of redness of the wound and not infrequently a small mass. The area is usually easily identified and opening the wound quickly corrects the problem with resolution of the infection.

A wound infection forming below the fascia and behind the pubis appears at a later time than those developing above the fascia. The patient has malaise and a low-grade temperature for several days, and often a slightly elevated pulse rate. As the number of bacteria multiply in this area, the clinical picture progresses to one with spiking fever, and tenderness above the pubis with very little induration in the area of the wound. These patients appear to be sicker than those in whom the wound infection is above the fascia. Incision and drainage of the abscess cavity is followed by rapid improvement. Cultures should be taken immediately, and an antibiotic regimen started. The opening must be large enough to insure good drainage.

A depressed immune defense (such as is seen in patients with malnutrition, a long hospitalization, obesity, shock, the administration of chemotherapeutic or cytotoxic drugs, old age, and malignancy) plays an important role in the development of wound infections.

The clinical syndromes commonly seen with infections in the compromised host reflect a specific immune defect of the particular host. Greater awareness of the types of immune defects seen in various disorders and the characteristic recurrent infections should allow more prompt diagnosis and precise therapy.

Disorders of host defense related to specific types of infection include: 1) the humoral defense system where there is an antibody deficiency. Complement deficiency often accompanies the humoral defense deficiency. Disorders in this group usually include bacterial infections such as sinusitis, pneumonia, or bacteremia; 2) the phagocytic defense system, which includes neutropenia, intrinsic chemotaxis defect, intrinsic phagocytic defect, and intracellular microbicidal defect. Disorders related to this imbalance include cellulitis, pharyngitis, urinary tract infections, pararectal abscesses, and pneumonia; 3) the lymphocytic defense system, which includes the B-cell functional defect with intact T-cell, and T-cell defect with intact B-cell, as well as combined B-cell and T-cell defect. Disorders in those groups manifest themselves as sinusitis, bacteremia, pneumonia, skin infections (especially with *Candida*), hepatitis, tuberculosis, and fungal pneumonia; 4) other defense defects such as impaired vascular profusion, abnormal drainage, integumental damage, and iatrogenic insults. This group includes a variety of metabolic disorders, such as diabetes mellitus, nephrotic syndromes, sickle cell anemia, cystic fibrosis, ureteral obstruction, as well as the improper use of antibiotic therapy and nosocomial infections. These defects are manifested by skin ulcers, cellulitis, osteomyelitis, pneumonia, urinary tract infections, bacteremia, and fungal as well as viral infections.

Malnutrition affects several aspects of the immune system. It may cause a deficit in neutrophil function, may reduce complement levels and activity of complement, may inhibit antibody synthesis, and may impair delayed hypersensitivity responses. This is important to realize when dealing with patients who are, or who are potentially, malnourished, since many of these can be corrected quickly.

Almost 1% of all patients admitted to acute care hospitals die with gram negative septicemia. This amounts to approximately 50,000 deaths annually, which is more than the incidence of death from automobile accidents, and about equals the incidence of death from respiratory malignancy. Thus, the introduction of various effective antibiotics has remarkably changed the spectrum of organisms with which we deal, but it has by no means eliminated the problem. While waiting for cultures, the drug of choice for suspected gram negative infections should be given. This is usually gentamicin. When a diagnosis of *Pseudomonas* septicemia is made, it is best to use a combination of gentamicin and carbenicillin. Clindamycin is the drug of choice for the treatment of *Bacteroides* infection. Rarely, *Salmonella* is the cause of gram negative septicemia, and chloramphenicol is the best form of treatment for this type of bacteremia.

SEPSIS AND SEPTIC SHOCK

The clinical picture of septic shock represents neglect of systemic effects of circulating bacterial toxins which, by virtue of their action on the pre- and postcapillary sphincters, lead to a multiorgan hypoperfusion and cellular anoxia. Prognosis depends upon early recognition and aggressive treatment. Despite this, mortality remains high. The incidence of gram negative shock is twice that of gram positive shock. With gram negative sepsis there is a substantial reduction in tissue perfusion, an increase in arterial resistance, and a sharp reduction in cardiac output. Gram positive sepsis results in vasodilatation; cardiac output is minimally decreased, if at all, and sometimes substantially increased, and arterial resistance is decreased.

Septic shock is defined as that condition observed in a patient with an apparent infection, temperature either above or below normal, thready pulse, pulse of 110 or more, hypotension (usually systolic 80 mmHg or below), and a decrease in urinary output below 20 ml per hour.

The pathophysiology relates to the hemodynamic consequences in septic shock, relating to the effect of circulating endotoxin on the circulatory system, especially alpha receptors, and to the release of various vasoactive substances (histamine, serotonin, epinephrine, and kinin). In the beginning there is a constriction of both the pre- and postcapillary sphincters, and this produces the early stage of ischemic anoxia at the cellular level. This stage is also characterized by the onset of arterial venous shunting. As anaerobic metabolism and, consequently, lactic acidosis dominate, the precapillary sphincter relaxes in a stage of stagnancy, and anoxia becomes established. This stage marks the onset of profound capillary pooling and increased vascular permeability. Despite an increased cardiac output, severely diminished peripheral vascular resistance persists, and multiorgan hypoperfusion and cellular anoxia continue. Critically affected target organs include: the lungs, with resultant adult respiratory distress syndrome (ARDS); the kidney, with resultant acute tubular necrosis; and the hematologic system, with resultant disseminated intravascular coagulation. As with other forms of shock, the central nervous system is also critically affected as manifested by rapid changes in the sensorium.

Shock is an emergency situation, no matter whether it is due to severe injury with blood loss, severe infection, heart failure, or other causes. The situation must be dealt with immediately, or cellular injury and death will soon progress to organ failure, followed by death of the patient.

Bacteremic shock is one of the true emergencies of medicine. It carries a mortality rate of 80%, which is higher when *Proteus* or *Clostridium welchii* is the infecting organism. The gram negative organisms most frequently seen in this group are: *E. coli* (most common), *Proteus mirabilis, Pseudomonas,* and *Aerogenes.* Pulmonary edema is more likely to occur in patients with gram negative shock if the colloid osmotic pressure declines. Also, as colloid osmotic pressure declines from normal ranges to less than 10.5 mmHg, there is a significant decrease in survival rates.

Among the most frequent gram positive bacteria cultured are *Enterococcus, Anaerobic streptococcus, Bacteroides, B. welchii,* and *Clostridium perfringens. B. welchii* and *Clostridium* secrete exotoxins. Infections due to *Bacteroides* are now being reported with increasing frequency. Gas in the tissues, as well as foul smelling purulent material, is almost always diagnostic of an anaerobic infection. Septic complications following surgery of the colon or uterus may be caused by anaerobes, as may pelvic thrombophlebitis and septic pulmonary emboli. Complications of aspiration pneumonia such as empyema and lung abscesses are usually associated with anaerobic organisms. In one retrospective study of patients with positive blood cultures on the general surgery and trauma services, the most common organisms cultured were *Bacteroides fragilis, Enterococcus, Klebsiella,* and *E. coli.* Anaerobic infections are generally caused by the host's own microflora, which extend beyond their normal confines as a result of a breech in the mucosal barriers, aspiration, or concurrent local disease processes. The recovery of anaerobic bacteria from infected sites is highly desirable but may prove difficult in many situations; for example, in conditions such as lung abscess, diverticulitis, and endometritis, there is no readily available culture source. Even when proper specimens are collected, the physician may not have access to a laboratory that can perform adequate microbiologic tests for anaerobes. Also, anaerobic bacteria tend to be slow growers as compared to common aerobic pathogens. Several days may be required to isolate and identify anaerobes, and the final culture report may not be available until long after important decisions regarding antimicrobial therapy are required. Therefore, a presumptive bacteriologic diagnosis must often be made on the basis of clinical observation. Clinical clues that specifically suggest anaerobic infection include the following: 1) infections associated with mucosal surfaces that normally harbor anaerobes as indigenous flora, 2) infections characterized by tissue necrosis and abscess formation, 3) putrid discharge (which is considered diagnostic of anaerobic infection), 4) the presence of gas production and infected sites, 5) failure to recover likely pathogens with routine aerobic cultures, especially when direct gram stains show the presence of bacteria, and 6) gram stains of exudate that show either polymicrobial flora or bacteria that have the morphologic features of certain anaerobes. The latter applies particularly to *Clostridia* and anaerobic gram negative bacilli; anaerobic gram positive cocci generally cannot be distinguished from their aerobic counterparts.

Shock is noted especially in conjunction with infected abortion, premature rupture of membranes (chorioamnionitis), pyelonephritis, especially in pregnancy, and diffuse peritonitis. It may be associated with gynecologic cancer or following extensive radical surgery. Sepsis and septic shock may follow chemotherapy for pelvic malignancy or trophoblastic disease. Although the entire mechanism has not been completely elucidated, most physicians accept the theory that the basic physiopathology is generalized intravascular clotting, initiated by the release of endotoxins (lipopolysaccharide) by the above-named gram negative bacteria.

Currently two main mechanisms have been evoked to explain the findings in endotoxic shock: 1) selective vasospasm and, 2) disseminated intravascular coagulation (DIC). The pathophysiology can be attributed to both these mechanisms as well as to reduced myocardial response to sympathetic stimuli.

The clinical syndrome is characterized by: 1) a change in the sensorium, 2) a sudden drop in blood pressure, below 70 mmHg systolic, 3) a weak, thready pulse, 4) respiratory disturbances (respiratory alkalosis), and 5) changes in arterial blood gases, such as diminished PaO_2, and diminished $PaCO_2$, which is secondary to severe shunting and hyperventilation. An elevated $PaCO_2$ may occur in late stages of septic shock.

With electrolyte defects and urine suppression the usual laboratory findings are a rise in a hematocrit, SGOT, SGPT, LDH, catecholamines, BUN, blood amylase, and blood sugar. Metabolic acidosis occurs later. The importance of the triad of hyperventilation, mental confusion, and fever in making an early diagnosis cannot be overemphasized. The drug of choice for gram negative infections is usually gentamicin. When a diagnosis of *Pseudomonas* septicemia is made, the combination of gentamicin and carbenicillin is given. Clindamycin is the drug of choice for the treatment of *Bacteroides* infection. Rarely, *Salmonella* is a cause of gram negative bacteremia and then chloramphenicol is the treatment of choice. When gentamicin is used, it should be given in a dose of 1.5 mg/kg of body weight, intravenously, over a three-minute period every eight hours. A combination of gentamicin, clindamycin, and penicillin is effective in patients with gram negative or gram positive septicemia and septic shock. Combined penicillin and chloramphenicol would be reasonable to use in bacteremic patients on an obstetrical and gynecological service.

Volume replacement is an important part of the therapy of gram negative sepsis. Two indications for the use of conventional vasopressor agents in the management of gram negative septicemia are an increased urinary output and an increased coronary perfusion pressure. However, these agents also have significant hemodynamic disadvantages and are unlikely to improve survival. Their routine use is discouraged. Norepinephrine and epinephrine are now rarely used, and isoproterenol is only used in specific situations. The best catecholamine with which to begin treatment of shock is dopamine. Dopamine is essentially three drugs in one, depending on the dosage used and the patient's response. Very small doses (2 to 5 μ/kg per minute) produce a dopaminergic response, ie, specific dilation of intestinal and renal vessels to increase blood flow to essential viscera. Moderate doses (5 to 30 μ/kg per minute) have, in addition, an inotropic effect (increased heart force) that increases cardiac output. Very high doses (greater than 30 μ/kg per minute) cause vasoconstriction that is just as powerful as that of norepinephrine or epinephrine. In other words, very high doses of dopamine have the same pressor effect as norepinephrine. All catecholamines act very rapidly, within 30 seconds after intravenous injection. Isoproterenol is used in patients with an inappropriately slow pulse, and also in small doses (1 to 2 μ/minute) for bronchodilatation. Isoproterenol is unsafe in patients with acute myocardial infarction. Corticoids, in experimental studies on animals, produce increased cardiac output, increased tissue perfusion, increased oxygen uptake, and maintained lysosomal integrity.

WOUND DEHISCENCE AND EVISCERATION

Wound dehiscence is more common in patients treated surgically for a malignancy than those treated for benign disease. Protein deficiency, anemia, chronic debility, vomiting, distension, malignancy, and wound infection are all contributing factors to dehiscence. The patient can usually be handled by opening the skin, irrigating the wound, and packing the area open. Dehiscence merely refers to a separation of the wound, but not below the fascia.

Evisceration is a more serious condition and involves the complete separation of the wound, exposing the bowel, peritoneum, and fascia. If the condition of the patient permits, the wound should be closed in the operating room with through-and-through interrupted wire or nylon sutures. Occasionally, it is necessary to irrigate the wound, pack it, and strap it closed until it is possible to perform a secondary closure.

THROMBOEMBOLIC DISEASE

The incidence of peripheral thrombophlebitis and pulmonary embolization in the postoperative period has not changed during the past decade, despite the fact that early ambulation is carried out routinely. One to 2% of all surgical patients develop thrombophlebitis postoperatively, and 0.5% experience pulmonary emboli. The exact mechanism for the venous thrombotic complications in postsurgical patients has not been defined, although many interesting theories, ie, platelet adhesiveness, have been suggested. Stasis, precipitated by immobility, is a factor in the high incidence of postoperative thrombotic complication. Many of these start in the operating room. Dehydration may also predispose to a thrombotic complication.

Pulmonary embolization follows thrombophlebitis in 5% to 10% of the cases, and the mortality rate is as high as 30% in some series. Thrombophlebitis is not uncommon in general gynecologic surgery, and is more frequent when the operation is carried out for the treatment of malignancy. Many cases of thrombophlebitis are not diagnosed, and even cases of pulmonary embolization escape notice. When thrombophlebitis develops, it is usually between days 5 and 10 postoperatively. Most reports indicate that phlebitis probably starts in the operating room. Thromboembolic disease may have an insidious onset with few, if any, clinical signs or symptoms until pulmonary embolization occurs. Superficial phlebitis is not dangerous, and fatalities result only from deep venous thrombi. The use of the terms phlebitis, phlebothrombosis, and thrombophlebitis has been a source of confusion in the past. The term phlebitis would indicate inflammation of a vein with no accompanying thrombosis. However, phlebitis cannot exist for very long without inciting the formation of a thrombus on the inflamed endothelium. Conversely, the term phlebothrombosis would indicate a venous clot with no inflammation present in the vein wall. However, some inflammatory reaction usually does occur, although it cannot be detected clinically. Therefore, the preferred term is thrombophlebitis, which indicates the existence of both thrombosis and inflammation. The term chronic thrombophlebitis is a misnomer, since healing invariably takes place once the acute inflammatory reaction has subsided. The common factors in the etiology of thrombophlebitis are stasis, hypercoaguability, and injury of the endothelium of the vein. Clinical and autopsy studies indicate an almost linear increase in the occurrence of thrombophlebitis with increasing age. Superficial thrombophlebitis in a middle-aged or older patient, especially if recurrent, should suggest occult malignancy.

Pulmonary embolism may be the first and only sign that thrombophlebitis is present. Other signs of phlebothrombosis and thrombophlebitis include: 1) tenderness of the foot, particularly on the medial side, 2) painful dorsiflexion of the foot (Homan's sign) — a very unreliable sign and one that is difficult to evaluate, 3) an ascending "stepladder" pulse associated with temperature elevation and increased respiration, 4) pain and swelling of the affected leg, and 5) over a period of several hours the entire extremity becomes swollen and mildly to moderately painful, and has a reddish cyanotic hue. The skin is warm, superficial veins are distended, and tenderness along the involved vein is noted. The patient's temperature rarely exceeds 101°F and chills are usually not present.

Tests for detection of clots in the lower extremity are the Doppler ultrasound technique, fibrinogen ^{125}I uptake test, and an impedance phlebophleborrhaphy. All of these tests are noninvasive and yield a reported 70% to over 90% accuracy, although all have some shortcomings. Indications for a venography include: 1) suspicion of thrombophlebitis in a patient without classic clinical findings, 2) suspicion of pulmonary embolism in a patient with equivocal findings on lung scan, and 3) strong suspicion of pulmonary embolism in a patient with negative findings on lung scan.

Cranley (1979) has developed phleborheography (PRG) as an accurate method of diagnosing thrombophlebitis. Phleborheography (PRG), defined as a tracing of moving currents within a vein, has been considered an accurate term to designate plethysmography for diagnosing deep vein thrombosis of the lower extremity. The technique is practical and highly accurate, and has become a standard clinical test. It is noninvasive and very accurate in diagnosing deep venous thrombosis of the lower extremity. Phleborheography can be performed by a technician in the laboratory, at the bedside, or in the office. It has taken the guesswork out of diagnosing deep vein thrombosis.

In the management of thrombophlebitis, bed rest with elevation of the involved extremity is advisable until the tenderness of thrombophlebitis subsides. However, only in unusual circumstances should the patient be kept in bed more than 7 to 10 days. Anticoagulant drugs are seldom indicated in the treatment of *superficial* thrombophlebitis. They are used if the thrombus progresses proximally despite treatment, or if the segment involved by thrombosis is near the deep venous system at the groin. Anticoagulant drugs should be used in the management of *deep* thrombophlebitis unless urgent contraindications are present. The usefulness of anticoagulants in preventing pulmonary embolism has been convincingly approved. Inferior vena caval interruption should be considered only when pulmonary embolism occurs in spite of adequate anticoagulant therapy, or when anticoagulation is absolutely contraindicated for a patient with *deep* thrombophlebitis or a pulmonary embolus. If edema is present when the patient becomes ambulatory after thrombophlebitis, adequate support with stockings or elastic bandages is the most important measure in the prevention of chronic venous insufficiency.

In the past few years prophylactic heparinization has been established as a method of treatment on many services, and it has proved most rewarding. The minidose heparin (1000 units of heparin and 1000 ml of infusions run over 8 hours) is started the evening before surgery, and is continued during surgery and during the first few days postoperatively. It has been reported to be more effective by this route of administration than if it were started in the operating room or in the immediate postoperative period.

PULMONARY EMBOLISM

Pulmonary embolism is one of the three more common causes of death. It is currently estimated that more than 500,000 patients suffer nonfatal episodes of pulmonary embolism, and approximately 140,000 patients die from the disorder each year in the United States. Pulmonary embolization is thought to cause 50% of sudden deaths, and this form of pulmonary vascular obstruction is found in 24% of general autopsy series. It is also found in 60% of autopsies of patients who succumb to heart failure. The incidence of pulmonary embolism increases markedly after the age of 40, and is particularly high in the elderly who have sustained an injury.

Pulmonary emboli usually consist of thrombi that originate in the peripheral venous system, but they may rarely be composed of nonblood constituents such as fat, bone marrow, liver, fatty tissue, amniotic fluid, or trophoblastic disease that embolize to the lung. Most pulmonary emboli (95%) arise from the vascular system below the renal veins. Predisposing factors include thrombophlebitis, varicose veins, surgery of the pelvis, carcinoma, pregnancy, and the adjustment in blood constituents in vessel walls that follow general surgery.

Every year about 47,000 deaths occur in America directly attributable to pulmonary embolism, and it is estimated that there were at least three times that number of nonfatal episodes. The true incidence of pulmonary embolism is probably higher than reported. Pulmonary embolism is a feared complication following pelvic surgery for a malignant condition. It occurs most frequently after coughing, sneezing, and squeezing on bed pans, when the glottis closes, followed by a sudden release of pressure. The embolization may be sudden and dramatic, resulting in death, or it may progress from minor symptoms. The patient may faint and have an acute pain in the chest followed by cyanosis and respiratory distress, or she may have an unexplained tachycardia for a few days with a slight elevation of temperature. The presenting signs and symptoms include: 1) dyspnea, 2) tachycardia and tachypnea, 3) chest pain, 4) apprehension, 5) phlebitis and/or thrombosis, 6) hemoptysis, 7) rales, and 8) rubs.

A high index of suspicion is most important in making the diagnosis. The triad of an elevated serum glutamic oxalic transaminase, bilirubin, and serum lactic dehydrogenase are helpful, as is the elevation of the arterial blood gases. The arterial blood gases are usually decreased with the pO_2 below 70 mmHg, and $PaCO_2$ normal or below 35 mmHg. The chest x-ray may be normal but, on the other hand, may reveal pleural effusion, elevation of the diaphragm, atelectasis, areas of radiolucency, and wedge-shaped defects. Fibrin split products have been recently demonstrated to be elevated in acute pulmonary embolism, and may become a useful noninvasive screening test. Lung scans have some value, but the most specific test in making this diagnosis is pulmonary angiography.

The differential diagnosis of pulmonary embolism includes all causes of chest pain, dyspnea, hemoptysis, and shock. Common problems which must be ruled out are pneumonia, asthma, acute myocardial infarction, pericarditis, pneumothorax, and intraabdominal processes such as subphrenic abscess.

The initial treatment of a patient with pulmonary embolism is supportive. Supplemental oxygen should be given as soon as the initial blood gases are drawn, or before that, if the patient is in respiratory distress. The patient should be supported with fluids and cardiopulmonary resuscitation if necessary. The main thrust of therapy of pulmonary embolism is prevention of further embolization and propagation of emboli already present. This is accomplished by anticoagulation with heparin. Heparin is given intravenously either by bolus or constant infusion. A bolus of 15,000 units of heparin is given immediately, followed by 4000 to 7000 units every four hours, or a dosage to maintain the APTT at 1½ to 2 times normal. It should be repeated at three-hour intervals. The continuous method is to give 300 to 600 units per kilogram per day by constant infusion.

SHOCK LUNG

The shock lung syndrome is characterized by acute respiratory failure after an episode of profound hypotension caused by hemorrhage, gram negative, or endotoxic shock. It is classically seen as a severe disease. Mortality rates 60% to 90% during the first 48 hours have been reported.

The signs and symptoms of respiratory failure are varied and nonspecific. At times they may be misleading, resulting in delayed diagnosis and treatment. The signs and symptoms of acute respiratory failure include: altered levels of consciousness, confusion, asterixis, papilledema, cyanosis, shock, tachycardia, headache, diaphoresis, and shallow respirations. The shock lung has three distinguishing characteristics: 1) gross intrapulmonary shunting with relative or absolute hypoxemia, 2) reduced pulmonary compliance, and 3) diffuse bilateral pulmonary edema. It occurs following hemorrhage or shock, and develops 18 to 48 hours after the profound hypotensive episode.

The prime example of noncardiogenic pulmonary edema is the entity of shock lung, sometimes referred to by a "catchall" term of adult respiratory distress syndrome (ARDS). The diagnosis of shock lung should be restricted to that episode of respiratory failure associated with shock, trauma, and postoperative state. Other causes of acute respiratory failure can usually be ascribed to such problems as aspiration, fat emboli, and specific drugs, including oxygen.

Patients with shock lung have intrapulmonary shunting, decreased pulmonary compliance, and radiographic findings consistent with pulmonary edema. In contrast, shock lung syndrome is not associated with any of these causes, and is always preceded by hemorrhagic or septic shock. Also, therapy directed to shock lung syndrome may not be beneficial in the conditions that comprise acute respiratory distress syndrome.

Three conditions that commonly lead to shock lung are systemic sepsis, massive fluid replacement, and a period of hypotension. Some of the many etiologic factors are lack of surfactant, disseminated intravascular coagulation (DIC), overtransfusion or overinfusion, heart failure, low osmolarity of blood, direct lung injury, fat embolism, transfusion embolism, oxygen toxicity, damage to respiration, increased antidiuretic hormone, and vasospasm.

The shock lung has often been confused with such pathologic diagnoses as bronchopneumonia, patchy atelectasis, and agonal changes.

In the acute state, the lung grossly shows edema, congestion, hemorrhage, heaviness, and relative airlessness. The lungs are liver-like, consolidated, and markedly saturated with fluid, literally oozing fluid onto their surface. Lungs from shock lung at autopsy may weigh as much as 2000 g (combined weight), and only rarely do they weigh less than 1000 g. Lungs from patients who have died during the first few days after an insult show primarily edema, congestion, perialveolar hemorrhage, and alveolar collapse. Lungs from patients who survive longer show, in addition, diffuse bronchopneumonia with microabscesses and hyaline membrane disease. Thick, succulent material fills the alveoli, respiratory ducts, and terminal bronchioli. Thromboemboli, unrelated to the time of death, are seen in the lungs of many patients. These same lungs often have small infarctions as well. The incidence of fat emboli is low, even in the lungs taken from patients with femoral fractures and gunshot wounds of the long bones.

Microscopically, the alveoli, interstitial spaces, and capillaries are diffusely involved. Hyaline membrane can be seen on surfaces from which damaged epithelial cells have sloughed. The septum between the alveoli are markedly edematous and disrupted. Alveolar collapse is widespread. There is evidence of intra- and interalveolar fluid sequestration with an eosinophilic-staining, fibrin-like material collected in the capillaries and alveoli. Leukocytes have infiltrated the lungs, and the white blood cells and platelets adhere to the vessel walls, forming thrombi. Diffuse hemorrhage and many red blood cells in the microscopic fields indicate marked breakdown and consolidation of pulmonary parenchyma. Patchy atelectasis and bronchopneumonia with their accompanying changes are present. Few areas of normal parenchymal tissue remain.

The clinical picture is characterized by apprehension, tachypnea, air-hunger, and sepsis, but cyanosis may not be present. Expiratory wheezes are almost pathognomonic of impending shock lung, but bronchial rales and signs of consolidation may not be present early in the disease.

A roentgenogram taken immediately after operation or injury may be clear and give no indication of impending shock lung. A repeat roentgenogram taken 36 to 48 hours later shows a characteristic snow field, patchy pneumonitis, and pulmonary edema.

Radioisotope techniques such as the use of macromolecular albumin particles, other reactive radioactive particles, and inspired xenon gas give a differential picture of ventilation and perfusion. These are valuable in a research setting, but their present clinical usefulness is slight.

Serial measurements of blood gases and tidal volumes are diagnostic and prognostic. Early in the disease, serum pO_2 ranges from 50 to 60 mm Hg, and serum pCO_2 from 20 to 30 mmHg. The pH is often alkaline. Later, the pO_2 declines further, but the pCO_2 rises or remains normal, and the pH becomes acidotic. These measurements give an indication of the ability of the lungs to utilize oxygen, and the degree of arterial venous shunting. When arterial pO_2 is low after the patient has inspired 100%

oxygen for 30 minutes, there is a high degree of shunting, and the chances for survival decrease. The prognosis is also poor when lung compliance is low, and decreases progressively. In the latter instance, functional residue capacity decreases as minute volume increases. The colloid osmotic pressure (COP) is very important because the relationship between it and the hydrostatic pressure, which is measured by pulmonary arterio-occlusive pressure, is significant in guiding therapy. In general, one wants to keep the colloidal osmotic pressure at least 3 to 5 mmHg higher than the pulmonary arteriooocclusive pressure (PAOP). Diuretics may increase the colloidal osmotic pressure and may reverse pulmonary edema, even when it is not due to heart failure.

Shock lung is a progressive, unrelenting disease, which may kill healthy young individuals who otherwise would have survived. To prevent this tragedy, treatment must be aggressive and must be started early, even when shock lung is suspected, but not yet proved. Treatment, as well as prevention, is based on: 1) a clear understanding of the factors that precipitate shock lung, and 2) serial measurements of certain physiologic variables in the patient with shock lung.

The treatment must be aggressive and start early. The patient should be placed in a high semi-Fowler position, and should be turned frequently. The absence of cyanosis is no assurance that she is ventilating well. Therefore, serial measurements of blood gases, tidal volumes, functional residual capacity, and vital capacity are essential during treatment. The treatment should include maintenance of a positive end expiratory pressure (PEEP), large amounts of steroids, infusion of albumin and diuretics, administration of broad spectrum antibiotics, restriction of fluid to levels that can be handled by a compromised cardiopulmonary system, and careful filtration of all fluids given to decrease the chances of particles forming microemboli in the lungs. If carried out in a carefully controlled manner, these measures may greatly decrease the incidence of death from this disease. The end expriatory pressure is first set at 8 cm of water and gradually increased to 18 to 20 cm, a level that maintains arterial pO_2 at the desired level of 60 to 90 mmHg on a minimum percentage of inspired oxygen. The positive end expiratory pressure should be maintained in the patient with shock lung until all signs of this disease has disappeared.

Serum salt poor albumin (50 g over a one-hour period), or low molecular weight dextran enhances the colloidal osmotic pressure of the pulmonary perfusate. This helps to prevent pulmonary edema. Two diuretics are useful: furosemide (60 to 90 mg), or ethacrinic acid (50 to 100 mg), given approximately 15 to 20 minutes after the albumin or dextran has been started.

Fluid therapy is monitored by urinary output, which gives some indication of tissue perfusion, as well as by either central venous pressure or the Swan-Ganz catheter. Central venous pressure (CVP) is not an infallible indicator of myocardial efficiency. Its use should be accompanied by frequent auscultation of the lungs to determine the presence of moist rales, and of the heart to determine the presence of protodiastolic gallop sounds. Central venous pressure monitoring measures only the function of the right side of the heart. Pulmonary arterial pressure (PAP) and pulmonary wedge pressure (PWP) monitoring by means of a Swan-Ganz catheter give an index of the left ventricular competence. The introduction of the Swan-Ganz catheter has been a tremendous boon to patients who have limited left ventricular competence. Probably the most important thing that we can do in the initial resuscitation of patients with bacterial shock is to provide systematic fluid challenge, in which we administer aliquots of between 50 and 200 ml of fluid every ten minutes. The manner in which this fluid is infused is very important. In patients who have an indication of limitation in left ventricular competence, which can usually be judged by clinical methods, including routine electrocardiography and chest x-ray, a pulmonary artery catheter is mandatory, at least for the measurement of pulmonary diastolic and, preferably, pulmonary wedge pressure. A rule to follow is to infuse fluid at a rate of 200 ml, if the central venous pressure is less than 12 cm of water. Then infuse 100 ml if the central venous pressure is less than 16 cm of water. Routinely, 50 ml is infused if the central venous pressure is greater than 16 cm of water. Even a patient who has an apparent increase in central venous pressure may have a deficit in volume. Following infusion of fluid, the central venous pressure may in fact decline as coronary perfusion is improved.

When this volume of fluid is infused the following rule should be observed. If the central venous pressure rises by more than 5 cm during any ten-minute period during the infusion which, incidentally, is measured through the site other than the site of pressure measurements, then that means that the cardiac competence has been exceeded. If it rises by more than 2 cm but by less than 5 cm, there should be a waiting period of ten minutes until the central venous pressure declines to within 2 cm or less from where it started. It is then time to keep on challenging. At any time that 2 cm is exceeded during any ten-minute period, it is wise to wait ten minutes. If there is no increase to more than 2 cm during any one period of time, the operator simply continues to challenge. The end point of the challenge, of course, is reversal of the shock state with reestablishment of normal mentation, normal arterial blood pressure, normal urine flow, osmolar clearance, and reversal of lactacidemia. The same rule applies to the pulmonary artery pressure, ie, if the pulmonary artery pressure rises by more than 3 mmHg during a ten-minute infusion period, there should be a waiting period of ten minutes. At any time that it rises in excess of 7 mmHg, the infusion should be slowed down.

In summary, the critically ill patient should be managed by one doctor who writes all the orders. A multidisciplinary team is desirable, but it must be coordinated by a single individual. More than one doctor writing the orders leads to confusion and, because of the labile nature of these patients where the condition changes from hour to hour, it jeopardizes the patient's chance for recovery. In the critically ill patient, the auscultation of blood pressure by the cuff measure is inaccurate, and it is better to cannulate a peripheral artery and connect it to a strain-gauge transducer measuring device. This also affords easy access for a sequential arterial blood gas determination and other laboratory blood samples.

Fluid replacement is adequate when either urinary output returns to adequate levels (more than 40 ml per hour), or CVP or PWP rise rapidly. If urinary output is not reestablished by fluid loading, furosemide (80 mg) or ethacrinic acid (100 mg) is given intravenously. In most patients, arterial blood pressure (CVP, PWP), urinary output, and pulse pressure will be restored to normal or near normal levels with these measures alone. However, if the urinary output does not return to adequate levels, indicating adequate perfusion, the patient should be rapidly digitalized.

Regulation of breathing with a machine that can maintain a positive end expiratory pressure (PEEP) is perhaps the most important treatment, and can be given to the patient when the shock lung syndrome develops. The end expiratory pressure is first set at 8 cm of water and gradually increased to 18 to 20 cm of water, a level that maintains arterial pO_2 at the desired level of 60 to 90 mmHg on a minimum percentage of inspired oxygen. A volume cycle respirator is more useful in these patients than the traditional pressure cycle ventilators.

In patients with gram negative or endotoxic shock, it has been recommended that methylprednisolone at a dose of 30 mg per kilogram of body weight be given once or twice. This has been used in the treatment of shock lung syndrome as a single dose or repeated after two to four hours. However, if methylprednisolone is to improve pulmonary blood flow, stabilize the endothelium of small pulmonary vessels, and slow the leakage of protein-containing fluid, then adequate tissue levels of the agent must be continued long enough to maintain these effects, not merely initiate them. The dosages that Lillihei indicated may be beneficial in the pure shock states and are probably adequate to maintain the hypothesized therapeutic action of the steroid on the lung when repeated every six hours. It, therefore, seems reasonable to begin early treatment of patients who have shock lung syndrome with methylprednisolone, 30 mg/kg, every six hours for 48 hours after the onset of the syndrome, in an attempt to determine whether such therapy might be beneficial in improving arterial oxygenation and resolving the pulmonary edema. Of course, this drug must always be used as an adjunct to therapies directed at the cause of the shock, since its only action is on the damaged lung; it does not correct the shock.

Mortality from this complication ranges up to 80%. The condition is supposedly reversible if support can be continued for a sufficient period of time and, for this reason, many investigators have attempted long-term support with membrane oxygenators and partial right heart bypass in cases where ventilatory failure is eminent despite conventional modes of therapy. Reported series are small, but some successes have been noted. Awareness of potential pulmonary complications, combined with adequate therapy, contributes to the preservation of lives that just a few years ago were considered hopeless.

DISSEMINATED INTRAVASCULAR COAGULATION (DIC)

Disseminated intravascular coagulation has been referred to as an insidious culprit. DIC is now recognized as a cause of symptoms and many clinical disorders. Intravascular deposition of fibrin is observed in allograft rejection, the cause of symptoms and autoimmune disorder, and is suspected as a factor in atherosclerosis and the aging process. Fibrin, which lines tumor emboli, may make tumors resistant to treatment and contribute to the development of metastases. The study of coagulation has become a complex and somewhat confusing subspecialty of hematology; however, the principles of coagulation and the interpretation of more basic coagulation tests are essential requirements to the understanding of disseminated intravascular coagulation.

Normal coagulation can be divided arbitrarily into three broad categories: 1) local vascular factors, 2) plasma coagulation proteins, and 3) platelets, both number and function. Bleeding, then, can be a result of problems in any one of these areas.

The commonly employed coagulation tests include: one-stage prothrombin time, partial thromboplastin time, activated clotting time (ACT), fibrinogen level, platelet count, IV bleeding time, and some measurement of fibrin monomers or fibrinogen degradation products.

When confronted with a patient who is bleeding, it is important to have a very careful history about the primary disease states, the drugs that are being taken, and a very careful examination of the entire body to back this up. Having done this, the results of the PT, ACT, PTT, platelet count, fibrinogen level, fibrin split products, and peripheral blood smear should be evaluated. The classic laboratory picture of disseminated intravascular coagulation is: 1) prolonged prothrombin time, 2) prolonged partial thromboplastin time, 3) low platelet count (usually below 100,000, but any fall in platelet numbers is suspicious), 4) low fibrinogen level, 5) presence of fibrin split products as circulating fibrin monomers, and 6) microangiopathic red cell morphology. The diagnosis of DIC can be established if a compatible laboratory profile is accompanied by clinical features that match.

The mechanism for production of DIC is the most common etiologic agent for shock lung, and has been intensely studied. DIC demands two conditions: 1) slowing of capillary flow as promoted by arteriolar vasoconstriction and opening of arteriovenous shunts, and 2) availability of a thromboplastic agent in the blood. These are numerous and include bacterial toxins, hemolysins, and massive tissue injury. Both conditions are always present in severe and refractory shock. DIC results in two important events: 1) onset of consumptive coagulopathy, and 2) occlusion of capillaries by thrombi. Patients developing shock lung usually have a consumptive coagulopathy indicative of DIC.

Successful management of DIC is dependent upon early laboratory diagnosis, recognition of clinical signs, identification and aggressive management of the underlying precipitating factors, and the correction of the bleeding diathesis. The primary treatment of DIC is dependent upon the successful treatment of the underlying illness. Having eradicated this, it is then possible to address the immediate management of the bleeding diathesis. Primary treatment consists of a heparin bolus (50 units/ kilograms), followed by 100 units per hour, administered by continuous infusion. This helps alleviate the underlying thrombotic aspects of the disease. The use of fresh frozen plasma and platelet donor packs is recommended as an adjunct to therapy. Reports indicate that it is advisable to replace 25% of circulating plasma volume with fresh frozen plasma in order to increase circulating fibrinogen. Fibrinogen concentrates should be withheld because of the risk of hepatitis. If the patient continues to bleed severely, then and *only* then (unless primary fibrinolysis is initially proved) should one consider the use of an antifibrinolytic agent. The currently used agent is aminocaproic acid (Amicar). The intravenous dose is usually 5 g immediately, followed by 1 g every hour for a total of 12 g (may be repeated every 12 to 24 hours until hemorrhage stops).

ACUTE RENAL FAILURE

The constellations of signs and symptoms that result from renal failure comprise the syndrome of uremia, which is an ancient term that literally means retention of urine in the blood. In the early descriptions of this state, there was an association with poisoning by-products of endogenous metabolism, and with the functional inability to maintain chemical hemostasis because of lack of renal compensatory adaptation. The syndrome of acute renal failure encompasses a broad category of various disorders which result in progressive azotemia and alteration of urine flow, most commonly oliguria (less than 40 ml of urine per 24 hours), anuria (less than 100 ml of urine per 24 hours), and occasionally polyuria (more than 1500 ml of urine per 24 hours).

In pathophysiology it is useful to have a classification dividing renal failure into three main categories: prerenal causes, renal causes, and postrenal or obstructive causes. The prerenal causes are seen when there is a state of depleted volume, such as dehydration, blood loss, gastro-intestinal fluid loss, diabetic ketoacidosis, peritonitis, bowel obstruction or Addisonian crisis, congestive heart failure, hypotension, or renal artery compromise. Renal causes include acute tubular necrosis (ATN), glomerular disease, end-stage chronic renal failure, interstitial disease, hepatorenal syndrome, and bilateral cortical necrosis. The postrenal causes include acute and chronic urinary tract obstruction, as well as renal vein thrombosis.

The two most common causes encountered in the critically ill patient are acute tubular necrosis and prerenal azotemia. Of these, acute tubular necrosis is, perhaps, the one seen more frequently in the treatment of the gynecologic cancer patient. Acute tubular necrosis may be due to rapid hypotension (in which case acute renal failure is both prerenal and renal in origin), extensive crush injuries and burns, hemolysis and hemo-globinuria, mild globinuria, transfusion reactions, nephrotoxic drugs and chemicals (including sulfonamide, colestipol, cephaloridine), and septic shock.

There are two basic pathophysiologic mechanisms responsible for the pathogenesis of acute tubular necrosis, ischemia and nephrotoxicity. In the latter, there is necrosis of the tubular epithelium but, for the most part, preservation of the basement membrane allows epithelial regeneration. In ischemic tubular necrosis, there is greater basement membrane damage with a patchy distribution of necrosis, possibly due to variable arteriolar constriction during a shock insult.

The stages of renal failure are characteristically classified as: 1) renal impairment (clearance 50 ml/min or higher), 2) renal insufficiency (clearance 20 ml/min to 50 ml/min with azotemia, mild anemia, and compensated deficits), 3) renal failure (clearance 50 ml/min to 20 ml/min with uncompensated chemical derangements), and 4) uremia (symptomatic renal failure). The uremic patient requires an aggressive search for potentially reversible causes unless there is certainty of chronicity. The best evidence of acute, possibly reversible, renal failure is documented normal renal function in the patient's recent past, absence of stigmata of chronic renal disease (pallor, pigmentation, bone disease, Terrey's nails, anemia), and rapid rise in creatinine (daily or weekly). Uremia which results from acute renal failure is usually heralded by sudden oliguria (less often, fixed polyuria), rapid decrease in glomerular filtration rate (GFR), and normal-sized kidneys as seen on an intravenous pyelogram with tomographic cuts.

Before the physician can assume a renal cause for renal failure, a vigorous approach to rule out prerenal and postrenal causes is mandatory. This approach involves correction of any volume defects (intra-vascular), cardiac compensation, and catheterization of the bladder. If anuria is present, either ureter should be catheterized to the renal pelvis to rule out obstruction of the ureters. Renal failure is most commonly first noted by a fall in urinary output to less than 30 ml of urine per hour over several hours, followed later by a rise in BUN. On occasion, polyuria can occur in both the acute and in the recovery phase of the acute tubular necrosis. The diagnosis of the etiology of acute renal failure is a prerequisite to rational therapy. This can be done by a brief history obtained from the patient, medical records, and nursing personnel. A very rapid but thorough physical examination may reveal the cause for the acute renal failure.

No single test is completely satisfactory in distinguishing prerenal from renal azotemia, but certain diagnostic studies can be initiated rapidly. Provided there is no strong evidence of postrenal obstruction, such as sudden, complete anuria (in which case the patency of the urinary tract must be proven by intravenous pyelogram, retrograde pyelography, or ureteral catheterization), one rapid way of distinguishing prerenal from renal azotemia is the patient's response to one of the following trials: 1) rapid infusion of 500 to 1000 ml of normal saline over 30 to 60 minutes, 2) 25 g of mannitol given intravenously if infused in ten minutes or less, 3) 80 mg of furosemide intravenously by the "push" method. If the patient responds to this treatment, it is obvious that the condition is not renal or postrenal failure.

In acute tubular necrosis, there are characteristically numerous pigmented casts, epithelial cells, a urine sodium concentration greater than 60 mEq/liter, a urine-osmolality to plasma-osmolality ratio of less than 1.2, a urine-urea to plasma-urea ratio of 3 or less, and urine-creatinine to plasma-creatinine ratio of 10 or less. Urinalysis is also definitive in identifying the rare but important acute renal failure caused by mild globinuria and hepatorenal syndrome. The hepatorenal syndrome refers to a specific failure. In this syndrome the patient with prior normal renal function develops severe oliguria with a concentrated urine that contains virtually no sodium, and progressive uremia that is invariably fatal unless liver function improves. The cause is unknown but the kidneys promptly function normally if transplanted to another patient.

Early sensitive signs of uremic encephalopathy include tremulousness, mild clonus, asterixis, and dysarthria consisting of thick, slurred, and slowed speech. The early signs of uremic neuropathy include decreased vibratory sense and loss of deep tendon reflexes, affecting the ankles more than the knees. Muscle weakness and development of foot-drop are other frequent signs. The major cardiovascular symptoms are related to extrafluid volume excess (congestive heart failure, pulmonary edema, and hypertension) and electrolyte disturbances (dysrhythmias from potassium and calcium derangements). Uremic pericarditis occurs in up to one third of uremic patients, and is more likely to be associated with rapidly progressive renal failure than with any particular level of urea. The uremic lung is a typical form of pulmonary edema of perihilar, butterfly distribution that is readily relieved by removal of fluid. Most likely, the

514

uremic lung results from extracellular volume excess alone, although altered pulmonary capillary permeability has not been entirely excluded as another cause. In uremia, hyperphosphatemia and hypocalcemia are usual, unless modified by medical maneuvers. The most frequent symptom of calcium and phosphorus derangement is severe pruritus. Pruritus commonly occurs when the calcium to phosphate product (serum calcium times serum phosphorus) is 60 or greater for any length of time, in which case metastatic calcification follows. In the skin, this metastatic calcification presents as small papules with a whitish center that may be so pruritic that patients shave them off.

The laboratory diagnosis of acute renal failure should include the following: urine (routine and microscopic), SMA-12, CBC, differential, crossmatch, EKG, serum electrolytes, BUN, serum creatinine, urine and serum osmolality, urine for specific gravity, 24-hour urine for creatinine clearance, protein and electrolytes, abdominal flat film for kidney size, ureteral calculi, and renal calcification, and residual bladder urine volume. The treatment of acute tubular necrosis can be divided into two stages, the oliguric phase, lasting from several hours to several weeks (average two weeks), followed by the diuretic or polyuric phase. Urine output varies from 100 to 400 ml per 24 hours during the oliguric phase, followed either by stepwise increments in urine output or sudden rapid increases in urine flow during the polyuric phase. The complete treatment is beyond the scope of this presentation and must be sought from more specific therapeutic manuals.

BIBLIOGRAPHY

Abel RM, Beck CH Jr, Abbott WM, et al: Improved survival from acute renal failure after treatment with intravenous essential L-amino acids and glucose. *N Engl J Med* 288:695, 1973.

Artz JS, Vinocur B, Sampliner J, et al: Application of a critical care monitoring program in the diagnosis and management of critically ill patients in a community hospital. *Crit Care Med* 2:42, 1974.

Ayres SM, Gianelli S Jr, Mueller HS, et al: *Care of the Critically Ill,* ed 2. New York, Appleton-Century-Crofts, 1974.

Balows A (ed): *Anaerobic Bacteria: Role in Disease.* Springfield, Ill, Charles C Thomas, 1974.

Barber HRK: Fluid and electrolyte problems, in Barber HRK, Fields DH, and Kaufman SA (eds): *Quick Reference to Ob-Gyn Procedure,* ed 2. Philadelphia, J.B. Lippincott Co, 1979, pp 237–250.

Barber HRK: Acidosis and alkalosis, in Barber HRK, Fields DH, and Kaufman SA (eds): *Quick Reference to Ob-Gyn Procedures,* ed 2. Philadelphia, J.B. Lippincott Co, 1979, pp 251–258.

Barber HRK: Fluid, electrolyte and nutritional management of the gynecologic patient, part I, in Goldstein DP, Leventhal J (eds): *Current Problems in Obstetrics and Gynecology.* Chicago, Year Book Medical Publishers, Inc, Vol II, No 12, Aug 1979, pp 3–32.

Barber HRK: Fluid, electrolyte and nutritional management of the gynecologic patient, part II, in Goldstein DP, Leventhal J (eds): *Current Problems in Obstetrics and Gynecology.* Chicago, Year Book Medical Publishers, Inc, Vol III, No 1, Sept 1979, pp 3–35.

Berk JL, Sampliner JE, Artz JS, et al: *Handbook of Critical Care.* Boston, Little, Brown and Company, 1976.

Bird B: *Talking with Patients,* ed 2. Philadelphia, J.B. Lippincott Co, 1973.

Burgess A (ed): *The Nurse's Guide to Fluid and Electrolyte Balance.* New York, McGraw-Hill Book Company, 1970.

Burke JE: Preventive antibiotics in surgery. *Postgrad Med* 58:65, 1975.

Canizaro PC, Shires GT: Fluid and nutritional management, in Schwartz SI (ed): *Principles of Surgery.* New York, McGraw-Hill, 1974.

Collins JA: Problems associated with massive transfusion of stored blood. *Surgery* 75:274, 1974.

Cranley JJ: Thromboembolic venous disease in obstetrical and gynecological patients. *Am J Obstet Gynecol* 1:29, 1979.

Dalen JE (ed): *Pulmonary Embolism.* New York, MedCom Press, 1973.

Dane EW, Fujikaws K: Basic mechanisms in blood coagulation. *Ann Rev Biochem* 44:799, 1975.

Flamenbaun W: Pathophysiology of acute renal failure. *Arch Intern Med* 131:911, 1973.

Goldfarb JW, Yates AP (eds): *Critical Care Medicine.* Pittsburgh, Synapse Publications, 1977.

Goldhirsch H: Postoperative psychosis. *Ohio State Med J* 69:375, 1973.

Heird WC, Dell RB, Driscoll JM Jr, et al: Metabolic acidosis resulting from intravenous alimentation mixtures containing synthetic amino acids. *N Engl J Med* 287:943, 1972.

Hills AG: *Acid-Base Balance.* Baltimore, Williams & Wilkins, 1973.

Kakkar VV, Nicolaides AN, Field ES, et al: Low doses of heparin in prevention of deep vein thrombosis. *Lancet* 2:669, 1971.

Laver MB: Acute respiratory failure: More questions, fewer answers. *Anesthesiology* 43:611, 1975.

Linfman H, Lalezari B: A plan of management of unexpected bleeding problems related to surgery. *Pacific Med Surg* 75:362, 1967.

Mazzara JT, Ayres SM, Grace WJ, et al: Extreme hypocapnia in the critically ill patient. *Am J Med* 56:450, 1974.

McCabe WR: Gram-negative bacteremia. *DM,* December 1973.

McCracken GH Jr, Eichenwald HF: Antimicrobial therapy. Therapeutic considerations. *J Pediatr* 85:297, 1974.

McDougal WS, Persky L: Renal function abnormalities in postunilateral ureteral obstruction in man: A comparison of these defects to postobstructive diuresis. *J Urol* 113:601, 1975.

Mitchell JP: Current concepts; trauma to the urinary tract. *N Engl J Med* 288:90, 1973.

Mitchell JC III: Axioms on uremia. *Hosp Med* July 1978, p 6.

Owen CA Jr, Bowie EJ, Thompson JH Jr, et al: *The Diagnosis of Bleeding Disorders,* ed 2. Boston, Little, Brown, 1974.

Powers SR Jr, Mannal R, Neclerio M, et al: Physiologic consequences of positive end expiratory pressure (PEEP) ventilation. *Ann Surg* 178:265, 1973.

Robinson AL: Computers: First the maxi, then the mini, now it's the micro. *Science* 186:1102, 1974.

Ryan JA Jr, Abel RM, Abbott WM, et al: Catheter complications in total parenteral nutrition. *N Engl J Med* 290:757, 1974.

Shapiro BA: *Clinical Application of Blood Gases.* Chicago, Year Book Medical Publishers, Inc, 1973.

Silver D: Coagulopathies and surgeons. *J Surg Res* 16:429, 1974.

Silver D, McGregor FH Jr: Nonmechanical causes of surgical bleeding. *Curr Probl Surg* January 1970.

Slefamini M: Disseminated intravascular coagulation: How to recognize an insidious culprit. *Mod Med* 2:31, 1974.

Sussman LN: The clotting time—an enigma. *Am J Clin Pathol* 60:651, 1973.

Swan HJC, Ganz W, Forrester J, et al: Catheterization of the heart in man with use of a flow-directed balloon-tipped catheter. *N Engl J Med* 283:447, 1970.

Thompson GE: Acute renal failure. *Med Clin North Am* 57:1579, 1973.

Thompson WL: Introduction: A perspective. *The Cell in Shock.* Kalamazoo, The Upjohn Co, 1974.

Vanatta JC, Fogelman MJ (eds): *Moyer's Fluid Balance: A Clinical Manual,* ed 2. Chicago, Year Book Publishers, Inc, 1976.

Weil HM, Shubin H (eds): *Critical Care Medicine: Current Principles and Practices.* Hagerstown, Md, Harper & Row, 1976.

19 Basic Principles of Radiation Therapy

Hugh R. K. Barber

In order to understand the modus operandi of a radiotherapy department, it is desirable to have a basic acquaintance with a few aspects of modern physics. This is not difficult and requires no in-depth knowledge of mathematics. The medical radiotherapist must be qualified in radiologic physics and works with professional physicists for treatment planning, dosage estimation, calibration of equipment, etc. Radiotherapy can be defined as treatment by ionizing rays (radiation — ionization). These rays are of two kinds, waves and particles. The biologic effects of ionizing radiation represent the efforts of living things to deal with the energy remaining in them after an interaction of one of their atoms with an ionizing ray or particle. For any living system, this energy will be in excess of the system's requirements for normal function; it will be a deviation from the proper energy relationships within that system. Radiation biology is the study of the sequence of events within organisms following the absorption of energy from ionizing radiation. It is the study of the efforts of organisms to restore proper energy relationships within themselves, and of the damage to them which may be produced by excess energy.

The three subatomic building blocks of nature are closely related to, and in certain instances are, members of a group of penetrating ionizing radiations which are of major importance in the control of cancer. These three particles are fundamental to all material structures, including man. Their actions and interactions account for all the known elements, and there are hundreds of isotopes, both stable and unstable. The laws of chemistry and nuclear physics depend upon the movements of these particles. In fact, they hold the secret of life.

Roentgen rays, radium, and radioactive elements owe their origin and energy to the electron, the proton, and the neutron. All types of penetrating and ionizing radiations ultimately impart their energies by virtue of the electron, the positron, the proton, and the alpha particle. The energy transfer may be by ionization, excitation, or collision. A large proportion of this energy ultimately assumes the form of heat. Among the different types of radiation discussed, a quantitative, but not a qualitative, difference in their action is noted.

All matter is made up of chemical substances which can be divided into two kinds—elements and compounds. An element is a distinct kind of matter which cannot be decomposed into two or more simpler kinds of matter. A compound is formed when two or more elements combine chemically to produce a more complex kind of matter. All matter—solids, liquids, and gases—is composed of basic chemical materials or elements. For example, hydrogen and oxygen are both elements; neither can be decomposed into simpler kinds of matter. They can combine to make a more complex kind of matter, eg, water, which is a compound of hydrogen and oxygen. About 99% of the earth's crust consists of oxygen, silicone, aluminum, iron, calcium, magnesium, sodium, and potassium. Almost the whole of organic living matter is composed of only four elements—carbon, oxygen, hydrogen, and nitrogen.

Each different element consists of huge numbers of tiny identical units called atoms. An atom is too small to be observed visually. The diameter of an atom is 10^{-8} cm, a convenient way of stating that 100 million atoms side by side would occupy a length of 1 cm. Atoms are the smallest particles of an element, and can exist without losing the chemical properties of that element. Molecules are the smallest particles of a compound that can exist without losing the chemical properties of that compound. They are combinations of atoms. For example, a molecule of water is composed of two atoms of hydrogen and one of oxygen; this fact underlies the law of chemical combination, in which elements combine together in simple proportions.

All material substances, whether animal, vegetable, or mineral, whether a mushroom or an airplane, are composed of multiples of three primary subatomic particles, ie, the electron, the proton, and the neutron. Under certain circumstances, each of these three particles may become a form of radiation energy.

Our present concept of the structure of the atom is based on the work of Rutherford and Bohr early in the twentieth century. This provides a simple picture of the atom as an electrical structure having three basic units, the proton, the neutron, and the electron, and it is adequate for the discussion of most phenomena in radiological physics.

The simplest atom is one of the element, hydrogen. This consists of a central nucleus comprising one proton around which an electron moves in a shell or orbit. The proton is a heavy particle carrying a positive electrical charge. The electron is a very much lighter particle, having a mass of only 1/1840 of the mass of the proton. It has a negative charge of exactly equal magnitude (but of opposite sign) to that of the proton. Consequently, almost all the mass of the atom is in the nucleus, and the positive charge of the nucleus is balanced by the negative charge of the electron to make the atom as a whole electrically neutral.

The next simplest atom is one of the element, helium. In this, the nucleus is comprised of two protons and two neutrons, with two orbital electrons moving around the nucleus. A neutron is a particle with a mass approximately equal to that of a proton, but with no electric charge. The nucleus of the helium atom, therefore, has a positive charge of two units (due to the two protons) and a mass of approximately four units. Also, the two positive charges of the nucleus are balanced by the two negatively charged electrons around the nucleus.

In essence, the atom consists of a massive central portion, the nucleus, which contains the positive protons and the uncharged neutrons. All atoms of a given element have the same number of positive nuclear charges; the neutrons add mass but no charge to the nucleus. Because of their similarity of mass, neutrons and protons are called neucleons. Since a neucleon (proton or neutron) has about 1860 times the mass of an electron, it is obvious that the mass of an atom is concentrated in its nucleus. The nucleus is surrounded by negatively charged electrons which are found in discrete orbits at relatively great distances from the nucleus. In the normal atom, the number of protons is equal to the number of electrons; the atom is electrically neutral.

Radiation may have sufficient energy to remove an electron from an atom completely and produce an electrical charge (ionization), or perhaps only to move an electron to an orbit further from the nucleus (excitation). These processes, particularly ionization, are responsible for the biologic damage produced by ionizing radiations.

In addition to protons and neutrons, the nucleus contains a variety of particles, the nature and function of which are, as yet, poorly understood. Of interest in this connection are the mesons. Several types of mesons have been identified, but at present the most abundant are the pi mesons with a mass 273 times that of the electron, and the mu mesons with a mass 270 times that of the electron. Both types may have either positive or negative charges, or they may be neutral. The pi mesons are radioactive, decaying to mu mesons. Physicists believe that the pi meson in some way holds the nucleus together by favoring traction among the nucleons (protons and neutrons) through a sharing process.

An element can be identified either by its atomic number (Z) or by its name. The atomic number of an element is the number of protons in the nucleus (which is equal to the number of electrons around the nucleus) of an atom of that element. In going from hydrogen to helium, for example, the number of protons in the nucleus (and also the number of orbital electrons) has increased from 1 to 2; thus the atomic number of hydrogen is 1 and that of helium is 2. The atomic number of an element determines its chemical properties because they depend on the number of electrons present and on the way in which they are arranged around the nucleus. The electrons are arranged in circular rings, each ring representing an energy level shell. The shells are identified by the letters of the alphabet, the innermost being the K shell, the second L, the third M, and so on. The maximum number of electrons permitted in the various shells are as follows: K shell, 2 electrons; L shell, 8 electrons; M shell, 18 electrons; N shell, 32 electrons; O shell, 18 electrons; P shell, 8 electrons; Q shell, uncertain.

The mass number of an atom is the total number of protons and neutrons in the nucleus, and gives a measure of the mass of the nucleus. Protons and neutrons are known collectively as nucleons because they are found in the nucleus. When it is necessary to indicate the values of the atomic number and the atomic mass, they are often added to the chemical symbol for the element as prefixes, the mass number being placed above the atomic number. Thus the helium described is represented as $_2\mathrm{He}^4$. This is an example of a nuclide. The atomic mass is written above as a superscript and to the right. A nuclide is a particular variety of atom characterized by a given atomic number and a given mass.

An isotope is a chemical element having the same atomic number as another (ie, same number of nuclear protons), but possessing a different atomic mass (ie, different number of nuclear neutrons). An isobar is a term applied to two or more substances that have the same atomic weight but different atomic numbers. A radionuclide is an atomic nucleus which will decay spontaneously into some other nuclear species, accompanied by the liberation of energy — a nuclear species that is radioactive.

Bremsstrahlung (Brems rays) is the term applied whenever high-speed electrons, regardless of their source, are abruptly slowed down and their energy converted to electromagnetic radiation. If the energy is large enough, the electromagnetic radiation is in the area of x-rays, and the resulting x-ray spectrum is continuous. This is best exemplified by the white radiation emitted by the target of an x-ray tube, consisting of a continuous range of wavelengths produced during deceleration of high-speed electrons by multiple collisions with the target atoms. This type of x-radiation, produced by the slowing down of high-speed electrons, is termed Bremsstrahlung, a German word which means "braking radiation." In a similar manner, high-energy beta particles, passing close to atomic nuclei, undergo deceleration and also give rise to Brems radiation.

TYPES OF RADIATION EMITTED

Radiation is the process of emission of energy by atoms, and the passage of this energy through space. There are two types of radiation:

1. Wave (electromagnetic) — x-rays and gamma rays. Transport of energy waves associated with vibrating electric charges characterize this type of energy.
2. Corpuscular — streams of particles including alpha particles, beta particles, neutrons, positrons, pi mesons, and others (certain aspects of wave radiation require assumption that waves are accompanied by discrete energy corpuscles; photons or quanta).

The sources of radiation are:

1. Atomic nuclei — a) alpha particles (helium nuclei), b) beta particles (fast electrons), c) gamma rays, d) neutrinos, e) positrons
2. Atomic orbits — a) electrons, b) x-rays.
3. Brems rays — arising during deceleration of energetic electrons, as in x-ray tube.
4. Annihilation radiation — combination of positron and negatron which immediately disappear and give rise to two gamma ray photons.
5. Cosmic rays — remote stars.

These radiations, whether natural or artificial radioisotopes, are of three kinds, named after the first three letters of the Greek alphabet — 1) alpha rays (or particles), 2) beta rays (or particles), and 3) gamma rays (energy). Alpha particles are streams of high-speed helium nuclei (two protons and two neutrons packed tightly together) that have been ejected from radioactive substances. Beta rays are streams of fast-moving electrons (particles) ejected from radioactive substances with velocities that may be as high as 98% of the velocity of light. In soft tissue, beta rays can travel distances ranging from small fractions of a millimeter up to about 1 cm, producing ionization in their path. The beta particles come from a neutron in the nucleus. Neutrons change into a proton and an electron. The electron is then ejected from the nucleus. Emission of the beta particle from the nucleus (beta decay) does not change the mass number (the total number of particles in the nucleus) but does increase the atomic number by 1, ie, $15^{P^{32}} \rightarrow 16^{P^{32}} \pm$ beta 0. Gamma rays come from radioactive substances. When they are produced by electrical machines, we call them x-rays. They differ fundamentally from alpha and beta radiations as they are not particles but waves of the same type as light and radio waves, but with different properties of their very much shorter wavelength.

Heavy nuclei are the nuclei of ordinary atoms whose electrons have been stripped away, yielding a very highly charged particle. They are artificially produced and are given high energy in an accelerator. Their large mass confers upon them the capability of colliding with nuclei in the absorber, and accelerating them (a reaction analogous to the production of high-speed electrons). Neutrons, since they are uncharged particles, are not affected by and cannot themselves affect charged objects (atomic nuclei or electrons). Since their interactions must depend upon chance collisions with atoms, they are able to penetrate matter of all kinds for great distances. Neutrons are classified by their distinctive property—their energy. Dependent on that factor, they are usually considered as fast or slow. Fast neutrons lose energy mainly by collision with atomic nuclei. Since carbon, oxygen, nitrogen, and hydrogen are the major components of soft tissue, their interaction with fast neutrons is of importance to radiobiology. Because hydrogen atoms are the most numerous in tissue of average water content (tissues are 70% to 80% water), and since the average energy transferred from a fast neutron to a hydrogen nucleus is much greater than the energy transferred to other nuclei, for practical purposes the major mode of energy loss of fast neutrons in soft tissue may be considered to be by the ejection of high-speed protons (hydrogen nuclei). The protons will have a variety of energies, depending upon the neutron energies, but all of them will be highly ionizing particles with a high linear energy transfer. Slow neutrons interact in matter mainly by the process of capture. The uncharged, slowly moving neutron actually enters the nucleus of an atom and matter, and loses its identity. It becomes just another nuclear neutron. The added neutron—and its energy—may put the atom in an unstable state; it may become radioactive itself and emit charged particles (protons, electrons, alpha particles) or gamma rays.

The interest in particles is obvious. First, the particles—neutrons, negative pi mesons (or pions), and accelerated heavy ions—produce a higher density of ionization in either x-rays or gamma rays. For this reason, they are called high linear energy transfer (LET) radiation, whereas electromagnetic radiation is called low-LET radiation. This difference in density of ionization is significant because it takes a certain number of ionization events within a cell to cause death; hence, low-LET radiation produces more misses. In other words, low- and high-LET radiation differ in their relative biologic efficiencies (RBE), so that high-LET is about three times more effective per rad than low-LET radiation. Thus, less high-LET radiation can be given to accomplish the same amount of tissue damage.

The pi meson, or pion, is a negatively charged particle produced when an accelerated proton beam strikes a graphite target. Conventional therapeutic radiation sources produce low-LET radiation. Pions act as a low-LET beam while passing through the tissues en route to the target tumor, then as a high-LET beam when they reach the tumor. Pions pass through tissue slowly, stopping at a depth determined by their energy levels. When a pion is captured by the nucleus of an oxygen, carbon, or nitrogen atom, it releases enough energy to produce a star effect in which the nucleus explodes into densely ionizing, cell destroying fragments.

Mesons are 200 times heavier than electrons. They were first found among cosmic rays. One difficulty about mesons is that they exhibited no absorption by atomic nuclei. This contradicted the notion that the meson was responsible for the binding force in the nucleus. Later, it was suggested that the mesons which had been observed were not ones which existed in the nucleus, but a lighter variety which represented a decay product from the heavier sort. According to this two-meson theory, the heavier mesons would be found at high altitudes in the earth's atmosphere where cosmic rays had knocked them out of the nuclei. The decay product of the lighter mesons would be found at lower altitudes. The heavier mesons, pi mesons, exist with a positive, negative, and neutral charge. They are 273 times heavier than electrons. The lighter mesons are called mu mesons, and are found to be positive and negative; there are no neutral mu mesons. They are 210 times as heavy as electrons. In open space, a positive and a negative pi meson decay into a positive or negative mu meson and a neutrino in about 1/250 millionth of a second. The mu meson decays into a positron or electron plus two more neutrinos in two millionths of a second. The neutral pi meson presents a special puzzle, since it decays into two high-energy photons or gamma rays. The K meson is lighter than the proton or the neutron. They are heavier than the pi mesons. There are four K mesons — positive, negative, and two types of neutral ones. A large atom smasher will produce positive or negative K mesons in pairs. These are high-energy K mesons. A low-energy positive K meson is produced along with a lambda or sigma.

RADIATION QUANTITIES AND UNITS

1. The unit for activity is the *curie.*
2. The unit of exposure is the *roentgen.*
3. The unit for absorbed dose is the *rad.*

Definitions

1. Roentgen (r) is a measurement of radiation exposure. It is defined as that amount of x- or gamma radiation such that the associated cor-

puscular emission per 0.001293 gram of air, produces in air, ions carrying one electrostatic unit of electricity of either sign. A milliroentgen is 1/1000 r.

2. Roentgen-equivalent-man (rem) is defined as that quantity of radiation which produces the same biological effect in man as 1 r.

3. The rad is a unit of absorbed dose. It is defined as an energy absorption of 100 erg per gram of any material (roughly equivalent to the roentgen).

4. Curie (C) is the quantity of any radioisotope which disintegrates at the rate of 3.7×10^{10} disintegrations per second. The subunits of the Curie unit are: millicurie (mCi) = 1/1000 of C; microcurie (μCi) = 1/1000 of mCi.

5. Milligram radium (mgRa). Used only for radium (1 mg radium = 1 mCi radium = 8.2 rhcm).

6. Milligram radium equivalent (mgRaeq). Used for gamma-emitting radioisotopes which are applied in radiation therapy as substitutes for radium or radon. Defined as the activity which produces the same ionization in air by gamma radiation as 1 mg of radium (1 mgRaeq = 8.25 rhcm).

7. Linear Energy Transfer (LET). This is the energy released (usually in keV) per micron of medium (tissue) along the tract of any ionizing particle.

THE INTERACTION OF PENETRATING
RADIATION AND MATTER

When an x-ray beam enters a body of matter, a part of the energy of the beam is absorbed and, at the same time, penetrating radiations are emitted from the body in all directions. The latter constitute the scattered and secondary radiations, arising from collisions of x-rays in the primary beam with the atoms of the body in the path of the beam. Secondary radiation is defined as the radiation emitted by the atoms that have been penetrated by x-rays. Scattered radiation refers to those rays that have suffered a change of direction after collision with atoms. The emission of secondary radiation goes hand-in-hand with x-ray absorption.

Some x-rays do not collide with atoms but pass through the body unchanged, because these rays are electrically neutral and therefore may penetrate matter for a considerable distance without encountering an atom. This accounts for the fact that a portion of the beam is not absorbed, but passes completely through the body.

The various types of collision between x-rays and atoms form a very interesting study. It is possible to simplify the concept as well as to make it more accurate scientifically if we assume that an x-ray beam consists of minute, discrete packets or chunks of energy travelling with the speed of light. Such a tiny unit of energy is called a photon or quantum. This may seem to contradict the electromagnetic wave theory of radiation discussed earlier but, actually, the phenomena of radiation absorption and emission can be explained only if one assumes that a given x-ray exists at the same time both as a wave and as a particle of energy. This permits an explanation of how characteristic radiation is produced in an x-ray tube when an electron drops from a higher to a lower energy level in the atom of the target metal. Such a characteristic ray is a quantum or photon of energy, and its energy content and wavelength are characteristic of the target element. Thus, an atom of a given element can emit rays of definite characteristic quantum, and these are different from those of any other element. The amount of energy in a given quantum represents the difference in the energy levels of the orbits between which the electron has jumped. On the basis of this concept, known as the *quantum theory,* an x-ray beam consists of showers of photons or bullets of energy travelling with the speed of light and having no electrical charge. This is also known as the *corpuscular theory* of radiation, and applies equally to other forms of electromagnetic radiation, eg, light and gamma rays.

Max Planck, a German physicist, established the following equation to represent the energy of a quantum: quantum energy = a constant × frequency $(E = h\nu)$. In this equation, h is known as Planck's constant $(6.625 \times 10^{-27}$ erg-sec) because it never varies, and the Greek letter ν represents the frequency of vibrations per second. From this equation, it is evident that the greater the frequency, the greater the quantum energy. This agrees with the observed fact that the penetrating power of x-rays increases as the frequency increases, and since the speed of x-rays is constant and equals frequency times wavelength, an increase in frequency is accomplished by a decrease in wavelength. Thus, highly penetrating x-ray photons have high frequency and short wavelength while, conversely, short x-rays have low frequency and low wavelength.

When x-ray photons penetrate a body of matter, there are three main types of interaction: 1) unmodified scattering, 2) photoelectric collision with true absorption, and 3) Compton collision with scattering absorption and pair production.

Unmodified Scattering

If an x-ray penetrates an atom of matter placed in its path, and happens to glance off the nucleus or strongly bound electron, the photon suffers no loss of energy because the atomic mass is tremendous compared with that of a photon. Since the energy of the photon is unchanged, it emerges with the same energy as it had when it entered the atom. In other words, the emerging photon has suffered no change in frequency or wavelength, although its direction has been changed. Thus, unmodified scattering merely changes the direction of the photon, but not its hardness. This type of interaction occurs chiefly with elements of higher atomic number than aluminum. It constitutes but a small fraction of the scattered radiation in clinical radiology.

Photoelectric Absorption:
A Low-Energy Phenomenon

When a low-energy photon collides with an orbital electron, the most likely result will be a transfer of all the photon's energy to the electron. The photon disappears entirely or is absorbed by the electron. The electron itself will be ejected from its orbit and from the atom. The process is, of course, ionization, and the result will be an ion pair. But not all orbital electrons are bound in their orbits by equal energies; those nearer the nucleus are bound more tightly than those more distant from it. The photon may have enough energy to remove an L or M electron from a particular absorbing atom, but not enough to remove the atom's K electron (the process cannot occur with electrons of a particular orbit if the photon energy is less than that of the orbit). Photoelectric interaction, then, depends on photon energy; ejection of an electron is most likely to occur when the photon has an energy slightly greater than the binding energy of the orbit. The probability of this interaction increases when the energy of the photon is slightly greater than that of the orbit, because all electrons of a given shell will be available to undergo photoelectric absorption. The probability of photoelectric interaction decreases with increasing photon energy. Higher photon energies will exceed those of the orbits, and the interaction becomes less likely to occur. In the photoelectric absorption process, the bombarding photon gives up all of its energy to the electron with which it interacts. All of the energy of the entering photon is used up in dislodging the electron from its orbit and giving it a high speed. The high-speed electron is called a photoelectron. As the vacancy is filled by outer electrons, this energy is irradiated as characteristic x-rays.

Compton Scattering:
A Medium-Energy Phenomenon

In contrast to photoelectric absorption, a Compton scattering, named after its discoverer, H.H. Compton, is a process in which higher energy photons interact with matter. In it the photons have only a portion of their energy absorbed in interacting with orbital electrons (they are not totally absorbed). The process is confined, for the most part, to interactions with outer, loosely bound electrons. Because these electrons are loosely bound, nearly all the energy exchanged to the electron will be in the form of electron kinetic energy (the binding energy of the orbit is essentially negligible). The photon itself will be deflected in the interaction; its direction will be changed. It is then said to have been scattered. The products of the interaction are: 1) a scattered, less energetic, degraded photon (some of its energy has gone to the electron it ejected); 2) a high-speed electron; and 3) an ionized atom. In the Compton collison with modified scattering, part of the photon's energy has been used up in removing an orbital electron. The dislodged electron is called a Compton electron or recoil electron. The emerging photon has less energy, and it has also undergone a change in direction. For photons in the range of 100 keV to 10 meV, Compton interaction is the most important photon interaction process in soft tissue.

Pair Production:
A High-Energy Phenomenon

Photon energy may be exchanged into matter by yet another mechanism (which differs from those already described) in two fundamental details: 1) It occurs exclusively with high energy photons, and 2) The intereaction is with the atomic nucleus and does not involve the ejection of orbital electrons. Photons with energy greater than 1.02 meV may interact with the electric force field of the highly charged nucleus so that their energy is converted to mass. The photon is changed into two particles, a positive and a negative electron (the process can occur in reverse; mass can also be converted to energy). Energy (E) and mass (m) are related to each other according to the Einstein formula, $E = mc^2$, where c is the velocity of light. Pair production cannot occur with photons whose energy is less than the combined mass of two electrons (0.51 meV per electron), a threshold energy of 1.02 meV. Photon energy in excess of the threshold value will be shared as kinetic energy between the two newly formed electrons. If there is no excess energy present, the electrons will immediately recombine (annihilation) and are converted back to energy. In the instance where threshold energy is exceeded, the electrons will move away from the point of formation. Both will move through matter, undergoing interactions with and ionizing other atoms in the substance until the excess kinetic energy is exhausted. In this way energy is ultimately transferred from the photon to matter. When the positive electron comes to rest, it will interact with an available negative electron. Annihilation will occur, the electrons will disappear, and the electron masses will be converted to two photons which share the energy. Pair production is dependent upon atomic number. The initial photon interaction is with the force field of the nucleus. Larger nuclei, having more protons, will have stronger force fields, thus increasing the probability of the occurrence of this process.

In summary, in pair production the photon interacts with the strong field near the nucleus, and a positron and electron are produced. The electron and the positron both give up their kinetic energy to the medium by ionizing and exciting other atoms. When the positron comes to rest, it combines with one of the abundant free electrons, annihilating each other, and two equal gamma rays (the energy equivalent of their masses) are given off in opposite directions.

The radiobiologic effects on the cell may be inhibition of cell division, chromosome mutation, or gene mutation. The energy of x-rays or gamma rays may cut through a chromosome, allowing the severed ends to join together with little change of function. The use of potentiating agents such as hydroxyurea or metronidazole may inhibit the chromosome from reforming. Particle radiation is so destructive that it tears large holes in the chromosomes and destroys them.

PHYSICAL BASIS OF RADIOBIOLOGY

Whenever ionizing radiation traverses body tissues (or any other material), it transfers energy to them by processes of atomic excitation and ionization. The magnitude of the resulting biologic effects depends on physical and biologic factors. These are: 1) the quantity of energy imparted by the radiation to a unit mass of tissue at the site of interest — the absorbed dose, and 2) the biologic effectiveness of the radiation, determined by the rate of energy loss (locally absorbed) per unit length of path by the ionizing particle — the linear energy transfer. It has been determined that the greater the transfer of energy to tissues per unit length of path, the greater will be the biologic effect. This concept is embodied in the term "linear energy transfer" — usually called LET — which is defined as the rate of energy lost (locally absorbed) per unit length of path by an ionizing particle traversing a material medium. Because of the variation in ion density along the track, an ionizing particle, increasing as the energy of the particle decreases, the LET may be averaged over the entire path of the particle.

LET is an extremely valuable concept. LET is the energy released (usually in keV) per micron of medium (tissue) along the track of any ionizing particle. Protons, helium ions, and heavy ions are heavy, charged particles. The particles pass through matter, travel in nearly a straight line, and come to a stop after passing through a certain depth of absorber, depending upon their initial energy. The rate of energy loss increases sharply near the end of the range. There the dose reaches a peak, known as the Bragg peak. The dose falls off very rapidly beyond the Bragg peak. Pions, unlike other heavy, charged particles, are unstable and have a very short half-life. They remain to be evaluated in gynecologic malignancy. Neutrons interact with tissue and release higher-ionizing, heavy, charged particles; most of the dose is contributed by recoiling protons from hydrogen in tissue. Current research with neutron therapy holds some promise, but has not added significantly to the survival rate at this time in the treatment of gynecologic cancer.

OXYGEN ENHANCEMENT RATIO (OER)

The presence of oxygen at the time of irradiation influences the response of many biological and chemical systems. The amount of ionizing radiation needed to produce a specific change may be two to three times as great in anoxia as in the presence of oxygen. Local oxygen tension in irradiated tissues has been manipulated, consciously or otherwise, almost since the inauguration of radiation therapy. The degree of oxygen's enhancement of radiation effects is expressed as the oxygen enhancement ratio, OER. It is determined by measuring the radiation dose required to produce a specific effect under conditions of full oxygenation and the fullest possible hypoxia, and expressing the result as a ratio. There is some variation, but the oxygen enhancement ratio of x-radiations and gamma radiations in mammalian cells commonly lies between 2 and 3, normally close to 3. This means that most mammalian cells are about three times as sensitive to x-radiation or gamma radiation under full oxygenation as under extreme hypoxia. The presence of oxygen in cells enhances the biologic effect of low-LET radiations. This effect occurs only when oxygen in cells is within a definite concentration range. As LET increases, OER decreases. As LET increases, survival curves show steeper slopes, become more exponential, and have values of nearly equal to one. With very high LET radiation, there appears to be little or no recovery between fractions. Dose rate influences radiation response. As dose rate decreases, survival increases. This is believed due to recovery between radiation interactions at low-dose rates. OER decreases as dose rate decreases. Oxygen enhances the magnitude of the radiation effect (an increase of two to three times), and concentrations of oxygen at tumor levels at the time of radiation is a critical factor. The effect of oxygen is exerted at the time of energy exchange, probably by drawing radiation-produced free radicals into destructive auto-oxidative reactions. The application of the oxygen effect in radiotherapy is dependent upon presumed hypoxic regions in tumors.

THE ROLE OF OXYGEN IN DIRECT ACTION

Oxygen may oxidize the free radicals produced by radiation from a target molecule.

$$RH \xrightarrow[\text{quantum}]{\text{energy}} R\cdot + H\cdot$$

$$R\cdot + O_2 \qquad RO_2\cdot$$

The target molecule RH is changed, and $RO_2\cdot$, the resulting free radical, is capable of numerous interactions to satisfy its electronic requirements. Beyond that, a back reaction, which is possible after radiation interaction and which would restore the target, may be blocked by oxygen.

$$RH \xrightarrow[\text{quantum}]{\text{energy}} R\cdot + H\cdot$$

$$R\cdot + H\cdot \qquad RH \quad \text{Restoration}$$

$$R + O_2\cdot + H \quad \text{Restoration blocked}$$

THE ROLE OF OXYGEN IN INDIRECT ACTION

A description of the reduction of oxygen by the hydrogen-free radical serves to show one means by which oxygen enhances indirect action.

$$H_2O \xrightarrow[\text{quantum}]{\text{energy}} H_2O^+ + e^-$$

$$e^- + H_2O \longrightarrow OH^- + H\cdot$$

$$O_2 + H\cdot \longrightarrow HO_2\cdot$$

$$RH + HO_2\cdot \; R\cdot + H_2O_2$$

RH, the target molecule, is changed and raised to a free-radical state, and becomes capable of a variety of reactions with other cellular substances. Reactions between free radicals and oxygen increase the probability that target molecules will be changed and lose function as a result of energy lost by radiation in another molecule.

PREDICTABILITY OF RADIORESPONSIVENESS

This is one of the most important current investigational areas. As yet, no good in vitro or in vivo model has been developed.

1. Histologic grading prior to therapy: a) Broder's classification (1926), b) nuclear grading. As a general rule, the more anaplastic the carcinoma, the better the radioresponsiveness, but this has many exceptions. It is important to recognize that not all radiosensitive tumors are radiocurable, eg, lymphosarcoma, and that not all radioresistant tumors are necessarily radioincurable, eg, carcinoma of the tongue.

2. Radiopathologic changes after test dose: a) Glucksman's analysis (1945) of carcinoma of the cervix, b) Glucksman's study (1952) of testicular and bladder tumors. In the above situations, Glucksman studied histopathologic sections after a test dose of radiation (1000 to 2000 rad) to predict whether the cancer was radiosensitive. This is a tedious procedure. The sections selected by biopsy may not be truly representative, and the method has not been widely used.

3. Cytologic tests: a) RR and SR of Graham in the cervix, b) A, B, T and R cells of Gusberg in the cervix, c) cell culture method of Pick and Marcus. None of these tests are widely accepted or currently used. The need for predictors and markers for radiation response is apparent.

DETECTION OF X-RAYS

There are a number of ways in which the presence of roentgen rays may be detected, though not necessarily measured.

1. Photographic effect—the ability of x-rays to affect a photographic emulsion so that it can be developed clinically.

2. Fluorescent effect—the ability of x-rays to cause certain materials to glow in the dark. Such materials include calcium sulfide, barium platinocyanide, calcium tungstate, and barium lead sulfate.

3. Ionizing effect—the ability of x-rays to ionize gases and discharge certain electrical instruments such as the electroscope.

4. Physiologic effect—the ability of x-rays to redden the skin, destroy tissues, and sterilize reproductive organs.

5. Chemical effects—the ability of x-rays to change the color of certain dyes.

GROSS EFFECTS OF INTRACAVITARY RADIATION

Erythema—1 week
Exudation—2 weeks
Slough—6 to 8 weeks
Scarring—6 months
Contraction—1 year

Radiobiological Effects on Skin

For 6000 r in 6 weeks, 250 keV, HVL 2 mm Cr. 10×10 cm^2 field. With supervoltage, approximately twice the dose is required to produce the same early effects.

Early Effects

> First week — Faint (first erythema after 6 to 12 hours, fading in 2 to 3 days)
> Second week — Sharply defined (second) erythema
> Third week — Deepening erythema
> Fourth week — Dry desquamation
> Fifth week — Beginning moist desquamation
> Eighth week — Complete moist desquamation
> Twelfth week — Complete healing

Late Effects

> 3 months to
> 1 year — Atrophy, telangiectasis, depigmentation, subcutaneous fibrosis

DATA ON PERMISSIBLE RADIATION EXPOSURE

Exposure in the United States for a 30-year period (reproductive life of average person)	Rad
For diagnostic radiology	4.1
For radioisotopes around us	1.4
For radioisotopes in body	0.8
For cosmic radiation	0.4
From luminous dial watches	0.4
From nuclear testing	0.1
Total	7.2

RADIATION CONTRIBUTION OF ROENTGENOGRAPHIC DIAGNOSTIC PROCEDURES

Procedure	Skin Doses	Female
Chest film 14 in $\times$ 7 in	100 mR	0.07 mR
Chest photofluoroscopic film	1000 mR	0.70 mR
Pyelogram	1200 mR	1300 mR
Pelvimetry	12,000 mR	1300 mR

POINT AT WHICH RADIATION
EXPOSURE DAMAGES FETUS

Fetal Damage (Month of Gestation)	Rad
First	40
Second	90
Third	140
Fourth	200
Fifth	250
Sixth	350
Eighth	500
Tenth	600

DEVELOPMENT OF REGULATIONS FOR
MAXIMAL PERMISSIBLE DOSE TO THE WHOLE BODY

1931	1000 mR per week	50 R per year
1935	500 mR per week	25 R per year
1946	300 mR per week	15 R per year
1958	100 mR per week	5 R per year

Currently, 100 mR per week; 15 times as much for hands and feet; 1/10 as much for nonradiation workers.

RADIOISOTOPES

Isotope	Symbol	Half-life	Alpha	Beta	Gamma
Radium-226	^{226}Ra	1620 years	+	+	+
Cesium-137	^{137}Cs	26.6 years	−	+	+
Cobalt-60	^{60}Co	5.4 years	−	+	+
Iridium-192	^{192}Ir	74.4 days	−	+	+
Phosphorus-32	^{32}P	14.3 days	−	+	−
Iodine-125	^{125}I	60.0 days	−	−	+
Radon-222	^{222}Rn	3.8 days	+	+	+
Gold-198	^{198}Au	2.7 days	−	+	+
Yttrium-90	^{90}Y	2.7 days	−	+	−

EVALUATION OF MACHINES
FOR EXTERNAL RADIATION THERAPY

Units of Measurement

1 electron volt = 1 eV
1 thousand electron volts = 1 kiloelectron volt = 1 keV
1 million electron volts = 1 meV
1 billion electron volts = 1 beV

MEGAVOLTAGE

Advantages

1. Less skin reaction due to lower surface dose. This is the most important advantage of megavoltage and permits radiation therapy without bothersome skin reactions.
2. Greater depth doses, especially for small and medium fields. This permits a simple set-up—usually opposing megavoltage fields are satisfactory as multiple fields or rotational therapy with kilovoltage.
3. Less dose in bone, and less bone "shadowing." Less side scatter.

Disadvantages

1. Much higher cost for machine and installation.
2. Beam shaping more difficult.
Megavoltage is essential for up-to-date curative and palliative radiation therapy.

Cobalt-60 vs Cesium-137

Isotope	Half-life	Gamma Lines
Cobalt-60	5.24 years	1.7 and 1.33 meV
Cesium-137	26.6 years	0.67 meV

Advantages of Cobalt

1. Better skin sparing (surface dose about one half that of Cesium-137).
2. Better field shaping (source diameter about one half that of Cesium-137).
3. Higher output.

Disadvantages of Cobalt

1. Source replacement every two to five years.
2. Room shielding more difficult.
3. Cobalt-60 is preferable.

X-ray and Gamma Rays vs Electrons

1. Advantages of x-rays and gamma rays:
   a. Better skin sparing.
   b. Larger beams.
2. Disadvantages of x-rays and gamma rays:
   a. Depth sparing more difficult.
   b. Lower output.
   c. Megavoltage electron-beam therapy is worthwhile only for very large institutions.

SUMMARY

The three subatomic building blocks of nature are closely related to, and in certain instances are, members of the group of penetrating and ionizing radiations which are of major importance in the control of cancer.

Roentgen rays, radium, cesium, and radioactive elements owe their origin and energy to the electron, the proton, and the neutron. They function by ionizing radiation and by transferring their energy to the tissue through which they pass. The different types of radiation differ as a quantitative concept but not as a qualitative one.

The biologic results subsequent to exposure to various penetrating and ionizing radiation depend upon the energy absorbed from the radiations by the biologic media through which they pass. The energy types of radiations, such as x-ray and gamma radiations, will pass through a chromosome and cut it as though it were cut with a Gigli saw. These chromosomes often join up and show no ill effects from the radiation. The use of potentiators inhibits the chromosome from reforming and therefore adds to the effect of the radiation therapy. Radiation particles, such as neutrons, protons, and pions, are more destructive and act like cannon balls as they project through the chromosome, causing a great deal of destruction. The energy types of radiations, such as x-ray and gamma radiation, need oxygen for maximal effect, whereas the particle radiation does not need oxygen to the degree that the energy type of radiation does.

The sensitivity of any particular type of radiation is dependent upon many factors: the mitotic activity, the life span of the adult cell, the

536

oxygen supply, vascularity, metabolic state, intensity of radiation, and total dosage.

The mechanisms through which the effects occur include the role of oxygen in direct action and also its role in indirect action. Reactions between free radicals and oxygen increase the probability that target molecules will be changed and lose function as a result of energy loss by radiation in another molecule.

BIBLIOGRAPHY

Abbe R: Radium and radioactivity. *Yale Med J* June 1904, p 433.

Barber HRK: Radiation therapy in gynecology, in Barber HRK, Fields DH, Kaufman SA (eds): *Quick Reference to Ob-Gyn Procedures,* ed 2. Philadelphia, J.B. Lippincott Co, 1979, pp 312–320.

Broder AC: Grading and practical application. *Arch Pathol* 2:376, 1926.

Buschke F: Radiation therapy: The past, the present, the future (Janeway Lecture). *Am J Roentgen* 108:236, 1970.

Buschke F: Clinical application of supervoltage radiation. *The Cancer Bulletin, Texas* 8:12, 1956.

Case JT: History of radiation therapy, in Buschke F (ed): *Progress in Radiation Therapy,* vol 1. New York, Grune & Stratton, 1958.

Cleaves MA: Radium therapy. *Med Res* 64:601, 1903.

Cohn CJ, Gusberg SB: Radiosensitivity testing—A modern adjuvant in the treatment of cervical cancer. *Clin Obstet Gynecol* 12:335, 1969.

Comas F, Brucer M: First impression of therapy with cesium-137. *Radiology* 69:231, 1957.

Delario AJ: *Roentgen, Radium and Radioisotope Therapy.* Philadelphia, Lea & Febiger, 1953.

Demy NG: Beam localization and depth dose determination. *Radiology* 51:89, 1948.

Glucksman A: Response of human tissues to radiation with special reference to differentiation. *Br J Radiol* 25:38, 1952.

Glucksman A, Spear FG: Qualitative and quantitative histological examination of biopsy material from patients treated by radiation for carcinoma of the cervix uteri. *Br J Radiol* 18:313, 1945.

Graham JB, Graham RM: Sensitization response in patients with cancer of the uterine cervix. *Cancer* 13:5, 1960.

Hay GA, Hughes D (eds): *First Year Physics for Radiographers.* Baltimore, The Williams & Wilkins Co, 1972.

Kaplan HS: Radiobiology's contribution to radiotherapy: Promise or mirage? *Radiat Res* 43:460, 1970.

Kligerman MM: Potential for therapeutic gain similar to pions by daily combinations of neutrons and low-LET radiations. *Med Hypoth* 5:257, 1979.

Kligerman MM, Sala JM, Wilson S, et al: Investigation of pion treated human skin nodules for therapeutic gain. *Int J Radiat Oncol Biol Physics* 4:263, 1978.

Kligerman MM, Sternhagen CJ: Radiation oncology, in Homburger F, Karger S (eds): *The Physiopathology of Cancer,* vol 2. Basel, Basel Publishers, 1976.

Kligerman MM: Present status of combined radiation therapy and chemotherapy, in Buschke F (ed): *Progress in Radiation Therapy,* vol III. New York, Grune & Stratton, 1965, pp 183–199.

Lightfoot DA: The physics of radiation therapy for gynecologic malignancy, in McGowan L (ed): *Gynecologic Oncology.* New York, Appleton-Century-Crofts, 1978.

Pizzarello DJ, Witcopki RL: *Medical Radiation Biology.* Philadelphia, Lea & Febiger, 1972.

Puck TT, Marcus PI: Action of x-rays on mammalian cells. *J Exp Med* 103:653, 1956.

Raju MR, Richman C: Negative pion radiotherapy: Physical and radiobiological aspects. Current topics in radiation. *Res Quarterly* 8:159, 1972.

Selman J: *The Basic Physics of Radiation Therapy.* Springfield, Ill, Charles C Thomas, 1960 and 1973.

Walter J: *Cancer and Radiotherapy.* Edinburgh, Churchill Livingstone, 1973.

Wharton JT, Smith JP, Delclos L, et al: Irradiation therapy for gynecologic malignancies, in *Davis' Gynecology and Obstetrics,* vol II. Hagerstown, Md, 1972, chap 73.

20 Chemotherapy

Hugh R. K. Barber

In the 1950s, chemotherapy was in its embryonic phase and generally given only to terminal patients, hopefully for some palliation and relief of symptoms. In the early 1960s, it assumed a more active role as a palliative measure and, in the late 1960s was progressing into the stage where it was being tried as an adjuvant type of therapy. During the 1970s, chemotherapy had effected profound changes in the outlook for patients with disseminated cancer. Physicians everywhere are now eager to make chemotherapeutic agents available to their patients. The specialty of medical oncology has been developed and has now assumed the status of a subspecialty, certified by a specialty board examination. The gynecologic oncologist manages the genital tumors of the pelvis and usually supervises the administration of the chemotherapeutic agents.

Chemotherapy is now the key factor responsible for long-term survival in at least ten types of widespread cancer occurring largely in children, adolescents, and young adults. There are at least ten other tumors that have shown fairly good response to treatment. The diseases that are highly responsive to chemotherapy include Burkitt's lymphoma, choriocarcinoma, acute lymphatic leukemia, Hodgkin's disease, lymphosarcoma, mycosis fungoides, embryonal testicular cancer, Wilms' tumor, Ewing's sarcoma, rhabdomyosarcoma, and retinoblastoma.

Chemotherapeutic agents for the treatment of neoplastic diseases are varied in their mechanism of action; however, they all have the common end point of cell destruction. This is accomplished by interfering in one or more of the sequences of replication which all cells undergo. Since, without exception, agents used in cancer chemotherapy are cell poisons, without particular specificity for malignant cells, their toxic effects will extend to normal cells. Briefly, it can be said that the goal of this type of drug therapy is the complete destruction of rapidly multiplying malignant cells with little or no damage to normal cells.

Generally, the maximal tolerated dose of these agents is given in a specified drug protocol. These protocols may consist of cytostatic agents (agents which directly interfere with cell division), cytotoxic agents, anti-inflammatory agents (such as corticosteroids), immunosuppressants, and immunologic stimulants (such as levamisole). The doses and routes and order of administration of these agents are carefully tailored to the patient, taking into consideration elements such as the patient's age, preexisting disease states, competency of excretory systems, and the type and extent of malignancy to be treated.

The most common toxic and side effects noted with these agents are bone marrow depression with leukemia, thrombocytopenia, aplastic anemia, disturbances of the digestive tract (stomatitis, nausea, vomiting), fever, and anorexia. Liver damage and neurologic dysfunction have been reported with some agents. Toxicity of some nature and degree should be anticipated in all patients receiving these preparations. Side effects may occur after their administration (particularly gastric symptoms), and may be delayed for several weeks (as with bone marrow depression), or several months (for example, azospermia after treatment with cyclophosphamide or loss of ova from the ovary). Thus, patients who have received these agents should be continually monitored for such acute or delayed problems.

Many of these agents are direct tissue irritants and may cause phlebitis and necrosis on administration. This is particularly true of doxorubicin, actinomycin D, vinblastine, vincristine, mitomycin, and nitrogen mustard. Special care must be taken with most anticancer agents to avoid these problems from developing. Carefully placed infusion lines, evenly flowing infusions, and prophylactic antiemetic preparations will help to alleviate problems which may cause severe patient discomfort with drug administration.

GENERAL PRINCIPLES

In contrast to surgery and radiation therapy, chemotherapy — the treatment of cancer with drugs or hormones — can be used effectively for disseminated as well as localized cancer. Chemotherapy has become a reality only in the past 30 years. Each of these three decades has seen important advances in the number of compounds available and in the spectrum of their usefulness. Within the last decade it has become clear that, although chemotherapy had long been considered largely a palliative procedure, capable of extending but not saving lives, certain kinds of cancer can now be cured by chemical treatment. A major goal of current cancer chemotherapy is to achieve cures by prompt and vigorous treatment.

Combinations of chemotherapeutic agents have been used with substantial success, particularly when each of the drugs acts on the cancer cells in a different way. A major improvement in the treatment of certain types of cancer has been achieved by using several of the active drugs simultaneously, as well as the use of different drugs in sequence.

The armamentarium of the oncologist has grown dramatically in the last three decades. In the last ten years alone, the National Cancer Institute has screened some 250,000 substances for potential anticancer activity, and it is probable that more than twice that number have now been examined in the world effort to find more effective agents.

Several disseminated human tumors have been cured with drugs alone, giving ample testimony to the proposition that selective toxicity does exist and that a potential for cure is available. Efforts must be extended to understand the interactions of drug, host, tumor, oncogenic agent, and host defense mechanism in this equation. The determination of which drugs to give for which tumors, in what combinations, and when in the course of the disease (before operation, after operation, with radiotherapy, after widespread metastases, etc), are areas of great importance.

There is no unique or specific difference between a cancer cell and a normal cell. Recent information regarding certain recorded biochemical differences; ie, reverse transcriptase, may represent the first recognized, concrete difference between a normal and a cancer cell. There is no specific action of a chemotherapeutic agent on cancer cells which will not affect normal cells; therefore, host-toxicity predictability occurs. Thus, the beneficial effects of chemotherapy are due to quantitative, not qualitative, differences between cancer cells and normal cells.

Structure of the Cell

Cancer is a disease of the cell. With the use of the electronmicroscope it has been possible to study the fine details and structures within the cell. Many of the important structures have been identified and their functions have been studied and tested.

The cell consists of the nucleus, which contains the chromatin, chromosomes, and genes, and the cytoplasm. The cell is enclosed by a porous type of membrane which allows materials to pass in and out of it.

This membrane provides the initial contact with the cell's external environment. The actions of hormones start to affect the cell at this point, and it has been shown that there are a variety of antigens on the surface of the cell membrane.

The nucleus contains the master chemical, deoxyribonucleic acid (DNA) in the chromosones; the nucleolus found in the nucleus is considered the storehouse of DNA, as well as the transport mechanism for messenger RNA (mRNA). The nucleus also contains the chromatin, chromosomes, and the genetic material.

The cytoplasm, once considered less complex than the nucleus, is taking on increasing importance as the inner secrets of the cell are probed and identified. It contains the protein-making sites or ribosomes. The endoplasmic reticulum is the network to which the ribosomes adhere. Mitochondria are the sites of energy metabolism, and probably have a limited production of protein. The Golgi complex is thought to play a key role in the intracellular synthesis and mobilization of certain proteins and carbohydrate components.

Through a complex but well integrated system, the DNA instructs messenger RNA to enter the cytoplasm and carry a message to transfer RNA, which in turn brings nucleic acid molecules to the ribosomes. At this point proteins are assembled, which serve as the enzyme system that controls the complex mechanisms of the integrated components of all cells.

The plasma membrane is a complex structure through which material passes in and out of the cell. It is the area of contact of a cell with its neighbors; it permits the passage of ions and molecules, influences movement of the cell, and probably plays an important role in controlling growth.

Of all components of the cell that theoretically may become transformed in malignancy, the cell surface is currently the most suspect. It has been shown that somatic cells of higher organisms express surface glycoproteins which are potentially immunogenic to other members of the same species. These surface markers are inheritable and are called histocompatible antigens. Each individual possesses a relatively unique array of surface markers. Thus, if tissue from one individual is grafted to another individual, the transplanted cells bearing these surface cell antigens are recognized as being foreign. A cell-mediated response ensues and the graft is rejected. A tissue transplant from one individual to a genetically different individual of the same species is called an allograft. The chromosomal region that encodes for the glycoproteins which function as strong histocompatibility antigens includes other genetic loci as well.

In mice, genes exist that determine whether the animal makes little or a great amount of antibody in response to certain kinds of antigens. Genes that appear to govern the level of immune responsiveness to antigens in this manner are called Ir genes (immune response). Analysis of segment populations of mice has shown that some Ir genes are closely linked to the genes for coding the major histocompatibility antigens, giving rise to the concept of a major histocompatibility complex (MHC).

Certain viruses are known to cause cancer in the mouse. It has been found that susceptibility to viruses that cause cancer (oncogenic viruses) is determined by genes within the major histocompatibility complex. The latter, therefore, includes several different kinds of genes: those that encode for histocompatibility antigens important in allograft immunity, those that govern the amount of antibody produced in response to antigenic challenge, termed Ir genes, and genes that govern susceptibility to oncogenic viruses.

Changes in the cell surface control the uptake and release of material from the cell, as well as controlling adhesiveness and cohesiveness. These properties may include invasion and metastases. It is not surprising that cell surface transplantation antigens are altered in malignancy. Although such tumor-specific antigens are not confined to the surface, it is on the surface of the intact cell that they are most readily detected. The tumor-specific transplantation antigens (TSTA) are present on the cell surface, and are responsible for and sensitive to the immune response in the host. This may result in tumor destruction.

Cell Kinetics or Cell Division

Only a portion of tumor cells are in an active growth cycle at any one time, and the synthesis of critical cellular constituents occurs during specific phases of that cycle. Much deeper understanding of selective toxicity during different phases of the cell cycle is needed, in addition to elucidation of the natural death of cells within the tumor, the fraction of cells in the tumor which can reproduce, and the techniques of killing cells which are not in the critical phases of synthesis. These types of information are required, particularly for slow growing, spontaneous neoplasms in experimental animals and in man.

Tumor cells watched at a distance from the closest capillary or beyond the blood brain barrier, may enjoy a pharmacologic sanctuary where adequate drug concentrations cannot reach them to exert lethal effects. Experimental and clinical research of this problem is required.

It is now well established that all renewing cells which are synthesizing DNA go through a series of phases. At the completion of mitosis, the cells spend a variable period of time in a resting phase (G1). During G1, DNA synthesis for cell replication apparently is absent, but does proceed for repair purposes, and RNA and protein synthesis continue normally. In late G1 (G1 minus synthesis conversion), an unknown signal initiates a burst of RNA synthesis. Shortly thereafter, the DNA synthesis (S phase) begins, and the cell is committed either to undergo division or remain polyploid. Next, the cells cease DNA synthesis during the G2 phase before entry into mitosis, although RNA and protein synthesis continue. Then, in mitosis, the rates of protein and RNA synthesis diminish abruptly, while the genetic material is segregated into daughter cells. An additional resting phase (G0) of the cell cycle has also been identified and described.

In summary, cellular reproduction (cell division cycle or cell kinetics) is divided into five phases:

1. Growth 1 (G1), which is postmitotic and takes up at least one-half the cell cycle of the cell.
2. Synthesis (S), in which the DNA content is doubled and takes up about 29% to 30% of the life cycle of the cell.
3. Growth 2 (G2), which occurs just before mitosis and takes up about 19% to 20% of the life cycle of the cell.
4. Mitosis (M), which takes up about 1% of the cell cycle.
5. Growth 0 (G0), the resting and undividing phase of the cell. This phase is variable and depends upon the type of cancer.

Tumor growth is dependent upon the proliferating pool (growth fraction) of the cells in the tumor mass. This concept of the proliferation pool or growth fraction can be briefly summarized as follows.

The rate of growth and the doubling time of small tumors is largely, but not entirely, dependent upon the percentage of cells in a mitotic cycle. Particularly in larger tumors, the rate of growth is also contingent upon the number of tumor cells spontaneously dying, or perhaps, becoming differentiated. The susceptibility of tumors to anticancer drugs is related to growth kinetics. Small tumor cell populations have a high proportion of cells in active cellular anabolism, leading to cell division (high-growth fraction). As a tumor mass increases, the growth fraction decreases. Many anticancer drugs are effective only against proliferating cells. Therefore, micrometastases that have a high-growth fraction should be much more susceptible to the killing effects of drugs, and this is clinically apparent in tumors. Moreover, experimental data are available to demonstrate this principle in a variety of animal tumor systems.

Based on this, the cell types in any individual tumor mass can be represented in three compartments (Figure 20-1). Compartment A includes the cells and cycle that are susceptible to most anticancer drugs, regardless of their mechanism of action. The cells in compartment B are in G0 or prolonged G1, and can convert to compartment A; however, while they remain in compartment B, they are relatively insensitive to agents ordinarily effective during cell division. Compartments A and B are interchangeable, but cells in either or both can enter compartment C, which comprises permanently nondividing cells destined ultimately to die. Most likely, tumor cell populations resemble the renewing population of normal cells. Some cell differentiation may be associated with inability to divide beyond one or two cell divisions, and thus tumor cells would be continually renewed from a tumor stem cell or clonogenic pool.

Such a model would explain current cytogenetic information, suggesting that cancer cells are not totally unresponsive to growth control mechanisms. While cell population kinetics provides an understanding of drug susceptibility in some tumors, it does not explain all successes and failures of drug therapy.

PHARMACOKINETICS

The reasons for success or failure are, in the final analysis, probably related to the pharmacologic disposition of drugs in patients. Even if the tumor is susceptible to a drug, it cannot influence the tumor in a favorable way unless it reaches the tumor site and remains there in tumoricidal concentration for a long enough period to kill the tumor cells. In general, the purpose of pharamcologic studies is to inform the physician how to get effective concentrations (C) of the drug to the target site for a long enough period of time (T) to bring about the desired effect. This is often referred to as the optimal C × T, and, in most diseases, can be approximated in man by studies in animals of the delivery of drugs to organs or tissues of interest. What makes cancer different is the need to relate optimal C × T to the phases of the cell cycle. The effectiveness of an antitumor agent is directly related to its C × T, which is markedly affected by dose and schedule. The tumor cells, and to some degree the critical normal tissues, present variable and fluctuating targets.

Knowledge of cell kinetics of normal tissue, which should remain relatively constant, and of tumor populations, can help determine the most effective means of obtaining an optimal C × T by the most ap-

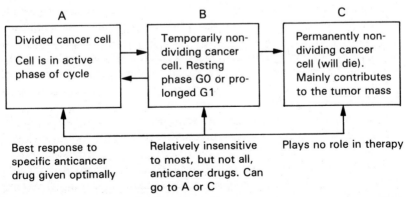

Figure 20-1 Conceptual model of types of cell growth in a tumor. Basic mechanism of cell vulnerability to anticancer drug therapy.

propriate doses and schedules. The optimal C × T should kill the maximal number of tumor cells with minimal lethality to cells of normal tissue.

Studies on cell kinetics reveal that certain anticancer drugs have a more predictable effect on different phases of the cell. For example, the alkylating agents attack cells in all phases of the cell cycle; antimetabolites attack the cell in the S phase, as does actinomycin D. Vincristine is a mitotic inhibitor and is most effective in the late G2 phase. Bleomycin has its most significant effect in the G2 phase.

The cell is relatively resistant to attack by anticancer drugs during the resting phase (G0). Many cells in a tumor population are at one time or another in phase G0, are at rest, and do not divide until some stimulus triggers the mitotic mechanism of cell division. Therefore, depending upon the nature of the cytotoxic agent, cells in the G0 phase are not susceptible to the drug's action. The reserved compartment of the hematopoietic system consists of cells in phase G0. Most of the drugs now used to treat cancer have little effect in the G0 phase.

Approximately 40% to 80% of the marrow stem cells are in phase G0 at any given time. When chemotherapeutic agents cause a decreased leukocyte count, the resting marrow cells temporarily enter the cell cycle and proliferate rapidly. This is a definite advantage when antineoplastic drugs are given.

Basis for Rational Cancer Chemotherapy

A single cancer cell following Gompertzian growth characteristics will eventually kill the host. Conversely, cure of cancer is possible only when the last lethal cell is eliminated from the body.

One of the principles of modern anticancer chemotherapy is the use of drugs in relation to the cell cycle or cell kinetics, in order to insure maximal therapeutic response and minimal toxicity. Currently, no single treatment, whether with one or several drugs, eliminates all neoplastic cells. Nevertheless, anticancer drugs reduce a constant percentage of tumor cells. This reduction is constant regardless of the number of cells present at the time of therapy. This means that cell destruction by drugs follows first-order kinetics. Most chemotherapeutic agents in any given dose kill the same *percentage,* not the same *number* of the cells.

As an example, take a chemotherapeutic agent with a 90% cell kill rate. It should be pointed out that, unless 90% of the cells in cycle are killed with each treatment, it is not possible to bring about a remission. Let us start with one million tumor cells. After the first injection, 900,000 cells are killed and 100,000 remain alive. After a second injection, 90,000 are killed and 10,000 remain alive. Eventually, for the last 10 cells, the same amount of drug must be used to reduce the tumor population by 90% or 9 cells. Thus, for ultimate therapeutic cure the same amount of drug is required with a low tumor cell burden as with a high one. Applying this principle, it is just as easy to reduce a million cancer cells to 10,000 as it is to reduce 100 cancer cells to 1. Both represent a 99% reduction. The ultimate goal of cancer chemotherapy is to eradicate the last cancer cell.

This is theoretically possible with constant chemotherapy. General toxicity, however, is a limiting factor. Cancer cells may eventually become resistant to the drugs as a result of selection from a mixed cell population. Resistance has been shown to result from the loss of activating enzymes, from the induction of synthetic enzymes, or from an increase in repair processes. Resistance can be minimized by the use of suitable drug combinations.

CELLULAR KINETICS

Cellular kinetics is the biological basis of cancer chemotherapy. Cancer cell population studies have demonstrated that each tumor cell divides into two cells, one for each generation time, the time for one entire division cycle. The time required for this cycle is about the same for all cells in a given population of cells. Since each tumor cell divides into two cells at each generation time, it is evident that by ten generations a single cell proliferates into a thousand (10^3) cells. Therefore, the growth of many cells following this pattern will result in a thousandfold increase every ten generations.

This growth pattern is referred to as exponential or logarithmic. When log cells are charted against time, the pattern is a smooth curve. It is possible to gain some insight into the effects of drugs on cancerous and normal cells by comparing the growth characteristics of each type. In order to be detected, the tumor must have a volume of at least 1 cc ($1 \times 1 \times 1$ cm) consisting of about one billion cells. The volume of cells necessary to kill a patient (critical volume) is 1000 cc ($10 \times 10 \times 10$ cm), or about 10^{12} power of cells (one trillion). Since these values are a thousandfold (10^{30}) apart, their separation in time represents ten generations of growth.

Cell Kill Hypothesis

Drugs used in the treatment of cancer are aimed at achieving selective kill of tumor cells. The survival of an animal with leukemia is inversely related either to the number of leukemia cells inoculated or the number remaining after treatment. Currently, well prescribed anticancer chemotherapy can reduce the population of lymphocytic leukemia cells from 10^{12} to 10^6 in acute lymphatic leukemia of childhood. Although the patient is not cured at this time, the disease is in remission. The goal of anticancer chemotherapy is to reduce the last million cells (10^6) to zero. It is accepted that 100% cell kill of leukemic cells is necessary to achieve cure. The assumption is based on work with the mouse leukemic cell. A single leukemic cell implanted into a mouse can multiply and eventually cause the death of the animal. The mouse leukemic cell reproduces in about 12 hours. After an interval of 20 days, one cell can multiply to approximately one billion cells, which is enough to kill the mouse. Since one cell can rapidly become a lethal number of cells, it is probably necessary to kill every leukemia cell to achieve a cure.

Studies have shown that a given dose of drug kills the same percentage of cells, no matter how many are present. For example, the same dose will kill 99% of 100,000 leukemia cells or 99% of 100 cells, whichever number of leukemic cells is present in the animal. Therefore, one million cells can be reduced to 10,000, 10,000 reduced to 100, 100 to 10 or less, and 10 cells to zero.

In leukemic mice, cures can be produced if the drug is administered on an intermittent schedule to allow for recovery of normal cells, if the dose is large enough so that the percentage of the cell population killed outpaces the multiplication of surviving leukemia cells. If the anticancer chemotherapy does not reduce the cell population by at least 75%, each day's multiplication of surviving cancer cells will outpace the inhibiting effect of the drug and will soon kill the animal.

Similar observations in leukemia in the human subject have been recorded. Estimates of the doubling time of human leukemic cells have ranged from two to eight days, but four-day doubling time has been more often assumed. Further calculations indicate that it takes about 160 to 170 days for one cell, doubling every four days, to reach one trillion cells, the number considered lethal for man.

Differences Between Cancer Growth and Normal Tissue Growth

1. All living things have an inherent capacity to multiply, and they cease multiplication for a variety of reasons. Cellular break is required to prevent overgrowth for the benefit of the community of cells. In vitro, this appears to be controlled by an unknown feedback mechanism, probably resulting from contact phenomena when cells are crowded.

2. In cancerous growth, cells no longer cease multiplying when they reach a critical mass, and the uncontrolled growth leads to death of the host.

3. Normal tissue is comprised of three types of cell populations as described above. After proliferation and embryonic life, a steady state of growth is reached in response to normal regulatory mechanisms.

4. A fundamental principle of all biologic systems is that, when a

certain cell mass is reached, there is cell die-off. The curve becomes more and more *asymptotic* with that seen in the steady state of normal tissue.

5. This curve, first described by Gompertz over 100 years ago, is known as the Gompertzian curve. As the tumor mass grows, tumor growth becomes less and less logarithmic. That is to say, initially it is logarithmic, like normal tissues, but then it becomes less so. As the tumor mass increases, the time it takes to double the volume increases.

6. Several kinds of cells are theoretically present in each tumor, ie, cells that are growing logarithmically and are very sensitive to the best drugs when optimally used, and cells that have temporarily stopped dividing and are partially or completely insensitive to drugs. These cells may grow actively, or the actively growing cells can move into the group that has temporarily stopped dividing. There is also a group of cells that are permanently nondividing, are not sensitive to drugs, and are no longer of concern to the chemotherapist. They are, however, of concern to the patient because they contribute to the tumor mass.

Skipper Model or Hypothesis

Drugs used in the treatment of cancer are designed to achieve selective kill of tumor cells. This concept is based on the cell kill hypothesis of Skipper and his colleagues (1964). It includes:

1. Survival of animals as inversely related to either the number of cells inoculated or to the number remaining after therapy.
2. A single underlying leukemic cell (or cancer cell) is capable of multiplying and killing the host.
3. A given drug kills a constant fraction (percentage) of cells, not a constant *number*, regardless of the number of cells present at the outset of therapy.
4. Drug dose and the ability to eradicate cancer cells are related.

Conclusion Improved results will occur if therapy is started before the volume of tumor is overwhelming.

Commonly Used Criteria for Objective Response and Disease Progression in Solid Tumors

Complete response Complete disappearance of all demonstrable disease.

Partial response More than 50% reduction in the sum of the products of the longest perpendicular diameters of discrete measurable disease, with no demonstrable disease progression elsewhere.

No response   No change in the size of any measurable lesion, or less than 50% reduction of measurable disease as defined above.

Progression   More than 50% increase in the sum of the products of the largest perpendicular diameter of any measurable lesion.

By cure is meant that the life expectancy of the treated cancer patient is the same as normal life expectancy; specifically, the same as that of the matched cohort in the general population.

IMMUNOTHERAPY VS CHEMOTHERAPY

The utilization of immunotherapy as an adjunct to surgery and/or radiotherapy rests on many of the same assumptions outlined for chemotherapy. The critical differences between immunotherapy and chemotherapy at this time within the framework of this strategy are as follows:

1. Immunotherapy is postulated to kill tumor cells by zero order of kinetics (fixed number).
2. Immunotherapy is postulated to be able to control only small numbers of cells.
3. Regression of advanced disease cannot be utilized as a predictor for adjuvant choice.
4. The correlation of tests which measure immune response enhancement with immune modulation, and tumor cell control is still not established.
5. The question of disease specificity with various tools for immune modulation remains to be established.

CLINICAL TRIALS

Preparations for Clinical Trials

After the development of an idea and synthesis of a new drug, or after the first evidence of activity of a compound isolated from a natural source, several steps are necessary before the drug can be used in cancer patients. Confirmation of the antitumor activity in the same screening system is essential, as well as a broad scale study and other known biologic screening systems. These include transplanted carcinomas, sarcomas, leukemias, those both sensitive and resistant to conventional chemotherapeutic agents, and miscellaneous tumors in mice, rats, and sometimes hamsters, guinea pigs, and rabbits which allow comparison of the biologic effects with that of other known compounds which have previously been tested in these systems.

After the activity of the compound has been confirmed, two general types of study ordinarily follow. One is undertaken to determine what the compound does and how it does it, and the other to test its effect on animals, which may predict some of its effects in man. Investigation of the mechanisms of action involve studies in cells and biochemical systems in vitro, as well as studies in the whole animal.

Preclinical Pharmacology

In preparation for use of a compound in man, it is critical to determine the drug's general metabolic characteristics and effects on other species. For this purpose the drug is tested in mice to determine that the dose of the compound which is lethal, and the relative ratio of the lethal dose to the therapeutic dose for several different tumor systems. Similar observations are made in rats and sometimes in other small animals.

A compound is administered by several routes, either orally, intravenously, subcutaneously, intramuscularly, or intraperitoneally, to determine differences in the rates of achieving high concentration in the blood and duration of drug activity.

Special test system While these studies are in progress, experimental therapy with unique animal systems is often in progress. Such studies as combinations of agents, treatment of tumors known to be resistant to particular agents, treatment in spontaneous tumors, combination therapy with surgery or radiation in animals, and the different selected schedules of drug administration, all may contribute information of value for clinical extrapolation.

Phase 1 trials and clinical pharmacology The first study of a new compound in man requires major skill in clinical pharmacology. One of the critical problems in a phase 1 study is how to reach the maximal tolerated dose (MTD) in the safest and most efficient fashion. Given the heterogeneity of anticancer drugs, it is not surprising that, although a variety of approaches have been tried, no current system can insure that the fewest number of patients receive either inordinately low or excessively toxic doses. The theoretical goal of a phase 1 study is to reach a single maximal tolerated dose for a particular dosage schedule. In actual practice, the maximal tolerated dose reached is often a function of the extent of prior therapy to which patients have been exposed. For example, patients with extensive prior chemotherapy or radiotherapy tolerate smaller doses of the drug, particularly those that are marrow suppressants, than patients with extensive prior treatment. When analyzing the results of a phase 1 study it is imperative to be aware of this patient selection factor before deciding upon the dose for further clinical investigation.

Phase 2 trials and combination therapy Phase 2 studies are investigations that determine whether a new drug has antitumor activity worthy of further clinical evaluation. The phase 2 trial is not planned to give definitive answers as to the ultimate value or role of a given drug. This is the purpose of the larger, phase 3 studies. In a sense, a phase 2 trial is a screen for antitumor activity and has the imperfections of any screening system. This phase concerns itself with the establishment of optimal dosage schedules and combinations of chemotherapeutic agents. This type of clinical investigation has produced such outstanding achievements as increasing the cure rate of metastatic choriocarcinoma from practically zero to greater than 75% and, in well-controlled centers, as high as 90+ % (in Burkitt's tumor from 0% to 50%). By the use of more rational dosage schedules in combination, the median survival rate in acute lymphoblastic leukemia has been increased from four months to 30 months, and the rates for five-year survival with no evidence of disease from 0% to as high as 20% or more in some series. These results emphasize the need for further imaginative studies in this area.

Phase 3 trials These are large scale trials to compare the efficacy of different applications of the various therapeutic modalities. Each of these requires extensive evaluation by critical observation in many patients with proper controls and in different institutions. For example, one such study now in progress has been undertaken to compare surgery plus 5-fluorouracil with surgery alone in surgically resectable large bowel cancer.

For a new drug, a phase 3 trial classically is a study in which the drug is given to large numbers of patients to determine if 1) the activity seen in phase 2 can be confirmed, 2) if unexpected events, such as new types of activity or adverse effects, occur, and 3) if the drug has any value in relation to other potential treatments.

Phase 3 is a major challenge. It is much more than an attempt to confirm the findings of phases 1 and 2; it is an attempt at total identification of the drug. What is not always appreciated or realized in phase 3 studies, is the amount of effort necessary to generate and retrieve essential information. In most cases, phase 3 trials are controlled clinical trials.

Drug dosage and schedules The optimal drug dosage is a critical variable in the management of patients with cancer. The treatment objective is to provide the patient with the maximal therapeutic benefit and the minimal amount of morbidity. Since anticancer drugs are only relatively selective for neoplastic cells as compared to host cells, most of the agents have a narrow therapeutic index.

The cancer chemotherapist must choose dosages within a narrow range because of the dose response relationship and the low therapeutic index for most antitumor drugs. The determination of the most appropriate dose is a complex clinical judgment that should be based on the therapeutic goal, the patient's anticipated tolerance to chemotherapy, and the characteristics of the drug to be used.

The therapeutic goal may be expressed as a risk and/or risk-to-benefit ratio; the morbidity of the treatment must be balanced with its potential benefits. In a patient with advanced cancer, who will die in a short period of time if untreated, highly aggressive use of the drug is warranted if a significant survival potential exists. If survival without treatment can be expected to be prolonged, then greater caution must be exercised with the drugs. In adjuvant trials, where drugs are given to some patients who have already been cured of their tumor, there must be cognizance of both acute toxic effects and long-term side effects. The clinician must make a judgment of the individual's potential tolerance to chemotherapy and decide upon a dosage schedule.

Substantial progress in the chemotherapy of cancer has been made, particularly over the past ten years. Further advances may be expected, but only after continuing research in basic pharmacology, biochemistry, and toxicology. Continued cooperation among all disciplines involved in clinical cancer care will be essential to organize and carry out carefully structured clinical trials for evaluation of new drugs, new drug combinations, and administration schedules. No matter how attractive the theory and the results of animal studies, only human clinical trials can provide the evidence of success.

Principles of chemotherapy   Prior to initiation of antineoplastic chemotherapy:

1. Establish a histologic diagnosis.
2. Evaluate the virulence of the tumor.
3. Reduce tumor burden.
4. Identify and measure residual disease from previous therapy.
5. Quantitate tumor markers.
6. Restore nutritional and metabolic balance.
7. Tailor the drug therapy to the type of tumor and the needs of the patient.
8. Inform the patient and/or his family of toxicity and complications of therapy.
9. Evaluate the performance of the patient's activity (as shown at the end of this chapter).

A brief outline of the principal groups of anticancer drugs used in the practice of gynecology and obstetrics is shown below.

A normogram for the determination of body surface area from height and weight is available from any pharamaceutical company marketing anticancer chemotherapy drugs.

When doses are expressed in mg/kg, the following formula can be used to convert to mg/m^2: mg/kg $\times$ 40 = mg/m^2. Depending on the drug, there may be an upper limit to the single dose given to patients weighing more than 70 kg.

ANTIMETABOLITES

Folic Acid Antagonists

Chemistry These are derivatives of folic acid. Folinic acid is 5-formyl tetrahydrofolic acid, a metabolically active reduced form of folic acid. It is also known as citrovorum factor.

Mechanism of action It blocks folic acid reductase to prevent availability of the single-carbon fragment. This in turn blocks purine ring biosynthesis. By a lesser action, it inhibits methylation of deoxyuridylic acid to thymidylic acid, blocking pyrimidine synthesis. It acts by relatively irreversible binding to dehydrofolate reductase, the enzyme that reduces folic acid to tetrahydrofolic acid. This depletes the cell of tetrahydrofolate, an important compound in one-carbon transfer, needed for the biosynthesis of thymidylic acid, an inosinic acid (part of RNA synthesis). Malignant cells have a high mitotic index requiring increased nucleic acid synthesis, and are thus affected to a greater extent than normal cells by the action of methotrexate. It is a cell-cycle specific for the S phase. The block in dehydrofolate reduction can be bypassed clinically by the use of folinic acid.

Drug interactions Weak organic acids, including salicylates, may delay renal excretion of this drug and thus lead to increased accumulation. Drugs with similar pharmacologic activity, such as pyrimethamine, should not be given to patients while they are receiving methotrexate.

Toxicity* mouth lesions, diarrhea, bone marrow depression, susceptibility to infection, alopecia, hyperpigmentation, teratogenesis, renal tubular necrosis, and osteoporosis.

Administration and dose 2.5–5 mg daily, by mouth, 0.4 mg/kg (maximum dose 25 mg) intravenously, daily for 4–5 days, 0.4 mg/kg intravenously, twice weekly. A large dose of methotrexate is currently followed by citrovorum factor rescue. Intravenous infusion of 20 to 300 mg/kg can be given every two to three weeks. From 2 to 12 hours after completion of the infusion, the patient is given leucovorin calcium, 6–16 mg/m^2, either intramuscularly or orally, repeated every 6 hours for 72 hours. The rationale is that the very high concentrations of intravenous methotrexate will result in preferential destruction of tumor cells. Citrovorum factor may then selectively enter and rescue normal cells.

Uses Choriocarcinoma, cancer of the ovary, cancer of the breast, and in combination with other anticancer drugs for treating cancer of the cervix.

---

*Renal function must be adequate and the urine output maintained, as well as normal hepatic function, prior to the start of treatment.

Pyrimidine Antimetabolites (Fluorouracil [5-FU])

Mechanism of action   Fluorouracil is a pyrimidine antimetabolite which acts by three possible mechanisms: 1) may block thymidylate synthetase, 2) may become incorporated to a small extent into RNA, producing a fraudulent RNA, 3) may inhibit utilization of pre-formed uracil in RNA synthesis by blocking uracil phosphatase. It must be metabolized to the nucleotide in vivo to be active, and is cell-cycle specific for the S phase.

Administration and dosage   12.5 mg/kg intravenously, daily for 3–5 days every four weeks; 15 mg/kg intravenously, weekly for six weeks.

Toxicity   Myelosuppression, stomatitis, gastrointestinal ulceration, nausea and vomiting, alopecia, and cerebellar ataxia.

Uses   Breast carcinoma, gastrointestinal tract adenocarcinoma, ovarian carcinoma, and experimental: other solid tumors.

Polyfunctional Alkylating Agents

Mechanism of action   An alkylating agent is one of many chemically active, chemically quite diverse, compounds that are employed for their cytotoxic (antineoplastic and immunosuppressive) activity. Over 700 compounds have been synthesized. In broad terms, they are all classified as cell-cycle nonspecific agents. Important sites of action appear to be on nucleic acids probably within the nucleus. This is suggested by the following observations that they: a) are mutagenic, b) are carcinogenic, c) preferentially deactivate DNA-containing viruses, d) inactivate the pneumococcal and *H. influenzae* transforming principles. Alkylation (insertion of an alkyl group) may interfere with synthesis of cross-linking in a number of places. This prevents H-bonding between chains of DNA. A monofunctional compound produces nuclear energy by a sheet mass effect. Polyfunctional agents are 50 to 100 times more active than monofunctioning agents. a) They are cross-linking agents. b) Reactive atoms bridge across two chromosomal strands and will react at two points on a chromosome. The specific mechanism of action of the alkylating agents stems from their ability to contribute a spontaneously derived, unstable alkyl group.

Toxicity   Delayed deaths may occur three to seven days after exposure to LD 50; decrease in antibody production; increased susceptibility to infection; diarrhea; ulceration of the gastrointestinal tract; hemorrhagic cystitis; involution in size of lymph nodes, thymus, and spleen; progressive fall in leukocytes and platelets in the peripheral blood; decrease in spermatogenesis; decrease in the number of ova; teratogenesis; alopecia.

Administration

Drug	Dosage
Mechlorethamine hydrochloride	0.4 mg/kg, intravenously single or divided doses
Chlorambucil	0.1–0.2 mg/kg/day, orally; 6–12 mg/day
Melphalan	0.2 mg/kg/day x 5, orally; 2–4 mg/day for maintenance
Cyclophosphamide	200 mg/day IV x 5, intravenously 50 mg bid, orally
Triethylenethiophosphoramide (thiotepa)	0.2 mg/kg x 5 days, intravenously
1,4 Dimethanesulfonyloxybutane	2–6 mg/day, orally (150–250 mg/course)
Nitroso-urea alkylating agents	
A. Carmustine (BCNU)	100 mg/m^2 every 6 weeks, intravenously. Next course in 4–6 weeks
B. Lomustine (CCNU)	120–150 mg/m^2 every 6 weeks, orally

Uses Carcinoma of the ovary, Hodgkin's disease, lymphoma, Burkitt's tumor, multiple myeloma, cancer of the breast, neuroblastoma, carcinoid, leukemia, and choriocarcinoma.

Antibiotics

Mechanism of action These agents form a complex with DNA involving selective binding at the guanine-cystosine segments, with a specific block in the DNA-dependent RNA synthesis (inhibits formation of messenger RNA [mRNA]).

Toxicity Damage to bone marrow and intestinal epithelium, nausea and vomiting, diarrhea, skin eruption, and skin necrosis.

NB Patients should be advised not to wear anything tight around their wrists, ankles, waist, or neck while they are taking these drugs because of the possibility of hyperpigmentation with necrosis.

Uses Lymphoma, leukemia, solid tumor, embryonal tumor, trophoblastic disease, carcinoid, and low calcium level (mithramycin).

Administration

Drug	Dosage
Actinomycin or Dactinomycin	0.01 mg/kg/day x 5 or 0.04 mg/kg weekly, intravenously
Daunorubicin hydrochloride	0.8–1.0 mg/kg/day x 3–6 days, intravenously. Total dose not to exceed 25 mg/kg
Mitomycin	0.06 mg/kg twice weekly if blood count permits
Doxorubicin	50–70 mg/m² in single or divided doses every 2 weeks
Mithramycin	25 μg/kg every other day for 3–4 days

Doxorubicin

Administration and dosage   60–75 mg/m², intravenously, single dose, every three weeks; 30 mg/m², intravenously, single dose, days 1– 3 inclusive, every four weeks. Doxorubicin is administered through a running intravenous infusion. Avoid giving this drug to patients with significant heart disease; reduce dosage in patients with impaired hepatic function.

Mechanism of action   Intercalation between base curves of DNA; inhibition of DNA-dependent synthesis.

Toxicity   Nausea and vomiting, diarrhea, stomatitis. Hematologic: leukopenia occurs 10–15 days after administration. The leukocyte count returns to normal approximately 21 days from the date of administration. Cardiac: EKG changes such as sinus tachycardia, ST-segment depression, voltage reduction, and arrhythmias, are indications to stop or defer treatment, congestive cardiac failure secondary to diffuse cardiomyopathy mandates discontinuation of treatment. Alopecia, which develops between the third and fourth week from the initial dose. Hair usually regrows completely within 2 to 5 months of cessation of therapy. Red urine (*not* hematuria).

The total cumulative dose of doxorubicin should not exceed 550 mg/m² since the risk of congestive heart failure increases markedly above this level. The patient should be observed for EKG abnormalities and signs of heart failure. Discontinue the drug if any of these appear. In multiple drug regimens it is probably preferable to keep the dose below the level of 500 mg/m².

Major indications   Ovarian cancer and sarcomas in the pelvis.

Bleomycin

Mechanism of action   This drug inhibits incorporation of thymidine into DNA and results in DNA fragmentation and strand scission. It is cell-cycle specific (reported to block the premitotic [G2] and mitotic [M] phase).

Administration and dosage   10–15 mg/m², intravenously or intramuscularly, once or twice weekly for a total dose of 300–400 mg. Use with caution in the presence of renal or pulmonary disease.

Toxicity   Nausea and vomiting; anorexia; stomatitis; allergic reactions such as fever, chills, hypotension, hyperpyrexia, cardiorespiratory collapse; dermatologic reactions such as desquamation of hands, feet, and pressure areas, hardening and tenderness of the tips of the fingers, ridging of the nails and, occasionally, bullous formation over pressure points, particularly the elbows, as well as alopecia, hyperpigmentation, and pruritic erythema. Pulmonary fibrosis: lung function should be monitored during treatment. The drug should be discontinued immediately if impairment of lung function is demonstrated, or if pulmonary changes are detected radiologically. The first signs and symptoms include cough, dyspnea, and bilateral basilar rales. Chest x-ray shows bilateral basilar and parahilar reticulonodular infiltrates with fibrosis. These changes may occur up to a month after the drug has been discontinued. Pulmonary function tests reveal a decreased vital and diffusion capacity. If the vital capacity decreases by more than 30% to 40% within four months, the drug must be discontinued. Myelosuppression.

Major indications   Esophageal cancer, cancer of the cervix, cancer of the vulva, squamous cell cancer of the head and neck, and testicular carcinoma.

MITOTIC INHIBITORS

Vinca Alkaloids

Chemistry   These drugs are extracted from the periwinkle plant.

Mechanism of action   They arrest mitosis in metaphase by destruction of spindles.

Toxicity   Nausea and vomiting, diarrhea, leukopenia, neurotoxic parasthesias, palsies, peripheral neuritis, alopecia, ileus, and syndrome of inappropriate secretion of antidiuretic hormone.

Administration and dosage   Vinblastine: 0.1–0.15 mg/kg, intravenously, weekly. Vincristine: 0.03–0.075 mg/kg, intravenously, weekly.

Indications   Choriocarcinoma, lymphoma, leukemia, Hodgkin's disease, ovarian cancer, Wilms' tumor, sarcomas (general), and rhabdomyosarcoma.

Enzymes (Asparaginase)

Mechanism of action   Asparaginase is an enzyme that catalyzes the hydrolysis of asparagine to aspartic acid and ammonia. Since asparagine is an essential amino acid and many tumors are deficient in the enzyme asparagine synthesis, asparaginase interferes with protein synthesis and tumor cell systems by its specific asparagine-depleting action.

Preparations are obtained from cultures of either *E. coli* or *Erwinia casotovora* and possess about 3% glutaminase activity. In addition to decreasing protein synthesis, a delayed but definite decrease in DNA and RNA synthesis is seen. It is cell-cycle specific for the postmitotic (G1) phase.

Normal cells can synthesize their own supply of asparagine. It appears that asparagine-deficient cells lack an enzyme (asparagine synthetase) which in normal cells converts aspartic acid to asparagine. Certain types of leukemia, such as acute lymphoblastic, have an asparagine dependence. This provides an explanation for the effect of asparaginase. The anti-tumor activity of asparaginase is also noted in transplanted rat tumors and in primary dog lymphosarcoma. The specific indications for the use of this agent in the treatment of malignancy remains to be determined.

Administration and dosage   50–200 IU/kg/day or 200–1000 IU/kg, intravenously, for 3–7 days each week for 28 days. Serum should be monitored for antibody to the drug prior to each dose.

Indication   Acute lymphoblastic leukemia.

Toxicity   Hypersensitivity reactions, neurotoxicity, hepatotoxicity, decreased protein synthesis, hyperglycemia, pancreatitis, and myleosuppression.

NONALKYLATING AGENT THERAPY

Hexamethylmelamine

Mechanism of action   Unknown. Although hexamethylmelamine structurally resembles triethylenemelamine, a known alkylating agent, it is not presently thought to act as an alkylating agent. Its activity is more like that of an antimetabolite, since it inhibits the incorporation of thymidine and uridine into DNA and RNA. Prolonged exposure of cells to hexamethylmelamine also inhibits protein synthesis. It is cell-cycle specific for the S phase.

Administration and dosage   12 mg/kg, orally, daily for 21 days, with a 4-week rest period. Alternatively, a low dose regimen of 8 mg/kg/day for periods of up to 90 consecutive days. The total daily dosage should be divided into four parts and given 1–2 hours after each meal and at bedtime. This may avoid some of the gastrointestinal side effects commonly seen with the use of this drug.

Toxicity Nausea and vomiting; may be severe. Hematologic, leukopenia, thrombocytopenia, anemia. Neurologic: A small percentage of patients will complain of paresthesias, numbness, sleep disturbances, and hallucinations. Ataxia, petit mal, and epilepsy-like seizures have been noted. Skin rashes, pruritus, and eczematous skin lesions have been reported infrequently. Alopecia, and skin rashes.

Major indications Ovarian carcinoma and bronchogenic carcinoma.

Cis-platinum

Mechanism of action Unknown. This is one of the many new platinum compounds being investigated for antitumor activity. Upon loss of a chloride atom, the drug binds to DNA, high molecular weight RNA, and transfer RNA. The resultant inhibition of DNA synthesis persists for several days following administration of the drug. It is a cell-cycle nonspecific agent.

Rosenberg (1975) reported that platinum complexes may disrupt antigenic masking on animal tumor cells, exposing what he thought might be new antigens at the cell surface, which generate a host immune reaction. He noted the appearance of densely stained patches associated only with the tumor cell membranes but not with normal cell membranes, and identified these as possibly masking antigens containing DNA.

Administration and dosage 80 mg/m², intravenously, every three weeks. Use a lower dosage in patients with any evidence of impaired kidney damage: 15–20 mg/m², intravenously, for five days, repeated every three weeks. Then, 50 mg/m², intravenously, as a single dose each week. Sixty to seventy-five mg/m², intravenously, every three weeks. Consult the specific protocol upon which the patient has been entered.

Toxicity Nausea and vomiting. Hematologic: leukopenia, thrombocytopenia, anemia. Renal toxicity: with doses above 3 mg/kg, the incidence of irreversible elevations of the serum creatinine is greater than 50%. At lower dosages, adequate hydration and mannitol will induce diuresis and help to prevent any significant renal toxicity. High frequency ototoxicity, characterized by tinnitus and hearing loss.

Major indications Ovarian cancer, testicular cancer, and bladder cancer.

NEWER AGENTS AND OTHER AGENTS THAT HAVE NOT BEEN EVALUATED IN GYNECOLOGIC CANCER

1. Cytembena
2. Porfiromycin
3. Porcarbazine

4. F Torafur
5. Streptozotocin
6. DTIC

DISCUSSION

It appears from a review of the literature on cures of cancer by chemotherapy, that this modality today stands about where infectious disease therapy stood in 1937, at which time it was established that chemotherapy could cure certain systemic streptococcal infections. There are now drugs that will cure more than 50% of patients with a few types of disseminated tumors. As in 1937, when infectious disease chemotherapists had nothing effective against staphylococcus, gram negative bacilli, streptococci, or viruses, the cancer chemotherapist now has only palliative rather than curative therapy available for most of the carcinomas and other slow growing tumors. Once the curative potential of antimicrobial therapy was established against a few infections, a massive research program was mounted, and it was only a relatively few years until the majority of bacterial infections were brought under chemotherapeutic control. Similarly, the significant percentage of cures achieved in the few previously mentioned metastatic tumors, leukemias, and gynecologic cancers demonstrates the potential curability of widespread neoplastic disease by chemotherapy.

As was the case in bacterial infections in 1937, the potentiality of chemotherapeutic cure of cancer has now become apparent, and there is sufficient technical knowledge to begin to mount a large scale chemotherapeutic program against other forms of widespread neoplastic disease.

The following steps must be taken when anticancer chemotherapy is employed:

1. Measure volume of any remaining tumor
2. Assess patient's physiologic state
3. Decide when to stop treatment or change drugs
4. Observe patient throughout her life

SCALE OF PERFORMANCE STATUS

Karnofsky Performance Status

100 = Normal; no complaints; no evidence of disease
90 = Able to carry on normal activity; minor signs or symptoms or disease

562

80 = Normal activity with effort; some sign or symptoms of disease
70 = Cares for self, but unable to carry on normal activity or do active work
60 = Requires occasional assistance, but is able to care for most personal needs
50 = Requires considerable assistance and frequent medical care
40 = Disabled; requires special care and assistance
30 = Severely disabled; hospitalization indicated, although death not imminent
20 = Very sick, hospitalization necessary; active supportive treatment necessary
10 = Moribund; fatal process progressing rapidly
0 = Dead

Zubrod Status

0 = No symptoms
1 = Symptoms, fully ambulatory
2 = Requires nursing assistance or equivalent, bedridden < 50% of normal day
3 = Bedridden > 50% of normal day
4 = Bedfast

BIBLIOGRAPHY

Barber HRK: Editorial Comments, in Barber HRK, Graber EA (eds): *Surgical Disease in Pregnancy,* Philadelphia, WB Saunders Co., 1974, p 718.

Baserga R: The relationship of the cell cycle to tumor growth and control of cell division. *Cancer Res.* 25:581, 1965.

Blum RH, Carter SK: Adriamycin, a new anticancer drug with significant activity. *Ann Int Med* 80:249, 1974.

Blum RH, Carter SK, Agre K: A clinical review of bleomycin—a new antineoplastic agent. *Cancer* 31:903, 1973.

Bruce WR, Meeker BE, Valeriote FA: A comparison of the sensitivity of normal hematopoietic and transplanted lymphoma colony forming cells to chemotherapeutic agents administered in vivo. *J Natl Cancer Inst* 37:233, 1966.

Carter SK, Slavik M: Investigational drugs under study by the United States National Cancer Institute. *Cancer Treat Rev* 3:43, 1976.

Carter SK: Study design principles for the clinical evaluation of new drugs as developed by the chemotherapy program of the National Cancer Institute, in Staquet M (ed): *The Design of Clinical Trials in Cancer Therapy,* Brussels, Editions Scientifiques Europeenes, 1972, pp 242–289.

DeVita VT, Wasserman TH, Young RC, et al: Prospectives on research in gynecologic oncology. Treatment protocols. *Cancer* 38:161, 1976.

Feinstein AR, Pritchett JA, Schimpff CR: The epidemiology of cancer therapy. The clinical course: data, decision and temporal demarcations. *Arch Int Med* 123:323, 1969.

Frytak S, Moertel CG, Schutt AJ, et al: A phase I study of cytembena. *Proc Am Assoc Cancer Res* 16:36, 1975.

Gehan EA, Schneiderman MA: Experimental design of clinical trials, in Holland JE, Frei E, III (eds): *Cancer Medicine.* Philadelphia, Lea and Febiger, 1973.

Gehan EA, Freireich EJ: Nonrandomized controls in cancer clinical trials. *N Engl J Med* 290:198, 1974.

Hammond CB, Borchert LG, Tyrey L, et al: Treatment of metastatic trophoblastic disease: Good and poor prognosis. *Am J Obstet Gynecol* 115:451, 1973.

Hersh EM, Carbone PP, Freireich EJ: Recovery of immune responsiveness after drug suppression in man. *J Lab Clin Med* 67:566, 1966.

Krakoff JH: *Cancer chemotherapeutic agents.* Professional Education Publication Monograph, New York, American Cancer Society, 1977.

Pinkel D: The use of body surface area as a criterion of drug dosage in cancer chemotherapy. *Cancer Res* 18:853, 1958.

Potter VR: Sequential blocking of metabolic pathways in vivo. *Proc Soc Exp Biol Med* 76:41, 1951.

Rosenberg B: Possible mechanisms for the antitumor activity of platinum coordination complexes. *Cancer Chemother Rep* Part 1, 59:589, 1975.

Sartorelli AC: Some approaches to the therapeutic exploitation of metabolic sites of vulnerability of neoplastic cells. *Cancer Res* 29:2292, 1969.

Schneiderman MA: How do you know you've done any better? *Cancer* 35:64, 1975.

Silver RT, Lanper RD, Jarowski CI: *A Synopsis of Cancer Chemotherapy.* New York, Dun-Donnelley Publishing Co, 1977.

Skipper HE: Clowes Memorial Lecture. *Cancer Res* 31:1173, 1971.

Skipper HE, Schabel FM, Wilcox WS: Experimental evaluation of potential anticancer agents. On the criteria and kinetics associated with "curability" of experimental leukemia. *Cancer Chemother Rep* 35:1, 1964.

Tan C, Rosen G, Ghavini F: Adriamycin in pediatric malignancies. *Cancer Chemother Rep* 6:259–266, 1976.

Wampler GL, Mellette SJ, Kuperminc M, et al: Hexamethylmelamine in the treatment of advanced cancer. *Cancer Chemother Rep* 56:505, 1972.

Wiltshaw E, Kroner T: Phase II study of cis-diamine-dichoro-platinum in advanced adenocarcinoma of the ovary. *Cancer Treat Rep* 60:55, 1976.

Young RC: Chemotherapy of ovarian cancer: Past and present. *Semin Oncol* 2:267, 1975.

Zelen M: Keynote address on biostatistics and data retrieval. *Cancer Chemother Rep* 4:31, 1974.

Zubrod CG, Schneiderman M, Frei E, et al: Appraisal of methods for the study of chemotherapy of cancer in man: Comparative therapeutic trial of nitrogen mustard and triethylene thiophosphoramide. *J Chron Dis* 11:7–33, 1960.

21 Infectious Disease in Gynecologic Oncology

W. David Hager

Recent emphasis on the study of infectious disease in obstetrics and gynecology has encompassed all of the subspecialty areas, including gynecologic oncology. The purpose of this chapter is to indicate what is known in the field, but even more to point out what is deficient in our fund of knowledge since there are so few well-designed studies available.

PATHOGENESIS

Postoperative infections of the pelvis are caused by organisms that comprise the normal cervicovaginal flora (Ohm et al 1975). These organisms are opportunistic, and any change in the inoculum of organisms, their virulence, or a reduction in host resistance may allow these commensals to become the pathogens of severe pelvic infections.

There are data to indicate that patients with invasive carcinoma of the cervix have an altered cervicovaginal flora that is very similar to that of immunosuppressed renal transplant patients (Mead 1978). This change in flora results in a decrease in lactobacilli, *Staphylococcus epidermidis* and enterococci with a concomitant increase in *Escherechia coli* and anaerobic gram negative bacilli. The patient with cervical cancer who is treated with surgery or radiation is thus exposed to this altered flora of potential pathogens. These data confirm the fact that preoperative culturing is of little value in determining what the postoperative pathogen may be. They do offer guidance in selecting an appropriate antibiotic(s) for treatment of patients with postoperative and postirradiation infections since aerobic, gram-negatives and anaerobes are the most frequent causative organisms.

Patients with gynecologic malignancies are at risk for the development of posttreatment infections due to several predisposing factors including: altered immunity, surgical manipulation, chemotherapy, and radiation therapy. An increased risk of pelvic infection following radiation therapy has been documented by Kottmeier (1964), and Frick and co-workers (1960) in spite of the evidence by Blythe (1978) that radiation of itself does not alter the normal vaginal flora. Active pelvic infection contraindicates radiation therapy due to the decreased efficacy of treatment in poorly oxygenated tissues, and the increased risk of radiation complications in this group of patients (van Nagell et al 1977).

TYPES OF POSTOPERATIVE INFECTIONS

There are a number of different categories of postoperative and postirradiation infectious morbidity. It is essential that the diagnostic criteria for these entities be well defined and adhered to since the treatment and necessity for surgical intervention varies among the diagnoses.

1. *Cuff cellulitis* — Fever, leucocytosis, inflammation, and induration of the vaginal cuff along with purulent exudate from the cuff.
2. *Cuff abscess* — Fever, leucocytosis, and a tender, fluctuant mass involving the vaginal cuff.
3. *Wound infection* — Erythema, purulent exudate, and breakdown of the incision. Dehiscence may be superficial or involve the fascia.
4. *Pneumonia* — A chest x-ray consistent with the diagnosis or a positive sputum culture.
5. *Urinary tract infection* — A positive sterilely collected urine culture.
6. *Pyometra* — Fever, leucocytosis, uterine tenderness, and purulent exudate from the endocervix.
7. *Septic pelvic thrombophlebitis* — A diagnosis of exclusion with persistent fever in spite of antibiotic therapy for pelvic infection and pulse that is asynchronous with temperature.

DIAGNOSIS

Any patient with a pelvic malignancy is at risk for pelvic infection due to the proximity of the malignant focus to the altered vaginal flora previously mentioned. Whenever such a patient develops fever, tachycardia, leucocytosis, and pelvic tenderness, a diagnosis of pelvic infection must be considered. After careful evaluation of all body systems, attention should be directed to the pelvis. A Gram's stain of any material obtained from the infected site should be done in order to determine if there is a predominant pathogen present. This information may be useful in the selection of an antibiotic(s) for treatment of the infection. When obtaining material for culture, aspirated specimens are preferred since swab specimens are less satisfactory for accurate anaerobic results. There are several double-lumen techniques being evaluated for obtaining specimens from the pelvis. Blood cultures should be obtained using appropriate sterile technique. After diagnosis and initial treatment, it is essential that culture results and sensitivity patterns be evaluated so that appropriate changes in therapy may be made if necessary. The use of minimal inhibitory concentrations (MIC) is beneficial in the determination of sensitivity and appropriate dosage.

THERAPY

There is a need for well-designed, randomized, controlled, double-blind studies to evaluate treatment of cancer-related infections. Pelvic infections are often polymicrobial with a predominance of gram-negative aerobes and anaerobes. Antibiotic selection should take into account the most predominant pathogens. Single-agent therapy may include ampicillin, a cephamycin or a third-generation cephalosporin. Multiple-agent therapy may include: 1) penicillin or a cephalosporin/aminoglycoside/anaerobic coverage, 2) an aminoglycoside/clindamycin or chloramphenicol, or 3) ampicillin or cephalosporin/metronidazole. Since more than 90% of pelvic abscesses are anaerobic in etiology, the presence of such an abscess necessitates treatment with an agent effective against anaerobes, and often requires surgical drainage or extirpation. The diagnosis of septic pelvic thrombophlebitis will require the addition of heparin to the antibiotic therapy.

Antibiotics should be administered parenterally, in adequate recommended dosages when treating serious pelvic infections. Toxicity of the antibiotic must be monitored carefully in order to prevent the development of serious side effects. The patient should be treated until she is clinically improved and afebrile for 48 to 72 hours. The antibiotics may then be discontinued or an oral antibiotic substituted and continued for seven to ten days.

568

Patients who develop a pyometra are best treated by drainage of the uterine infection by sounding the endometrium or removal of the radiation implant. Antibiotics should also be used in treating such patients.

ANTIBIOTIC PROPHYLAXIS

There is a paucity of well-designed, randomized, controlled, double-blind studies evaluating the use of prophylactic antibiotics to prevent serious infectious morbidity in women undergoing radical surgery in gynecologic oncology. Data from studies evaluating prophylaxis in vaginal hysterectomy have indicated a beneficial effect in reducing febrile and infectious morbidity. Unpublished data (Spence) also indicates a beneficial effect of single-dose antibiotic prophylaxis in women undergoing radical hysterectomy for carcinoma of the cervix. Antibiotics should be administered just prior to or within two hours of making the incision (Burke 1961). Guidelines for administration have been detailed by Ledger et al 1975. Guidelines for the use of prophylactic antibiotics in

Table 21-1
Guidelines for Use of Prophylactic Antibiotics in Gynecologic Surgery

1. Limit to situations of high risk.
2. Cover the most common pathogens.
3. Establish tissue levels before the incision.
4. Use short course (less than 48 hours).
5. Use a single agent.
6. Reserve valuable antibiotics.
7. Toxicity of antibiotic less than risk of infection.
8. Use to prevent serious infection, not just fever.

BIBLIOGRAPHY

Blythe JG: Cervical bacterial flora in patients with gynecologic malignancies. *Am J Obstet Gynecol* 131:438–445, 1978.

Burke JF: The effective period of preventive antibiotic action in experimental incisions and dermal lesions. *Surgery* 50:161, 1961.

Frick HC, Taylor HC, Guttmann RH, et al: A study of complications and radiation therapy of cancer of the cervix. *Surg Gynecol Obstet* 111:493–496, 1960.

Kottmeier HL: Complications following radiation therapy in carcinoma of the cervix and their treatment. *Am J Obstet Gynecol* 88:854–866, 1964.

Ledger WJ, Gee C, Lewis WP: Guidelines of antibiotic action in experimental incisions and dermal lesions. *Am J Obstet Gynecol* 121:1038–1045, 1975.

Mead PB: Cervical-vaginal flora of women with invasive cervical cancer. *Obstet Gynecol* 52:601–604, 1978.

Ohm MJ, Galask RP: Bacterial flora of the cervix from 100 prehysterectomy patients. *Am J Obstet Gynecol* 122:683–687, 1975.

Spence MR: Unpublished data.

van Nagell JR, Parker JC, Maruyama Y: The effect of pelvic inflammatory disease on enteric complications following radiation therapy for cervical cancer. *Am J Obstet Gynecol* 128:767–771, 1977.

22 Total Parenteral Nutrition

Charles T. Van Buren
Stanley J. Dudrick

Intravenous hyperalimentation (IVH) has been used successfully in the management of many patients who cannot eat due to anatomic or functional disruption of the alimentary tract. The success of this regimen in supporting patients suffering from gastrointestinal malignancy has been ascribed to nutritional restoration of individuals whose tumors mechanically obstructed, or otherwise interfered with normal digestion. Extension of this experience to patients with other malignancies, however, has revealed that the incidence of malnutrition may be higher than anticipated in individuals who suffer from disseminated extra-alimentary cancer. Furthermore, as combined oncologic regimens of multiple drug chemotherapy, aggressive radiotherapy, and extirpative surgery have been used more frequently, especially in some of the later stages of ovarian carcinoma, the scope of patients who may benefit from aggressive nutritional therapy has expanded. Those clinically experienced in the management of patients with advanced ovarian or endometrial cancer can attest to the high frequency with which malnutrition afflicts these patient populations. However, because such individuals may be more malnourished than previously realized, the advantages of an intravenous rather than an enteral means of therapy and the attendant risks must be reviewed critically.

Enthusiasm for the use of IVH in the treatment of cancer patients has not been very great until recently. This is because of the concern that the growth of the malignancy might be accelerated by the provision of concentrated nutrients, and that the risk of sepsis may be increased in a group of immunocompromised patients. Moreover, the risk of infection is accentuated by the neutropenia induced by chemotherapy, or the loss of T-lymphocyte responsiveness associated with extensive radiotherapy, as initially documented in patients with Hodgkin's disease (Fuchs 1976). Furthermore, in patients with disseminated gynecologic tumors who are often likely to develop both ascites and malignant pleural effusions, fluid overload as a consequence of aggressive IVH poses yet another concern. In order to balance properly the risk of IVH in patients having gynecologic malignancies with the benefit to be obtained from such nutritional intervention, the specific needs and problems of this group of patients must be examined. One must consider both the metabolic burden imposed by the spreading malignancy, and the natural history of the disease in order to help determine the most opportune and effective means of nutritional therapy.

The primary objective of IVH is to provide exclusively by vein those essential nutrients that are required for the maintenance of optimal nutrition in patients who cannot meet these requirements by oral intake. Objective evidence for success in such therapeutic ventures has been the establishment of positive nitrogen balance, or an anabolic state in individuals who have suffered erosion of their endogenous energy stores. In order to understand which patients might benefit most from total parenteral nutrition, one must define the host stresses resulting from disseminated malignancies, the nutrient requirements of both tumor and host, the host-tumor interaction and its modulation by the nutritional state, and the special stresses imposed by treatment programs of chemotherapy, radiation therapy, and extirpative surgery.

A prominent feature of patients harboring an occult malignancy is the history of recent weight loss. Although such a sign associated with gastrointestinal malignancy may result from interference with normal mechanical or physiologic function of the gut, the explanation for this common complaint of patients suffering with cancer is much more complex. Fundamental alterations in cellular metabolism are often linked to the transformation of neoplastic cells. Warburg (1931) observed that anaerobic glycolysis was increased in neoplastic cells, and hypothesized that tumor cells had an inherent defect in cellular respiration. More recent investigations have revealed that the dependence of a cell upon glycolysis and anaeorbic metabolism for its energy metabolism is determined by the rate of growth of the tumor. Slow growing, well-differentiated tumors demonstrate normal respiration and aerobic glycolysis. However, virtually all tumors that have been studied have increased activity of key glycolytic enzymes, decreased activity of the key gluconeogenic enzymes, and increased synthesis of isoenzymes that are less responsive to nutritional and endocrine regulation (Weber 1977). All of these transformational events result in neoplastic cells competing favorably with normal tissue for a limited energy substrate.

These alterations in metabolism are not limited to glycolysis and gluconeogenesis. Activity in the pentose phosphate pathway is increased in neoplastic cells. Tumor purine biosynthesis and utilization is increased compared with normal tissue, whereas activity of nucleotide catabolic enzymes is decreased. Thus, tumors are less dependent upon the availability of nucleotides from the environment, or on hormonal activity for their biosynthesis than are normal tissues. The elevated level of serum uric acid in patients with rapidly growing malignancies is an index of the increased rate of purine catabolism in cancer patients. Such neoplastic transformation makes possible maximal tumor growth (Weber 1977).

As one might anticipate, such biochemical changes result in an increased metabolic rate in patients who have malignancies. The basal metabolism of cancer patients is elevated 10% to 15%, compared with control populations having similar degrees of activity (Holroyde 1975). This increment presumably reflects the increased energy required by the rapidly growing neoplastic cell population. Fever due to the release of endogenous pyrogens, a feature of some lymphoproliferative malignancies, imposes an additional energy burden, and leads to increased gluconeogenesis in order to meet the body's energy needs.

While experimental animals who have been inoculated with tumors often gain weight as their tumor burden grows in proportion to the weight of normal body tissue, patients manifest weight loss as a protean clinical manifestation of cancer. Not only are the energy needs increased in patients who are suffering from malignancies, but the oral intake is also diminished. This cachexia develops even if the tumor does not interfere with the function of vital organs, such as the liver or the intestine. Malnutrition may result from loss of appetite, perhaps secondary to as yet undefined tumor-induced changes in the normal physiologic response of the hypothalamus and central nervous system to hunger. Abnormalities in taste perception have been documented in patients with cancer (DeWys 1974). Anemia secondary to bleeding in the intestinal tract or decreased red blood cell production may contribute to the sense of malaise which prevents the cancer patient from carrying on normal activities. All of these factors lead to the nutritionally deprived state that seems to be a regular feature of patients with widespread malignancy.

The consequences of the weight loss and malnutrition found in patients suffering from cancer are great. The treatment of neoplasms through chemotherapy, radiation therapy, surgery, or a combination of these modalities can be a long and debilitating process. If the endogenous protein and energy stores in patients have already been depleted by the disease, the individual is at greater risk to develop a complication of the treatment of the tumor. The incidence of poor wound healing, infection, and mortality following definitive surgery for malignancies is higher in patients suffering from malnutrition prior to the operation (Copeland 1977). The anorexia and diarrhea which may result from radiation or chemotherapy add an additional period of starvation to patients who are already weakened by their disease. Unless normal intake of calories and protein is restored in these patients, they may develop medical complications which preclude completion of the treatment regimen for the malignancy. Finally, both experimental and clinical studies suggest that nonspecific immune responsiveness is depressed in cancer patients, and that successful treatment is contingent upon reversing this immunosuppression (Catalona 1973, Daly 1980).

Nutritional support of malnourished tumor-bearing rats that are anergic to challenge with an intradermally injected antigen, results in weight gain, restored immunocompetence, and longer survival when compared with control animals maintained on a protein deficient diet (Daly 1976). Tumor growth is not stimulated out of proportion to total weight gain in the animals that are restored nutritionally. Further animal studies reveal that rats nourished by IVH have a better response to a chemotherapeutic regimen than do orally fed control animals (Souchon 1975). Malnourished cancer patients were identified by three objective criteria: 1) a recent unintentional loss of 10% or more body weight, 2) a serum albumin concentration less than 3.4 gm/dl, 3) or a negative delayed cutaneous hypersensitivity response to a battery of five microbial antigens. In 406 cancer patients supported by IVH prior to, or during chemotherapy, radiation therapy, or extirpative surgery for their tumors, the average duration of IVH was 24 days, and the average weight gain during this period was five pounds. To document the incidence of catheter infections, all IVH catheters were cultured on removal. Pathogenic organisms were grown from 4.4% of all catheters; however, only 10 patients (2.3%) had simultaneously positive blood and catheter cultures. Another source of sepsis was identified in three of these ten patients, resulting in 1.6% of patients who developed IVH catheter-associated sepsis. No serious morbidity or mortality resulted from these infections, which resolved once the catheters were removed. This experience has been shared by the group at the Henry Ford Hospital, who have found no greater incidence of infectious complications in neutropenic cancer patients who are supported by IVH when compared with a similar neutropenic control population (Dindogru 1980).

Though the risk of treatment is small, the benefit accrued by patients supported by IVH can be significant. In a group of 22 malnourished patients with non-oat cell carcinoma of the lung, 10 of the patients were supported by IVH. Fifty percent of this IVH group responded to chemotherapy, while none of the remaining 12 non-IVH patients responded to the same chemotherapeutic regimen (Lanzotti 1975). In a prospective study of cancer patients who are anergic to recall skin test antigens, IVH improved response to chemotherapy. Patients who converted to a positive response to recall antigens while receiving IVH, had a 52% response to chemotherapy, while no patients who became anergic on IVH responded to treatment (Daly 1976). Cancer patients receiving chemotherapy experienced fewer episodes of neutropenia while receiving IVH when compared with a patient group receiving a similar treatment regimen (Issell 1978). The clinical information suggests that both the tolerance of toxic drug effects and the tumor response to chemotherapy are increased in patients supported by IVH.

Recent studies from this laboratory have suggested that defined diets alter the growth pattern of subcutaneously inoculated tumors in mice. The defined diets used are nutritionally comparable in some respects to the solutions used for IVH, raising the question of whether diets can be formulated which will specifically suppress tumor growth in both animals and man. As experience is gained with the use of formulated solutions in the treatment of patients with widespread malignancy, a better understanding of the influence of diet on tumor growth, chemotherapeutic drug metabolism, and on the interaction between tumor and host will be reached.

PREPARATION OF HIGH CALORIE SOLUTIONS

The basic hypertonic nutrient solution used for total parenteral nutrition consists of approximately 20% to 25% dextrose and 4% to 5% crystalline amino acids (Table 22-1). This solution provides 5.25 to 6 gm of nitrogen (32 to 37 gm of protein equivalent) and 900 to 1000 nonprotein calories/liter. Added to this solution are the minerals and vitamins based upon the requirements of the individual patient. These solutions can be prepared from commercially available stocks by a pharmacist or technician using strictly aseptic mixing technique. Kits containing the basic solutions and transfer apparatus have made possible the development of home hyperalimentation regimens for patients. Individual units of base solutions may be mixed aseptically in a laminar flow filtered air hood, adding 500 ml of 50% dextrose solution to 500 ml of 8.5% amino acid solution. Usually 40 to 50 mEq/liter of sodium chloride or acetate is added per liter of solution as well as 30 to 40 mEq of potassium as chloride, and/or acid phosphate. Sodium requirements are based upon the losses via urine or enteric drainage, while potassium is one of the major intracellular cations required for synthesis of lean body mass. Sodium requirements are decreased in patients with significant cardiovascular, renal or hepatic disease. Approximately 20 mEq of phosphate per 1000 calories is administered daily as well as 15 to 20 mEq of magnesium, as magnesium chloride. The requirements for phosphate, potassium, and magnesium may be decreased in patients with renal or hepatic dysfunction, and these additives will have to be modified according to individual patient needs. One ampule of parenteral water-soluble vitamins and one ampule of calcium gluconate are provided daily to meet adult requirements. Although the American Medical Association has recommended the addition of trace elements to all parenteral hyperalimentation regimens (*JAMA* 1979), this has not been common practice at the University of Texas Medical School at Houston. None of the reported trace element deficiency states have been documented at this institution, possibly due to the liberal use of fresh frozen plasma infusion, and the relatively short duration of therapy in oncology patients. Iron may be added to the solution daily or weekly in calculated doses to treat deficiency of this micronutrient. Zinc sulfate (5 mg/day) and copper (1 mg/day) may be added to solutions of patients on long term intravenous hyperalimentation. Folate (1 mg) is added to the solution daily, and 10 mg of vitamin K is delivered by intramuscular injection weekly. Vitamin B_{12} (1 mg) is administered monthly.

Controversy has arisen over the use of parenteral lipid preparations as a calorie source in patients supported totally by intravenous nutrition. Currently available lipid emulsions, such as Intralipid, and Liposyn, have the same caloric density (1 Cal/ml) as a standard hypertonic dextrose amino acid solution. Consequently, there is little or no advantage to infusing lipid emulsions to deliver more calories to patients. The available lipid emulsions are a more expensive calorie source than hypertonic dextrose, which has influenced this center to rely on lipid emulsions primarily as a source of essential fatty acids. Three times per week, 500 ml of 10% lipid emulsion is infused by piggyback administration through the IVH tubing. Using this regimen the complications of essential fatty acid deficiency have been avoided.

Modification of the standard IVH formula is required for treatment of patients with congestive heart failure, renal failure, or hepatic failure. Table 22-2 reveals the composition used for the treatment of patients with acute or chronic renal failure who require total parenteral nutrition. Base units consisting of 600 ml of 70% dextrose, 200 ml of 8.5% amino acid solution, and 200 ml of 5.4% essential amino acid solution are mixed in this pharmacy. The overall mixture contains approximately 28 gm of amino acids and 420 gm of dexrose per liter. Such a mixture provides the essential amino acid enrichment required by patients with renal failure. However, this formula offers enough nonessential amino acids to avoid the protein malnutrition ascribed as a consequence of restricted protein, high carbohydrate oral diets in patients with chronic renal failure (Kaye 1968). Magnesium, potassium, and phosphate are added to this mixture as needed. Patients who suffer from hepatic failure have been treated with

Table 22-1
Preparation of Adult Intravenous Hyperalimentation Solution

Base Solution	
50% dextrose in water	500 ml
8.5% crystalline amino acids	500 ml
Additives to Each Unit	
Sodium chloride	40-50 mEq
Potassium chloride	20-30 mEq
Potassium acid phosphate	15-30 mEq
(10-20 mM phosphorus)	
Magnesium sulfate	15-18 mEq
Additives to Any One Unit Daily	
Calcium gluconate 10%	4.5 mEq
Multivitamin infusion (MVI-12)	10 ml
Zinc sulfate	5 ml
Copper sulfate	1-2 mg
Imferon (iron dextran injection)	0.1 ml
Additive to Any One Unit Twice Weekly	
Vitamin K	10 mg
Optional Additives per Unit	
Insulin	5-50 units
Albumin	12.5-25 gm
Heparin	2000-6000 units
Cimetidine	300-800 mg
Carbohydrate calories	850 kcal/L
Protein calories	150 kcal/L
Fat calories	500-1000 kcal/L
Nitrogen	6.5 gm/L
Amino acids	40 gm/L

mixtures which are rich in branched chain amino acids (tryptophan and phenylalanine). Though such solutions have proven efficacious in treatment of hepatic coma (Fischer 1976), the solutions are of unproven benefit for the treatment of patients with chronic liver disease. Moreover, no evidence exists which supports the use of such solutions in the treatment of patients with liver failure secondary to hepatic tumor metastases. Generally, the dictum for treatment of patients with hepatic insufficiency is to restrict protein intake based upon clinical signs of hepatic insufficiency, elevated serum ammonia, and serum amino acid levels. Increased levels of aromatic amino acids in the blood stream should lead to the reduction of protein intake. Generally, in patients with severe hepatic disease, the dextrose content of the solutions is reduced to provide a mixture containing 15% to 20% carbohydrates. Reduction in the dextrose load appears to reduce the problem of hepatic fatty infiltration which is a greater risk in a patient with diminished hepatic function.

Table 22-2

Preparation of Intravenous Hyperalimentation Solution for Renal Failure Patients

Base Solution	
50-70% dextrose solution	600 ml
8.5% amino acid solution	200 ml
5.4% essential amino acid solution	200 ml
Additives	
Folate	1mg
Multivitamins	5 ml concentrate vial
MgSO	As needed
KHPO$_4$	As needed
NaCl	As needed
Calcium gluconate	As needed
ZnSO$_4$	5 mg/day
CuSO$_4$	1 mg/day
To be added as required by the individual patient	
Nonprotein calories	1020-1428 calories/liter
Nitrogen	4.45 gm/liter

Safe intravenous hyperalimentation is dependent upon careful monitoring of body weight, balance of intake and output, fractional urine sugar determinations, and measurements of blood glucose and serum electrolytes. Rapid gains in weight exceeding one pound per day usually reflect the acquisition of salt and water, rather than an increase in lean body mass. Such weight gain is usually treated either by reducing the sodium content of the solutions, or by initiating a diuresis with diuretics. Forced osmotic diuresis secondary to glycosuria is avoided by measurement of quantitative urinary glucose excretion. A urinary excretion of 2 gm/dl as measured by the nitroprusside reaction is treated by reducing the infused dextrose load, or by adding exogenous insulin to the IVH solution. Serum concentrations of glucose and electrolytes are determined daily. A complete blood count, serum bilirubin, serum glutamic-oxaloacetic transaminase (SGOT), serum glutamic pyruvic transaminase (SGPT), alkaline phosphatase, serum calcium, phosphate, and serum protein concentrations are performed weekly to confirm that there is no significant alteration in these values. Arterial blood gases and blood pH are monitored as clinically indicated. In patients with marked hypoproteinemia, albumin may be added to the intravenous hyperalimentation solution in order to restore normal plasma osmotic pressure. Patients who are anemic are transfused to normal levels with packed erythrocytes before the institution of parenteral hyperalimentation. Abnormalities in clotting factors are treated by transfusion with fresh frozen plasma. In order to utilize maximally and safely the substrates provided, the patient's hemodynamic status must be optimal. For this reason restoration of circulating blood volume with colloid and/or blood is essential to establish normal visceral blood flow before instituting hyperalimentation.

The safe delivery of IVH is dependent upon an accurate and infection-free means of access to the vascular system. Infusion of the hypertonic solution (1800 to 2400 mOsm/liter) is usually accomplished via a catheter directed into the superior vena cava following percutaneous insertion into the subclavian vein. This has been the most common means of access to the central venous system at this institution, and has proven to be both safe and effective. Either subclavian vein may be used for this technique unless there is a specific local contraindication, such as a radical neck dissection, local radiation therapy, or a history of thrombophlebitis in the upper extremities. In order to insert the central venous catheter, the patient is initially restored to a euvolemic status by infusion of crystalloid or colloid, as clinically indicated. The patient is then positioned with her head down 15°, in order to allow dilatation of the subclavian vein, enlarging the target. The shoulders are thrown back maximally, or hyperextended over a rolled sheet placed longitudinally under the thoracic spine. With the shoulder then depressed, and gentle traction on the hand ipsilateral to the insertion site, the head is turned toward the opposite side. The subclavian vein then becomes most easily accessible for percutaneous catheterization. The skin over the lower neck, shoulder, and upper chest is shaved, cleansed with either acetone or Freon in order to remove skin oil, and painted with a povidone-iodine solution. Using aseptic technique with sterile gloves and instruments, the area is draped with sterile towels, and local anesthetic is infiltrated into the skin, subcutaneous tissue, and periosteum at the inferior border of the midpoint of the clavicle. A 2-inch, 14-gauge needle attached to 2-ml, or 3-ml non-Luerlock syringe is inserted bevel down through the wheal, and advanced beneath the inferior margin of the clavicle in a horizontal plane. The needle tip is aimed at the anterior trachea at the level of suprasternal notch (See Figures 22-1, 22-2, 22-3, 22-4). With the needle and syringe barrel in a frontal plane, and adjacent to the anterior deltoid prominence, the needle enters the anterior wall of the subclavian vein. As the needle is advanced beneath the clavicle, slight negative pressure applied to the syringe will indicate venipuncture by the withdrawal of blood from the vein into the barrel of the syringe. The needle is then advanced a few millimeters further in order to ensure that the entire beveled tip of the needle is within the lumen of vein. The patient is asked to perform a Valsalva maneuver to increase venous pressure, and avoid air embolism; and the syringe is detached carefully with the needle held firmly in place. A 16-gauge, 8-inch radiopaque catheter is introduced immediately through the needle until its full length has been inserted. The catheter should advance easily if the needle tip is correctly positioned. If the catheter does not advance at this stage, the entire needle and catheter apparatus should be removed as one unit,

580

and another attempt at venous cannulation should be performed. One should never try to remove the catheter once it has been advanced beyond the tip of the needle, since this risks shearing off the tip of the catheter, and could result in catheter embolization into the heart or lung.

Once the catheter has been properly positioned, its proximal end is

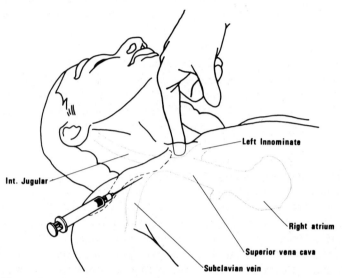

Figure 22-1   The 14-gauge needle is directed in a frontal plane toward a fingertip which is pressed firmly into the suprasternal notch. Accurate puncture of the subclavian vein is indicated by a flash-back of blood in the syringe. Reprinted with permission from Dudrick and Copeland (1973).

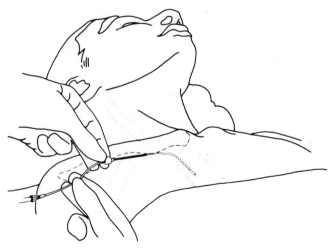

Figure 22-2   With the bevel of the needle directed caudally, a 16-gauge catheter is directed into the superior vena cava. Reprinted with permission from Dudrick and Copeland (1973).

connected with the solution by sterile intravenous tubing, and flushed with the solution; the needle is withdrawn from the patient; and the catheter is secured to the skin by a #3-0 silk or nylon suture placed laterally to the skin puncture site. At this point, the solution bag or bottle is momentarily lowered below the bed level to ensure free flow of blood

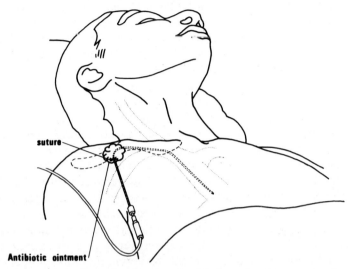

Figure 22-3 The catheter is sutured to the skin lateral to the puncture site to prevent in and out motion of the catheter at the skin entrance site. Reprinted with permission from Dudrick and Copeland (1973).

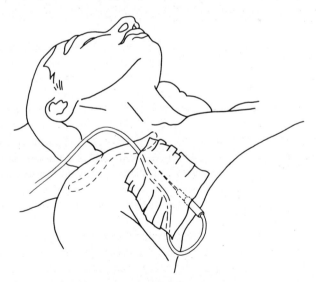

Figure 22-4 An occlusive, water-repellent sterile dressing covers the catheter entrance site and secures the infusion tubing. Reprinted with permission from Dudrick and Copeland (1973).

back into the tubing, an indication that the catheter has been properly placed within the vena cava. A guard is placed on the tip of the needle in order to avoid the inadvertent shearing of the catheter by the needle. A broad spectrum antimicrobial ointment is placed around the puncture site, and an occlusive sterile dressing is secured over the catheter insertion site with tincture of benzoin and adhesive tape. To prevent accidental disengagement of the intravenous tubing from the catheter, the tubing-catheter connection is carefully reinforced with adhesive tape. A loop is made in the intravenous tubing which is secured again with tape to guard against accidental traction upon the catheter itself. Prior to the infusion of hypertonic solution, a chest x-ray should be obtained to verify the position of the catheter in the vena cava.

Percutaneous cannulation of the subclavian vein is the preferred access to the superior vena cava for intravenous hyperalimentation. Catheters inserted into the internal jugular vein via supraclavicular insertion, or via the external or internal jugular vein are usually more difficult to dress and to maintain than those placed by the subclavian approach. In our experience, long venous catheters advanced into the superior vena cava by surgical cannulation of the brachial vein have been associated with a higher incidence of thrombophlebitis and infection than subclavian catheters. In order to achieve safe long-term central venous access, compulsive and meticulous care of the catheter is as important as proper insertion. Every two to three days the intravenous tubing is changed, and the dressing over the puncture site is removed. Using aseptic technique and sterile gloves, the area is again defatted with acetone or Freon, and painted with povidone iodine. Antimicrobial ointment is reapplied at the catheter insertion site, and a sterile occlusive dressing is secured. Withdrawal or administration of blood through the subclavian catheter should be avoided since these practices significantly increase the risk of contamination, or clotting of the catheter. Antibiotics, heparin, or steroids are not routinely added to the solutions, but may be administered through Y-tubing attached to the intravenous catheter. The measurement of central venous catheter pressure through a central venous feeding catheter should be avoided since manipulation of IVH catheters has been associated with an increased incidence of catheter or solution contamination. It has not been the practice of our center to use an in-line membrane filter with hyperalimentation solutions, since an acceptably low rate of catheter contamination has been achieved without filters using meticulous aseptic technique.

The solution is usually delivered continuously to the patient by means of pump infusion. The rate of delivery is increased from 1 liter daily to 2 to 3 liters daily, depending upon the energy requirements and fluid restrictions of the individual patient. Each solution bag is clearly marked by the pharmacy, indicating the composition of the solution, the additives present, the rate of infusion, and the duration of the IVH therapy to date.

In this fashion the physician may confirm that the solution being delivered to the patient is that which has been ordered.

An expanding population of patients has been found who require intravenous hyperalimentation outside a hospital setting. Most patients who require this type of support have anatomic or functional defects of the gastrointestinal tract that preclude adequate oral intake for indefinite periods of time. In addition, patients who are receiving prolonged courses of chemotherapy which interfere with adequate oral intake have been included in this home IVH population. Patients wear custom-made, lightweight, polyester mesh vests to which are attached the plastic bags for continuous infusion of hyperalimentation solution (Figure 22-5). This vest fits under a loose fitting shirt or blouse, and enables the patient to work or carry on her daily home activities. The solution is infused by a light-weight, battery-operated pump which is held in a vest pocket. The patient can mix the IVH solution at home for daily use (upon completing training in the Ambulatory Hyperalimentation Center at the University of Texas), or can obtain the solution from a convenient hospital pharmacy. Tubing is changed daily with this system, and initially the patients are seen weekly to confirm that there are no problems with the continuous delivery system. Follow-up visits decrease in frequency as patient experience and competence increase.

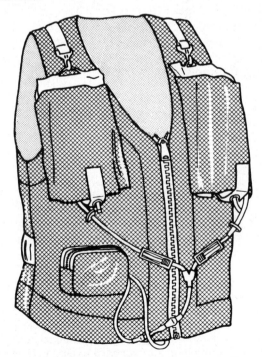

Figure 22-5 Schematic drawing of polyester mesh hyperalimentation vest for ambulatory patients. Reprinted with permission from Dudrick et al (1977).

Approximately 60 patients have been treated by this means over the past five years (Figure 22-6). There have been no serious technical complications of outpatient hyperalimentation that could not be easily remedied, and the infection rate, consisting of only one episode of infection per 1000 catheter days, has not led to IVH associated mortality or significant morbidity. Most catheter contamination episodes can be traced to specific violations of aseptic technique by the patient or family.

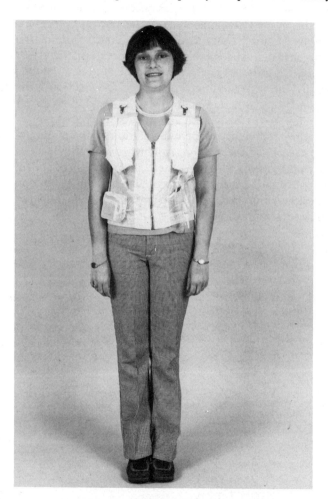

Figure 22-6   This 27-year-old woman with a nine-year history of Crohn's disease eventually lost almost all of her small bowel and colon, leaving her with 18 inches of proximal jejunum and an end-jejunostomy. She gained more than 40 pounds on ambulatory home hyperalimentation wearing this tailor-made vest which carried two 500 ml bags of nutrient solution, a 1¼ lb battery-operated pump, and specially designed Y-infusion tubing connected to her implanted silicone rubber central venous feeding catheter. She has required intravenous hyperalimentation for more than five years, and will require it supplemental to oral feeding for life.

The hallmark of a successful hyperalimentation program is the prevention of infection and sepsis secondary to catheter contamination while an anabolic state is attained. This is especially important in oncology patients who are immunosuppressed by the nature of their disease, and who are often myelosuppressed by the treatment of their cancer. The incidence of catheter sepsis is negligible if aseptic and antiseptic principles are conscientiously observed during insertion and maintenance of central venous catheters. Should a fever occur without obvious cause, the IVH solution which is being infused, and the attached tubing are promptly replaced, and specimens of the blood and solution are cultured. If the fever persists following the replacement of solution and tubing, the infusion is terminated, and a blood culture is drawn through the catheter prior to removal. The subclavian catheter is removed, and the tip is immediately placed in thioglycolate broth and sent for culture. Depending upon the clinical circumstances, another catheter may be inserted into the opposite subclavian vein or administration of isotonic dextrose may be started by peripheral vein to prevent rebound hypoglycemia. Long-term antibiotic therapy is rarely required. Broad spectrum antibiotic therapy may be started at the time of catheter removal and modified when specific sensitivity testing is completed. The latter course of action is most judicious for patients who are myelosuppressed at the time they become febrile.

The presence of fever or sepsis prior to the institution of IVH is not necessarily a contraindication to the use of the technique. In critically ill patients, sepsis further increases the need for adequate nutrition. Patients who are septic are less capable of using the fat stores of their body as an energy source, and have increased requirements for glucose and amino acids. Antibiotic therapy has already been instituted in many such patients. Although seeding of the indwelling catheter by circulating microorganisms is a possibility, this has been a rare occurrence in our experience. Successful treatment of the systemic infection has occurred frequently during the period of hyperalimentation. Whenever the physician is concerned that the febrile course of the patient might be caused or aggravated by IVH, the hyperalimentation catheter should be removed and cultured promptly.

Myelosuppression in patients with gynecologic malignancies often results from chemotherapy. Neutropenia is not a contraindication to hyperalimentation. Generally, the risk of sepsis is no greater in neutropenic patients who are treated with hyperalimentation than in comparably neutropenic patients supported by enteral feeding. Prophylactic antibiotics may be required in IVH patients during the nadir of the marrow suppression, and granulocyte transfusions have been used in some patients on a therapeutic or prophylactic basis. Similarly, if the patient has thrombocytopenia as a manifestation of myelosuppression, percutaneous cannulation of the subclavian vein may be accomplished following platelet transfusion. There has not been an increase in bleeding complications of subclavian vein catheterization, if platelet transfusions and fresh frozen plasma have been used to correct any clotting abnormalities present prior to catheterization.

Although thrombophlebitis is a potential complication of long term indwelling catheters for hypertonic solution infusion, superior vena cava thrombosis has rarely been observed in more than 3000 patients studied. The high blood flow in the superior vena cava dilutes the hypertonic solution to reduce the chance of septic thrombophlebitis. If the patient develops clinically apparent thrombophlebitis, indicated by swelling of the arm ipsilateral to the subclavian catheter insertion site, and tenderness over the ipsilateral supraclavicular fossa, the catheter should be removed and cultured. Rare cases of aseptic thrombophlebitis have occurred, particularly in patients in whom the catheter tip was misdirected into the external jugular, internal jugular, or axillary vein.

Technical complications of IVH such as inadvertent air embolism, catheter embolism, and catheter sepsis can be avoided by adherence to the principles and techniques previously described. A thorough knowledge of anatomy of the subclavian vein and adjacent structures, combined with common sense and strict adherence to the established techniques of percutaneous subclavian catheterization, should minimize the risk of accidental pneumothorax, hydrothorax, hemothorax, subclavian artery puncture, injury to the thoracic duct, or brachial plexus injury. The risk of pneumothorax is often greater in patients who have emphysema and bullous transformation of the apices of the lung. Examination of the lateral chest film will identify those patients who are at higher risk for this complication.

Hyperosmolar nonketotic hyperglycemia may be precipitated by infusion of an excessive dextrose load causing a marked osmotic diuresis, serum electrolyte aberrations, dehydration, and central nervous system obtundation. Such a complication is best avoided by close monitoring of serum and urinary glucose levels. Hyperglycemia should be treated by decreasing the rate of dextrose administration, or increasing the delivery of exogenous insulin to facilitate intracellular glucose utilization. A decrease in glucose tolerance during IVH may result from pancreatitis, renal insufficiency, or chromium deficiency; or it may be a harbinger of sepsis. Once hyperosmolar hyperglycemia develops, its treatment consists of aggressive infusion of isotonic or half normal solutions of saline, along with small amounts of insulin while obtaining frequent measurements of urine output, urine sugar, central venous pressure, serum electrolytes and blood sugar.

Metabolic hyperchloremic acidosis is a described complication of IVH usually associated with the use of solutions which contain a preponderance of synthetic amino acids as either chloride or hydrochloride salts. Recent conversion to amino acid solutions which are more balanced in the total titrable acid content, or addition of acetate to the IVH mixture, has decreased the incidence of this complication. The usual treatment of hyperchloremic acidosis is the administration of bicarbonate acutely to correct the metabolic acidosis, and conversion to acetate and acid phosphate salts of the various cation additives to the hyperalimentation solution.

In patients with gynecologic malignancies, fluid overload is a risk with IVH. Close monitoring of daily weight and careful physical examination for increased ascites, increased weight, peripheral edema, or evidence of pleural effusion is important in patients with disseminated ovarian or uterine malignancies. Weight gain exceeding 0.5 lb daily usually is due to an increase in total body water. If the patient's avidity for salt and water limits the calories which can be delivered, one may either use more concentrated dextrose solutions with a reduced rate of IVH infusion, or one may administer diuretics. The salt in the formulations given to such patients can be reduced appreciably, or omitted as indicated.

Parenteral nutrition has developed into an important therapeutic modality in the support of patients with disseminated malignancies. It has made possible the extension of the benefits of chemotherapy, radiation therapy, or extirpative surgery to patients who previously would not have been able to withstand such extensive treatment because of poor nutritional status. The seriously ill patient requires increased nutritional support for the restoration of normal body tissues and metabolism. Cancer patients have increased metabolic needs which might not be met because of the anorexia and decreased oral intake associated with the malignancy.

Increased resting body metabolism, periods of intraoperative stress, or catabolic periods following oncologic therapy demand aggressive nutritional therapy. By judicious intravenous administration of adequate basic nutrients, tissue synthesis, weight gain, and restoration of immunity can be achieved to benefit gynecologic oncologic patients who cannot, should not, or will not eat at all, or cannot eat enough to maintain homeostasis.

BIBLIOGRAPHY

AMA Department of Foods and Nutrition, Guidelines for essential trace element preparations for parenteral use. *JAMA* 241:2051–2054, 1979.

Catalona WJ, Chretian PB: Abnormalities of quantitative dinitrochlorobenzene sensitization in cancer patients: correlation with tumor stage and histology. *Cancer* 31:353–356, 1973.

Copeland EM, Daly JM, Dudrick SJ: Nutrition as an adjunct to cancer treatment in the adult. *Cancer Res* 37:2451–2456, 1977.

Copeland EM: Intravenous hyperalimentation as an adjunct to cancer patient management. *Cancer Bull* 30:102–108, 1978.

Daly JM, Dudrick SJ, Copeland EM: Effects of protein depletion and repletion on cell mediated immunity in experimental animals. *Ann Surg* 188:791–796, 1976.

588

Daly JM, Dudrick SJ, Copeland EM: Intravenous hyperalimentation: Effect on delayed cutaneous hypersensitivity in cancer patients. *Ann Surg* 192:587–592, 1980.

DeWys WD: Abnormalities of taste as a remote effect of a neoplasm. *Ann NY Acad Sci* 230:427–434, 1974.

Dindogru A, Pasick S, Rutkowski Z, Vinson B, Vaitkevicius V: Total parenteral nutrition in leukopenic cancer patients. *JAMA* 244:680–681, 1980.

Dudrick SJ, Copeland EM: Parenteral hyperalimentation. *Surg Ann* LM Nyhus (ed), New York, Appleton-Century-Crofts, 1973, pp 72–73.

Dudrick SJ, Englert DM, MacFadyen BV, et al: A vest for ambulatory patients receiving hyperalimentation. *Surg Gynecol Obstet* 148:587–590, 1977.

Fischer JE, Rosen HM, Ebeid AM, et al: The effect of normalization of plasma amino acids on hepatic encephalopathy in man. *Surg* 80:77–91, 1976.

Fuchs ZV, Stroeber S, Bobrove AM, et al: Long term effects of radiation on T and B lymphocytes in peripheral blood of patients with Hodgkin's Disease. *J Clin Invest* 58:803–814, 1975.

Holroyde CP, Gabuzda RG, Putnam RC, et al: Altered glucose metabolism in metastatic carcinoma. *Cancer Res* 35:3710–3714, 1975.

Issell BF, Valdiveso M, Zaren HF, et al: Protection of chemotherapy toxicities by intravenous hyperalimentation. *Cancer Treat Rep* 62:1139–1142, 1978.

Kaye M, Comty C: Nutritional repletion during dialysis. *Am J Clin Nutr* 21:583–589, 1968.

Lanzotti VM, Copeland EM, George SL, et al: Cancer chemotherapeutic response and intravenous hyperalimentation. *Cancer Chemother Rep* 59:437–439, 1975.

Souchon EA, Copeland EM, Watson P, et al: Intravenous hyperalimentation as an adjunct to cancer chemotherapy with 5-Fluorouracil. *J Surg Res* 18:451–454, 1975.

Warburg O: *The Metabolism of Tumors* New York, R.R. Smith, 1931.

Weber G: Enzymology of cancer cells. *N Engl J Med* 3:486–493, 1977.

Weber G: Enzymology of cancer cells. *N Engl J Med* 10:541–551, 1977.

23 Tumor Immunology

Hugh R. K. Barber

Immunology is the study of immune responses. It is a relatively new discipline of medicine. However, the concept of immunity is an ancient one and is properly termed the study of "resistance to infection." The term "immunity" has now taken on a more sophisticated and expanded role. It is the property whereby the lymphoreticular system makes a memorized response to an antigenic stimulus. This may result in a state of positive reaction known as *sensitization,* or in one of negative reaction known variously as *immunological tolerance* or *enhancement.* The immune response is a continuum, going from sensitization to tolerance. For those working in the field of oncology, all energies are directed to producing a sensitization, whereas those working in reproductive immunology are attempting to produce a state of tolerance or enhancement. Immunity is a complex state arising from the properties of the individual, of the community, of the race, and of the species; but the most striking thing about it is the specific nature of its enhancement in individuals after recovery from infection.

The immune response does not often involve a single process. Lymphocytes, phagocytic cells, the vascular system, antibody, complement, and other components of the body have complex interactions, which cannot be understood by studying only one or two facets of this intertwining maze.

The ability to distinguish between self and nonself, and the capacity to acquire reactivity characterized by memory with specificity, are the hallmarks of the immune response. Immunity requires an immune response of sufficient magnitude and speed to prevent serious disease or death from an invading biologic agent. Since ancient times it has been known that persons who recover from certain infectious diseases do not develop those diseases again. Immunity is associated with an individual's ability to mount an anamnestic response to a pathogenic agent. The immune response to a foreign substance has four characteristics: it is acquired, remembered, specific, and transferable.

Modern immunology started when Jenner discovered that inoculation with cowpox crusts protected mankind against smallpox. He published his monumental work on vaccination for the prevention of smallpox in 1798, and in the following 175 years both immunology and medicine grew at an increasingly rapid rate. Jenner's recognition that the shiny-faced milkmaids did not develop smallpox because they had previously been infected with cowpox was revolutionary. Since the initial exposure to a serious disease entails considerable risk, infection is not an ideal method of immunization.

Jenner noted that his patients who contracted cowpox (a very mild disease) developed immunity to smallpox as well. Apparently, the causative microorganisms are closely related and differ mainly in their pathogenicity for humans. It was fortuitous that he selected cowpox which acted as an attenuated virus and was effective for the stimulation of active immunization.

In Turkey, a different form of variolation (smallpox was then known as variola) was observed by Lady Montagu, wife of the British ambassador. There, pustular material was taken from the lesions of a person with a mild case of smallpox and transferred by a common needle into a vein or tissue of the person desiring the immunization. Hopefully, a mild form of smallpox would develop, and apparently did, with sufficient regularity for Lady Montagu to have her own children vaccinated in this manner. In 1718, she introduced this procedure to England, and she is credited with introducing the method to the Western world. From these early beginnings in immunology, progress toward the control of infection led the increasingly common advances in medicine.

The next advancement in immunology was made through the contributions of Louis Pasteur. His chance observation that aged cultures of chicken cholera bacillus would not cause the expected disease in chickens led to the development of methods for reducing the virulence of pathogenic microorganisms, a process called attenuation. The protection given to animals by preinoculation of such attenuated organisms led to the widespread use of the method for purposes of immunization. Microorganisms that are passed through an unnatural host (such as the infection of rabbits with rabies virus) may then induce immunity in a natural host without causing disease. The introduction of microorganisms that have been treated to make them harmless for the purpose of eliciting an immune response, is called vaccination. Although it was accepted that this was a great advance, there was some uneasiness that the use of attenuated organisms carried an inherent risk; the organisms might revert to their original virulent form. This difficulty was resolved, in part at least, by the observations that heat-killed organisms still retained their immunological potential, but did not cause the disease that they were intended to prevent. Despite the validity of these discoveries, the nature of immunity remained unknown.

The next step in our knowledge was made when it was discovered that not only the toxins of diphtheria, but that injection of the toxin into laboratory animals resulted in the appearance of a neutralizing substance in the blood of the injected animal. This neutralizing substance was called antitoxin. Thus the idea grew that, when the body was invaded by microorganisms, it would produce antibodies which would serve to neutralize the effect not only of the currently invading organisms, but of future invading organisms of the same type. Futhermore, it was shown that antitoxin could be taken from one animal and injected into another, thereby conferring passive immunity on the second animal. This principle found its greatest application in the prevention and treatment of diphtheria.

In 1895, Héricourt and Richet attempted passive immunization with antiserum produced in animals injected with human tumors; the results were highly unpredictable. In addition, Richet had shown that, in certain instances, repeated antigenic stimulation, far from protecting the animal, actually killed it. This is what Richet called anaphylaxis. But in those days anaphylaxis was a phenomenon seen almost exclusively in laboratory animals; it rarely occurred in man, so it did not excite much attention. Bashford, in 1906, claimed that prior inoculations of tumor and whole blood in mice prevented the growth of transplants of a mammary adenocarcinoma, and that established transplants of spontaneous cancers were not affected. Southam and Brunschwig, approximately 50 years later, demonstrated the same thing in humans.

In the early part of the twentieth century, Paul Ehrlich (1906) proposed the humoral theory of antibody formation. He also hypothesized that malignant neoplasms were antigenic and, as such, could be recognized by the host as being foreign to it. This concept was easily adapted to his previous observations but, in actuality, the completion of his work escaped him. Following his death, his students turned their attention to carcinogens, and his ideas lay dormant for several decades. In addition, Ehrlich indirectly suggested the theory of immunological surveillance in

1908. At that time, he stated that in the enormously complicated course of fetal and postfetal development, aberrant cells become unusually common. Fortunately, in the majority of people, they remain completely latent, thanks to the organism's positive mechanisms. The latter, Ehrlich implied, was immunity. He also provided the key factor of the theory that a depressed immune response allows the rapid, parasitic growth of (neoplastic) cells. It is interesting to speculate why his provocative idea failed to stimulate research during his lifetime. Perhaps medical history will some day supply the answer. Currently, the concept of immunological surveillance as formulated by Thomas (1961) and elaborated by Burnet (1970) into a theory, is being challenged. However, at this time, there seem to be as many pros as cons, as far as the acceptance of the immunologic surveillance theory is concerned.

Landsteiner introduced a new era and a new field in immunology with the discovery of the ABO blood group system, and then, later, the discovery of the Rhesus factor. At the turn of the century, Landsteiner discovered the ABO blood group system. In 1939, in collaboration with Wiener, Landsteiner discovered what history may decide is the greatest of all discoveries in this field — the Rhesus factor. This opened up the whole field of immunohematology.

At the turn of the century, considerable effort had already been expended to define differences between normal and neoplastic cells that can be used as a point of attack in tumor diagnosis, prophylaxis, and therapy. Even if no qualitative differences exist, quantitative differences may be large enough to serve the same purpose. The hope was held that there was a dissimilarity between normal and neoplastic cells, and that this difference could be demonstrated by immunological methods. The next logical step would be to establish a method of early diagnosis by this method, as well as producing a vaccine against cancer. This view was based on experiments in which the growth of transplanted animal tumors could be prevented by immunization of recipients of transplants in various ways. These were performed in non-inbred animals. The graft recipients rejected the neoplastic cells not only because there was an immunity to tumor specific antigens, but, more importantly, because of sensitization to those normal alloantigens that were present in the animal in which the transplanted tumor originated (and therefore in the tumor), but not in recipients.

When it was recognized that the many claims of tumor-specific antigenicity were based on experiments in which an immunity to normal alloantigens, rather than tumor-specific antigens, had been demonstrated, the field of tumor immunology came into disrepute. A common view was that tumor-specific antigens could not possibly exist, since they confer a selective disadvantage on the cells that carry them, and lead to their immediate elimination by immunologic mechanisms. For the next 40 years there were only sporadic attempts to identify antigens that were related to tumors.

Present Status

The advances made in the last few decades offer hope for curing certain cancers and the opportunity for early diagnosis in others, all within the foreseeable future. Cancer-specific antigens were first identified in a little-quoted study by Gross in 1943. Resistance to transplants of a chemically induced sarcoma in a pedigreed strain of mice was first demonstrated in 1943. Gross had inbred strains of mice for many generations and called them pedigreed mice, but in reality they represented the inbred strain that we know today and call syngeneic strains. Mice immunized by intradermal inoculation of tumor cells rejected a subcutaneous transplant of the same tumor while nonimmunized animals did not. Unfortunately, Gross performed his experiment on a small number of animals and did not supply a sufficient number of controls. His report was ignored at that time because it was published in a little known publication, and the other important consideration was that we were more interested in building an atomic bomb than pursuing this type of scientific work.

Similar results were reported in 1953 by Foley and in 1955 by Baldwin. However, the rebirth of tumor immunology as an active field of research may be said to have occurred in 1957 when Prehn and Main observed that mice immunized against syngeneic methylcholanthrene (MCA)-induced fibrosarcomas by inoculation of living sarcoma tissue, followed by surgical removal of the growing tumor, were resistant to subsequent grafts of the same tumor. In addition, immunization with normal tissue did not confer resistance to the tumor grafts. The mice that had become resistant to the tumors still accepted skin grafts from the primary hosts of these tumors. Different methylcholanthrene (MCA)-induced sarcomas were found to have individually distinct antigens; mice that were immune to one tumor still accepted grafts of other tumors. Additional projects were carried out, and these studies were extended by the demonstration that tumor-specific immunity against methylcholanthrene-induced sarcomas can also be induced in the primary, autochthonous host by repeated inoculation with heavily irradiated sarcoma cells after surgical removal of the primary tumor. Since the tumor-specific antigens were detected by transplantation techniques, they were referred to as tumor-specific transplantation antigens (TSTA). The tumor antigens are now referred to as tumor-associated antigens (TAA), since they are generally found in more than one tumor and occasionally even in normal tissue. Tumor-specific antigen is reserved for those situations in which the antigen has been identified with only one tumor.

A normal cell and a tumor cell in the same host have similar histocompatible antigens. The cancer cell has histocompatibility identical to HL-A antigens of the normal cell of the same host, since this is characteristic of the organism. In addition, the cancer cell has a new antigen called tumor-associated antigen (TAA). Antigenic differences represent the first known qualitative distinctions between cancer cells and their normal counterparts. Modern tumor immunology began with this finding.

Definitions

As a scientific discipline, immunology encompasses *immunity,* dealing with the adaptive response to infective agents; *immunochemistry,* concerned with the chemical nature of antigens and antibodies; and *immunobiology,* which deals with the activity of cells with the immune system and the relation to each other and their environment.

ANTIGENS

An antigen is a substance that is capable of binding to an antibody. The ability of a molecule to be bound in a specific fashion at the combining site of an antibody is termed antigenicity. An immunogen is a substance that is capable of initiating an immune response. It is possible for a substance to be antigenic, but not immunogenic. Some substances are capable of binding to antibody but, by themselves, are incapable of inducing antibody production. It should be noted that substances that are immunogenic are always antigenic. But substances that are antigenic are not necessarily immunogenic. Substances that are antigenic but not immunogenic are called haptens. Haptens are usually small molecules (molecular weight less than 1,000 daltons) that are incapable (by themselves) of activating the cellular machinery of the immune response.

Although the words antigen and immunogen really are not the same, in current practice they are used interchangeably. Antigens are usually protein, but may also comprise carbohydrate and lipid and have the following properties: 1) molecular complexity with rigid chemical structures called antigenic determinants (epitope); 2) adequate molecular size (not critical); and 3) susceptibility to at least partial degradation in the responding organism.

Tumor Antigens

Tumors have been found to have antigens present on the surface of the tumor cell. They have been designated as tumor-specific transplantation antigens (TSTA) because they were demonstrated by transplanting the tumor into another inbred animal. More recently they have been called tumor-associated antigens (TAA). Tumor antigens have been divided into two groups, ie, unique antigens or common antigens. Until recently, it was reported that a tumor would have one or the other, but not both, depending on the agent that initiated the response. It is now generally accepted that a tumor may have one or both types of antigens.

Unique Antigens

Animal tumors induced by chemical carcinogens have individual specificity with unique antigens. The same chemical carcinogen painted on different places in the same animal will produce different tumors. Each new tumor has its own specific antigenicity that is not shared with other tumors. The action of the chemical carcinogen appears to be mainly a random interaction with the native cell DNA, resulting in a tumor with unique antigens.

Common Antigens

Virally induced tumors appear to carry antigens common to all tumors induced by a given virus, even in animals of different species. Although this is generally true, recent studies indicate that there may be some cross-reacting, some virus tumors having unique antigens as well as common ones, and some chemically induced tumors having common antigens. In some instances, depending on the techniques used, either the common or the individually unique antigens were detected.

The association between viruses and animal tumors has long been appreciated. Nevertheless, despite a great amount of work, there is no documented instance of a virus origin for a tumor. The isolation of the enzyme, reverse transcriptase, may solve this problem. Using this enzyme system, progress has been made in studying myelogenous leukemia.

ANTIBODIES

An antibody is a substance produced in response to an antigen. An antibody is commonly, if not always, a gamma globulin. Currently, the word immunoglobulin is a collective noun to include all the globulins that have antibody activity. It also includes similar proteins that have no such activity. The antibody portions of the serum globulins are referred to as immunoglobulins. The most important immunoglobulins are G (IgG), M (IgM), A (IgA), D (IgD), and E (IgE). Most, if not all, immunoglobulins are the products of plasma cells, which secrete these products into the serum and tissue fluids.

Immunity is associated with an individual's ability to mount an anamnestic response to a pathogenic agent. The ability to eliminate foreign substances more rapidly on subsequent exposure than on the first encounter is evidence of an anamnestic response. The anamnestic response is specific for previously introduced substances. The immune response to a foreign substance has four characteristics: it is acquired, remembered, specific, and transferable.

Blocking or Enhancing Antibodies

A blocking antibody is a term used to describe the antibody that reacts (coats) with the antigens on the surface of the cell and prevents an attack by a cytotoxic antibody and/or a reactive killer T cell. The existence of F (ab')$_2$ fragments of IgG, which have blocking activity, have been described in the sera of cancer patients. These fragments were able to inhibit cell-mediated immune reactions in vitro.

Unblocking Antibodies

Certain sera taken from either animals or human patients during the period of tumor remission have been found to increase the cytotoxic effect of immune lymphocytes. The mechanism of the potentiation effect (unblocking or deblocking) is unknown, as are the molecules mediating it. If it is correct to assume that the blocking factor is an antigen-antibody complex, the "unblocking" effect of certain sera could be due to antibodies that are bound to the blocking complexes. They could be different from the antibodies of the blocking complexes, or they could be the same antibodies in excess. An antibody may also act as an antigen, and if the antibody acting as an antigen is a blocking antibody, it is conceivable that it may produce an unblocking antibody. The blocking factors are considered antigen-antibody complexes (and occasionally free antigen), and, therefore, it is anticipated that antibodies to the antigen in such a complex would be unblocking antibodies. The unblocking antibodies may interfere with the attachment of blocking factors to the target cells or to the lymphocytes, may alter the blocking factors, or depress their formation by feedback inhibition. Lymphoid cells may produce unblocking antibodies. The unblocking or deblocking factor may provide a method for monitoring the patients and would be superior to monitoring the blocking factor. This is predicated on the assumption that the disappearance of unblocking serum would occur before the blocking factors are detected. Recently, it has been shown that certain sera can "arm" lymphoid cells from nonimmune donors, so that they become specifically cytotoxic for syngeneic tumor cells. A similar "arming" has been reported in systems involving normal alloantigens rather than tumor-specific antigen.

IMMUNE REFLEX ARC

The immune response is divided into three phases. The first begins with the administration of the antigen and ends when antigen encounters antigen-reactive lymphocytes; this is called the *afferent limb*. The afferent limb is the means by which the stimulus (the antigen) is delivered to the central processing mechanism which, in turn, manufactures the effectors of the immune response: antibodies and specifically sensitized cells. The dissemination of the effectors throughout the body defines the afferent limb of the immune reflex arc. The afferent limb delivers the antigen to the *central processing mechanism* which is usually a lymph node, and at this point the effectors of the immune reflex are manufactured. Since there are plasma cells and lymphocytes present in the central processing area, the processed antigen comes in contact with a plasma cell and gives rise to the immunoglobulins, whereas if the processed antigen comes in contact with a previously sensitized lymphocyte, specifically sensitized cells are produced. The former make up the humoral mechanism and the latter make up the cell-mediated immune mechanism. These effector cells are carried throughout the body by the efferent limb of the immune reflex arc.

For most antigens, central processing involves both B and T lymphocytes. Clonal expansion and differentiation of B lymphocytes into memory cells and antibody forming cells require the assistance of helper T cells. Antigens that require these two cell types for the production of antibody are called T dependent antigens. Irrespective of the presence of B lymphocytes, clonal expansion of T lymphocytes in response to antigen also occurs during central processing. The result of this event is the elaboration of effector T cells. Thus, central processing achieves the production of two kinds of effector modalities: antibody and specifically sensitized cells.

CELLULAR EVENTS IN AN IMMUNE RESPONSE

The cellular events in an immune response are fundamental in understanding the basic mechanisms relative to the development of both cell-mediated and humoral immunity. The macrophage represents the keystone in the development of an immune response. The mononuclear phagocyte is a macrophage. The macrophage in blood is called a monocyte, in connective tissue is called histiocyte, and in the spleen, lymph nodes, and thymus, is called a sinus lining macrophage or a reticulum cell. It is obvious that the macrophage has wide distribution. The antigen (any substance foreign to the host) is processed by the macrophage if an immune response is to occur. The antigen is now a processed antigen. Following contact between the antigen and a macrophage, the latter sends out a message in the form of an RNA or RNA-antigen complex. The uncommited lymphocytes are transformed into lymphoblasts. The transformed blasts give rise to sensitized lymphocytes as well as plasma cells. The plasma cells in turn produce a variety of immunoglobulins; five have been identified, ie, IgM, IgG, IgE, IgA, and IgD. The sensitized lymphocytes proliferate into the so-called killer lymphocytes that have the ability to destroy cancer cells, produce lymphokines and produce delayed hypersensitivity.

The B cell apparently must receive a stimulus from the antigen plus one from the antigenically simulated T cells if it is to mature into a plasmocyte. This helper function of the T cell appears to depend in large measure on the T and B cells sharing certain products of the major histocompatibility locus.

When the sensitized lymphocyte comes in contact with the antigen that sensitized it, the lymphocyte is stimulated to form an immunoblast which produces at least four mediators of cellular immunity, including transfer factor (TF), lymphocyte transforming activity (LTA), migration inhibition factor (MIF), and lymphotoxin (LT).

ORIGIN OF T AND B CELLS

Thymus-dependent (T cells) and thymus-independent (B cells) probably arise from a common stem in the bone marrow. The exact mechanism by which each cell is processed at the central level to form a T or B cell has not been completely elucidated. When it is fully developed, the lymphoid system consists not of a single cell type, but of two distinct cell types clearly separable from one another in the process of differentiation.

Pluripotent stem cells originally arise in the yolk sac and, during fetal to postnatal life, progressively move from the yolk sac to fetal liver to the adult bone marrow. These pluripotent cells differentiate into the precursor stem cells of all the major hematopoietic elements. Lymphoid stem cells can function as prethymic cells and are processed in the thymus under the influence of thymosin (thymopoietin) to differentiate into T cells. Lymphoid precursor cells are processed by an alternate pathway in a poorly defined organ in man, but they have been extensively studied in birds (in the bursa of Fabricius), in some mammals (in the fetal liver, probably under the influence of another hormone-like substance, bursin), and they differentiate into B lymphocytes. In response to antigenic stimulation, B cells differentiate into lymphocytes that secrete and synthesize antibody, immunoglobulins, and totally differentiated plasma cells. These cells are relatively sessile cells and represent about 8% to 10% of circulating lymphocytes. These B lymphocytes in the plasma cell reside in the bone marrow, in the lamina propria of the gastrointestinal tract, in Peyer's patches, in the pharyngeal tonsils, and in the far cortical areas of the lymph nodes. They make up the majority of cells in the medullary cord of the nodes and red pulp of the spleen. A subpopulation of thymus-dependent T cells are called helper T cells, which have a direct effect on immunocompetent B cells and the suppressor T cells which act as an influence to control the number of helper T cells. In addition, there are tolerant T cells and memory T cells.

Previously, a subpopulation of thymus-independent lymphocytes (B cells) had been detected which mediate cytotoxic reactions on antibody and coated target cells in the absence of complement. They are called killer cells, or K cells. In addition to the above three classes of lymphocytes, there is another population of circulating lymphocytes that had been identified with the characteristics of both T and B lymphocytes. These double (D), often called null cells, represent 2% to 3% of circulating lymphoid population. Their origin, function, and role in tumor immunology remain to be determined. Currently, the thinking has changed relating to the K and to the D cells. Null lymphocytes are cells that cannot be recognized as either B cells or T cells. For example, B lymphocytes are determined by fluorescent antibody techniques to look at surface immunoglobulin content. Lymphocytes having demonstrable surface immunoglobulin with this fluorescent technique are classified as B cells. T cells are evaluated by a technique of looking for E (sheep erythrocyte) rosette formation. T lymphocytes have receptor sites that interact with the cell membrane of sheep erythrocytes; the sheep red cells form a ring (rosette) around each T lymphocyte. Lymphocytes that do not have demonstrable surface immunoglobulin and do not produce rosettes with sheep red blood cells are considered null cells.

The average B cell population of a normal person is about 8%, the average T cell population is about 68%, and the remaining 24% of lymphocytes are considered null cells.

Null cells may be precursors of either B or T cell lines, or they may be killer lymphocytes or intermediate stages of B or T cells. B and T lymphocytes do not function autonomously. They interact. This is why a patient having a complete absence of one cell line usually has altered function of the other group. Whether this interaction goes through a specific null cell or whether null cells are a mixture of lymphocytes with many potential functions, is not known.

Sometimes the so-called K cells are referred to as null cells because they lack markers characteristic for T or B cells. The best surface marker for these cells is that they form rosettes with human Rh-D positive cells that have been coated by apparent monovalent antibodies against Rh-D antigens. Such antisera were originally identified in a patient whose name was Ripley, and the rosettes formed with the third population cells are sometimes called Ripley rosettes. This third population of lymphoid cells lacks demonstrable surface IgG, but the cells may carry highly avid membrane receptors for C3 and the Fc portion of the IgG molecule, and may kill target cells sensitized with IgG antibody (antibody-dependent, cell-mediated cytotoxicity). They are not phagocytic. The tests used to differentiate T, B cells and macrophages are listed in Table 23-1.

Table 23-1
Tests Used to Differentiate T Cells, B Cells, and Macrophages

Test	T Cells	B Cells	Macrophages
Surface immunoglobulin	$(-)$	$(+)$	$(\pm)$
"E" rosette formation	$(+)$	$(-)$	$(-)$
Latex particle phagocytosis	$(-)$	$(-)$	$(+)$

IMMUNOLOGIC DEFICIENCY DISEASES

Immunodeficiency disorders are classified as defects of stem cells, T cells, or B cells. More than 30 phenotypic patterns of immunodeficiency have been recognized in humans.

Any deviation in nature supplies valuable material for studying normal mechanisms. Nature has supplied such an experiment to study the role of the humoral and cell-mediated response.

Deficiency of Cell-Mediated Immunity (T Cell)

In the Di George syndrome there is hypoplasia or dysplasia of the thymus and absence of parathyroid glands. The patient has no resistance to virus or other agents that are controlled by cell-mediated immunity systems, such as tuberculosis, brucella, leprosy, and certain parasitic diseases. They do not have the immunologic capacity to develop a delayed hypersensitivity reaction. They are unable to reject grafts of foreign tissue. However, they can produce circulating antibodies and have the ability to respond to bacterial vaccines by developing normal circulating antibodies.

Deficiency of Humoral Immunity (B Cell)

In the human patient with Bruton type of agammaglobulinemia, there is a deficiency of immunoglobulin synthesis in which IgG is decreased tenfold, and IgA and IgM about a hundredfold. These patients do not give a normal circulating antibody response to bacteria, and are therefore susceptible to pyogenic infections. These patients do not respond with normal circulating antibody to bacterial vaccines. The lymphoid tissue in the appendix and Peyer's patches is somewhat reduced, and patients do not develop plasma cells or germinal centers in the lymph nodes. Nevertheless, the cell-mediated immunity mechanisms function normally in these patients, and they can reject grafts and exhibit delayed hypersensitivity to the tuberculin skin test.

Combined Deficiency of T and B Cells

In the Swiss type of agammaglobulinemia, which is an X-linked disease of male children, both cell-mediated and humoral mechanisms are deficient. There is almost complete absence of lymphoid tissue in the body, the thymus is very small, and the lymphoid tissues of the appendix and Peyer's patches are absent. These children cannot make humoral antibodies (immunoglobulins) or develop cell-mediated immune reactions. They suffer from progressive bacterial or viral infections and die within the first two years of life.

The clinician today is being offered ways of treating serious immunodeficiency diseases that until a few years ago were impossible to treat and were fatal. It is now feasible, first, to determine just what is lacking in the patient's immune system, and then to make up that lack. This is outlined in Table 23-2.

Table 23-2
Primary Immunodeficiency States

Deficiency	Infection	Treatment
B cell (eg, Bruton's)	Pyogenic Bacteria Pneumocystis carinii Candida	Gamma globulin
T cell (eg, Di George's)	Certain viruses Candida	Thymus graft
Stem cell (eg, Swiss type)	All of the above	Bone marrow graft

AUTOIMMUNE DISORDERS

Clinical and experimental observations show that individuals can sometimes respond immunologically to certain of their own antigens (self-antigens). These important exceptions to the principle of self-tolerance help analyze its fundamental mechanisms, and they are frequently associated with disease. It is often not clear, however, whether these anomalous responses cause, or are the result of, disease; hence, it is necessary to emphasize the distinction between an autoimmune response, in which an individual makes antibodies or becomes allergic to a self-antigen, and an autoimmune disease, which is a pathological condition arising from an autoimmune response. Autoimmune reactions can be both antibody- and cell-mediated.

Autoimmune diseases and disorders include clinical disorders resulting from an immune response against self-antigens (autoantigens). To fit this definition, a disease should: a) show evidence of an immune response against self-antigens; b) show lesions, with the presence of immunologically competent cells, that are related to the distribution of such antigens; c) be reproducible in experimental animals following injection of the relevant antigen, and be transferable from such animals to normal animals by passive transfer of lymphocytes or antibody.

The term is also used loosely for diseases associated with the presence of autoantibodies, even when these are not of known significance in the pathogenesis.

An imbalance in autoimmunity occurs as a consequence of genetic, viral, and environmental mechanisms acting singly or in combination.

The pathogenicity for autoimmunity is found in the central mechanism where there is an excess of helper T cell activity and/or a deficiency of suppressor T cell activity. Whenever the B cell is overstimulated by the helper T cell activity and there is no feedback control by suppressor T cell activity, there is an imbalance that leads to the development of autoantibodies. In the New Zealand mouse, it has been shown that continued overstimulation will result not only in the development of autoantibody but will eventually lead to the development of a lymphoma. This shows the progression from overstimulation through the production of autoantibodies on to the development of a neoplasm. It is well known now that autoimmune diseases are associated with an increased development of neoplastic processes. This is also true for the immunodeficiency diseases.

HYPERSENSITIVITY

Hypersensitivity is a state of the previously immunized body (to alter the reactivity of a host to an antigen by exposing it to that antigen in such a way that it produces an immune response), which results in tissue damage from an immune reaction to a further dose of that antigen. Hypersensitivity reactions may be antibody- or humoral-mediated as in immediate hypersensitivity, or they may be a reaction of cell-mediated immunity as in delayed hypersensitivity. The term hypersensitivity implies a heightened reactivity to an antigen, but it is difficult to define all hypersensitivity reactions, particularly cell-mediated reactions, in such terms.

The immediate type of hypersensitivity reaction may be defined as an inflammatory reaction mediated by antibodies. Immediate type, or antibody-mediated, hypersensitivity fall into three categories: 1) Anaphylaxis occurs when immunoglobulins of the IgE class interact with the antigen and thereby cause the release of vasoactive substances which induce an immediate inflammatory response; 2) Cytotoxic hypersensitivity results when antibodies bind to self-antigens and destroy the host cell; 3) Immune-complex hypersensitivity occurs when antigen-antibody complexes are deposited at tissue sites and a subsequent destructive inflammatory response ensues. Despite its designation, immediate type (antibody-mediated) hypersensitivity is not always immediate. The symptoms of anaphylaxis appear dramatically, often within ten minutes, following administration of the inciting antigens, but symptoms of cytotoxic and immune complex hypersensitivity may take days or weeks to appear.

The immediate type of hypersensitivity reaction are antibody-mediated, types 1 through 3, while type 4 is a cell-mediated delayed hypersensitivity type of reaction.

Type 1 – Anaphylactic

The antibody IgE is bound to cells that cause release of vasoactive substance on contact with the antigen. The immunoglobulin IgE possesses the ability to bind to the surface of basophils and mast cells, and this property is a function of the Fc portion of the molecule. Some antigens may produce anaphylactic type reactions in allergic individuals. Intravenous administration may produce vasomotor collapse and shock. Cutaneous administration elicits the characteristic wheal and flare reaction. Common allergies such as hay fever are attributable to air-borne pollen whose antigenic determinants bind to IgE antibodies. Since these antigens produce immediate inflammatory reactions in allergic individuals, the pollen is considered to be an allergen. Examples of anaphylactic reaction are seen in asthma, hay fever, and severe penicillin reactions.

Type 2 – Cytotoxic

When antibodies bind and destroy host cells, this type of immediate type hypersensitivity is classified as cytotoxic hypersensitivity. This type is seen more frequently now than formerly because of the potency of the newer drugs being administered. These drugs adhere to the red cells and produce foreign tissue or, at least, tissue that is not identified as self. As a result, an antibody response is stimulated, and, when complement is present, there is a resulting agglutination and lysis of the red blood cells. Examples of this are blood transfusion reaction, hemolytic disease of the newborn, and the hemolytic crisis that is a result of the administration of drugs.

Type 3 — Immune Complex Hypersensitivity

When tissues are damaged by the deposition of antigen-antibody complexes such as in serum sickness, this type of immediate hypersensitivity reaction is called the immune complex hypersensitivity. The Arthus reaction is a local manifestation of immune complex hypersensitivity. Repeated cutaneous injections of antigen build up high titers of specific antibody in the serum and locally. Characteristically, further cutaneous administration of antigen produces an inflammatory reaction marked by edema and erythema within 3 to 8 hours. The event that initiates the inflammatory reaction is the local formation of antigen-antibody complex. The Arthus reaction develops optimally when antibodies specific for the inciting antigen are present in moderate excess and insoluble complexes form at or near the site of administration. The Arthus phenomenon is a localized inflammatory reaction, whereas there is a generalized inflammatory reaction called serum sickness, which coincides with the appearance of large numbers of antigen-antibody complexes in the blood stream. A generalized inflammatory reaction, characterized by inflammation of blood vessels, joints, and kidneys, and resulting from the formation of circulating antigen-antibody complexes, is termed serum sickness. Serum sickness, unlike the Arthus reaction, occurs optimally at the region of moderate antigen excess and can be produced by a single, large dose of antigen. Serum sickness expresses itself symtomatically in the vasculature, joints, and kidneys.

Delayed Type — Type 4 — Cell-Mediated

Delayed hypersensitivity is an immunologic process. It is an acquired and transferable capacity which exhibits memory and specificity for the antigen. Lymphocytes that have been previously sensitized by contact with a specific antigen are stimulated on repeated contact by releasing lymphokines. These lymphokines are pharmacologically very active agents and include the transfer factor (TF), migration inhibition factor (MIF), blastogenic transformation factor (LBTF), and cytotoxic factor (LCF).

This type of hypersensitivity reaction is encountered in the rejection of transplanted tissue and in attacking viruses or intracellular bacteria, parasites, as well as malignant cells. It is the basis for the skin test used to evaluate the host cell-mediated status. In the early days of immunology, it was discovered that the injection of tuberculin into healthy guinea pigs cause no reaction. However, the same injection given to a guinea pig with tuberculosis caused something to happen. The animal showed no change for about 24 hours after the injection. Following this, there was a systemic manifestation, with fever and listlessness as well as a local reaction at the site of the injection. Since it took time to develop, it was called a delayed reaction.

COMPLEMENT

Complement is an enzymatic system of proteins that is activated by many antigen-antibody reactions and which is essential for antibody-mediated immune hemolysis and bacteriolysis. It also plays a part in several other biological reactions, eg, phagocytosis, opsonization, chemotaxis, and immune cytolysis. It consists of a system of at least 11 proteins found in different concentrations in normal serum, and serves primarily to amplify the effects of the interaction between specific antibody and antigen. Complement is a naturally occurring group of serum proteins. Immunization is not required for the presence of the 11 complement proteins in serum.

In the late nineteenth century it was reported by Bordet that the serum of immunized guinea pigs destroyed *Vibrio cholerae* organisms in vitro, whereas the serum of unimmunized animals did not. He observed further that the capacity of the immunized serum to lyse the microorganism, which was lost when the serum was heated to 56°C for 30 minutes, could be restored by the addition of unheated and unimmunized guinea pig serum. It was concluded that lysis requires at least two different components: one that was produced by immunization (antibody), and a second that was heat-labile and was normally present even without immunization. Since the heat-labile component seemed to complement the protective function of antibody, it was termed complement. It was then determined that two serum components responsible for the lysis of *Vibrio cholerae* organisms were antibody and complement.

The antibodies react with antigen on the surface of the invading cell, and the classical cascade complement chain commences. It ends with the destruction of the cell. In the classical complement pathway, an inciting agent stimulates an antigen-antibody response which in turn stimulates production of C1, C4, and C2 in the presence of calcium and magnesium, which in turn stimulates C3, leading to the production of C4 on through to C9 (chemotaxis). This is called a cascade effect. An alternate pathway has been proposed and supported by recent work. This method is called either the alternative pathway or the properdin pathway. This pathway starts with a polysaccharide or an endotoxin, which, in the presence of magnesium, leads to the production of properdin C3 proreactor. Enhanced phagocytosis follows production of C3. From C4 to C9, the steps are the same as in the classic pathway. The alternate pathway has given rise to the theory of nonspecific resistance mechanism against infection.

FAILURE OF THE IMMUNE RESPONSE

If tumor cells possess antigens on their surface capable of stimulating a specific immune response, why does cancer continue to grow in the presence of a mechanism designed to control its growth? The explanation may be that the rate of growth exceeds the capacity of the immune response. However, from studies in animals, more specific reasons are known for the failure of the immune response to prevent the start and growth of cancer. These are discussed below.

Immunosuppression

There are many factors which contribute to this. Among these are aging, the neoplastic process itself, anticancer drug therapy, radiation therapy, genetic defects, neonatal thymectomy, and, to a lesser extent, antibiotics, anesthetics, analgesics, and hypnotics. In reality, it is often difficult to separate the contributions of drugs and disease in bringing about this state of immunosuppression.

Immunologic Tolerance

In a broad sense, this may represent a specific form of immunosuppression. It is usually associated with the exposure to an antigen during embryonic or early neonatal life before the immune system has matured. The latter then fails to recognize the antigen as nonself and is not capable of mounting an immune response to it. Since cancer is considered to rise from a single cell clone, the tolerance theory for the progress of cancer is offered as an explanation. Research on choriocarcinoma bears out this theory. When this occurs, the host is not immunologically tolerant in general, but only for the specific tumor antigen.

Acquired Tolerance

Acquired tolerance is induced by injecting very small or very large doses of antigen, persisting so long as the antigen remains in the body. In clinical practice, immune tolerance has been suggested to occur in the host with large tumors. Following the removal of such a large tumor mass, the host exhibits resistance to the reimplantation of its own tumor cells. This suggests that the intrinsic failure of the immune response was not the cause of the original lack of immune reaction. Rather, the temporary paralysis observed was due to the fact that the system was unable to cope with too large a challenge.

Immunologic Enhancement

This results in an increased growth of the tumors in animals. The observation was made in animals transplanted with grafts of foreign cancer cells and then given injections of antiserum against the cancerous cells. It was anticipated that the grafts of foreign cancer cells would be promptly rejected. However, it was found that not only were the cancer cells tolerated, but often were found to grow more rapidly. How can this be explained? It is conceivable that the antibody produced and then injected was an enhancing or blocking antibody as opposed to a cytotoxic or cytolytic antibody. These antibodies may have coated the tumor in the same manner as could be done by covering the tumor with a layer of cream. This would prevent the killer lymphocytes from attacking the tumor. The protective coating (by blocking or enhancing antibodies) would serve to protect the tumor. The process of immunologic enhancement is more complicated than described, but was presented in this manner for a simplistic explanation.

Immunologic tolerance has indirecly been shown to play a role in humans with choriocarcinoma.

Immunoselection

Cancer develops from a clone of cells. The cell has tumor antigens on the surface and, as the tumor grows, the bulk of cancer cells have the same type of antigens. During the course of many generations, mutations may occur, and certain cells may have more of the original antigen present, stimulating a greater antibody production. These cells will attract more antibodies and may be eliminated from the cell population, leaving cells with weaker antigens as survivors. The result may be a colony of cells with weak antigens, followed by a relatively slow growth of tumor at first. It is conceivable that this may even lead to tolerance as described earlier. After a period of time, the tumor cells develop autonomy and progressively greater invasive properties.

Antigen Modulation

This is a temporary change in antigenicity reflecting an adaptational alteration in an entire population of cells. In summary, it can be stated that as soon as antibody is present, cancer cells of certain animal leukemias cease synthesizing antigens. As a result, the immunologic defense becomes ineffective. In humans, this response has not been documented.

Unknown Factors

The tumor-bearing host may possess factors that depress the immunologic reactivity in a nonspecific way, or possibly they may lack factors that are important for such reactivity. This has been suggested by the poor response that the tumor-bearing host develops when tested for delayed hypersensitivity reactions to a variety of antigens. In vitro studies in this group have also shown a decreased ability to transform lymphocytes after stimulation with phytohemagglutinin.

IMMUNOTHERAPY AND IMMUNOPOTENTIATION

Cancer immunotherapy, the treatment of cancers by immunologic methods, is still only in its experimental phases. Knowledge acquired only very recently suggests that there are many different ways by which immunotherapeutic methods can be developed. Some are already being tried clinically; others are as yet mere possibilities, which should await either further evaluation in animal models or, in particular, unequivocal evidence of the involvement of specific viruses in human cancer.

The most efficient cures conceived by our philosophy involve the potentiation of normal, biophysical, or biochemical processes, or the countering of abnormal processes which lead to or accompany disease. Cancer presents a few examples of this ideal at present, but studies of what has become known as host resistance are clearly an early step in this apparently logical direction. There are many factors such as intercellular communication, metabolic peculiarity, biochemical selection, and hormonal requirement possibly involved in host resistance. The immune activities of the lymphoreticular system have received the greatest attention and will be the main topic of this discussion.

For orientation purposes an outline for the immunotherapy of cancer is presented as follows:

    I. Active immunization against cancer
        A. Active immunization against oncogenic virus
        B. Active immunization against cancer cells
            1. Autochthonous or autologous cells
            2. Allogeneic cells
            3. Attenuated cells
            4. Soluble tumor antigens
        C. Modification of antigenicity
   II. Passive immunization against cancer
        A. Passive immunization
        B. Adoptive immunization
            1. Allogeneic lymphocyte transfer

2. Transfer factor
3. Immune RNA
4. Autologous lymphocytes stimulated in vitro with a mitogen, phytohemagglutinin (PHA)
5. Bone marrow transplant
6. Thymosin

III. Nonspecific and miscellaneous
   A. Coley's toxin
   B. BCG (bacille Calmette Guérin)
   C. Vaccinia, pertussis vaccine, poly-IC
   D. MER (methanol extraction residue of BCG)
   E. Maruyama vaccine
   F. Cornybacterium parvum
   G. Levamisole
   H. DNCB (dinitrochlorobenzene)
   I. Chalones
   J. Interferon and interferon inducers
   K. Deblocking factor
   L. Neuraminidase, Vibro cholerae (VCN)
   M. Concanavalin A (Con A)
   N. Viruses
   O. Bone marrow transplants

ACTIVE IMMUNIZATION AGAINST ONCOGENIC VIRUSES

Immunization is usually a preventive measure rather than a treatment. However, active immunization against DNA oncogenic viruses in animals (such as polyoma virus) is not preventive in the usual sense since, when it is given after infection with the virus, it still inhibits the appearance of tumors. It is completely protective if given early in the period elapsing between infection with the virus and the time tumors start developing. Vaccination of chickens against Marek's lymphomatosis, which fully prevents the disease, has been a much applauded scientific victory. The virus of the herpes group that causes Marek's disease is related to some of the viruses implicated in human cancer, which include the Epstein-Barr virus that was isolated from Burkitt's tumor.

ACTIVE IMMUNIZATION AGAINST CANCER CELLS

Active immunization against cancer cells has been attempted. A variety of antigenic stimuli have been used including: 1) preparations made from the patient's own tumor cells, killed by physical or chemical means, 2) similar preparations from tumors of the same histologic type removed from other individuals, and 3) cell extracts from different kinds.

Since the antigens capable of stimulating a cytotoxic immune response are part of the cell surface, the best source of immunizing material may ultimately be a fraction of the cell containing cell surface membrane, or just purified soluble antigen. Such materials are now being tested with tumors in animals.

MODIFICATION OF ANTIGENICITY

Attempts are being made to increase the inherent capacity of tumor antigens to elicit an immune reaction.

Many cancer antigens may be so similar to normal cell constituents as to be relatively ineffective in eliciting immune reactions. Modifying the cancer cell surface by a variety of means, including the coupling of foreign proteins, polysaccharides, or chemicals, may serve to increase its immunogenicity. An effective antigen for immunotherapy may well be purified cancer cell surface components to which a strongly immunogenic substance has been coupled.

Another method for increasing antigenicity is being developed using hybrid cells. These cells are formed between normal cells of different species, which are strongly antigenic, and cancer cells, which are presumably weekly antigenic. Such hybrids, it is believed, will be less malignant than cancer cells, are completely nonmalignant, yet high antigenic, and thus capable of stimulating tumor rejection.

PASSIVE IMMUNIZATION AGAINST CANCER

Passive immunization is the administration of preformed antibody that has been tried against leukemias induced by vertically transmitted viruses in mice. If cancer is vertically transmitted (from parent to offspring), passive immunization will have more to offer than active immunization. The carcinogenic agent in vertical transmission would resist the effects of active immunization due to immunological tolerance. The use of antiserum for passive immunization has certain drawbacks, that is, serum sickness may result, the antibody may be enhancing rather than cytolytic, and there may not be enough complement to complete the antigen-antibody reaction that is needed in the humoral mechanism.

ADOPTIVE IMMUNIZATION

In its strict and original usage, adoptive immunization described the colonization of a recipient by live and viable immunocompetent cells from an immune dose. It has now been extended to include transmission of the immune state through cell fractions derived from immune cells such as immune RNA and transfer factor. The response is usually predictable and effective. Success is achieved by the frequent development of an immune response directed against the recipient when intact live lymphocytes are used. Unless there is a close tissue-matching, a graft-versus-host reaction may result. This does not occur when transfer factor and immune RNA are administered. Since the recipient is immunodeficient, the donor cells (live lymphocytes) may stimulate an antibody response to the antigens of the recipient, producing a graft-versus-host syndrome (characterized by anorexia, diarrhea, wasting, loss of hair, skin rash, leukopenia, anemia, thrombocytopenia, and often death of the recipient). The graft-versus-host response may occur in young animals, and, if they avoid death, their course is characterized by poor growth, susceptibility to infections, and diarrhea (runt disease). Subcellular extracts (transfer factor and immune RNA) have been demonstrated to transfer immunity to the recipient without initiating a graft-versus-host syndrome. When sensitive lymphocytes are cultured in the presence of antigens, at least four mediators of cellular immunity are produced, including transfer factor. Immune RNA has recently been isolated. It is a hot phenol extract of immune lymphoid cells that can transfer specific tumor immunity. Its action is quite similar to transfer factor, although they are not identical, and their ultimate relationship is unknown.

NONSPECIFIC AND MISCELLANEOUS

Coley, in the early part of this century, working at New York's Memorial Hospital, noted the regression of a malignancy in a patient whose course was complicated by erysipelas. He began to treat patients with various bacterial toxins (streptococcus and *Serratia marcescens*). Although there were a few very promising results, there was no predictable cure rate among the patients treated with bacterial toxins.

Among the nonspecific methods of immunotherapy, *bacille Calmette-Guérin* (BCG) and *Cornybacterium parvum* have received the most extensive clinical trial. Nonspecific immunotherapy has been reported to promote both cell-mediated immunity and antibody protection, and may be effective in partially reversing the immunosuppressant effects of both the tumor and the conventional therapy. BCG requires a certain number of live bacteria whereas *Cornybacterium parvum* does not require live bacteria to be present to produce an immunologic response. In order to eliminate the disadvantages of BCG, immunotherapeutic trials of MER, a rather crude methanol extractable residue of BCG, are now in progress. Each method has certain complications, both local and systemic. The remaining types of nonspecific immunotherapy that are listed have had only limited application and will not be discussed.

TUMOR MARKERS*

All vertebrates have a defense mechanism, the immune defense system, that protects them from disease-causing microorganisms. Its delicate exploitation has conquered many infectious diseases and has been a major achievement of medical science in terms of preventing suffering and saving lives.

Cancer cells, like bacteria and viruses, have their own characteristic antigens. An antigen is defined as a substance—usually a protein or polysaccharide—that the body recognizes as foreign and in whose presence it reacts by forming antibody. Antigenic differences represent the first known qualitative distinction between cancer cells and their normal counterparts.

These qualitative differences between normal and cancer cells had escaped other methods of investigation but were revealed by immunologic techniques—techniques that take advantage of the extraordinary power of discrimination of the immune defense mechanism itself. This mechanism is capable of distinguishing even minute differences between protein molecules, probably as little as one different amino acid in a chain of several thousand.

It is obvious that the human body arises from a single cell, and present in the cell are all the things it needs in its journey through life, or at least the machinery to produce it. There are many antigens that appear on the surface of the cell during the lifetime of an individual. Recently it has been reported that chorionic gonadotropins, using the new sensitive radioimmunoassay methods, have demonstrated a positive reaction in 40% of all tumors, including squamous and adeno type of tissue in both females and males, and that among embryonal tumors this figure climbed to over 90%.

The carcinoembryonic antigen (CEA) has been demonstrated in the fetal gut in the first and second trimesters, but disappears in the third trimester. Later, it can be identified in certain endodermal cancers, cirrhotics, and heavy smokers. The question that is raised is: what represses the gene controlling this antigen in the third trimester and depresses the gene later in life?

Stolbach (1969) has reported work from his laboratory with the Regan alkaline phosphatase isoenzyme. He found this isoenzyme in the serum of 30% to 40% of patients with ovarian cancer and in 50% to 70% of malignant fluids from patients with carcinoma of the ovary.

In the laboratory at New York's Lenox Hill Hospital, a common antigenic component has been identified among the common epithelial ovarian cancers, using a double immunodiffusion technique and im-

---

* See also Chapter 24.

munofluorescence methods. Heterologous antiserum produced by pools of ovarian carcinoma tissue have reacted consistently and specifically with tissues of origin in immunodiffusion and immunofluorescence tests. Fresh ovarian tissue was taken directly from the operating room, homogenized, and the tissue homogenates were then mixed with complete Freund's adjuvant and emulsified by sonication at 4°C. This emulsion was injected into New Zealand, white, virgin female rabbits. The sera was collected after an appropriate time. The highly absorbed sera showed no reaction with normal ovarian tissues, normal human serum components, and various other neoplasms. These investigations have suggested the presence of a specific antigenic component in carcinoma of the ovary. This antigen did not crossreact with the carcinoembryonic antigen, ferratin, and was not revealed in fetal tissues.

It has been repeatedly reported that a piece of tumor removed from the parent tumor and explanted close to it, will probably grow, but the same piece of tumor explanted at a distance from the parent tumor may or may not grow. It is obvious that the tumor explanted close to the parent tumor was protected. Evidence indicated that a cloud of antigen-antibodies surrounded the parent tumor and served as enhancing or blocking antibodies. A study of peritoneal fluid was undertaken to isolate these factors. Peritoneal effusion of patients with ovarian cancer contains sizable amounts of free and complexed immunoglobulins. Each new antibody preparation is first tested by nephelometry, over a wide range of dilutions, against a pool of soluble antigen from ovarian carcinomas to determine its level of reactivity. Those showing reaction curves indicative of substantial levels of activity are screened at an appropriate dilution against a panel of soluble antigen extracts from a variety of normal, benign, and malignant tissues.

By lowering the pH to 2.5, it was possible to elute, from the surface of the ascitic cancer cell, candidate antigens and antibodies. The antibody has been identified as an IgG antibody and is immunoelectrophoretically pure. An immunoadsorbent column was prepared by linking the autologous antibody to a matrix (Afigel 10 by Biorad) and, after antigen-loading and washing, the column was eluted with pH 2.8 glycine hydrochloride buffer. Recently, 8M urea has been used to dissociate the immune complexes and yield almost complete dissociation. It does not interfere with the separation of dissociated antibody from antigen by ion exchange chromatography. Protein recovered from the column is currently being analyzed by polyacrylamide gel electrophoresis to determine its heterogeneity and the molecular weight range of its components. Hopefully, this material can be used to raise a high affinity, monospecific antiserum in animals. Recently, the antibody linked to a staphylococcus protein A has been reacted with a fluorescein-tagged candidate antigen, and gives a very specific immunoelectrophoretic positive response. A blocking test has been devised where the antibody is linked to a staphylococcus protein A,

614

is then reacted with the candidate antigen, and later with the candidate antigen that has been tagged with fluorescein. This results in a negative immunofluorescent response. By diluting the candidate antigen, reacting it with the antibody bound to the staphylococcus protein A, and then reacting this with the candidate antigen that has been tagged with the fluorescence, it is possible to reach a dilution where the candidate antigen is no longer present. Hopefully, the blocking test will add one more step in the goal to isolate the ovarian cancer antigen in a very pure form.

AREAS OF PROMISE

1. Development of tests for the identification of specific immune deficiencies, the evaluation of immune reaction potential, and the monitoring of cancer patients.
2. Naturally occurring immune deficiencies and their relationship to cancer.
3. Immunosuppression associated with aging.
4. Basic events in all forms of immune response at the cellular and molecular levels.
5. Cell surfaces, their different receptor and antigenic sites, and their structural, biochemical, and functional properties.
6. Cancer antigens — their relatedness, structure, and function.
7. Serological tests for the detection and identification of cell-associated and circulating antigens.
8. Selective immunochemotherapy.
9. Delayed hypersensitivity, its mechanisms, and use in diagnostic and prognostic tests.
10. Origin, nature, function, and chemical composition of complement.

BIBLIOGRAPHY

Alexander JW, Good RA: *Fundamentals of Clinical Immunology.* Philadelphia, WB Saunders Co., 1977.

Alper CA, Rosen FS: Genetic aspects of the complement system. *Adv Immunol* 14:252, 1971.

Baldwin RW: Immunity to methylcholanthrene-induced tumors in inbred rats following implantation and regression of implanted tumors. *Br J Cancer* 9:652, 1955.

Barber HRK: *Immunobiology for the Clinician.* New York, Wiley, 1977.

Barlow JJ, Bhattacharya M: Tumor markers in ovarian cancer: Tumor-associated antigens. *Sem Oncol* 2:203, 1975.

Bashford EF: Report of the General Superintendent. Fourth Annual Report of the Imperial Cancer Research Fund. London, 1906, p 5.

Bernier GM: Structure of human immunoglobulins. *Prog Allergy* 14:1, 1970.

Bordet J: *Traite de L'Immunité dans les Maladies Infecienses,* ed 2. Paris, Maison Publishing, 1937.

Burnet FM: The concept of immunological surveillance, in Schwartz RA (ed): *Progress in Experimental Tumor Research. Immunological Aspects of Neoplasia.* Basel, Switzerland, S. Karger, 1970, p 1.

Cochrane CG: Initiating events in immune complex injury, in Amos B (ed): *Progress in Immunology.* New York, Academic Press, 1971, p 143.

Coley WB: Treatment of malignant tumors by repeated innoculations of erysipelas with a report of ten cases. *Med Res* 43:60, 1893.

Coley WB: The treatment of malignant tumors by repeated inoculations of erysipelas, with a report of original cases. *Am J Med Sci* 105:487, 1893.

Coley WB: Late results of the treatment of inoperable sarcoma with mixed toxins of erysipelas and Bacillus prodigiosus. *Trans Am Surg Ann* 19:27, 1901.

Currie GA: Eighty years of immunotherapy: A review of immunological methods used for the treatment of human cancer. *Br J Cancer* 26:141, 1972.

DiSaia PJ, Rutledge FN, Smith JP, et al: Cell-mediated immune reaction to two gynecologic malignant tumors. *Cancer* 28:1129, 1971.

Dorsett BH, Ioachim HL, Stolbach L, et al: Isolation of tumor specific antibodies from effusions of ovarian carcinomas. *Int J Cancer* 16:777, 1975.

Dumonde DC: Tissue specific antigens. *Adv Immunol* 5:30, 1965.

Ehrlich P: On immunity with special reference to cell life. *Proc R Soc Lond (Biol)* 66:424, 1906.

Foley EJ: Antigenic properties of methylcholanthrene-induced tumors in mice of the strain of origin. *Cancer Res* 13:835, 1953.

Fudenberg H: Primary immunodeficiencies. Report of World Health Organization Committee. *Pediatrics* 47:927, 1971.

Fudenberg H, Stites DP, Caldwell JL, et al: *Basic and Clinical Immunology.* Los Altos, Cal., Lange Medical Publishers, 1976.

Gewurz H: The immunobiologic role of complement, in Good RA, Fisher DW (eds): *Immunology.* Stamford, Conn., Sinauer Associates, Inc., 1971.

Gross L: Intradermal immunization of C3H mice against a sarcoma that originated in animals of the same line. *Cancer Res* 3:326, 1943.

Gupta S: Cell surface markers of human T and B lymphocytes. *NY State J Med* 76:24, 1976.

Hellström KE, Hellström I: Cellular immunity against tumor antigen. *Adv Cancer Res* 12:167, 1969.

Héricourt J, Richet C: De la serotherapies dans le traitement du cancer. *CR Acad Sci [D] (Paris)* 121:567, 1895.

Israel L, Halpern B: Le Corynebacterium parvum dans les cancers avances: Premier evaluation de l'activité therapeutique de cette immuno-stimuline. *Nouv Press Med* 1:19–23, 1972.

Landsteiner K: *The Specificity of Serological Reactions.* Springfield, IL, Charles C Thomas, 1936.

Lepow IH, Rosen FS: Pathways to complement systems. *N Eng J Med* 286:942, 1972.

McKhann CF, Yarlott MA: Tumor immunology. *CA* 25:187, 1975.

McKhann CF, Gunnarsson A: Approaches to immunotherapy. *Cancer* 34:1521, 1974.

Naff GB: Editorial: Properdin—Its biologic importance. *N Eng J Med* 287:716, 1972.

Oettgen HF, Hellström KE: Tumor immunology, in Holland JF, Frei E III (eds): *Cancer Medicine.* Philadelphia, Lea & Febiger, 1973.

Prehn RT, Main IM: Immunity to methylcholanthrene-induced sarcomas. *J Natl Cancer Inst* 18:769, 1957.

616

Roitt J: *Essential Immunology*. London, Blackwell Scientific Publications, 1972.

Sell S: *Immunology, Immunopathology and Immunity*. New York, Harper & Row, 1972.

Southam CM, Brunschwig A, Levin A, et al: Effect of leukocytes on transplantability of human cancer. *Cancer* 19:1743, 1966.

Stolbach LK, Krant NJ, Fishman WH: Ectopic production of an alkaline prostatase isoenzyme in patients with cancer. *N Engl J Med* 281:757, 1969.

Streilein JW, Hughes JD: *Immunology—A Programmed Text*. Boston, Little, Brown and Company, 1977.

Terethia SS, Katz M, Rapp F: New surface antigen in cells transformed by simian papovavirus SV-40. *Proc Soc Exp Biol Med* 119:896, 1965.

Thomas L: *Discussion in Cellular and Humoral Aspects of Hypersensitivity States*. New York, Hober Medical Division, Harper & Row, 1961, p 529.

Wier DM: *Immunology For Undergraduates,* 3rd ed. Baltimore, Williams and Wilkins, 1976.

Yunis EJ, Greenberg LJ: Immunopathology of aging. *Fed Proc* 33:2017, 1974.

24 Tumor Markers in Gynecologic Cancer

John R. van Nagell, Jr.
Edward J. Pavlik
E. C. Gay

In realistic terms, a tumor marker can be defined as a substance which is selectively produced by a tumor and which is then released into the circulation in detectable amounts. Ideally, the majority of cells within a tumor should produce the marker, so that its concentration will accurately reflect the amount of viable tumor present in the host. Disappearance of the marker should indicate eradication of the tumor, whereas an increase in marker concentration should be indicative of tumor growth.

In order to understand fully the biologic potential of an antigenic marker, one should know the concentration of the antigen in tumor and normal tissues, the levels of the antigen in the plasma or serum, and, finally, the sites of antigen metabolism and excretion. Conceptually, an exemplary tumor marker could be used as: 1) a reliable immunodiagnostic test for cancer, 2) a target for radiolabeled antibodies which could be used in photoscanning techniques for tumor staging, and 3) a method for monitoring the response of tumors to therapy. At the present time, there is no marker for gynecologic cancers which can successfully be used in all

617

three of these roles. However, there is a variety of markers which can be used clinically. These markers can generally be defined as oncofetal antigens, carcinoplacental proteins, and tumor-associated antigens.

In this chapter, present knowledge concerning the use of these markers in patients with gynecologic cancers will be reviewed. Specific sections will be devoted to oncofetal antigens, hormonal markers, and to the more specific tumor-associated antigens. In addition, guidelines for the effective clinical use of these markers will be discussed.

ONCOFETAL ANTIGENS

The expression of specific embryonic proteins by a tumor cell is thought to be related to a loss of regulator gene function, and has been associated with rapid cellular growth. These antigens are often produced by normal embryonic tissues during fetal life, but antigenic expression is inhibited as these normal tissues mature. With neoplastic transformation, the cellular production of these markers is activated or derepressed. In gynecologic cancer, the two most extensively studied oncofetal markers are carcinoembryonic antigen (CEA) and alpha-fetoprotein (AFP).

Carcinoembryonic Antigen

Carcinoembryonic antigen was first described by Gold and Freedman (1965) in adenocarcinoma of the colon and in embryonic digestive tissues during the first two trimesters of pregnancy. Hence, it was given the name "carcinoembryonic" antigen. This antigen is a glycoprotein with a molecular size of approximately 200,000 daltons and beta-globulin mobility on electrophoresis. Since its initial description, CEA has been detected in the tumors and plasma of patients with a variety of gynecologic neoplasms (Khoo and MacKay 1973, DiSaia et al 1975, van Nagell et al 1975, 1978). The incidence of elevated plasma CEA levels in patients with gynecologic cancer and in control groups of healthy volunteers and patients with benign gynecologic disease is presented in Table 24-1. Plasma CEA levels are elevated in approximately 50% of patients with gynecologic cancer, as compared to 18% in patients with benign gynecologic disease and 11% in healthy volunteers. The highest frequency of elevated plasma CEA concentrations has been reported in patients with cervical and ovarian malignancies. The incidence of elevated plasma CEA is related both to tumor CEA content and to the stage or extent of disease. Likewise, CEA metabolism by the host affects the level of circulating CEA. Shuster and co-workers (1973) have shown that CEA metabolism in experimental animals is related directly to liver function, and this observation has been confirmed in human studies. Likewise, Lurie and colleagues (1975) have reported that biliary tract obstruction can produce elevated plasma CEA levels.

Table 24-1
Plasma Levels of Carcinoembryonic Antigen in Gynecologic Cancer

	No. of Patients	CEA Levels > 2.5 ng/ml
Healthy volunteers	176	19 (11%)
Benign gynecologic disease	95	17 (18%)
Carcinoma of the cervix	592	313 (53%)
Carcinoma of the endometrium	279	103 (37%)
Carcinoma of the ovary	203	95 (46%)

Data obtained from Barrelet and Mach (1975), DiSaia et al (1975), Donaldson et al (1976), Kjorstad and Orjaseter (1977), LoGerfo et al (1971), Reynoso et al (1972), Seppala et al (1975), and van Nagell et al (1975, 1977, 1978a, 1978b).

In patients with ovarian cancer, plasma CEA levels have also been related to cell type. For example, van Nagell and colleagues (1978) reported that plasma CEA levels were elevated in 53% of patients with mucinous cystadenocarcinomas of the ovary, as compared to only 31% in patients with serous ovarian malignancies. In patients with cervical cancer, elevated plasma CEA values have been observed most frequently in patients with mucin-producing endocervical adenocarcinomas and keratinizing squamous cell carcinomas (van Nagell 1978). Although the incidence of elevated plasma CEA is significantly higher in patients with each of the major types of gynecologic cancer than in the control groups of normal volunteers and patients with benign gynecologic disease, the lack of tumor specificity of this antigen has limited its diagnostic usefulness.

The major clinical role of CEA is as a monitor of disease status in patients whose tumors or plasma contain high antigen concentrations prior to therapy. The effect of surgical treatment on plasma CEA levels was first reported by Khoo and MacKay (1973). These investigators found that plasma CEA concentrations decreased to normal within four to eight weeks following complete surgical excision of uterine and ovarian tumors. In contrast, CEA levels remained abnormally high in patients with incomplete surgery or persistent disease. Barrelet and Mach (1975) also noted a progressive decline in plasma CEA levels within seven weeks following excision of ovarian, endometrial, and cervical carcinomas.

It should be emphasized that plasma CEA levels have not shown consistent patterns of decline during radiation therapy of gynecologic tumors. Van Nagell and colleagues (1978) reported that CEA levels often rose during radiation therapy, presumably due to the prolonged release of membrane-bound antigen into the plasma from radiation-damaged tumor cells. Following completion of radiation therapy, there is a gradual decline of plasma CEA to normal values, but this decline often takes up to 16 weeks (Donaldson et al 1976).

The value of serial plasma CEA in the follow-up of selected patients with cervical and ovarian cancers has been emphasized by several investigators. Van Nagell and co-workers (1979) reported that progressively rising CEA values accurately predicted recurrent cervical cancer in over 80% of patients whose tumors stained immunohistochemically for CEA. In approximately one-half of these patients, rising plasma CEA determinations preceded the clinical diagnosis of recurrent cancer by one to five months. In contrast, serial plasma CEA values correlated positively with disease status in only 28% of patients whose tumors were devoid of CEA. Khoo and co-workers (1979) studied the accuracy of serial plasma CEA values in predicting the clinical status of over 200 patients with ovarian cancer. These investigators reported that serial CEA determinations reflected disease status in over 95% of patients with minimal residual disease following surgical debulking. However, predictive accuracy fell to 62% in patients with extensive disease in whom complete surgical excision was impossible.

Recently, Primus and associates (1975) reported the successful localization of CEA in tissue sections of gynecologic and other tumors using a modified immunoperoxidase technique. Heald and co-workers (1979), using this method, noted that CEA was present most consistently in mucinous ovarian tumors. Similarly, van Nagell and colleagues (1978a) reported that CEA was detectable in a significantly higher percentage of mucinous ovarian carcinomas than in serous cystadenocarcinomas. In cervical cancer, keratinizing squamous cell carcinomas and endocervical adenocarcinomas have most consistently demonstrated CEA staining. In all gynecologic tumors, CEA has been identified almost exclusively on the cell membrane, and isolated nuclear staining has been absent.

A theoretical use of CEA in human cancer is as a target for radiolabeled antibodies used in tumor photoscanning experiments. Radioimmunodetection of gynecologic cancers using radiolabeled anti-CEA antibodies was first reported by Goldenberg and colleagues (1978). These investigators reported photoscan localization of primary and metastatic CEA-producing tumors using affinity purified ^{131}I-labeled antibodies to CEA. Effective localization occurred despite high circulating levels of plasma CEA. Included in these tumors were cervical and ovarian malignancies. In a subsequent study, van Nagell and colleagues (1980) noted that primary ovarian tumors could be localized using this method. Sites of metastatic ovarian cancer were reliably detected in approximately 67% of the cases.

Alpha-Fetoprotein

Alpha-fetoprotein (AFP) is a glycoprotein with a molecular weight of approximately 70,000 and alpha$_1$-globulin mobility on electrophoresis.

This marker was originally described by Abelev (1963) in the sera of mice bearing transplantable hepatocellular carcinomas. Since that time, this antigen has been detected in human hepatocellular carcinomas and in testicular and ovarian germ cell tumors (Abelev et al 1967, Tatarinov 1964). In addition, the synthesis of AFP has been demonstrated in vitro by cells of the fetal liver and yolk sac. In gynecologic malignancies, elevated serum levels of AFP (>20 μg/ml) have been confined to patients with ovarian germ-cell tumors, although preliminary observations may indicate the presence of small amounts of this antigen in certain epithelial tumors of the cervix and ovary (Donaldson et al 1980). Specifically, serum AFP has been markedly elevated in virtually every case of ovarian endodermal sinus tumors prior to surgical removal of the tumor (Kurman and Norris 1976a, 1976b, Gallion et al 1979). Elevated serum levels of AFP have also been reported in patients with ovarian teratocarcinomas (Table 24-2). It is not clear, however, if endodermal sinus elements were actually present in these tumors. Serum concentrations of AFP have been shown to be increased in a variety of non-neoplastic diseases such as acute viral hepatitis (Akeyama et al 1972), liver cirrhosis (Abelev 1971), ataxia-telangiectasia (Waldmann and McIntire 1972), and obstructive jaundice (Abelev 1971). Therefore, elevated serum concentrations of AFP cannot be interpreted as pathognomonic for cancer. However, markedly elevated serum AFP levels in a patient with an ovarian tumor strongly suggests the presence of endodermal sinus or teratocarcinomatous elements.

Although the number of patients studied is small, there is substantial evidence to indicate that serial AFP determinations reliably reflect the clinical disease status in patients whose tumors contain high antigen concentrations (Gallion et al 1979). For example, Sell and colleagues (1976) reported that serial AFP levels accurately predicted the extent of disease

Table 24-2
Serum Alpha-Fetoprotein in Germ-Cell Tumors of the Ovary According to Tumor Type

Tumor Type	Cases	Elevated Serum AFP (> 20 μg/ml)	AFP Concentration μg/ml
Endodermal Sinus Tumor			
Tsuchida et al (1973)	3	3	>10,000
Wilkinson et al (1973)	3	3	—
Talerman and Haije (1974)	1	1	4,000
Norgaard-Pedersen et al (1975)	3	3	950–7,100
Sell et al (1976)	6	6	590–19,200
Teratocarcinoma			
Esterhay et al (1973)	1	1	23,000
Talerman and Haije (1974)	1	1	—

in five of six patients with endodermal sinus tumors of the ovary who were treated with radiation therapy or chemotherapy. It is apparent from these data that a patient suspected of having a malignant germ-cell tumor of the ovary should have a serum sample obtained for AFP determinations. Should the tumor or serum contain high antigen levels, it is probable that serial AFP determinations will provide an accurate reflection of its response to therapy. In malignant ovarian germ-cell tumors which contain several histologic components, the disappearance of serum AFP may indicate only a selective response of the endodermal sinus elements to therapy, despite persistence of other extra-embryonal components.

Recently, AFP has been used as an adjunct to confirm the histologic diagnosis of ovarian endodermal sinus tumor. In a review of 71 ovarian germ-cell tumors from the Armed Forces Institute of Pathology, Kurman and Norris (1976a, 1976b) reported that endodermal sinus tumors could be reliably differentiated from embryonal cell carcinomas on the basis of marker production. Endodermal sinus tumors were found to produce only AFP, whereas embryonal cell carcinomas contained both AFP and hCG. Alpha-fetoprotein was demonstrated in the hyaline droplets, cytoplasm, and intercellular spaces of these tumors. It is suggested, therefore, that immunohistochemical staining for AFP and hCG be performed on all germ-cell tumors of the ovary. The localization of specific antigens in these tumors will not only help identify the appropriate marker for serum determinations, but may also aid in making the correct pathologic diagnosis.

Radioimmunodetection methods, utilizing radiolabeled anti-AFP antibodies, have been recently reported both in experimental animals and in humans. Koji and co-workers (1980) reported the localization of transplanted rat hepatomas utilizing ^{131}I-labeled antibodies to AFP and total body scintigraphy. Microautoradiograms of tissue sections showed specific localization of radioactivity in the tumor, but not in adjacent normal tissue. Similarly Kim and co-workers (1980) reported the effective photoscan localization of diverse AFP-producing human tumors and their metastases using ^{131}I-labeled goat immunoglobulin-G prepared against AFP. Included in these tumors was an endodermal sinus tumor of the ovary. Localization was most effective when the tumor/nontumor AFP ratio was highest.

CARCINOPLACENTAL PROTEINS

The second class of markers of clinical importance in gynecologic tumors is the carcinoplacental proteins. These proteins are not normally produced in the absence of pregnancy, and their presence in the serum of nonpregnant patients is often indicative of neoplastic growth. These hormones are ectopically produced by rapidly dividing tumor cells through selective expression of the cancer cell genome. Human chorionic gonadotropin (hCG), human placental lactogen (hPL), and the Regan isoenzyme of placental alkaline phosphatase (RI) are three carcinoplacental proteins which have been studied in gynecologic tumors.

Human Chorionic Gonadotropin

Human chorionic gonadotropin is a glycoprotein with a molecular weight of approximately 39,000. It consists of two dissimilar subunits, the alpha and beta chains, which are noncovalently linked. The alpha chains of human chorionic gonadotropin (hCG), human leuteinizing hormone (hLH), and thyroid stimulating hormone (TSH), have similar primary structures (Bellisario et al 1973). However, the C-terminal residues of the beta subunits of these hormones are different, and it is upon this difference that Vaitukaitis and co-workers (1972) developed a specific radioimmunoassay for the beta subunit of human chorionic gonadotropin. The first observation as to the possible role of hCG as a tumor marker in trophoblastic tumors was made by Li et al (1958). These investigators detected increased amounts of this hormone in the urine of patients with choriocarcinoma, and demonstrated the reliability of hCG determinations as a criterion tumor response to chemotherapy (Hertz et al 1961). Subsequently, human choriocarcinoma in tissue culture was shown to produce hCG (Patillo et al 1968). Rapid radioimmunoassays for the measurement of hCG were developed (Wilde et al 1967), but it was not possible to distinguish low levels of hCG from pituitary hLH until the development of the specific radioimmunoassay by Vaitukaitis (1972). This assay has enabled numerous investigators to evaluate hCG as a tumor marker not only in trophoblastic neoplasms, but also in other gynecologic tumors.

Although hCG is not a tumor-specific antigen, it is quantitatively increased in trophoblastic tumors. The increased production of hCG by choriocarcinoma cells has been quantitated both in vitro and in vivo (Braunstein et al 1973). In a normal pregnancy, hCG is produced by the blastocyst, but is usually not detected until after ovum implantation. Following implantation, serum hCG concentrations increase rapidly with a doubling time of approximately two days. Peak serum hCG values of 10,000–100,000 mIU/ml occur near the end of the first trimester. Although a single hCG determination alone cannot reliably differentiate trophoblastic disease from pregnancy, hCG values in excess of 300,000 mIU/ml, particularly in the presence of low serum hPL concentrations, are highly suggestive of trophoblastic disease.

The reliable production of hCG by the syncytiotrophoblast and the predictable release of this marker into the serum, has allowed formation of treatment regimens for patients with trophoblastic tumors based solely on the serum concentration of hCG. Specifically, complicated tropho-blastic disease requiring adjunctive chemotherapy is defined by: 1) a failure of hCG levels to decline to normal by eight weeks following evacuation of trophoblastic tissue from the uterus, 2) a plateau in serum hCG levels for two or more weeks after therapy, or 3) a rise in serum hCG levels following therapy. More recently, a serum hCG concentration in excess of 40,000 mIU/ml, in the presence of metastatic trophoblastic disease, has placed the patient in the "poor prognosis" category, necessitating treatment with combination chemotherapy (Hammond et al 1980). Finally, serum hCG levels have so accurately reflected clinical disease status that the absence of detectable hCG for three consecutive weeks is indicative of complete remission, thereby allowing cessation of additional chemotherapy.

In a sense, hCG is an optimal tumor marker. Both diagnostic and therapeutic decisions can be made on the basis of serum marker concen-trations alone, and patients with trophoblastic malignancies are spared the complications of more invasive diagnostic techniques.

The incidence of elevated serum hCG levels in patients with non-trophoblastic gynecologic malignancies is illustrated in Table 24-3. Serum hCG concentrations are more often increased in patients with ovarian and cervical malignancies than in those with endometrial cancer (Rutanen et al 1978). These clinical data confirm previous reports demonstrating the production of hCG by both cervical and ovarian cancer cell lines in tissue culture (Kanabus et al 1978). The presence of hCG in the serum of a small percentage of patients with benign gynecologic disease (Carenza et al 1980) has prevented its use as an immunodiagnostic method in non-trophoblastic gynecologic malignancies. However, serial serum hCG determinations do reflect disease status, particularly in ovarian germ-cell tumors having choriocarcinomatous or embryonal cell elements.

Immunohistochemical staining procedures have indicated that a very high percentage of trophoblastic tumor cells produce hCG (Yorde et al 1979). In addition, hCG expression by ovarian epithelial tumors has

Table 24-3
Elevated Serum Levels of Human Chorionic Gonadotropin in Patients With Non-Trophoblastic Gynecologic Cancers

	No. of Patients	Elevated hCG
Controls	317	9 (3%)
Cervical Cancer	318	111 (35%)
Endometrial Cancer	185	34 (18%)
Ovarian Cancer	156	59 (38%)

Data from Carenza et al (1980), Dash et al (1978), Donaldson et al (1980), Fishman et al (1975), Goldstein et al (1974), Rosen (1975), Rutanen and Seppala (1978), and Stanhope et al (1979).

recently been reported. Recently, Kurman and Norris (1976b) noted the presence of hCG in every embryonal-cell carcinoma of the ovary tested by the immunoperoxidase method. It is highly likely, therefore, that hCG will be a useful marker in germ-cell tumors of the ovary containing either choriocarcinomatous or embryonal-cell elements.

Photoscan localization of hCG-producing tumors and their metastases has not been attempted in a significant number of patients. However, preliminary studies have indicated successful localization of trophoblastic tumors using radiolabeled antibodies to hCG (Goldenberg et al 1980).

Human Placental Lactogen

Human placental lactogen (hPL) is a polypeptide hormone with a molecular weight of approximately 22,300. This hormone was described initially by Josimovitch and MacClaren (1962) in the normal human placenta, but has since been detected in a very high percentage of trophoblastic tumors. Also, Weintraub and Rosen (1971) noted elevated (>1 ng/ml) levels of hPL in the serum of patients with ovarian or testicular choriocarcinomas. This marker is not specific for any particular type of gynecologic cancer. However, determinations of hCG and hPL have been useful in distinguishing pregnancy from trophoblastic disease. In trophoblastic disease, serum hCG is characteristically higher and serum hPL significantly lower than that found in normal pregnancy. Immunohistochemical staining for hPL has not been studied extensively. However, preliminary studies have indicated that detectable concentrations of hPL are present in ovarian epithelial tumors. Therefore, it is possible that serum hPL may be an effective marker in trophoblastic disease, and in germ cell tumors of the ovary containing choriocarcinomatous elements. Also, hPL may be clinically useful as a marker in selected patients with ovarian epithelial cancers. To date, radioimmunodetection procedures using antibodies radiolabeled to hPL have not been performed in patients with gynecologic cancer.

The Regan Isoenzyme

The Regan isoenzyme (RI) is a type of placental alkaline phosphatase which has a molecular size of approximately 120,000 daltons (Rosen et al 1975). This carcinoplacental marker was initially detected in the tumor tissue and serum of a patient, Mr. Regan, with lung cancer—hence, the name Regan isoenzyme. A serum specimen is considered positive when it contains more than 0.2 placental isoenzyme units of alkaline phosphatase per 100 ml as confirmed by electrophoresis (Fishman et al 1975). Elevated serum levels of RI have been observed in approximately 25% of patients with cervical and ovarian malignancies, and in 10% of patients with endometrial cancer (Kellen et al 1976, Fishman et al 1975). The Regan isoenzyme also has been produced by Hela cells in tissue culture. In patients with cervical and endometrial malignancies, the incidence of elevated RI levels has not been directly related to stage of disease. In fact, Kellen and co-workers (1976) reported that the highest elevations of serum RI occurred in cervical cancer patients with stages Ia and Ib disease. Enzyme levels were lower in patients with more advanced cervical cancer. In contrast, RI levels seemed to correlate more directly with extent of disease in patients with ovarian cancer. Serum levels of this marker have been reported to reflect response to therapy accurately, and decrease to normal within three months following complete tumor excision. However, the presence of this enzyme in the sera of patients with a variety of benign inflammatory conditions such as hepatitis and colitis, has prevented its use as a reliable immunodiagnostic method.

Histochemical methods do exist for the localization of this enzyme in tumor tissue. However, these methods are not antibody directed, and immunodetection procedures using this enzyme as a target for radiolabeled antibodies have not been developed.

TUMOR-ASSOCIATED ANTIGENS

With recent advances in the technology of antigen isolation and purification, much effort has been directed toward the search for markers which are specific to one type of gynecologic cancer. Presumably, these tumor-associated antigens are newly expressed at the time of malignant transformation or are previously undetectable normal tissue antigens which are produced in increased amounts by rapidly proliferating tumor cells. In order to be clinically useful, these markers must be produced by a significant percentage of the cells within a tumor, and then released into the circulation in amounts detectable by radioimmunoassay.

Tumor-associated antigens that have been detected in gynecologic cancer are illustrated in Table 24-4. Although there is a relatively large number of these antigens associated with both ovarian and cervical carcinomas, radioimmunoassays have been developed for only three of them. Two of these are ovarian cancer-associated antigens, and one is a cervical cancer-associated antigen.

The first of these antigens is the ovarian cystadenocarcinoma antigen (OCAA) reported by Bhattacharya and Barlow (1972, 1975). This antigen is a high molecular weight mucoprotein with an electrophoretic mobility in the beta region. It is composed of approximately 60% protein and 40% carbohydrate (Bhattacharya and Barlow, 1979). Ouchterlony diffusion testing indicated the presence of OCAA in 26 of 37 serous ovarian

Table 24-4
Tumor-Associated Antigens in Gynecologic Cancer

Investigator	Site	Histology	Radioimmuno-assay
Witebsky et al (1956)	Ovary	Mucinous Cystadenocarcinoma	−
Levi et al (1969)	Ovary	Serous Cystadenocarcinoma	−
Dorsett and Ioachim (1973)	Ovary	Mucinous and Serous Cystadenocarcinoma	−
Bhattacharya and Barlow (1973, 1975, 1978, 1979)	Ovary (OCAA)	Mucinous and Serous Cystadenocarcinoma	+
Order et al (1975)	Ovary	Mucinous and Serous Cystadenocarcinoma	−
Knauf and Urbach (1974, 1977, 1978)	Ovary (OCA)	Mucinous and Serous Cystadenocarcinoma	+
Burton et al (1976)	Ovary	Mucinous and Serous Cystadenocarcinoma	−
Imamura et al (1978)	Ovary (OCV$_2$)	Mucinous and Serous Cystadenocarcinoma	−
Dawson et al (1980)	Ovary	Mucinous and Serous Cystadenocarcinoma	−
Levi et al (1971)	Cervix	Squamous Cell	−
Gall et al (1973)	Cervix	Squamous Cell	−
Kato et al (1979)	Cervix (TA-4)	Squamous Cell	+

cystadenocarcinomas and in 7 of 7 mucinous cystadenocarcinomas. It was not present in normal ovarian tissue, and was immunologically distinct from CEA, AFP, and normal histocompatibility antigens. Also, this antigen was not present in other malignancies. The absence of OCAA in extraovarian malignancies has been used by these authors as a diagnostic aid in differentiating primary ovarian tumors from tumors metastatic to the ovary from other primary sites such as the gastrointestinal tract or breast. In addition, these investigators developed a radioimmunoassay for the detection of OCAA and designated a serum antigen concentration in excess of 10 ng/ml as abnormally high. Elevated levels of circulating OCAA were observed in over 60% of patients with stages II and III disease, and 80% of patients with Stage IV ovarian cancer. Serum levels of OCAA usually returned to normal within three weeks following tumor excision, and correlated quite well with response to treatment. There were patients with known active disease, however, who never had elevated serum levels of OCAA. Similarly, the sera of patients with extensive colonic, cervical, and breast cancers often showed cross-inhibition in the OCAA radioimmunoassay. This antigen is presently not specific enough to be used as a diagnostic method for ovarian cancer. However, it was proven to be reliable as a biochemical monitor for disease status in patients undergoing treatment for epithelial ovarian cancer. At present, this antigen has been evaluated mainly by one group of investigators, and the promising clinical results they have reported await confirmation in multi-institutional trials.

A second ovarian cancer associated antigen for which there is a reliable radioimmunoassay is the ovarian cancer antigen (OCA) described by Knauf and Urbach (1974). These investigators, using immunodiffusion techniques, reported the isolation of a high molecular weight glycoprotein which was present in extracts of epithelial ovarian cancer, but was absent in normal ovarian tissue and normal human serum. This antigen was soluble in perchloric acid and differed from CEA in electrophoretic mobility. A double-antibody radioimmunoassay for OCA was developed (Knauf and Urbach 1978), and a plasma level above 1.8 ng/ml was defined as abnormally elevated. Using this definition, 57% of patients with ovarian cancer had elevated plasma OCA levels compared to 14% in patients with benign gynecologic disease. This antigen was more specifically associated with ovarian cancer than was CEA in the population studied. However, the presence of OCA in patients with benign gynecologic disease has precluded its diagnostic efficacy. Although OCA has not been evaluated in large numbers of patients, it has correlated quite well with clinical disease status.

The only cervical tumor-associated antigen that has received clinical trials is the squamous cell carcinoma antigen (TA-4). This antigen was initially described by Kato and Torigoe (1977) in cervical cancer tissue using immunodiffusion methods. This antigen was not present in extracts of normal cervical tissue, normal liver, or normal kidney. These investigators developed a double-antibody radioimmunoassay for the detection of this antigen, and a serum level above $4\mu U/ml$ was considered elevated. Elevated serum levels of antigen were present in 27 of 35 patients (78%) with cervical cancer and varied directly with the stage of disease. All patients with stages III and IV disease had elevated serum concentrations of TA-4. In a later study (Kato et al 1979), the specificity of this antigen was tested in a coded panel of sera from the NCI-Mayo Clinic Serum Bank. Thirteen of 25 patients with cervical squamous cell carcinoma showed positive serum antigen levels while only 1 of 58 control cases had detectable TA-4 in the serum. Serum levels of this antigen correlated extremely well with clinical disease status. Thirteen patients with positive TA-4 serum levels prior to therapy underwent complete tumor resection, and antigen values returned to normal in all cases within 14 days following surgery. In contrast, nine patients had tumor progression during therapy, and serum TA-4 levels demonstrated a consistent rise in all cases.

THE CLINICAL USE OF TUMOR MARKERS

Although the advances in tumor immunology may allow future investigators to isolate truly tumor specific antigens, the lack of specificity of the antigens previously reviewed have prevented their use in the diagnosis of gynecologic malignancies. At the present time, the major clinical role of tumor markers in patients with gynecologic cancers is as a biochemical monitor of disease status following therapy. A question of fundamental importance, however, is how to determine the most appropriate marker for each particular tumor. It is relatively easy to identify the correct marker in certain gynecologic tumors such as trophoblastic disease (hCG) or endodermal sinus tumor of the ovary (AFP). However, the majority of gynecologic tumors may contain several nonspecific markers such as CEA or hCG as well as tumor-associated antigens, and it is often quite difficult to determine which of these markers is most clinically useful. In this regard, it is important to emphasize that a marker must be present in significant concentrations in tumor tissue if it is to reflect disease status. Too often, studies have concluded that a particular marker is not clinically useful because tumor recurrence was noted without a corresponding rise in plasma marker concentrations. In many of these investigations, there was no evidence that the specific marker studied was ever present in the tumor itself. It must be remembered that less than 50% of cervical, endometrial, or ovarian cancers contain detectable concentrations of one specific marker. Therefore, it is useless to measure plasma marker concentrations serially in all patients with gynecologic cancers.

Clearly, what is needed is a tissue screening test which reliably identifies the antigenic profile of each tumor. On the basis of this antigenic profile, the appropriate marker can then be selected for serial plasma determinations as a means to monitor therapeutic response. One approach is to measure the antigen concentration in tumor tissue extracts by radioimmunoassay. Unfortunately, this method is subject to significant sampling errors, and is not well suited for screening large numbers of tumor specimens.

At the present time, a most reliable tissue antigen screening method is immunohistochemical staining. In this method, an enzyme tracer is chemically coupled with antibodies prepared against a specific marker, and the site of immunological reactivity is identified by a histochemical reaction (Nakane and Pierce 1966, 1967). The most commonly utilized enzyme for tumor antigen localization has been peroxidase. The histochemical reaction is developed with diaminobenzidine, and the site of antigen production stains brown (Figure 24-1). Unlike immunofluorescence, formalin-fixed specimens stained by immunoperoxidase are permanent and can be counterstained with conventional histologic stains, thereby permitting direct observation of antigen location within morphologic structures of the tumor (Primus et al 1978). In addition, the simplicity and convenience of immunoperoxidase methodology makes it readily adaptable to the rapid screening of tissue sections as they are processed for histopathology. Using this method, a number of different nonspecific markers including CEA, hPL, hCG, and AFP have been localized in gynecologic tumors. The importance of this technique is that it can reliably predict those patients who should benefit most from serial plasma antigen determinations.

As has been previously mentioned, van Nagell and co-workers (1979) reported that serial plasma CEA values correlated with clinical disease status in over 80% of cervical cancer patients whose tumors were shown to contain CEA by immunohistochemical staining. In contrast, plasma CEA was predictive of disease status in only 28% of patients whose cervical tumors were devoid of antigen. This accuracy could be further increased by the development of a more quantitative assessment of the extent of immunohistochemical staining. It is not sufficient to characterize a tumor as antigen-positive or antigen-negative. Rather, the number and distribution of tumor cells staining positively for a specific antigen should be noted. It is apparent that plasma determinations of a marker will most effectively reflect the number of tumor cells within a host if the majority of those tumor cells produce the marker that is measured. Such is the case in trophoblastic tumors which characteristically contain a high percentage

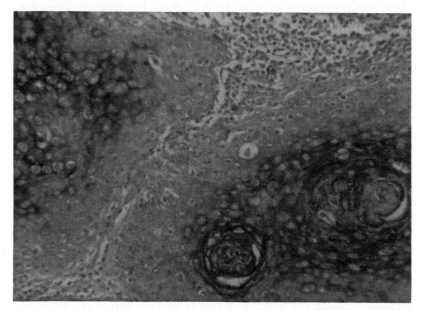

Figure 24-1 Immunohistochemical staining for CEA in keratinizing squamous cell carcinoma of the cervix. Note intense antigen staining in areas of keratin production. (Hematoxylin counterstain, 250 × magnification)

of hCG-producing cells. Conversely, it is quite unlikely that plasma marker levels will reliably reflect clinical disease status if a tumor contains only minimal numbers of marker-positive cells. Further investigation should be undertaken to determine the relationships between the percentage of marker-producing cells within a tumor and the ability of serial plasma marker values to predict clinical disease status. At the present time, it is suggested that histochemical tumor tissue staining be utilized to develop a tumor antigen profile before obtaining serial plasma determinations of a specific marker. Although histochemical staining alone cannot guarantee that a marker will accurately reflect disease status, it can aid in the selection of an antigen that has the highest probability of success. Similarly, it can identify those tumors which contain no detectable marker substances, thereby sparing the patient unnecessary plasma marker determinations.

One area in which our present knowledge is incomplete is antigen metabolism. It has been demonstrated both in experimental animal studies and in humans that the metabolism of CEA, hCG, and hPL is related directly to liver function. In fact, liver disease itself may cause elevated serum levels of these markers (Shuster et al 1973, Lurie et al 1975). Metabolic clearance rates for these antigens have been defined. However, the quantitative distribution of these substances within various normal tissues as a function of time has not been thoroughly studied. Antigen distribution both in normal and malignant tissues is obviously of extreme importance when one considers the theoretical use of these tumor associated markers as sites for antibody-directed therapy either with radiopharmaceutical or chemotherapeutic agents.

Two areas of experimental interest in marker research include: 1) the use of markers as targets for radiolabeled antibodies which can localize both primary and metastatic cancer, and 2) antibody-directed therapy. The effective use of radioimmunodetection procedures to localize tumors is based on the general concept that antibodies directed against tumor-associated antigens will selectively accumulate in tumors. If these antibodies can then be radiolabeled with a suitable gamma emitting source, their preferential accretion in neoplastic tissue would allow tumor localization using external scintillation imaging. In 1953, Pressman reported the successful localization of rat lymphosarcomas using radiolabeled anti-lymphosarcoma antibodies. Somewhat later, Spar and co-workers (1967) reported that diverse human tumors could be localized using ^{131}I-labeled antibodies to human fibrin. With recent advances in antigen purification methods and isotope subtraction techniques, localization of both ovarian and cervical tumors using anti-CEA radioantibodies has been achieved (Goldenberg et al 1978, van Nagell et al 1980). Briefly, affinity-purified goat anti-CEA antibodies were labeled with [131]I. The antibodies were tested for pyrogenicity, and a test dose was administered to potential subjects to rule out a possible anaphylactic reaction. In addi-

632

tion, Lugol's solution was administered to the patients prior to injection of the radiolabeled antibody to prevent thyroid uptake of [131]I. The radioiodinated anti-CEA antibodies were then administered intravenously (Goldenberg et al 1978). To subtract blood pool activity, [99m]TcO4 and ^{99m}Tc-labels were given prior to the administration of anti-CEA antibodies. Images of the chest and abdomen were obtained with a gamma scintillation camera and data were stored on a computer capable of generating digital images of the ^{131}I-labeled antibody minus the technetium components (Figure 24-2).

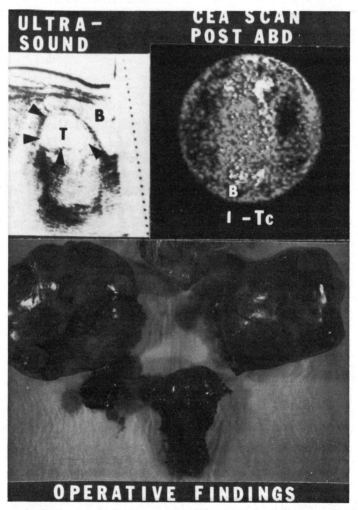

Figure 24-2 Photoscan utilizing radiolabeled anti-CEA antibodies in a patient with stage II serous cystadenocarcinoma of the ovary and extensive omental metastases. Both primary tumors and omental metastases are localized using this technique.

Using this methodology, Goldenberg and colleagues (1978) reported the successful localization of diverse CEA-producing tumors, including cervical and ovarian cancers. Both primary and metastatic sites were detected, thus confirming the histochemical observation that primary and metastatic tumors have the same patterns of marker production. Radio-immunodetection procedures have also been successful in localizing gynecologic tumors which produce both AFP and hCG. Kim and co-workers (1980), for example, reported the detection of embryonal cell carcinomas of the ovary and testis using radiolabeled anti-AFP antibodies. Circulating serum AFP levels in these patients varied from 800 μg/ml to 18,000 μg/ml, and did not interfere with tumor localization. Likewise, Goldenberg and colleagues (1980) reported the radioimmunodetection of hCG-producing ovarian germ-cell tumors and trophoblastic tumors using anti-hCG radioantibodies. At present, a major deficiency in these detection procedures is that they have not reliably identified tumor nodules less than 2 cm in diameter (van Nagell 1980). However, it is hoped that this deficiency will be rectified by methods which increase the specific activity of the radionuclide on the antibody, and by improved resolution of tomographic photoscanning techniques.

A second theoretical use of tumor markers is to provide targets for antibody-directed therapy. Both chemotherapeutic agents and radioactive sources can be coupled to antibodies which can then be directed to antigens on the tumor cell surface. The theoretical advantages of such an approach are obvious since therapy is directed specifically at marker-producing tumor cells, whereas normal cells are spared. Bale and Spar (1965), McCardle et al (1966), and Spar et al (1967) reported the therapeutic use of purified antifibrin antibodies conjugated with [131]I. These investigators reported that radiolabeled antifibrin antibodies produced occasional short-term remissions in a variety of fibrin-containing human tumors. However, no long-term remissions or curative results were obtained. More recently, Latif and colleagues (1980) reported that chlorambucil-antibody complexes were effective in the treatment of human myelosarcomas transplanted in nude mice.

Bale and colleagues (1980) have suggested prerequisites for the successful use of antibody-directed therapeutic agents. These are as follows: 1) the antibody molecule should not be functionally altered by the attached agent in such a way that it loses its specificity, 2) the antibody must carry a sufficient amount of the therapeutic agent to the tumor, and 3) the cytotoxic activity of the therapeutic agent must be preserved until it is bound to the tumor cell, and not destroyed by interaction with tissue or plasma components. Although antibody-directed therapy has been utilized in a number of animal systems, this form of treatment has not received clinical trials in patients with gynecologic malignancies.

A conceptual model of the clinical use of tumor markers is illustrated in Figure 24-3. A tumor antigen profile is established by histochemical

634

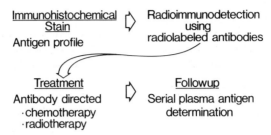

Figure 24-3 Conceptual model of the clinical application of tumor markers. Tumor antigen profile, as determined by histochemical staining, aids in selection of the most appropriate marker for photoscan localization studies and serial plasma measurements following therapy.

staining techniques, thereby defining the antigen or antigens which should be used as a marker for the particular tumor. That marker is then used for radioimmunodetection procedures which can complement conventional clinical staging methods. The same marker can then be used as a target for antibody-directed chemotherapy or radiotherapy. Finally, serial plasma marker determinations can then serve as a noninvasive method for monitoring disease status. At the present time, this model system is purely conceptual. Much additional work must be completed related to many of the basic aspects of tumor immunology and nuclear medicine. However, tumor-associated markers are already providing clinically meaningful data concerning many gynecologic cancers, and it is highly probable that they will be even more useful in the future.

BIBLIOGRAPHY

Abelev GI: Study of the antigenic structure of tumors. *Acta Un Intern. Cancer* 19:80–92, 1963.

Abelev GI, Assecritova V, Kraevsky NA, et al: Embryonal serum α-globulin in cancer patients: Diagnostic value. *Int J Cancer* 2:551–558, 1967.

Abelev GI: Alpha-fetoprotein in ontogenesis and its association with malignant tumors. *Adv Cancer Res* 14:295–358, 1971.

Akeyama T, Kayama T, Kamada T: Alpha-fetoprotein in acute viral hepatitis. *N Engl J Med* 287:989, 1972.

Bale WF, Spar IL: Fibrinogen and antibodies to fibrin as carriers of ^{131}I for cancer therapy, in Hoffman MG, Scheers DE (eds): *Radionuklide in der Klinischen und Experimentellen Onkoligic.* Stuttgart, F.K. Schattauer, 1965.

Bale WF, Contreras MA, Grady ED: Factors influencing localization of labeled antibodies in tumors. *Cancer Res* 40:2965–2972, 1980.

Barrelet V, Mach J: Variations of the carcinoembryonic antigen level in the plasma of patients with gynecologic cancers during therapy. *Am J Obstet Gynecol* 121:164–168, 1975.

Bellisario R, Carlsen RB, Bahl OR: Human Chorionic Gonadotropin: Linear amino acid sequence of the α subunit. *J Biol Chem* 248:6796–6801, 1973.

Bhattacharya M, Barlow JJ: Immunologic studies of human serous cystadenocarcinoma of ovary. *Cancer* 31:588–595, 1972.

Bhattacharya M, Barlow JJ: An immunologic comparison between serous cystadenocarcinoma of the ovary and other human gynecologic tumors. *Am J Obstet Gynecol* 117:849–853, 1973.

Bhattacharya M, Barlow JJ: A tumor-associated antigen from cystadenocarcinomas of the ovary. *Natl Cancer Inst Monogr* 42:25–32, 1975.

Bhattacharya M, Barlow JJ: Ovarian tumor antigens. *Cancer* 42:1616–1620, 1978.

Bhattacharya M, Barlow JJ: Tumor markers for ovarian cancer. *Int Adv Surg Oncol* 2:155–176, 1979.

Braunstcin GD, Grodin JM, Vaitukaitis J, et al: Secretory rates of human chorionic gonadotropin by normal trophoblast. *Am J Obstet Gynecol* 115:447–450, 1973.

Burton RM, Hope NJ, Lubbers LM: A thermostable antigen associated with ovarian cancer. *Am J Obstet Gynecol* 125:472–477, 1976.

Carenza L, DiGregorio R, Mocci C, et al: Ectopic human chorionic gonadotropin: Gynecological tumors and non-malignant conditions. *Gynecol Oncol* 10:32–38, 1980.

Dash RJ, Dutta TK, Purohit OP, et al: Prevalence of ectopic hCG production in non-endocrine malignancy. *Indian J Cancer* 12:23–27, 1978.

Dawood MY, Saxena BB, Landesman R: Human chorionic gonadotropin and its subunits in hydatiform mole and choriocarcinoma. *Obstet Gynecol* 50:172–181, 1977.

Dawson JR, Kutteh WH, Whitesides DB, et al: Identification of tumor-association antigens and their purification from cyst fluids of ovarian epithelial neoplasms. *Gynecol Oncol.* 6–17, 1980.

DiSaia PJ, Haverback BJ, Morrow CP: Carcinoembryonic antigen in patients with gynecologic malignancies. *Am J Obstet Gynecol* 121:159–166, 1975.

Donaldson ES, van Nagell JR, Wood EG, et al: Carcinoembryonic antigen in patients treated with radiation therapy for invasive squamous cell carcinoma of the uterine cervix. *Am J Roentgenol* 127:829–831, 1976.

Donaldson ES, van Nagell JR, Pursell S, et al: Multiple biochemical markers in patients with gynecologic malignancies. *Cancer* 45:948–953, 1980.

Dorsett BH, Ioachim HL: Common antigenic component in ovarian carcinomas: Demonstration by double diffusion and immufluorescence techniques. *Immunol Commun* 2:173–184, 1973.

Esterhay RJ, Shapiro HM, Sutherland JC, et al: Serum alpha-fetoprotein concentration and tumor growth dissociation in a patient with ovarian teratocarcinoma. *Cancer* 31:835–839, 1973.

Fishman WH, Inglis NR, Vaitukaitis J, et al: Regan isoenzyme and human chorionic gonadotropin in ovarian cancer. *Natl Cancer Inst Monogr* 42:63–73, 1975.

Forney JP, DiSaia PJ, Morrow CP: Endodermal sinus tumor. A report of two sustained remissions treated postoperatively with a combination of actinomycin D, 5-fluorouracil, and cyclophosphamide. *Obstet Gynecol* 45:186–189, 1975.

Frantz AG, Rabkin MT, Friesen HG: Human placental lactogen in choriocarcinoma of the male. Measurement by radioimmunoassay. *J Clin Endocrinol Metab* 25:1136–1139, 1975.

Gall SA, Walling J, Pearl L: Demonstration of tumor-associated antigens in human gynecologic malignancies. *Am J Obstet Gynecol* 115:387–393, 1973.

Gallion H, van Nagell JR, Powell DF, et al: Therapy of endodermal sinus tumor of the ovary. *Am J Obstet Gynecol* 135:447–451, 1979.

Gitlin D, Perricelli A, Gitlin GM: Synthesis of α-fetoprotein by liver, yolk sac, and gastrointestinal tract of the human conceptus. *Cancer Res* 32:979–982, 1972.

636

Gold P, Freedman SO: Demonstration of tumor specific antigens in human colonic carcinoma by immunological tolerance and absorption techniques. *J Exp Med* 121:439–462, 1965.

Goldenberg DM, DeLand F, Kim E, et al: Use of radiolabeled antibodies to carcinoembryonic antigen for the detection and localization of diverse cancers by external photoscanning. *N Engl J Med* 298:1384–1388, 1978.

Goldenberg DM, Kim E, DeLand FH, et al: Clinical radioimmunodetection of cancer using radioactive antibodies to human chorionic gonadotropin. *Science* 208:1284–1286, 1980.

Goldstein DP, Kosasa, TS, Skarim AT: The clinical application of a specific radioimmunoassay for human chorionic gonadotropin in trophoblastic and non-trophoblastic tumors. *Surg Gynecol Obstet* 138:747–751, 1974.

Goldstein DP: Chorionic gonadotropin. *Cancer* 38:453–459, 1976.

Hammond CB, Weed JC, Currie JL: The role of operation in the current therapy of gestational trophoblastic disease. *Am J Obstet Gynecol* 136:844–858, 1980.

Heald J, Buckley CH, Fox H: An immunohistochemical study of the distribution of carcinoembryonic antigen in epithelial tumours of the ovary. *J Clin Path* 32:918–926, 1979.

Hertz R, Lewis J, Lipsett MB: Five years' experience with the chemotherapy of metastatic choriocarcinoma and related trophoblastic tumors in women. *Am J Obstet Gynecol* 82:631–637, 1961.

Imamura N, Takahashi T, Lloyd KO, et al: Analysis of human ovarian tumor antigens using heterologous antisera: Detection of new antigenic systems. *Int J Cancer* 21:570–577, 1978.

Jones WB, Lewis JL, Lehr M: Monitor of chemotherapy in gestational trophoblastic neoplasm by radioimmunoassay of the β-subunit of human chorionic gonadotropin. *Am J Obstet Gynecol* 121:669–673, 1975.

Josimovitch JB, MacClaren JA: Presence in the human placenta and term serum of a highly lactogenic substance immunologically related to human growth hormone. *Endocrinology* 71:209–215, 1962.

Kanabus J, Braunstein GD, Emry PK, et al: Kinetics of growth and ectopic production of human chorionic gonadotropin by an ovarian cystadenocarcinoma cell line maintained in vitro. *Cancer Res* 38:765–770, 1978.

Kato H, Torigoe T: Radioimmunoassay for tumor antigen of human cervical squamous cell carcinoma. *Cancer* 40:1621–1628, 1977.

Kato H, Niyaughi F, Morioka H, et al: Tumor antigen of human cervical squamous cell carcinoma. Correlation of circulating levels with disease progress. *Cancer* 43:585–590, 1979.

Kellen JA, Bush RS, Malkin A: Placenta-like alkaline phosphatase in gynecological cancers. *Cancer Res* 36:269–271, 1976.

Khoo SK, MacKay EV: Carcinoembryonic antigen in cancer of the female reproductive system. Sequential levels and effects of treatment. *Aust NZ J Obstet Gynaecol* 13:1–7, 1973.

Khoo SK, Whitaker S, Jones I, MacKay E: Predictive value of serial characinoembryonic antigen levels in long-term follow-up of ovarian cancer. *Cancer* 43:2471–2478, 1979a.

Khoo SK, Whitaker SV, Jones ISC, et al: Carcinoembryonic antigen in patients with residual ovarian cancer. *Gynecol Oncol* 7:288–295, 1979b.

Kim EE, DeLand FH, Nelson MO, et al: Radioimmunodetection of cancer with radiolabeled antibodies to α-fetoprotein. *Cancer Res* 40:3008–3012, 1980.

Kjorstad KE, Orjaseter H: Studies on characinoembryonic antigen levels in patients with adenocarcinoma of the uterus. *Cancer* 40:2935–2956, 1977.

Kjorstad KE, Orjaseter H: Carcinoembryonic antigen levels in patients with squamous cell carcinoma of the cervix. *Obstet Gynecol* 51:536–540, 1977.

Knauf S, Urbach GI: Ovarian tumor-specific antigens. *Am J Obstet Gynecol* 119:966–970, 1974.

Knauf S, Urbach GI: Purification of human ovarian tumor-associated antigen and demonstration of circulating tumor antigen in patients with advanced ovarian malignancy. *Am J Obstet Gynecol* 127:705–711, 1977.

Knauf S, Urbach GI: The development of a double-antibody radioimmunoassay for detecting ovarian tumor-associated antigen fraction OCA in plasma. *Am J Obstet Gynecol* 131:780–786, 1978.

Koji T, Ishii N, Munehisa T, et al: Localization of radioiodinated antibody to α-fetoprotein in hepatoma transplanted in rats and a case report of α-fetoprotein antibody treatment of a hepatoma patient. *Cancer Res* 41:3013–3015, 1980.

Kurman RJ, Norris HJ: Endodermal sinus tumor of the ovary. *Cancer* 38:2404–2419, 1976a.

Kurman RJ, Norris HJ: Embryonal carcinoma of the ovary: A clinicopathological entity distinct from endodermal sinus tumor resembling embryonal carcinoma of the adult testes. *Cancer* 38:2420–2433, 1976b.

Latif Z, Lozzio B, Wust C, et al: Evaluation of drug-antibody conjugates in the treatment of human myelosarcomas transplanted in nude mice. *Cancer* 45:1326–1332, 1980.

Levi MM, Keller S, Mandl I: Antigenicity of a papillary serous cystadenocarcinoma tissue homogenate and its fractions. *Am J Obstet Gynecol* 105:856–861, 1969.

Levi MM: Antigenicity of ovarian and cervical malignancies with a view toward possible immunodiagnosis. *Am J Obstet Gynecol* 109:689–698, 1971.

Li MC, Hertz R, Bergenstal DM: Therapy of choriocarcinoma and related trophoblastic tumors with folic acid and purine antagonists. *N Engl J Med* 259:66–70, 1958.

LoGerfo R, Krupey J, Hansen HJ: Demonstration of an antigen common to several varieties of neoplasia: Assay using zirconyl phosphate gel. *N Engl J Med* 285:138–141, 1971.

Lurie BB, Oweinstein MS, Zamcheck N: Elevated carcinoembryonic antigen levels and biliary tract obstruction. *JAMA* 233:326–330, 1975.

McCardle RJ, Harper PV, Spar IL, et al: Studies with iodine[131]-labeled antibody to human fibrinogen for diagnosis and therapy of tumors. *J Nucl Med* 7:837–847, 1966.

Nakane PK, Pierce GB: Enzyme labeled antibody for the light and electron microscopic localization of tissue antigens. *J Cell Biol* 33:307–318, 1967.

Nakane PK, Kawaoi A: Peroxidase-labeled antibody. A new method of conjugation. *J Histochem Cytochem* 22:1084–1091, 1974.

Nathanson L, Fishman WH: New observations on the Regan isoenzyme of alkaline phosphatase in cancer patients. *Cancer* 27:1388–1397, 1970.

Norgaard-Pedersen B, Albrechtsen R, Teilum G: Serum alpha-fetoprotein as a marker for endodermal sinus tumour (yolk sac tumour) or a vitelline component of teratocarcinoma. *Acta Path Microbiol Scand* 83:573–589, 1975.

Order SE, Thurston J, Knapp R: Ovarian tumor antigens: A new potential for therapy. *Natl Cancer Inst Monogr* 42:33–43, 1975.

Patillo RA, Grey GO, Delfs E, et al: The hormone-synthesizing trophoblastic cell in vitro: A model for cancer research and placental hormone synthesis. *Ann NY Acad Sci* 172:288–298, 1971.

Pressman D, Koringold L: The in vivo localization of anti-Wagner osteogenic sarcoma antibodies. *Cancer* 6:619–623, 1953.

Primus FJ, Wang RH, Sharkey RM, et al: Detection of carcinoembryonic antigen in tissue sections by immunoperoxidase. *J Immunol Methods* 8:267–276, 1975.

Primus FJ, Sharkey RM, Hansen HJ, et al: Immunoperoxidase detection of carcinoembryonic antigen: An overview. *Cancer* 42:1540–1545, 1978.

Reynoso G, Chu T, Holyoke D, et al: Carcinoembryonic antigen in patients with different cancers. *JAMA* 220:361–365, 1972.

Rosen SW: Placental proteins and their subunits as tumor markers. NIH Conference. *Ann Int Med* 82:71–83, 1975.

Rutanen EM, Seppala M: The hCG-subunit radioimmunoassay in nontrophoblastic gynecologic tumors. *Cancer* 41:692–696, 1978.

Sell A, Sogaard H, Horgaard-Pedersen B: Serum alpha-fetoprotein as a marker for the effect of post-operative radiation therapy and/or chemotherapy in eight cases of ovarian endodermal sinus tumor. *Int J Cancer* 18:574–580, 1976.

Seppala M, Pihko H, Ruoslahti E: Carcinoembryonic antigen and alpha-fetoprotein in malignant tumors of the female genital tract. *Cancer* 35: 1377–1381, 1975.

Shuster J, Silverman M, Gold P: Metabolism of human carcinoembryonic antigen in xenogeneic animals. *Cancer Res* 33:65–68, 1973.

Spar IL, Bale WF, Marrack D, et al: Labeled antibodies to human fibrinogen. Diagnostic studies and therapeutic trials. *Cancer* 20:865–870, 1967.

Stanhope CR, Smith JP, Britton JC, et al: Serial determination of marker substances in ovarian cancer. *Gynecol Oncol* 8:284–287, 1979.

Stolbach LL, Krant MJ, Fishman WH: Ectopic production of an alkaline phosphatase isoenzyme in patients with cancer. *N Engl J Med* 281:757–762, 1969.

Talerman A, Haije WG: Alpha-fetoprotein and germ cell tumors: A possible role of yolk sac tumor in production of alpha-fetoprotein. *Cancer* 34:1722–1726, 1974.

Talerman A, Haije WG, Beggerman L: Serum alpha-fetoprotein (AFP) in diagnosis and management of endodermal sinus (yolk sac) tumor and mixed germ cell tumor of the ovary. *Cancer* 41:272–278, 1978.

Tatarinov JS: Presence of embryonal α-globulin in the serum of a patient with primary hepatocellular carcinoma. *Vop Med Khim* 1:90–91, 1964.

Tsuchida Y, Saito S, Ishida M, et al: Yolk sac tumor (endodermal sinus tumor) and alpha-fetoprotein. A report of three cases. *Cancer* 32:917–921, 1973.

Vaitukaitis, JL, Braunstein GP, Ross GT: A radioimmunoassay which specifically measures human chorionic gonadotropin in the presence of human luteinizing hormone. *Am J Obstet Gynecol* 113:751–756, 1972.

van Nagell JR, Meeker WR, Parker JC, et al: Carcinoembryonic antigen in patients with gynecologic malignancy. *Cancer* 35:1372–1376, 1975.

van Nagell JR, Donaldson ES, Wood EG, et al: The prognostic significance of carcinoembryonic antigen in the plasma and tumors of patients with endometrial adenocarcinoma. *Am J Obstet Gynecol* 128:308–313, 1977.

van Nagell JR, Donaldson ES, Gay EC, et al: Carcinoembryonic antigen in ovarian epithelial cystadenocarcinomas: Prognostic value in serial plasma determinations. *Cancer* 41:2335–2340, 1978a.

van Nagell JR, Donaldson ES, Wood EC, et al: The clinical significance of carcinoembryonic antigen in the plasma and tumors of patients with gynecologic malignancies. *Cancer* 42:1527–1532, 1978b.

van Nagell JR, Donaldson ES, Gay EC, et al: Carcinoembryonic antigen in carcinoma of the uterine cervix. 1. The prognostic value of serial plasma determinations. *Cancer* 42:2428–2434, 1978c.

van Nagell JR, Donaldson ES, Gay EC, et al: Carcinoembryonic antigen in carcinoma of the uterine cervix. 2. Tissue localization and correlation with plasma antigen concentration. *Cancer* 44:944–948, 1979.

van Nagell JR, Kim E, Casper S, et al: Radioimmunodetection of primary and metastatic ovarian cancer using radiolabeled antibodies to carcinoembryonic antigen. *Cancer Res* 40:502–506, 1980.

Waldmann TA, McIntire KR: Serum alpha-fetoprotein levels in patients with ataxia telangiectasia. *Lancet* 2:1112–1115, 1972.

Weintraub BD, Rosen SW: Ectopic production of human chorionic somato-mammatropin by non-trophoblastic cancers. *J Clin Endocrinol Metab* 32: 94–101, 1971.

Wilde CE, Orr AH, Bagshawe KD: A sensitive radioimmunoassay for human chorionic gonadotropin and luteinizing hormones. *J Clin Endocrinol* 27:23–35, 1967.

Wilkinson EJ, Friedrich EG, Hosty TA: Alpha-fetoprotein and endodermal sinus tumor of the ovary. *Am J Obstet Gynecol* 116:711–714, 1973.

Witebsky E, Rose NR, Schulman S: Studies of normal and malignant tissue antigens. *Cancer Res* 16:831–841, 1956.

Yorde DE, Hussa RO, Garancis JC, et al: Immunocytochemical localization of human choriogonadotropin in human malignant trophoblast: Model for human choriogonadotropin secretion. *Lab Invest* 40:391–398, 1979.

ab. Abbreviation for antibody.

Aberrant clone. The preferred term is forbidden clone. In a hypothetical clone of immunologically competent cells with specificity for self antigens which, according to the clonal selection theory, has been suppressed in fetal life and which may regain activity in adult life and cause autoimmune disease.

Ablastin. Antibody which inhibits reproduction of parasites.

Absorption. Removal of antibodies from solution as insoluble complexes, by combination with specific antigens; serum so treated is then said to be absorbed, and the absorbing antigen is called absorben.

Absorption of radiation. This term refers to "collision-like" interactions between the individual particulate or quantum components of a beam of radiation and the subatomic parts of matter that occur at random during irradiation. Each interaction may result in partial or complete transfer of energy. Partial transfer of energy usually results in redirection (scattering) of the beam component. The total number of interactions determines the fraction of the radiation absorbed and depends upon the type of radiation and thickness (total path length), density and atomic number of absorbing material. For some types of radiation, strategies to increase the absorption of radiation within cancerous tissue have been proposed, eg, magnetic containment of electron beams or loading of target with material with high probability for interaction with neutron beams.

Absorbed dose. The energy deposited per unit mass, strictly definable for a localized area, with a size neither too large nor too small for changes in it to influence the ratio. Absorbed dose is never perfectly uniform throughout a clinically irradiated volume. Successful results in radiation therapy are dependent upon delivery of an adequate absorbed dose to all tumor-bearing structures. The tolerance, expressed in units of absorbed dose of unavoidably irradiated normal tissue, frequently is the basis for cessation of treatment of various regions of the body. There is good correlation between absorbed dose and the fraction of the site that are ionized. The most common unit of absorbed dose is the rad (1 rad = 100 erg/gm = 0.01 J/kg).

Accelerator (particle). A device that imparts kinetic energy to charged particles, such as electrons, protons, deuterons, and helium ions. These particles may be used in medical irradiation either directly or indirectly (via the production of x-rays or neutrons).

Accessible antigens. Antigens of self that are in contact with antibody-forming tissues and with the host, which is normally tolerant.

Active immunization. Direct immunization of the intact individual or immunocompetent cells derived from the individual and returned to him.

Active immunotherapy. May be devided into two groups: specific immunogens and nonspecific adjuvants. Active specific immunotherapy is attempted by the immunization of a tumor-bearing patient with autologous tumor cells that have been altered chemically or by radiation. Nonspecific immunotherapy attempts to augment antitumor immunologic activity with nonspecific stimulants such as BCG or phytohemagglutinin.

Adaptation. The process whereby protection accorded to a foreign graft from the immune reaction of the recipient renders the graft less vulnerable to immunologic attack by the host.

Adenoacanthoma. Is a mixture of malignant glandular epithelium and benign squamous epithelium. Some authors feel that this squamous metaplasia is a protective development.

Adenosquamous (Adenoepidermoid). Unlike the adenoacanthoma which is characterized by a benign-appearing squamous component and a malignant appearing glandular component the mixed adenosquamous has both malignant-appearing squamous and glandular components. Examination with the electron microscope demonstrated keratohyalin-like granules and desmosomes with tonofilaments, structures regarded as characteristic of squamous cells.

Adoptive immunization. The transfer of immunity from one individual to another by means of specifically immune lymphoid cells or materials derived from such cells which are capable of transferring specific immunologic information to the recipients' lymphocytes.

Adjuvant. A substance which, when mixed with an antigen, enhances its antigenicity.

Afterloading technique. These techniques were introduced by Henschke. The use of applicators for brachytherapy so designed that they may be quickly loaded with radioactive sources after placement with the patient. Such techniques have the advantage of eliminating radiation exposure of personnel involved in the operative placement of the applicator. Loading is usually performed in the patient's room a few hours after applicator placement. The most commonly used afterloading technique is that used in the treatment of carcinoma of the cervix.

ag. Abbreviation for antigen.

Agglutinin. An antibody that produces aggregation or agglutination of a particulate or insoluble antigen.

Air dose. The absorbed dose that would be delivered to the center of an equilibrium mass of soft tissue which is situated at the point in question for the duration of treatment and otherwise surrounded by air only.

Allergy. The specifically altered state of reactivity of a host following exposure to an allergen. The term applies to either hypersensitivity or immunity.

Allogeneic. Pertaining to genetically dissimilar individuals of the same species or referring to tissues originating in different individuals of the same species or in members of a different inbred strain.

Allogeneic inhibition. In vitro damage to cells caused by contact with genetically dissimilar cells. When two antigenetically different lymphocytes are cultured in the presence of phytohemagglutinin (a substance which activates lymphocytes), there is a mutually damaging effect — the opposite of syngeneic preference.

Alpha fetoprotein (AFP). A serum protein synthesized in the fetus by perivascular hepatic parenchymal cells and found in a high percentage of patients with hepatomas and malignant teratomas, especially of the endodermal sinus type. It is present in concentrations up to 400 mg/100 ml in early fetal life, falling to less than 3 μg/100 ml in adults. Increased levels may be detected in the serum of adults with hepatoma (80% positive) and teratoma (40% positive) and may be used to follow the progress of the disease.

Alpha ray.   A stream of alpha particles, which are helium nuclei.

Amniography.   Radiography of the uterine contents after instillation of opaque media into the endometrial cavity.

Anamnestic response.   A recall mechanism; the accelerated response of antibody production to an antigen which occurs in an animal that has previously responded to the antigen; synonymous with secondary immune response.

Androgenesis.   The development of an ovum under the influence of a spermatozoon nucleus, with the original nucleus of the ovum being either absent or inactivated.

Anergy.   A deficiency in the response to agents which normally induce an immune response, especially delayed hypersensitivity.

Aneuploid.   Having a chromosome number that is not an exact multiple of the haploid number.

Antibody.   A specific globulin (immunoglobulin) produced in response to stimulation by an antigen and capable of reacting specifically with that antigen. A paratope is the site or area on an antibody molecule complementary to the epitope on the antigen molecule. The number of paratopes per molecule is the valency of the antibody.

Antigen.   A substance that is capable of inducing the production of specific immunity. The antigens may be extrinsic (an antigen that is not a constituent of the cell), intrinsic (an antigen that is a constituent of the cell), or occult (a self-antigen that does not reach antibody-forming tissues).

Antigen determinant (epitope).   The small three-dimensional configuration of the everted surface of the antigen molecule which combines with a specific antibody. The total number of antigen determinants per antigen molecule is the valence of that antigen.

Antiserum.   A serum containing antibodies and obtained from animals exposed to antigen(s) of a certain nature.

Atopy.   An hereditary predisposition to develop immediate-type hypersensitivity on contact with certain antigens (atopens or reagins).

Autoantigen.   A substance in a person's tissues to which he or she is immunologically sensitive.

Autochthonous.   Tissues of any sort originating in the same host or tumor borne by the host of origin.

Autologous.   Derived from the subject itself.

Axiom.   An established principle, for example, that a neoplasm is named from its most differentiated portion and graded from its least differentiated parts.

Backscatter.   Some of the radiation before entering the tissue will scatter back toward the surface. This portion of the radiation is called backscatter. Therefore, the peak absorbed dose may be equated to the air dose plus the backscatter dose.

B cell or B lymphocyte.   A bone marrow cell. These cells mediate humoral immunity and are thymus-independent cells. In the avian species, B cells are derived form the bursa of Fabricius. In man, no discrete bursa has been identified.

Beam shaping.   The use of special blocks, wedges, compensators, and other devices to create a treatment beam of the geometric proportions required for a treatment plan that is beyond the capabilities of the collimator.

Betatron. A megavoltage treatment machine capable of delivering high energy x-rays and, in some instances an electron beam. The electrons are accelerated in a circular orbit during a portion of the cycle of a low frequency alternating magnetic field.

Bergonie and Tribondeau 1906. The radiosensitivity of cells and tissues in proportion to their reproductive capacity and in inverse proportion to their degree of differentiation.

Binding site. Antibody-combining sites and other sites of specific attachment of macromolecules to one another.

Blast transformation. The transformation of small lymphocytes with minimal cytoplasm, condensed nuclei, and few cytoplasmic organelles into a lymphoblast characterized by abundant cytoplasm, numerous organelles, and a large nucleus with multiple nucleoli. Blast transformation may be induced by a number of mitogens.

Blocking factor (enchancement antibody). A humoral antibody or an antigen-antibody complex that acts as a noncytotoxic antibody. Instead of damaging the cell, it coats it with a protecive covering so that neither complement nor killer lymphocytes can attack the cell.

Bolus. A material of density nearly equivalent to tissue placed within the treatment beam to compensate for unevenness of body contour or to enhance the absorbed dose of the skin.

Bowen's disease. A specific histologic type of carcinoma in situ of the vulva.

Brachytherapy. (from the Greek *brachy* — short, and *therapy* — treatment). A term used to distinguish the therapeutic use of encapsulated radionuclides *close to* the tumor from their use *at a distance from* the tumor. For the latter, the term *teletherapy* (from the Greek *tele* — far) has been used.

Cancer. (From the Latin *cancri* — crab.) An inclusive term used to describe a variety of malignant neoplasms.

Cancerous growth. A cancerous growth measuring 1 cubic centimeter (approximately 1/16 cubic inch) and weighing about 1 gram (approximately 1/30 ounce) is about the smallest that can be detected by palpation or by x-rays, yet is contains about one billion cancer cells, each perhaps capable of originating a new focus of disease.

Carcinoembryonic antigen (CEA). An antigen found originally in fetal tissues of endodermal origin as well as in malignant tumors of adult tissues of endodermal origin. It probably results when a gene is derepressed by some stimulus. Since other tissues have been found to contain CEA, it is possible that the CEA molecule has more than one antigenic surface determinant.

Carcinoplacental proteins. Hormones normally produced by the placenta which may also be ectopically produced by rapidly dividing tumor cells.

Carcinoma. In modern medicine, all malignant tumors.

Carcinoma Puellarum Dysgerminoma. The "cancer of girls" or tumor of early life so named because it occurs most commonly in the first three decades of life.

Cell-mediated immunity (CMI).   Specific immunity that is mediated by small lymphocytes. They are thymus-dependent cells and are referred to as T cells, as opposed to the thymus-independent cells which are called B cells. The T cells are probably the most important cells in cancer immunity and organ rejection.

Cell Types in Invasive Epidermoid Carcinoma.   Keratinizing carcinoma. There is predominance of relatively large abnormal cells with a high degree of pleomorphism characterized by candate and elongated forms. The chromatin pattern is coarse and irregular. Macronucleoli are present. Nuclear degeneration characterized by an opaque nuclear mass is a distinct feature. The cytoplasm may be very abundant and is often eosinophilic or orangiophilic. Pearls or portions of pearls composed of malignant cells are sometimes found. A tumor background may not be present in this form of cancer. Large-cell non-keratinizing carcinoma. There are numerous syncytial masses as well as isolated relatively large, cyanophilic cells. The chromatin pattern is coarse and irregular, and there are several dense chromocenters of varying size and shape. The nuclei contain prominent macronuclei. Although the size of the cell tends to be uniform, there is a moderate degree of variation. The tumor background is useful for distinguishing these lesions from the large-cell carcinoma in situ. Small-cell non-keratinizing carcinoma. Relatively uniform small cyanophilic cells with a high nuclear cytoplasmic ratio predominate. The chromatin pattern is coarse and irregular, and there are several dense chromocenters of varying size and shape. Macronucleoli are prominent. The cells are usually associated with a tumor background.

Central venous pressure.   The following data have been helpful in interpreting central venous pressure (measured in centimeters of water), assuming there is no significant abnormality of cardiac output:

0–5 cm H_2O pressure = hypovolemia
6–12 cm H_2O pressure = normovolemia
over 12 cm H_2O pressure = hypervolemia

Cervical intraepithelial Neoplasia (CIN).   Richart reports that the various degrees of dysplasia or intraepithelial neoplasia are distinguished by the extent to which the full thickness of the epithelium is composed of undifferentiated neoplastic cells. If such cells occupy the lower one-third of the epithelium, the lesion is referred to as cervical intraepithelial neoplasia (CIN) Grade I or mild dysplasia, if they occupy up to two-thirds of the thickness of the epithelium, the term moderate dysplasia, or CIN Grade 2 is used and if the undifferentiated neoplastic cells reach almost to the surface, the lesion is referred to as severe dysplasia, or CIN Grade 3. When the entire epithelium is composed of undifferentiated neoplastic cells, it is generally diagnosed as carcinoma in situ, or CIN Grade 3. (See dysplasia.)

Cesium 137 tubes.   Used instead of radium for intracavitary insertions, especially in the treatment of carcinoma of the cervix. They are cylinders 2 cm in length and approximately 4 mm in diameter, usually calibrated as milligram equivalent of radium.

Chalones.   A group of naturally occurring substances which are sensitized by cells and appear to be importantly involved in the regulation of the cell division as well as in differentiation of such normal cell types. Since the antimitotic effect of these substances is tissue-specific and since they are essentially nontoxic, they would appear to represent an almost ideal group of substances for use in the suppression of growth of those tumors that have lost the ability to synthesize their own chalones but remain sensitive to their inhibitory effects.

Chimerism. A state in which two or more genetically different populations of cells coexist.

Chromosome. Carriers of genetic information composed of DNA on a framework of protein. They are in the cell nucleus and are visible in a dividing cell as deeply staining rod-shaped or J-shaped structures.

Citrate intoxication. Intoxication characterized by hypotension, a narrow pulse pressure, and elevated left ventricular end diastolic and central venous pressures.

Clonal selection theory of acquired immunity of Burnet. A theory which suggests that immunity and antibody production are functions of clones of mesenchymal cells. Each clone is able to react immunologically with a small number of antigens, and each cell is immunologically competent because it carries on its surface a receptor that is able to react with a given antigen.

Clone. A population of cells derived from a single cell by asexual division.

Cobalt 60. A radioactive isotope with a half-life of 5.3 years which emits beta and gamma radiations (1.17 and 1.33 meV) and is used as teletherapy.

Collimator. The part of the radiation therapy machine that controls the size of the radiation beam usually through the use of movable blocks of heavy metal attached to a manual or motor-driven cranking mechanism. Some collimators have removable inserts usually called cones or diaphragms.

Common epithelial ovarian cancers. These cancers are composed of one or more of several types of epithelium and stroma in a variety of combinations. They are generally considered to be derived from the surface epithelium (mesothelium) covering the ovary and from the underlying ovarian stroma. The work *common* has been applied because most ovarian tumors belong in this general category.

A. *Serous tumors* are composed of epithelium resembling that of the Fallopian tube or the surface epithelium of the ovary. Ciliated epithelium is found on the benign tumors but rarely in the presence of cancer. Psammoma bodies may be present and any mucus produced is extracellular.

B. *Mucinous tumors* are composed of tumors whose epithelial element includes a prominent component of mucin-filled cells. The epithelial may resemble endocervical or enteric epithelium, occasionally containing argentaffin cells and rarely Paneth cells. From time to time the question is raised whether these tumors should be included among the germ cell tumors as teratomas. The differential diagnosis should include metastatic adenocarcinoma from the large bowel.

C. *Endometrioid tumors* have the microscopic features of one of more of the typical forms of endometrial neoplasia. A small number of endometrioid tumors can be shown to arise in endometriosis, but the demonstration of such an origin is not required for the diagnosis. Endometrioid carcinomas may have a markedly papillary pattern, which is unusual in carcinomas of the endometrium.

D. *Clear cell (mesonephroid) tumors* are composed of cells containing glycogen and resemble those of the renal cell carcinoma and/or the hobnail or pig-shaped cells lining small cysts and tubules. Hobnail cells are characterized by scant cytoplasm and large nuclei that project into the lumen. The clear cell tumor must be distinguished from the endodermal sinus tumor, the dysgerminoma, and the lipid cell tumor.

Complement. A system of serologically nonspecific proteins present in fresh normal serum which are necessary for the lysis or death of cellular antigens in the presence of antibody.

Computer assisted tomography (CAT) scan. Scan based on x-ray analog data which has been digitalized and computer processed to show axial images.

Concomitant tumor immunity. The ability to reject a second tumor graft while the first tumor graft continues to grow. A piece of a tumor removed and implanted close to the original tumor will usually continue to grow, while the same piece of tumor transplanted at a distance from the original tumor may be rejected.

Conventional therapy. Treatment by x-ray beams other than supervoltage therapy.

Cryosurgery. Cryosurgery is the use of freezing by means of special probes cooled with liquid nitrogen, Freon gas or carbon dioxide.

Curie. The quantity of any radioisotope which disintegrates at the rate of 3.7×10^{10} disintegrations per second. Subunits of the curie (C) unit are the millicurie (mCi) = 1/1000 of a C; microcurie (μCi) = 1/1000 of a mCi; and millimicrocurie ($\mu\mu$Ci) = 1/1000 of a μCi.

Cyclotron. A circulate accelerator used to produce high-energy protons, deuterons, and other relatively heavy charged particles. Energies over 100 million eV may be achieved. Such particles may be used for basic physic research and to produce radionuclides for medical applications. They are sometimes used directly for experimental therapy or to produce neutron beams for therapy. The cyclotron utilizes high-frequency alternating voltage and a nonalternating magnetic field.

Cytophilic antibody. A globulin component of immune serum which becomes attached in vitro to certain normal cells in such a way that these cells are subsequently capable of specifically absorbing antigens.

Deblocking antibody. An antibody capable of overcoming the inhibitory effect of blocking factor, thereby permitting immunologic destruction of malignant cells.

Delayed hypersensitivity. See *Cell-mediated immunity.*

Depth dose. Dose at some specified depth or depths in tissue relative to the dose at a fixed reference point on the beam axis. Depth dose is usually expressed as a percentage.

Dinitrochlorobenzene (DNCB). A drug used to test for cell-mediated immunity. When applied to the skin it acts as a hapten attaching to a protein in the skin, producing an antigen that has the potential to sensitize lymphocytes. In 2 weeks the challenge produces a marked local response in patients with good cell-mediated immunity.

Disseminated intravascular coagulation (DIC). Characterized by a triad of thrombocytopenia, hypofibrinogenemia, and lysis of a blood clot within 2 hours.

Dosimetry. Strictly, the measurement of dose; in practice, calculations, measurements, and other activities required for determining the radiation dose delivered.

"Dysgerminoma with a lymphoid stroma." Makes an easily remembered rhyme. They are quite sensitive to irradiation.

Dysplasia. Cells present in dysplastic epithelium exhibit varying degrees of differentiation. The nucleus is always enlarged and hyperchromatic. 1) In mild dysplasia the cells are usually of the superficial type, rarely of the parabasal type. The chromatin pattern is uniform; there may be numerous small chromocenters. 2) In moderate dysplasia there is a group of cellular patterns intermediate between mild and severe dysplasia. 3) In severe dysplasia the cells are mainly of the parabasal and small intermediate type. The chromatin is dense and uniform, with many darkly stained, slightly enlarged chromocenters and no nucleoli.

Electrode. An x-ray tube component from which electrons emanate or to which they are attracted. The positive electrode is the anode and the negative one, the cathode.

Electron. The negatively charged part of an atom. When electrons strike a metal object at high energy, x-rays are produced.

Electron beam therapy. Treatment by electrons accelerated to high energies by a machine such as the betatron. Used mainly for lesions situated at or near the surface, electrons deliver maximum dose within the first few centimeters with the advantage, compared to x-rays, of rapidly diminished dose at greater depth. The depth of the high-dose region can be varied by varying the electron energy.

Electron Volt. A unit of energy equal to 1.602×10^{-19} joule.

Electrophilic atom. An electron-deficient atom, for example, a carcinogen. See *Nucleophilic atom.*

Enhancement antibody. See *Blocking factor.*

Epidemiology. Cancer epidemiology seeks to correlate differences in the incidence of different types of cancer with already established differences in the external or internal environments of the persons developing these cancers; for example, the relationship identified between cigarette smoking and lung cancer.

Epigenetic change. A change due to an alteration of a nongenetic biochemical process which sometimes affects the hereditary material. It is theoretically a reversible process.

Epithelial ovarian cancers. See *Common epithelial ovarian cancers.*

Epitope. See *Antigen determinant.*

Established tumor. In tests of substances for antigrowth activity against transplantable tumors in animals, the test substance is sometimes given before there is any visible growth of the tumor. If, on the other hand, the tumor implant is allowed to grow before the test substance is administered, it is referred to as *established.*

Etiology. Cancer etiology is the study of the causes of cancer. Its ultimate goal is cancer prevention. Three types of agents have now been shown to cause cancers: chemicals, radiation, and viruses. Of these, two (chemicals and radiation) clearly cause cancer in man, and the third (viruses) are highly suspect on the basis of present knowledge.

Ewing's histologic grading. Ewing influenced many pathologists when he presented his material using only three grades. In the Ewing-inspired grades, Broders' grades III and IV are combined and called grade III. The histologic classification is based on the uniformity or lack of uniformity of the cells, whether the nucleus is regular or not, the ratio between the nucleus and cytoplasm, the number and size of the nucleoli, and the number of mitoses per highpower field.

Exenteration. Essentially there are three types: anterior, posterior, and total pelvic exenteration. Total pelvic exenteration is a synthesis of three major procedures: 1) radical hysterectomy with bilateral pelvic node dissection and excision and bilateral salpingo-oophorectomy, 2) total cystectomy, and 3) combined abdominoperineal resection of the rectum. Anterior pelvic exenteration is employed to encompass disease that is located in the region of the bladder; it is a fusion of radical cystectomy, radical hysterectomy, bilateral pelvic node dissection, bilateral salpingo-oophorectomy, and partial vaginectomy. In those instances in which the malignant disease arises in the posterior part of the fornix and involves the rectovaginal septum and rectum, a posterior pelvic exenteration is indicated to excise the disease en bloc. In the posterior exenteration, which is merely an extended form of abdominoperineal resection, a radical excision of the lower bowel and rectum is carried out along with radical hysterectomy, bilateral pelvic node excision, bilateral salpingo-oophorectomy and vaginectomy.

Exit dose. The dose at the point where the axis of the beam emerges from the patient.

External irradiation. A method of irradiation in which the source of radiation is outside the body. The radiation beam must always traverse the skin and some normal tissue except with a superficial lesion.

Favored or privileged site. The anatomic region where foreign tissues tend to survive because of the diminished ability of an immunologic reaction to be incited there.

Filter. An insert, composed of various layers of different metals (aluminum, copper, tin), put in the x-ray beam to filter out the lower energy rays of the beam, and hence increase the half-value layer at the expense of the reduced beam intensity.

Forbidden clone. A hypothetical clone of immunologically competent cells with specificity for self-antigens which, according to the clonal selection theory, has been suppressed in fetal life and which may regain activity in adult life and cause autoimmune disease.

Fractionation. A technique of administering radiation therapy in multiple doses over a number of days or weeks to achieve a maximum therapeutic ratio.

Freund's adjuvant. *Complete:* Freund's water-in-oil emulsion of mineral oil, plant waxes, and killed tubercle bacilli used to incorporate with antigen to stimulate antibody production. *Incomplete:* Freund's mixture without tubercle bacilli.

Gene. An elementary germinal unit, situated in chromosomes, which carries an hereditary transmissible character. It is composed of distinctly arranged deoxyribonucleic acid chains. Histocompatibility genes are special entities, the nature of which determines the fate of grafts.

Genotype. The sum of the genes of an organism.

Germ cell tumors. Undifferentiated tumors; in some, extraembryonic structures predominate; in others the predominant structures are immature and/or mature structures which may be derived from any or all of the three embryonic layers—ectoderm, mesoderm, and endoderm.

A. *Dysgerminoma* is composed of germ cells that have not differentiated to form embryonic or extraembryonic structures. The tumor has a uniform appearance and is composed of large, rounded, clear cells which resemble primordial germ cells, both morphologically and histochemically. Its stroma is almost always infiltrated with lymphocytes and often contains granulomas similar to those of sarcoid.

B. *Teratomas*

1. *Extraembryonal forms* The endodermal sinus tumor is composed of embryonal cells lining a network of spaces. The most specific feature is the presence within some of the spaces of isolated papillary projections containing single blood vessels and having a peripheral lining of neoplastic cells. The tumor resembles the endodermal sinuses of the rat placenta. It contains intracellular and extracellular hyaline bodies resembling Russell bodies. When, on rare occasions, these vesicles form a major portion of the neoplasm, it is called a polyvesicular vitelline tumor.

2. *Choriocarcinoma* is a rare tumor composed of both cytotrophoblast and syncytiotrophoblast. It may be associated with precocious puberty.

3. *Adult teratoma* is composed exclusively of mature (adult) structures. It may be solid or cystic. The cystic is commonly called a dermoid. It is made up mainly of ectodermal elements but may contain endodermal and mesodermal tissue.

4. *Embryonal teratoma* is one that contains immature (embryonal) structures. Mature tissue may be present as well. The tumor is highly malignant and usually radioresistant. *Polyembryonic embryona* is a very unusual and poorly differentiated form of embryonal teratoma. Myriads of early embryos make up a large portion of the tumor.

5. *Struma ovarii* is a teratoma in which thyroid tissue is exclusively present or constitutes a grossly recognizable component of a more complex teratoma.

6. *Carcinoids* arises most often from respiratory or gastrointestinal epithelium in a dermoid cyst, but may develop within a solid teratoma or a mucinous cystic tumor.

C. *Gonadal stromal tumors*

1. *Female type:* The granulosal cell tumor is the most common. It may contain not only granulosa cells but also varying numbers of spindle-shaped, collagen-producing cells, elements resembling theca cells, and lutein cells. A variety of microscopic patterns may be encountered: microfollicular, macrofollicular, trabecular, cyclindromatous, insular, gyriform, solid-tubular, and sarcomatoid or diffuse.

2. *Male type:* The Sertoli-Leydig cell tumor contains Sertoli and Leydig cells of varying degrees of maturity; indifferent gonadal cells of embryonal appearance are present in certain cases. The designation *arrhenoblastoma* has been abandoned because not all of these tumors produce masculinization.

D. *Gynandroblastroma* is a very rare tumor in which collections of granulosa cells with typical Call-Exner bodies coexist with hollow tubules lined by Sertoli cells.

E. *Gonadoblastoma,* a rare ovarian cancer is composed of germ cells (dysgerminoma) and gonadal stromal cells (granulosa-Sertoli). Sex chromatin studies usually show a negative nuclear pattern (46 XY) or a sex chromosone mosaicism (XO/XY). Most patients are intersexual with phenotype female habitus, amenorrheic, and possibly virilized. The malignancy rate is very low.

Gold, radioactive (^{198}Au). A radioactive isotope with a half-life of 2.7 days which emits beta (960 keV) and gamma (412 keV) radiation; used in small sources in a colloidal form to suppress malignant serous effusions and to control free-floating cancer cells in the peritoneal cavity.

Graft-versus-host reaction. In the presence of an immune-deficient host, the graft may produce lymphocytes that react to the host antigen, producing hepatosplenomegaly, lymphopenia, diarrhea, and skin rash. In the very young a disease called *runt disease* (allogeneic disease), which develops after injection of allogeneic lymphocytes into immunologically immature experimental animals, produces a picture similar to the one outlined above plus the failure to thrive and often death.

Half-life. The time required for the radioactivity to reduce to one-half of the value present at the start of the time period. After 10 half-lives the radioactivity will be reduced by a factor of 1024. Complete decay of a 1 mC$_1$ sample to a single undecayed nucleus depends on the decay constant and requires about 40 to 80 half-lives for medically useful materials. The effective half-life of an ingested source is determined by both the decay and excretion characteristics.

Half value layer (HVL). The thickness of a specific material which reduces the flux of radiation by one-half; a function of voltage, filtration, and target material, it is used as a rough gauge of radiation quality.

Haploid. Having a single set of unpaired chromosomes in each nucleus, a characteristic of gametes.

Hapten. A partial antigen which contains at least one of the determinant groups of an antigen. It can react specifically with antibodies, but in itself it does not induce the formation of antibodies unless it is complexed with a carrier molecule such as a protein.

Helper factor. Sensitized T-lymphocyte subpopulations release a helper factor which enables immunocompetent B cells to respond to antigens which they would otherwise be unable to recognize. The stimulated B lymphocytes differentiate into plasma cells, which are the main producers of antibody. The helper factor also stimulates the B lymphocyte to produce a variant of the B cell, the *killer (K) cell,* which is able to attack tumor cells only after the tumor cells have been exposed to specific antibody. Complement is not required for this action. See *Killer cell.*

Hepatitis-associated antigen (Australian antigen). This antigen (Au antigen), first detected in the serum of an Australian aborigine, has been detected in the sera of patients during the incubation period and early clinical course of serum or transfusion hepatitis, but not in the sera of patients with a short incubation form of infectious hepatitis. The serum of patients carrying the antigen has been shown, under the electron microscope, to contain aggregates of pleomorphic particles and tubules. The aggregates have been interpreted to be antigen-antibody complexes, and the particles are thought to be antigen derived from the virus causing the infection.

Heterophil. Pertaining to antigenic specificity shared between species.

Heterozygosity. The occupancy of dissimilar genes in the same chromosome.

Histocompatibility. The ability to accept transplants of tissue from another animal of the same species. Such ability depends on the identical genetic constitution of donor and recipient.

Histologic grading. The Broders classification consisted of four numerical grades (I, II, III and IV) for both epidermoid and adenocarcinoma of the cervix. The basis for this classification is the well-known observation that the degree of malignancy keeps pace with the degree of cell differentiation, grade I being the most highly differentiated and grade IV the most immature. The original Broders grading method is cumbersome to apply, because as many as 13 different cytologic characteristics have to be observed and evaluated. The following factors are recorded for each grade: epithelial pearls, individual keratinized cells, intercellular bridges, tumor giant cells, and mitosis per high-power field. Most pathologists now use a simplified version. See *Ewing's histologic grading*.

Histologic type and grading. The parameters which classify the microscopic characteristics of the tumor.

Histologic grading. Grade 1 (G1) Highly differentiated adenomatous carcinoma. Grade 2 (G2) Differentiated adenomatous carcinomas with partly solid areas. Grade 3 (G3) Predominantly solid or entirely undifferentiated carcinomas.

HL-A antigen (human leukocyte antigen). A genetic locus containing two closely linked groups of several alleles, ie, subloci. It is present on the cell membranes of all nucleated cells and plays a major role in determining graft rejection.

Horizontal transmission of viruses. Transmission of viruses between individual hosts of the same generation. See *Vertical transmission of viruses*.

Hormone receptors. Although polypeptide and steroid hormones differ slightly in their mechanism of action in general they have more similarities than differences. Estrogen binding has been discussed most often and will be used as the model. Estrogens are carried bound to a plasma transport protein. Estrogens are able to enter the cytoplasm of all cells whether they are target tissue or not. However, in the cytoplasm of target tissue are found specific protein molecules that are termed receptors. These proteins can bind biologically active estrogens with great affinity and great specificity. Following the initial binding step, the steroid-receptor complex undergoes a temperature dependent activation. This activation allows the steroid-receptor complex to enter the nucleus of the cell and bind to the chromatin, the genetic information of the cell. Once bound to the chromatin, by a process which is poorly understood, the interaction of the steroid-receptor complex with the genetic information of the cell leads to an elaboration of new species of messenger RNA. These messenger RNA molecules can be translated on polysomes into new proteins, and it is these new proteins that lead to the induced effects of the steroid hormone.

Horror autotoxicus. Fear of self-poisoning, as related to the usual inability of an antigen to serve as an autoantigen.

Host. An organism whose body serves to sustain a graft; loosely interchangeable with *recipient*.

Human chorionic gonadotropin (hCG). A glycoprotein with a molecular weight of approximately 39,000 produced by trophoblastic tumors.

Human placental lactogen (hPL). A polypeptide hormone with a molecular weight of approximately 23,600 produced by a high percent of trophoblastic tumors.

Humoral immunity. Pertaining to the body fluids, in contrast to cellular fluids. It is initiated by the thymus-independent B cells. These B lymphocytes proliferate and differentiate into plasma cells that secrete immunoglobulins (IgG, IgM, IgA, IgD, and IgE).

Hybrid. An animal whose parents belong to different species. Ordinarily procreation is dependent on a fixed sexual role of one or the other species partners. When it occurs, regardless of the sexual identity of the mated species, the offspring is a reciprocal hybrid (mutual hybrid).

Idiotype. An antigen, unique to an individual or small group of individuals, as opposed to allotype.

Immune adherence.   Adhesive nature of antigen-antibody complexes to inert surfaces when complement is bound into the complex.

Immunoblast.   Cell intermediate between the lymphocyte and plasma cell.

Immunodiffusion.   Diffusion of soluble antigens and/or antibodies toward each other leading to their precipitation in gel.

Immunoelectrophoresis.   Electrophoretic displacement of antigen (S) or antibodies followed by immunodiffusion.

Immunogen.   An antigen that induces a specific immunologic response.

Immunologic surveillance.   Described by Sir F. MacFarlane Burnet, effective immunological surveillance depends on the presence of tumor-specific antigenic determinants on the surfaces of neoplastic cells, which enable these altered cells to be recognized as nonself and to be destroyed by immunologic reactions.

Immunoreaction.   Reaction between antigen and its antibody.

Incidence.   Number of new cases of a disease over a given time period, usually one year.

Interferon.   A protein released by cells in response to virus infection. It represents nonspecific immunity.

Inverse Square Law.   The rule that accounts for the differences in dose rate or exposure rate at various distances from a point source of radiation due to the divergence of the radiation and not including any effects or absorption of radiation. Dose rate or exposure rate is inversely proportional to the square of the distance from a point source.

In vitro.   In an artificial environment, such as a culture tube, outside the body.

In vivo.   Within the living body.

Isodose curve.   A curve on which all points receive an equal radiation dose. A series of them will map out the relative insensitivities of a radiation field in a phantom or patient.

Isotopes.   Atoms of identical chemical properties (same configuration of orbital electrons) but with a different atomic weight (different number of neutrons contained in the nucleus of the atom).

Karyolysis.   A form of degeneration in which the nucleus of the cell swells, gradually loses its chromatin and finally disappears.

Karyorrhexis.   Nuclear fragmentation.

Keratinization.   The formation of anucleate squares.

Keratinized carcinoma cell.   A malignant squamous epithelial cell that stain orange with the Papanicolaou stain.

Killer cell (K cell).   Sensitized T lymphocytes produce a helper factor that acts on the immunocompetent cell to produce a population of cells, possibly variants of the B cell, termed killer cells (K cells), which are able to attack tumor cells that have been exposed to a specific antibody. Unlike the usual humoral antibody (immunoglobulin) response, complement is not needed to destroy the cell.

Krukenberg tumor.   A metastasis of distinctive appearance characterized by the presence of mucus-filled signet-ring cells accompanied by a sarcoma-like proliferation of the ovarian stroma. This tumor is usually secondary to gastric cancer, but may originate in any organ in which mucinous carcinomas arise, including the breast and intestine. On rare occasions a tumor with the pattern of a Krukenberg tumor appears to be primary in the ovary.

Laser.   Is an acronym—stands for light amplification by stimulated emission of radiation. See maser.

LD 50/30.   A term that represents a single total-body irradiation lethal in 30 days to 50% of a group of animals. For man it is about 350 to 450 rad.

Lichen sclerosus.   Vulvar skin desorder characterized by thinning of the epithelial layer with loss of rete ridges and formation of a prominent hypocellular, subepithelial component.

Linear accelerator.   Essentially a pipe in which charged particles may be accelerated by applying a high-frequency potential difference during the transit along the pipe. In electron accelerators for radiotherapy, the pipe becomes a waveguide which may be a corrugated tube with continually increasing spacing between corrugations. Microwave frequency electromagnetic fields generated at one end travel down the waveguide in a wave of increasing velocity. A bunch of electrons injected at precisely the right time is accelerated by riding the crest of this wave. The electrons produce x-rays by striking a target at the far end of the tube.

Linear energy transfer (LET).   A measure of the average rate of energy loss along the track of an ionizing particle, expressed as energy units per unit track length. It is the energy released (usually in keV) per micron of medium (tissue) along the track of any ionizing particle.

Locus.   The precise location of a gene on a chromosome. Different forms of the gene (alleles) are always found at the same position on the chromosome. A complex locus is a locus within which mutation and recombination can occur at more than one site.

Lymphokine.   Substances released by sensitized lymphocytes when they come in contact with the antigen to which they are sensitized. There are at least four mediators of cellular immunity, including transfer factor (TF), lymphocyte-transforming activity (LTA), migration inhibition factor (MIF), and lymphotoxins.

Lysogeny.   A virus joins up with the DNA of the cell and is carried along through many generations. It is inactive unless some noxious agent stimulates it to become active. In *lysogeny*, the virus is part of the DNA of the cell, and, in *transduction*, some of the DNA is carried along as part of the virus.

Macrophage.   A large mononuclear phagocyte; in the tissues this cell may be designated a histiocyte and in the blood a monocyte. Macrophages in the spleen, lymph nodes and thymus are known as the sinus-lining macrophages (sometimes called reticulum cells). An antigen must contact or pass through a macrophage before it can become a processed antigen with the ability to encounter and then sensitize a small lymphocyte.

Macrophage activating factor (MAF).   The sensitized T lymphocytes release a nonspecific macrophage activating factor which creates a cytotoxic population of macrophages that appears to distinguish malignant from normal cells, killing only malignant ones.

Maser.   Stands for microwave amplification by stimulated emission of radiation.

Megavoltage radiation.   X or Y (gamma) radiation with peak photon energies in excess of 1 meV.

Melanoma.   Tumor composed of melanocytes.

Migration inhibition factor (MIF).   A lymphokine produced when a sensitized lymphocyte is cultured in the presence of an antigen to which it is sensitized. It inhibits the migration of these lymphocytes.

Mitogen.   A substance that induces lymphocytes to undergo blast transformation, mitosis, and cell division (causing mitosis or cell division).

Mixed lymphocyte (leukocyte) culture (MLC).   The transformation of small lymphocytes to blast cells, with synthesis of DNA, in mixed cultures of blood leukocytes from normal allogeneic individuals. The magnitude of the reaction reflects the degree of disparity between histocompatibility antigens of the two donors. In identical twins, neither set stimulates the other, whereas in unrelated pairs there is almost always stimulation of each cell by the other. The degree of stimulation is analyzed either morphologically by blast transformation or biochemically by measuring tritiated thymidine incorporation into newly synthesized DNA.

Mosaic.   An individual composed of two or more cell lines but from the same species. This can come about either through somatic mutation or by grafting cells between individuals of a very close genetic constitution, such as dizygotic twins.

Multiple-part treatment.   To deliver a high dose to the tumor volume at a depth without destroying the tissue near the surface, one may direct more than one radiation beam toward the tumor from different angles in order to increase the dose to the tumor relative to the skin.

NSD.   The normal standard dose. The tolerance of normal tissue is influenced by dose rate, protraction and fractionation, as well as total dose. Computation of the NSD yields a value (measured in rets) that may correlate sufficiently well with late complications to permit more meaningful evaluation of alternate radiation therapy techniques.

Nuclear grade.   The nuclei of the tumor cells were graded from 1 to 3 according to the classification of Black and Speer: grade 1, markedly enlarged, irregular in outline with chromatin clumping and prominent nucleoli; grade 2, intermediate degree of differentiation; grade 3, similar in size and appearance to each other and to normal ovarian tissue when present. It should be noted that in the histologic grading the better differentiated tumors are Grade I and Grade III is the least differentiated, whereas in grading the nuclei grade 1 is the most anaplastic and grade 3 the least anaplastic.

Nucleophilic atom.   An atom with excess electrons. The information-containing macromolecules of the cell (DNA, RNA, and protein) are relatively rich in nucleophilic sites and, in those cases that have been adequately studied, derivatives of chemical carcinogens have been found to be firmly bound to the DNA, RNA, and protein of target tissues. Furthermore, in some cases, susceptibility to cancer formation by chemical carcinogens has been correlated with the kinds and amounts of these macromolecule-bound carcinogens. See *Electrophilic atom.*

Nude mice (nu nu mice).   Mice born with a congenital absence of the thymus. The blood and thymus-dependent areas of the lymph nodes and spleen are depleted of lymphocytes. These mice are homozygous for the gene "nude" — which is abbreviated *Nu,* hence *nu nu* — and they have no hair. They should be distinguished from mice carrying other genes that cause a lack of hair, eg, shaven, *sha;* hairless, *hr;* bare, *br;* hair loss, *hl;* etc. All of these latter strains have normal thymuses.

Oncofetal antigens.　Antigens produced by normal embryonic tissues and tumor cells. Cellular production of these markers is indicative of rapid cellular growth.

Orthovoltage x-ray therapy.　X-ray therapy applied with a machine producing 140 to 600 kVp x-rays.

Ovary.　A *supernumerary ovary* is one which is independent of and equal in size to the normal ovary. It is extremely rare.

Accessory ovaries are usually attached to the normal gland by peritoneal bands in the mesovarium or adjacent part of the broad ligament, near the hilum of the ovary. They have clinical significance if they undergo pathologic changes or when bilateral oophorectomy is carried out; their presence may result in continued ovarian activity. Accessory ovaries *occur in about 3% of women.*

Ectopic ovaries may be congenital or acquired, but the acquired type is much more common. Congenital displacement may be due to nondescent, a phenomenon by which the ovary remains above the pelvic brim, or it may be due to the ovary having been pulled into the inguinal canal or large labia by the gubernaculum. The acquired type is common and may follow pregnancy with prolapse of the ovary into the cul-de-sac.

Overgrowth stimulating factor (OSF).　This factor can cause normal cells in culture to adopt the appearance and growth habit of the transformed cell. Stimulated cells revert to normal when the overgrowth stimulating factor is removed.

Oxygen enhancement ratio (OER).　The ratio of the radiation dose under anoxic conditions to the dose under fully oxygenated conditions required to produce an equivalent effect. The oxygen enhancement ratio (OER) for most mammalian cells is about 3.

Paget's cell.　Is of epidermal origin and represents an aberrant differentiation of epidermal stem cell. Paget's cell with ultra-structural characteristics of both secretory sweat-gland cells and squamous keratinocytes have been described. Histochemical stains show positive reactions for intracellular mucopolysaccharides in the Paget's cells and clearly distinguish them from the cells of the even more unusual superficial amelanotic melanoma.

Papovavirus.　Group of small DNA viruses, some of which are oncogenic or potentially oncogenic. These viruses have been associated with the production of vulvar epithelial abnormalities.

Paratope.　See *Antibody.*

Passive transfer of immunity.　The transfer of specific antibody from one individual to another.

Peak absorbed dose.　The highest value of absorbed dose on the central ray of a single radiation beam. The depth of peak absorbed dose ranges from several millimeters to several centimeters below the skin surface for megavoltage radiation beams. The exact depth depends on beam energy and yield size.

Penumbra.　The radiation just outside and adjacent to the full beam arising from the finite size of the source; its usage usually includes components from scatter in tissue or from incomplete beam collimation.

Phosphorus (^{32}P). A beta emitter with a maximum energy of 1.7 meV and a half-life of 14.2 days, which may be given orally, intravenously, or intraperitoneally. It is maximally incorporated into cells with short turnover times, and is used to suppress malignant serous effusions and to control free-floating cancer cells in the peritoneal cavity.

Photoscan localization. Process of using a radioisotope to localize various concentrations of a given substance within the body.

Phytohemagglutinins. Lectins extracted from the red kidney bean, *Phaseolus vulgaris* or *P. communis.* They can be purified to yield a glycoprotein mitogen, which stimulates lymphocyte transformation and causes agglutination of certain red cells. Phytohemagglutinins provide a method for estimating the pool of thymus-dependent lymphocytes (T cells).

Pions. Negative II mesons are negatively charged particles with a mass 273 times as great as the electron. They are produced by a complex process which necessitates a device such as synchrocyclotron, capable of accelerating protons to energies of around 700 meV. For radiotherapy, pions with energies between about 40 to 70 meV are of interest, since these particles have ranges in tissues of approximately 6 and 15 cm, respectively. The negative II meson loses energy like any other charged particle; this results in a Bragg peak at the end of the track just before the particle comes to rest. In addition, because of nuclear disintegrations confined essentially entirely to the end of the range of negative pions, additonal high-LET radiation is liberated in the region of the Bragg peak. If these densely ionizing peak portions of the negative pion tracks could be made to coincide with the position of a deep tumor with predictable certainty, extensive destruction of the tumor cell will result.

PMPO syndrome (postmenopausal palpable ovary syndrome). Palpation of what is interpreted as a normal-sized ovary in the premenopausal woman represents an ovarian tumor in the postmenopausal woman.

Pneumocystitis carinii. An example of a parasite of low-grade virulence which presents a clinical problem only in the *immunologically compromised* host. The organism induces a pneumonitis with characteristic clinical and pathologic findings. Three groups of susceptible hosts have been defined: 1) premature or debilitated infants, 2) individuals with primary immunologic deficiency disorders, and 3) individuals with a malignancy or who are receiving immunosuppressive therapy and who demonstrate an immunologic deficit. There is an increasing state of dyspnea, progressive cyanosis, and a dry, nonproductive cough. Most remarkable is the lack of systemic reaction to this infection, and many patients are usually dyspneic and cyanotic, even in the absence of fever, malaise, or anorexia. The laboratory findings include the demonstration of a ventilation perfusion deficit, with a relatively normal pH and pCO_2 and a low pCO_2. Serologic techniques for the diagnosis of the diseases are hindered in humans, because most affected individuals have immunologic deficiency states and are therefore incapable of an antibody response.

Point A. An imaginary point described by Todd and Meredith as being 2 cm lateral to the cervical canal and 2 cm above the cervical os. The point is supposed to be in the paracervical tissues.

Point B. A reference point that lies 3 cm lateral to point A and is used as a means of evaluating pelvic wall damage.

Pokeweed mitogen (PWM). A mitogen extracted from the pokeweed plant which can be purified to yield a glycoprotein. The pokeweed mitogen stimulates blast formation of both B and T cells.

Post film. A radiograph taken with the patient interposed between the treatment machine portal and an x-ray film. The purpose of this film is to demonstrate radiographically that the treatment field as externally set on the patient adequately encompasses the desired treatment volume and at the same time avoids adjacent critical structures.

Prevalence. Total number of cases of a disease at a specific time in a given area.

Primary beam. The direct radiation beam emanating from the head of the irradiating unit. Scattered radiation is produced during the absorption of this beam.

Prophylactic immunization. Immunization of an individual against a causative agent (eg, a virus) or tumor-specific antigen, before any natural encounter with the agent or tumor.

Quality. The penetrating power of a photon beam, described in terms of half-value layer.

Rad. A unit of absorbed dose of ionizing radiation equivalent to the absorption of 100 ergs per gram of irradiated material.

Radiation. The propagation of energy through space or matter. In radiology it can be divided into two main groups: charged particles (eg, electrons, protons, α (alpha) particles and electromagnetic (x-rays, gamma rays).

Radiation beam. A pathway of defined size and shape along which radiation is being propagated. The types of radiation involved include x-rays, γ-rays, electrons, and other particulate radiation.

Radioactivity. The property of certain nuclides of spontaneously emitting particles of γ (gamma) radiation, or if emitting x radiation following orbital electron capture, or if undergoing spontaneous fission.

Radioactivity, artificial. Emission of radiant energy arising from the breakdown of nuclei which are unstable in their natural states, for example, ^{60}Co and ^{137}C$_5$.

Radioactivity, natural. Emission of radiant energy arising from the breakdown of nuclei which are unstable in their natural states, for example, radium.

Radioimmunoassay. Determination of the concentration of an antigen or antibody by means of a radioactive-labelled substance that reacts with the substance to be tested.

Rays, Alpha. Alpha rays are streams of high-speed helium nuclei that have been ejected from radioactive substances.

Rays, Beta. Beta rays are streams of electrons ejected from radioactive substances with velocities that may be as high as 0.98 of the velocity of light.

Rays, Gamma. Gamma rays are electromagnetic radiations consisting of high-energy photons and resulting from a nuclear reaction.

Reagan isoenzyme. A placental type of alkaline phosphatase which may be elevated in the serum of patients with cervical and ovarian cancers.

REM (Roentgen-Equivalent-Man). Special unit of radiation protection quantity "dose equivalent." Dose equivalent is obtained by multiplying absorbed dose by a "quality factor," which has higher values for higher LET radiations. When dose is expressed in rads, dose equivalent is in rems.

Reverse transcriptase (RNA-dependent DNA polymerase). This recently isolated factor can transcribe the base sequence of a viral RNA onto a DNA strand, in vitro. It is now possible to test human cancers for association with any one of a number of RNA viruses.

Roentgen. A roentgen is the international unit of x or gamma radiation. It is the quantity of x or gamma radiation such that the associated corpuscular emission per 0.001293 gm or air produces in air ions carrying 1 electrostatic unit of electrical charge of either sign.

Rotation therapy. External beam teletherapy in which the source of radiation moves circumferentially around the patient while being centered in the volume of interest. Some devices allow the patient to rotate in the vertical plane within a stationary beam.

Second look operation. The reoperation of a patient at a stated time without evidence of any clinical disease.

Selective IgG deficiency. A deficiency associated with a variety of disorders, but most frequently with diseases of an autoimmune nature. The immunoelectrophoretic pattern shows absence of IgA. Cellular immunity is intact, and all other immunoglobulins are present, eg, IgG, IgM, IgD, and IgE. Selective IgG deficiency affects 1 in 700 individuals.

Sequestered antigen. Any antigen or antigenic determinant that is hidden from contact with immunologically competent cells or antibody and thus cannot stimulate an immune response. They may be intracellular antigens or hidden determinants on cell surfaces or on soluble molecules.

Serology. The study of antigen-antibody reactions in vitro.

Serum sickness reaction. A systemic allergy to the administration of a large amount of serum or purified foreign protein. Its appearance coincides with, and is caused by, the interaction of newly formed antibody with excess antigen circulating in the blood and tissue fluids.

Shock lung. An entity which has long been confused with such pathologic diagnoses as bronchopneumonia, patchy atelectasis, and agonal changes. Pulmonary edema can be the result of sepsis, fat embolism, cardiac failure, lung contusion, or oxygen toxicity. The resulting pulmonary insufficiency is a major cause of death in injured patients and patients receiving intensive care. A single cause for shock lung has not been described, and any or all of the above may be implicated.

Simulation film. X-ray films taken with the same field size, source-to-skin distance, and orientation as a therapy beam in order to mimic the beam and for visualization of the treated volume on an x-ray film.

Simulator. A radiation generator operating in the diagnostic x-ray range with the mechanical capability to orient a radiation beam toward a patient with parameters imitating that proposed for therapy, and affording direct x-ray fluoroscopic visualization and roentgenographic images of the area. Machine is not capable of delivering radiation therapy.

Skin sparing. Because of the build-up of the absorbed dose in supervoltage radiation deep to the skin, the skin surface does not receive the maximum dose delivered. The skin reaction is therefore much less than would be expected from conventional radiation.

Source-skin distance (SSD). The distance along the central ray from the source of radiation to the skin of the patient.

Specific stimulation. The utilization of tumor cells or their antigenic products for immunization directed specifically toward that tumor or other tumors sharing the same antigens.

Squamous cell. Basal cell. A small, rounded, cyanophilic cell derived from the basal layer. It has a centrally placed vesicular nucleus. The nuclear/cytoplasmic ratio is between 1:2 and 1:3.

Parabasal cell. A small, round, or oval, cyanophilic cell with thick dense cytoplasm and a vesicular nucleus. The nuclear/cytoplasmic ratio varies from 1:3 to 1:6.

Intermediate cell. A polygonal cell with cyanophilic cytoplasm. The nucleus is vesicular and has a diameter larger than 6 μm. The nuclear/cytoplasmic ratio is less than 1:6.

Staging of ovarian cancer. A clinically determined estimate of the extent of the disease and the size of the tumor, whereas histologic type and grading classify the cancer's microscopic character.

Stem (primitive) cell. A cell which is capable of proliferation and may give rise to differentiated cells.

Stromal reactions. Chabon, Takenchi, and Sommers have employed a stromal evaluation in a breast study and have adapted this method of grading for the ovarian cancers in this study. The stroma of each epithelial ovarian cancer was graded according to the number of lymphocytes, plasma cells, and polymorphonuclear leukocytes present. Lymphocytes, plasma cells and polymorphonuclear infiltration in the stroma and around small veins were graded 0 to 3: 0 = none, 1 = minimal, 2 = moderate, and 3 = marked.

Superficial therapy. Treatment with an x-ray machine of relatively low voltage, approximately 100 keV. Penetration is not large.

Supervoltage radiation. High-energy radiation with ill-defined limits usually extending beyond energies which no longer are preferentially absorbed in bone (ie, 500 keV) to peak energies of several meV.

Supervoltage therapy. Treatment with x-rays or γ-rays with energies in excess of 600 keV. Included greater than 600 kVp rays, cesium 137, cobalt 60.

Suppressor T cells. An important set of feedback controls, centered around sensitized T lymphocytes, though which inhibitory populations of these cells suppress the production of sensitized lymphocytes and antibody-forming cells.

Syngeneic. Pertaining to genetically identical or nearly identical animals such as identical twins or highly inbred animals.

Syngeneic preference. Unlike allogenic inhibition, syngeneic preference represents improved growth in syngeneic recipients.

Teletherapy. Treatment with the radiation source at a distance from the body. See *Brachytherapy*.

Template theory. An instructive theory of antibody production in which it was supposed that an antigen was taken into a cell and acted directly as a template that determined the shape of the combining site of the antibody which is produced by that cell. The theory was originally proposed by Haurowitz, Mudd, and Alexander.

Tests for evaluating a clotting disorder. *Bleeding time* can be unreliable because of variations in puncture technique; it may also be abnormal because of platelets deficient in number or function or because of von Willebrand's disease. Normal = *less than 4 minutes.*

Clotting time (glass) is an insensitive test. It does, however, test for all intrinsic coagulation factors except VII, XIII, and platelets. Normal = less than 15 and usually less than 10 minutes.

Prothrombin time (one-stage) is a reliable and sensitive test for the extrinsic system coagulation factors (V, VII, and X) as well as for fibrinogen (I) and prothrombin (II). Normal = less than 20 seconds (check control value).

Prothrombin consumption tests are reliable in testing platelet function (unlike bleeding time) and have acceptable sensitivity for the intrinsic system coagulation factors (unlike the clotting time). This test checks V, VIII, IX, X, XI, and XII. Normal = less than 20% (alternatively expressed as greater than 80%).

Partial thromboplastin time (PTT) (activated partial thromboplastin time) is a sensitive screening test for detection of alterations in coagulation mechanisms such as previously undiagnosed hemophilia, various coagulation deficiencies, and circulating anticoagulants, Normal = 20 to 45 seconds.

Thrombin time, when prolonged, indicates over-heparinization, defibrination, or fibrinolysis.

The quantity of platelets can be rapidly estimated from a smear. Platelet counts considerably below 100,000 may implicate massive bank blood transfusions as a cause of bleeding. Normal = over 100,000.

Tetraploid.   Having four times the haploid number of chromosomes.

Therapeutic immunization.   Any therapy initiated after the patient shows clinical manifestations of malignancy.

T lymphocyte (T cell).   Lymphocytes that have matured and differentiated under thymic influence are termed thymic-dependent lymphocytes. These cells are primarily involved in the mediation of cellular immunity, as well as in tissue and organ rejection.

TNM staging system.   System used in staging certain cancers which makes use of size and location of the primary tumor (T); involvement of lymph nodes (N); and presence or absence of metastases (M).

Tolerance.   Failure of the antibody response to a potential antigen following exposure to the antigen. Tolerance commonly results from prior exposure to antigens.

Tolerance dose.   The maximum radiation dose that may be delivered to a given biologic tissue at the specified dose rate and throughout a specific volume without producing an unacceptable change in the tissue.

Toluidine blue stain.   Nuclear stain used to locate areas of high mitotic activity for purposes of biopsy.

Total parenteral nutrition (TPN).   Method of providing protein, caloric, and total nutritional requirements to a patient in a parenterally administered solution.

Transcription stage.   The transcribing of genetic information from nucleus to cytoplasm, ie, from DNA to RNA by messenger RNA.

Transduction. This form of recombination depends upon bacteriophage for its completion. A phage particle can carry some DNA from the lysed cell in which it was formed to the new cell it infects. There, instead of multiplying, it remains inactive, and the transferred bacterial DNA may become incorporated into the DNA of the new host. Apparently only a small portion of the genetic material undergoes transduction at any one time. In *Salmonella,* a genus of bacteria to which many pathogenic intestinal bacteria belong, the ability to resist certain drugs can be transferred by transduction. See *Lysogeny.*

Transfer factor. A heat-labile, dialyzable extract of human lymphocytes that is capable of conferring specific antigen reactivity to the donor. See *Lymphokine.*

Transformation. The process that occurs when a bacteria absorbs the DNA of a dead bacterium and incorporates some of it into its own genetic constitution. The incorporated DNA is then transmitted to later generations. Usually only a small part of the genetic material is involved in transformation, and usually the process occurs only between members of the same species; however streptomycin resistance has been transferred in this way from pneumococci to streptococci.

Translation stage. The translation of the base sequence code in RNA into an amino acid sequence in proteins.

Treatment field. A plane section of a beam, perpendicular to the beam axis, as defined by the collimator of the treatment machine. Term often used synonymously with treatment port.

Tumor angiogenesis factor (TAF). The tumor angiogenesis factor represents the induction of the growth of blood vessels by a stimulant released by tumor cells. The growth of the tumor parallels the development of new blood vessels.

Tumor volume. That volume encompassing all known or presumed tumor.

Ultrasonography. Process using ultrasonic wave reflections to visualize structures deep to the surface of the body.

Vertical transmission of viruses. Transmission of viruses from one generation to the next, ie, from mother to offspring. See *Horizontal transmission of viruses.*

Xenogeneic (heterologous). Pertaining to individuals of different species.

INDEX